The Movement Disorders Prescriber's Guide to Parkinson's Disease

W0071768

Professor K. Ray Chaudhuri is Professor of Neurology/Movement Disorders at King's College Hospital and King's College London and the Medical Director of the Parkinson Foundation International Centre of Excellence at King's College.

Professor Peter Jenner is an expert on the pharmacology of drugs and treatment strategies used at all stages of Parkinson's disease. He has been involved in the development and marketing of most of the key therapies. Peter has published over 700 papers on the cause, treatment, and cure of Parkinson's disease.

Dr Valentina Leta is a neurologist movement disorder specialist interested in infusion therapies and autonomic dysfunction in Parkinson's disease. She has worked as principal/sub-investigator of numerous trials investigating the efficacy and safety of new drugs for Parkinson's disease. Valentina has been invited as a faculty at international conferences. She is author of over 55 peer-reviewed papers and book chapters on Parkinson's disease.

Ms Shelley Jones is a consultant pharmacist in neurosciences, with over 16 years' experience working with people with Parkinson's and helping them to manage their medications optimally. Shelley has worked in the Parkinson's Centre of Excellence and been involved in publication of book chapters, papers, and conference posters.

Dr Iro Boura is a neurologist specializing in movement disorders and a PhD candidate in neurogenetics. She is currently a clinical research fellow at the Neurology Laboratory at the University of Crete and she is also affiliated with King's College London and the Parkinson's Foundation Centre of Excellence at King's College Hospital. Iro has contributed to numerous publications on Parkinson's disease, including book chapters, peer-reviewed papers, and conference posters.

The Movement Disorders Prescriber's Guide to Parkinson's Disease

K. Ray Chaudhuri
King's College London

Peter Jenner
King's College London

Valentina Leta
King's College London

Shelley Jones
King's College London

Iro Boura
School of Medicine, University of Crete

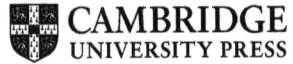

CAMBRIDGE UNIVERSITY PRESS

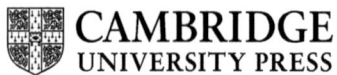
CAMBRIDGE
UNIVERSITY PRESS

Shaftesbury Road, Cambridge CB2 8EA, United Kingdom

One Liberty Plaza, 20th Floor, New York, NY 10006, USA

477 Williamstown Road, Port Melbourne, VIC 3207, Australia

314–321, 3rd Floor, Plot 3, Splendor Forum, Jasola District Centre,
New Delhi – 110025, India

103 Penang Road, #05–06/07, Visioncrest Commercial, Singapore 238467

Cambridge University Press is part of Cambridge University Press & Assessment,
a department of the University of Cambridge.

We share the University's mission to contribute to society through the pursuit of
education, learning and research at the highest international levels of excellence.

www.cambridge.org
Information on this title: www.cambridge.org/9781009222617

DOI: 10.1017/9781009222648

First published 2025

A catalogue record for this publication is available from the British Library.

A Cataloging-in-Publication data record for this book is available from the Library of Congress

ISBN 978-1-009-22261-7 Paperback

CONTENTS

CONTENTS

FOREWORD

Pharmacological therapy for Parkinson's disease, now regarded as a multi-system, multi-neurotransmitter dysfunction has become complex in spite of levodopa still being the gold standard of treatment across all stages of Parkinson's disease. Newer developments include advances in dopamine replacement therapies such as oral enzyme inhibitors like opicapone and safinamide whereas advanced therapies have evolved to clinical trials and licensing of subcutaneous foslevodopa/foscarbidopa preparations as well as newer delivery systems for apomorphine infusion of levodopa with entacapone. The non-dopaminergic aspect of Parkinson's disease is manifested by the evolving non-motor profile of Parkinson's disease with descriptions of non-motor subtypes, and management also, therefore, includes non-dopaminergic strategies as well as lifestyle changes. A comprehensive strategy encompassing implementation of these clinical strategies as well as attention to dopaminergic and non-dopaminergic drug use in Parkinson's disease and related side effects has been signposted in the recent publication of the Chaudhuri dashboard for Parkinson's disease. The complexity of pharmacological management of Parkinson's disease is further complicated by non-availability of many drugs in different countries around the world. In this short and concise book we aim to address these issues by providing a comprehensive guide to the different medication used for Parkinson's disease and the Parkinson syndrome. We hope healthcare professionals who care for people round the world with Parkinson's will find this book useful as a reference point.

Professor K. Ray Chaudhuri

ABBREVIATIONS

ACE	angiotensin-converting enzyme
ACh	acetylcholine
AD	Alzheimer's disease
ALT	alanine aminotransferase
ANC	absolute neutrophil count
APTT	activated partial thromboplastin time
ARDS	acute respiratory distress syndrome
AST	aspartate transaminase
AUC	overall plasma exposure
BID	two times a day
BUN	blood urea nitrogen
CAD	coronary artery disease
CADASIL syndrome	cerebral autosomal dominant arteriopathy with subcortical infarcts and leukoencephalopathy
CDC	Centers for Disease Control and Prevention
Cmax	maximum plasma concentration
CNS	central nervous system
COMT	catechol-O-methyltransferase
COPD	chronic obstructive pulmonary disease
CPAP	continuous positive airway pressure
CPK	creatinine phosphokinase
CR	controlled release
CrCl	creatinine clearance
CYP450	cytochrome P450
DaTSCAN	dopamine transporter scan
DAWS	dopamine agonist withdrawal syndrome
DBS	deep brain stimulation
DDI	dopa decarboxylase inhibitor
DDS	dopamine dysregulation syndrome
DLB	dementia with Lewy bodies
DOPA	dihydroxyphenylalanine
ECG	electrocardiogram
EMA	European Medicines Agency
EMC	Electronic Medicines Compendium (UK)
ER	extended release
FDA	US Food and Drug Administration
FoG	freezing of gait
FTD	frontotemporal dementia.
GABA	gamma-aminobutyric acid
GFR	glomerular filtration rate
GI	gastrointestinal
GP	general practitioner
HD	Huntington's disease
HDL	high-density lipoprotein
HIV	human immunodeficiency virus
ICD	impulse control disorder

IM	intramuscular
INR	international normalized ratio
IR	immediate release
IV	intravenous
LBD	Lewy body dementia
LCIG	levodopa/carbidopa infusion gel
LDH	lactic dehydrogenase
LDL	low-density lipoprotein
LID	levodopa-induced dyskinesias
MAO-A/-B	monoamine oxidase-A/-B
MAOIs	monoamine oxidase inhibitors
MCI	mild cognitive impairment
MDS EBM Committee	Movement Disorders Society Evidence-Based Medicine Committee
MI	myocardial infarction
MMSE	mini mental state examination
MPTP	1-methyl-4-phenyl-1,2,3,6-tetrahydropyridine
MRI	magnetic resonance imaging
mRS	modified ranking score
MSA	multiple system atrophy
NAION	non-arteritic anterior ischaemic optic neuropathy
NMDA	N-methyl-D-aspartate
NMS	neuroleptic malignant(-like) syndrome
NSAIDs	non-steroidal anti-inflammatory drugs
OCD	obsessive-compulsive disorder
ODT	orally disintegrating tablets
PDD	Parkinson's disease dementia
PEG	percutaneous endoscopic gastrostomy
P-gp	P-glycoprotein
PPI	proton pump inhibitor
PR	prolonged release
PSP	progressive supranuclear palsy
PT	prothrombin time
QID	four times a day
QoL	quality of life
RBC	red blood cell
RBD	REM sleep behaviour disorder
RCT	randomized controlled trial
REM	rapid eye movement
RLS	restless legs syndrome
SC	subcutaneous
SGOT	Serum glutamate-oxaloacetic transaminase
SIADH	syndrome of inappropriate antidiuretic hormone secretion
SNP	single nucleotide polymorphism
SNRI	serotonin and norepinephrine c inhibitor
SSRI	selective serotonin reuptake inhibitor
STN	subthalamic nucleus
TCA	tricyclic antidepressants

ABBREVIATIONS

TIA	transient ischaemic attack
TID	three times a day
Tmax	time to maximum serum concentration
TSH	thyroid-stimulating hormone
TTS	transdermal therapeutic systems
UK	United Kingdom
UNL	upper normal limit
UPDRS	unified Parkinson's disease rating scale
USA	United States of America
VAT	value-added tax
WBC	white blood cells
γGT	gamma-glutamyl transferase

ABBREVIATIONS

INTRODUCTION

The *Movement Disorders Prescriber's Guide to Parkinson's Disease* provides a comprehensive and succinct guide for all clinicians and health professionals involved in the treatment of people with Parkinson's disease. The guide provides practical information for use by clinicians and healthcare practitioners at all levels.

The chapters are alphabetical and follow the same format to enable quick retrieval of required information. Clinical experience of place in therapy and practice vignettes are included in each chapter.

General Notes
- All provided information applies to adult and not paediatric populations.
- 'Usual dosage range' under the section of 'Dosing and Use' refers to total daily dose, unless otherwise stated.
- Provided information applies for drug use in the context of Parkinson's disease (not other drugs indications), unless stated otherwise.
- The sections of drug-to-drug interactions refer to the most commonly used drugs in routine clinical practice; in case of doubt, consider consulting the marketed product provided information.
- In case of overdose always consult the relevant (local) poison control centre for the most up-to-date information.
- Provided costs only apply in the UK.

A

AMANTADINE

Therapeutics

Chemical Name and Structure

Amantadine (tricyclo[3.3.1.1]decan-1-amine, 1-adamantanamine, 1-aminoadamantane) is a white or nearly white crystalline, odourless, and bitter-tasting powder, with a molecular weight of 151.25 and an empirical formula of $C_{10}H_{17}N$. Amantadine is a tricyclic amine with two available preparations, amantadine hydrochloride, which is given orally, and the salt amantadine sulphate, which is administered either orally or IV.

Brand Names

- **Actison, Ampakine** (*Argentina*); **Amandin** (*Hong Kong*); **Amantex** (*Tunisia*); **Amantix** (*Poland*); **Amantrel** (*India*); **Atenegine** (*Japan*); **Amantix** (*Poland*); **Amantin** (*Ukraine*).
- **Enzil** (*Hong Kong*).
- **Gocovri** (*USA*).
- **Hofcomant** (*Greece*).
- **Kinestrel** (*Mexico*).
- **Lysovir** (*UK*).★
- **Mantadan** (*Italy*); **Mantadix** (*France*); **Mantidan** (*Brazil*); **Midantan** (*Russian Federation*).
- **Neomidantan** (*Russian Federation, Ukraine*).
- **Osmolex** (*USA*).
- **Parkadina** (*Portugal*); **PK-Merz** (*Austria, Czech Republic, Estonia, Germany, Hong Kong, Hungary, Israel, Lithuania, Malaysia, Mexico, Philippines, Russian Federation, Switzerland, Turkey, Ukraine*); **Prayanol** (*Chile*).
- **Symadin** (*South Africa*); **Symmetrel** (*Australia, Greece, Hong Kong, Japan, Netherlands, New Zealand, Singapore, South Africa, Switzerland, UK*).
- **Tregor** (*Germany*); **Trilasym** (*UK*).
- **Viregyt-K** (*Czech Republic, Hungary, Poland*).

★Not licensed for Parkinson's disease.

Generics Available

- Yes.

Licensed Indications for Parkinson's Disease

- Idiopathic Parkinson's disease, either as monotherapy or as an add-on to standard preparations (FDA, EMA, EMC), anti-dyskinetic action and used to manage levodopa-induced dyskinesias.

Licensed Indications for Other Conditions

- Post-encephalitic parkinsonism, symptomatic parkinsonism following CNS injury by carbon monoxide intoxication (FDA-only for immediate release tablet/capsule or syrup), drug-induced parkinsonism (FDA), parkinsonism cases (FDA, EMA).

A

- Herpes zoster, in elderly or debilitated patients at risk of developing a severe and painful rash in order to manage long-duration pain (EMC).
- Influenza A virus infection (prophylaxis, treatment) (FDA-only for immediate release tablet/capsule or syrup).*

*No longer recommended due to resistance (Centers for Disease Control and Prevention (CDC)).

Non-licensed Use for Parkinson's Disease
- Levodopa-induced peak dose and diphasic dyskinesias.

Non-licensed Use for Other Conditions
- Creutzfeldt–Jacob disease (limited early evidence).
- Triple therapy of amantadine, ribavirin, and interferon in chronic hepatitis C patients previously unresponsive to therapy.
- Intractable hiccups.
- Fatigue in multiple sclerosis.
- Fatigue in Parkinson's disease (investigational).

Ineffective
- Depression.
- Huntington's disease.
- Essential tremor.
- Tardive dyskinesia.
- Chronic hepatitis C patients, who are treatment-naïve or experience relapses.

Mechanism of Action
- Although the precise mechanism by which amantadine exerts anti-parkinsonian effects is poorly understood, it has been proposed to be due to increased dopamine release, prevention of dopamine reuptake and a direct, mild anticholinergic effect.
- Amantadine is a weak, non-competitive antagonist of NMDA glutamate receptors. Its anti-glutamatergic properties may explain the anti-dyskinetic efficacy.
- The antiviral mechanism seems to be unrelated to the amantadine effect in the context of Parkinson's disease.

Efficacy Profile
- The goal of amantadine therapy is to achieve better control of parkinsonian symptoms/signs, including levodopa-induced dyskinesias, plus minimizing adverse effects produced by increased levodopa dosage and improving patients' quality of life.
- According to the MDS EBM Committee:
  - amantadine is 'likely efficacious' and 'possibly useful', as an early monotherapy in Parkinson's disease;
  - amantadine is 'efficacious' and 'clinically useful' in treating dyskinesias.
  - there is 'insufficient evidence' to support amantadine use in the management of Parkinson's disease-related ICDs and related disorders.

THERAPEUTICS

3

- The beneficial effect of IR amantadine preparations has been demonstrated in numerous high-quality studies, while a multi-centre, double-blind RCT has shown that wash-out of amantadine in dyskinetic Parkinson's disease patients significantly worsened LID.
- Long-term efficacy of IR amantadine preparations (≥1 year) has been demonstrated in one RCT and one double-blind, placebo-controlled, non-randomized study.
- Three double-blind RCTs have demonstrated the efficacy of ER amantadine preparations on LID in Parkinson's disease patients, while an open-label extension study has found no long-term safety and tolerability issues for a 2-year follow-up period (EASE LID 1, 2 & 3, ALLAY-LID 2). A secondary benefit of reduction in OFF time was also noted.
- A double-blind crossover study with an open follow-up period has found that a small sample of Parkinson's disease patients abolished or reduced pathological gambling with amantadine use. Interestingly, a retrospective analysis of a large cross-sectional study (DOMINION) of ICDs in Parkinson's disease has shown that amantadine use was associated with occurrence of ICDs, including pathological gambling.
- According to a retrospective study, a longer duration of amantadine treatment may decrease the rate of FoG. Another small retrospective study has found a patient-reported subjective improvement in FoG after initiating amantadine, although this effect was transient on some occasions.
- Amantadine is less effective than levodopa in treating parkinsonian motor symptoms.
- It is probably equally effective to anticholinergic agents in treating parkinsonian symptoms. Addition of amantadine to anticholinergic agents might produce further improvement, although this is not a commonly encountered or recommended as a combination due to significant safety issues.
- Addition of amantadine to levodopa is expected to produce greater reduction in parkinsonian symptoms than amantadine or levodopa alone (in patients who cannot tolerate high levodopa doses).
- Amantadine's anti-dyskinetic action is expected to appear about 48 h after ingestion. In some countries (e.g. Austria) Amantadine is occasionally given IV to counter severe dyskinesias.
- Preliminary evidence based on primary cultures (neurons, microglia, and astroglia) has suggested a neuroprotective role of amantadine on dopamine neurons via an anti-inflammatory effect mediated by microglia and an enhanced expression of GDNF in astroglia.

Pharmacokinetics

Absorption and Distribution
- Oral bioavailability: 86–90%.
- Food co-ingestion: neither delays the rate, nor reduces the extent of absorption.

A

- Tmax: 2–4 h (IR preparations) and 12 h (ER preparations).
- Time to steady state: within 3 days.
- Pharmacokinetics: linear for doses up to 200 mg/day, higher doses may result in greater than proportional increase in maximum plasma concentrations.
- Protein binding: 67%.
- Volume of distribution: 1.5–6.1 l/kg (oral preparations).

Metabolism
- Metabolized to a minor extent, mostly by N-acetylation (5–15%). At least eight metabolites have been identified in the urine (unknown clinical significance).

Elimination
- Half-life in healthy adults is about 16 h (10–31 h).
  - Half-life may be at least two- or three-fold prolonged in impaired renal function (CrCl<40 ml/min/1.73 m^2).
- Amantadine is mostly (~80–90%) excreted unchanged in the urine after 4–5 days.
  - Urine acidification (including urine-acidifying drugs) may increase amantadine excretion, while an increased pH in the urine might have the opposite effect.

DRUG INTERACTION PROFILE

Drug Interaction Profile
Pharmacokinetic Drug Interactions
- Urine-acidifying drugs (e.g. *acetazolamide*) may decrease levels and effects of amantadine due to increasing its excretion rate.
- *Quinidine, sulfamethoxazole,* and *triamterene* may increase levels and effects of amantadine by decreasing renal clearance.

Pharmacodynamic Drug Interactions
- Co-medication with *abobotulinumtoxinA, onabotulinumtoxinA,* tricyclic antidepressants, neuroleptics, antimuscarinic agents used for overactive bladder (e.g. *solifenacin, oxybutynin*), antihistamines, MAOIs, and other agents with anticholinergic properties (e.g. *trazodone*) may enhance potential systemic anticholinergic effects (synergistic action), particularly in terms of inhibiting GI motility.
  - Co-administration with anticholinergic antiparkinsonian agents may provide additional therapeutic benefit in marginally treated patients compared to either agent alone, but may lead to adverse anticholinergic effects, including nightmares, confusion, and acute psychotic reactions.
- Co-administration with opiates may lead to anticholinergic-like effects (usually in opiate abuse, not in usual doses).
- Co-administration with alcohol might increase potential CNS effects, such as dizziness, somnolence, light-headedness, orthostatic hypotension and confusion.

A

AMANTADINE

- Co-administration with CNS stimulants may result in additive CNS stimulation, causing nervousness, irritability, insomnia, or even seizures or arrhythmias.
- Co-administration with *thioridazine* has been reported to worsen tremor in elderly Parkinson's disease patients.
- Co-medication with drugs causing electrolyte imbalance or increasing QT interval, such as Class IA and III anti-arrhythmics, antipsychotics (e.g. *haloperidol*, *phenothiazine derivatives*, *pimozide*), tricyclic antidepressants, certain antimicrobial agents (e.g. *moxifloxacin*, *erythromycin*), certain antihistamines (e.g. *astemizole*, *mizolastine*),, and others may lead to potentially fatal Torsade de Pointes arrhythmias and is considered a risk factor for sudden cardiac death.
- Co-medication with serotonergic agents, including SSRIs/SNRIs, tricyclic antidepressants, opioids, *lithium*, *buspirone*, amphetamines, MAOIs, and triptans may increase the risk of a potentially life-threatening serotonin syndrome.
- Co-administration with *bupropion* or *memantine* may lead to pharmacodynamic synergism and increased adverse effects from the CNS (e.g. agitation, dizziness).

Adverse Effects
How Drug Causes Adverse Effects
- The exact mechanism by which amantadine causes adverse effects has not been established, although acute toxicity may be attributable to its anticholinergic effects.
- It is generally well-tolerated with more side effects occurring with higher doses.
- Side effects usually appear within the first 2–4 days of treatment initiation and disappear 24–48 h after amantadine discontinuation.

Common Adverse Effects
- Very common (≥1/10):
  - IR preparations: oedema of ankles, livedo reticularis.
  - ER preparations: hallucinations, dizziness, dry mouth, peripheral oedema, constipation, falls, orthostatic hypotension, urinary tract infections.
- Common (≥1/100 to <1/10):
  - Neuropsychiatric: anxiety, elevation of mood, light-headedness, headache, lethargy, hallucinations, nightmares, ataxia, slurred speech, loss of concentration, nervousness, depression, insomnia, myalgia, hallucinations, confusion, nightmares.
  - Cardiovascular: palpitations, orthostatic hypotension.
  - GI: dry mouth, anorexia, nausea, vomiting, constipation.
  - Skin: diaphoresis.

- Uncommon (≥1/1,000 to <1/100):
  - Eye/ear: blurred vision.

Life-Threatening or Dangerous Adverse Effects
- Rare (≥1/10,000 to <1/1,000):
  - Suicidality.
  - Neuroleptic malignant-like syndrome.
  - Convulsions.
  - Psychosis.
  - Heart failure.
  - Urinary retention.
- Very rare (<1/10,000):
  - Leukopenia.
- Unknown frequency:
  - Delirium.

Rare and Not Life-Threatening Adverse Effects
- Corneal oedema
- Reversible elevation of liver enzymes.
- ICDs.
- Tremor, dyskinesia.
- Diarrhoea.
- Exanthema, photosensitization.
- Urinary incontinence.

Weight Change
- Not reported.

What to Do About Adverse Effects
- Discuss common adverse effects with patients or caregivers before starting medication, including symptoms that should be reported to the physician.
- In some cases, adverse effects subside after the first week of continued therapy.
- Some adverse events (especially CNS-related) are dose-dependent, so consider lowering the dose to 200 mg or 100 mg daily. If adverse effects are still troublesome or persist, consider withdrawing therapy completely.
- In case of newly developing adverse effects, consider excluding renal impairment or interactions with newly introduced medications.
- If patients on amantadine experience excessive drowsiness, somnolence, and/or episodes of sudden-onset sleep during activities that require active participation, they should refrain from driving or operating machines and inform their treating physician. Therapy discontinuation is generally advised.
  - Patients should be particularly vigilant, as they may not have any warning signs and they may feel alert just prior to falling asleep.

A

Dosing and Use

Usual Dosage Range
- IR: 100–400 mg daily (a dose of 400 mg/day should not be exceeded).
- ER: 137–274 mg daily (Gocovril).
- ER: 129–322 mg daily (Osmolex ER).

Available Formulations
- Capsules: 100 mg.
- Oral solution: 50 mg/5 ml.
- Capsules, ER: 68.5 mg, 137 mg (Gocovril).
- Tablets, ER: 129 mg, 193 mg, 258 mg (Osmolex ER).

How to Dose
- IR: 100 mg daily for at least one week; may increase to 100 mg twice daily and titrate accordingly against signs and symptoms without exceeding 400 mg/day in divided doses (gradual dose increase at intervals of at least 1 week).
- ER (Gocovril): 137 mg once at bedtime; increase to 274 mg once at bedtime after one week.
- ER (Osmolex): 129 mg once in the morning: may increase dose in weekly intervals up to 322 mg/day (one 129 mg + one 193 mg tablet).

Dosing Tips
- Amantadine IR or ER products are not interchangeable.
- Direct switching from conventional amantadine to ER preparations was found to be efficacious and well-tolerated.
- Doses exceeding 200 mg/day may provide some additional relief but have been associated with increased neuropsychiatric side effects.
- Amantadine may appear to lose efficacy within a few months of continuous treatment; effectiveness may be prolonged by withdrawal for 3–4 weeks.
- Avoid evening or bedtime dosing of amantadine to prevent insomnia, confusion, or hallucinations, especially among the elderly.
- Administer daily doses in two divided doses to decrease adverse CNS effects.
- No additional benefit is expected from amantadine therapy where optimized therapeutic doses of levodopa are administered.

How to Withdraw Drug
- Amantadine should be withdrawn gradually, e.g. half the dose at weekly intervals, in order to lower the risk of withdrawal symptoms.
  - Osmolex ER: gradually reduce dose from higher doses to 129 mg daily for 1–2 weeks before discontinuation.
  - Gocovri: to stop therapy in patients who have been on the drug for more than 4 weeks, the dose should be reduced by half if possible for their final week of dosing.

- Withdrawal symptoms may present as aggravation of parkinsonian features, delirium, agitation, delusions, hallucinations, paranoid reaction, stupor, anxiety, depression, or slurred speech.
  - Parkinsonian crises, manifesting as confusion, marked rigidity, urinary retention, and bulbar palsy, have been reported within 3 days after an abrupt amantadine discontinuation, even in the absence of apparent clinical efficacy of amantadine.
- In case of amantadine titration or discontinuation, close patient monitoring is advised; cases of NMS have been reported, especially in patients treated with neuroleptics.

Overdose
- May be fatal; the lowest reported acute lethal dose was 1000 mg.
- It can present as:
  - Cardiovascular: arrhythmia, tachycardia, hypertension, heart failure/arrest.
  - Respiratory: hyperventilation, pulmonary oedema, respiratory distress, ARDS.
  - Renal: urine retention, decreased CrCl, renal insufficiency.
  - CNS: hyperreflexia, restlessness, convulsions, torsion spasms, dystonic posturing, dilated pupils, dysphagia, confusion, disorientation, delirium, hallucinations, acute psychosis, myoclonus, lethargy, hyperthermia, coma.
  - Gastrointestinal: dry mouth, nausea, vomiting.
- There is no specific antidote. Close monitoring is advised.
- Vomiting induction and/or gastric aspiration (and lavage in conscious patients), administration of activated charcoal, or saline cathartic may be used according to clinical judgement.
  - Haemodialysis does not remove significant amounts of amantadine (~4%), possibly due to extensive tissue binding.
- In case of convulsions and/or excessive motor restlessness, consider administering anticonvulsants, such as diazepam IV, paraldehyde IM or per rectum, or phenobarbital IM.
- In case of acute psychotic symptoms, delirium, dystonic posturing, or myoclonus, consider administering physostigmine by slow IV infusion (1 mg in adults). Repeat as applicable.
- In case of urine retention, consider placing an indwelling bladder catheter, which can be maintained for the time required.

Tests and Therapeutic Drug Monitoring
- Assessment of renal function is advised at baseline and at regular intervals, especially in the case of new adverse events.
- Periodic monitoring for melanoma development is advised.

Other Warnings/Precautions
- Close monitoring is advised in patients with known cardiovascular disorders (including orthostatic hypotension, peripheral oedema, and

A

AMANTADINE

congestive heart failure) or eczematoid dermatitis, as amantadine may aggravate these conditions.
- Close monitoring is advised in patients with known psychiatric disorders, as amantadine may exacerbate psychosis (particularly the ER preparations), especially at initiation and after dose increases. An alternative therapeutic option should be used, if possible.
- Close monitoring is advised in case of conditions (including pharmacological agents) that alter the urine pH to more acidic or alkaline, as they will predispose to an increased or decreased excretion of amantadine, respectively. On the latter occasion, increased accumulation of amantadine may occur, increasing the possibility for adverse events.
- Co-administration with alcohol is not recommended. Alcohol may result in dose-dumping if co-administered with ER amantadine.
- Amantadine may be co-administered with the influenza virus vaccine, administered by intramuscular injection (inactivated vaccine), but not with the nasal flu vaccine (live attenuated vaccine).

Do Not Use (Contraindications)
- Known sensitivity to amantadine or to any of its excipients, including lactose.
  ◦ Patients with rare hereditary problems of galactose intolerance, total lactase deficiency or glucose–galactose malabsorption.
- History of gastric ulceration.
- Untreated angle closure glaucoma.
- History of seizures.
- Cholinergic subtype of Parkinson's disease where use of anticholinergics can be hazardous owing to worsening cognitive function.

Special Populations
Renal Impairment
- Elimination is almost exclusively via urinary excretion, even in renal failure, and amantadine may persist in the plasma for several days, causing severe side effects in the case of accumulation.
- Amantadine dosage should be individualized according to CrCl:
  - UK:
    - CrCl>35 ml/min: 100 mg daily.
    - CrCl 15–35 ml/min: 100 mg every 2–3 days.
    - CrCl<15 ml/min: not recommended.
  - USA:
    - CrCl 30–50 ml/min: 200 mg on the first day; 100 mg daily afterwards.
    - CrCl 15–29 ml/min: 200 mg on the first day; 200 mg on alternate days afterwards.
    - CrCl<15 ml/min or patients on haemodialysis: 200 mg every 7 days.
    - ER preparations are contraindicated in end-stage renal disease (CrCl<15 ml/min).

Hepatic Impairment
- The pharmacokinetics of amantadine are unaffected by hepatic function and dosage adjustments are not necessary in hepatic impairment.

Elderly
- Elderly patients are more susceptible to adverse effects due to age-related reductions in renal clearance; thus, the lowest effective dose should be used.
- Dosage can be guided by CrCl.
- Half-life may be prolonged in healthy geriatric adults, for example 29 h (20–41 h) in men 60–76 years old.

Pregnancy
- Amantadine is contraindicated during pregnancy and in women trying to become pregnant.
- Amantadine-related complications during pregnancy, including cardiovascular lesions of the fetus, have been reported.
- Adverse developmental effects (embryo lethality, high risk of malformations, reduced fetal body weight) have been found in animal studies with amantadine use.

Breastfeeding
- Amantadine is excreted in human milk.
- There is no available information on the effect of amantadine on milk production or the breastfed infant; however, potential undesirable effects cannot be excluded.
- Amantadine use is contraindicated in nursing mothers.

Costs
NHS indicative price (accessed on 31 October 2021):
- 56×100 mg caps £22.60+VAT.
- 150 ml of 50 mg/5 ml oral solution £140+VAT.

The Overall Place of Amantadine in the Treatment of Parkinson's Disease

Amantadine is fairly unique among the anti-parkinsonian drugs in combining glutamatergic, dopaminergic, and anticholinergic properties, although safinamide has multi-target action as well. The efficacy of amantadine on the core motor symptoms of Parkinson's disease (tremor, bradykinesia, rigidity) is considered modest. Despite being officially approved as early monotherapy in Parkinson's disease, it is usually administered as an adjunct therapy to levodopa, especially to mitigate levodopa-induced dyskinesias. ER preparations of amantadine have been recently developed with updated indications to address motor fluctuations, specifically levodopa-induced dyskinesias. Potential non-motor effects of

A

THE TREATMENT OF PARKINSON'S DISEASE

amantadine include a possible benefit in central fatigue. Clinical experience suggests poor efficacy for daytime sleepiness. Pivotal studies suggest that patients on IR formulations can be directly switched to ER preparations without interruption, which may provide dosing convenience benefits and additional clinical efficacy. Strong evidence is lacking on the effect of oral preparations of amantadine on FoG in the context of Parkinson's disease. Finally, although there is some evidence considering amantadine efficacy on pathological gambling in the context of dopaminergic medications, this effect remains largely controversial and needs to be further investigated. High doses of amantadine are usually avoided due to the risk of adverse events, with hallucinations and confusion being particularly common, especially among the elderly or individuals with renal impairment. Finally, a neuroprotective role of amantadine has been reported considering various neurological disorders, including Parkinson's disease; this notion guides many clinicians to introduce amantadine early in Parkinson's disease therapy; however, no robust evidence exists to conclusively support this practice.

Potential Advantages
• Amantadine is a globally available cheap therapeutic option with a good safety profile and numerous high-quality studies supporting its efficacy in different stages of Parkinson's disease.
• Maximum concentration of amantadine is reached more slowly and sustained for longer with ER preparations, thus reducing the rate of adverse events and rendering the drug more tolerable for patients. It, thus, constitutes a reasonable therapeutic option in the management of refractory LID, as it is less invasive than DBS or infusion regimens.
• ER amantadine formulations improve patients' adherence, which is particularly important for advanced Parkinson's disease patients who commonly follow complex drug schemes.

Potential Disadvantages
• Careful dosage increase is necessary to lower amantadine risk of psychotoxicity.
• Amantadine may exhibit anticholinergic adverse effects, especially in combination with other drugs with such properties.
• Extra caution is required when using amantadine in geriatric patients.

Clinical Box
A 65-year-old man with a 7-year history of Parkinson's disease on levodopa/benserazide 200/50 mg QID and transdermal rotigotine 12 mg/24 h presented with peak-dose, troublesome dyskinesias. He was prescribed amantadine IR 100 mg in the morning for 1 week and then increased to 100 mg BID (morning and afternoon avoiding night-time dosing). Marked improvement of dyskinesias was documented within 2 weeks after amantadine initiation.

A

Suggested Reading

Isaacson, SH, S Fahn, R Pahwa, CM Tanner, AJ Espay, C Trenkwalder, CH Adler, R Patni, R Johnson. Parkinson's patients with dyskinesia switched from immediate release amantadine to open-label ADS-5102. *Mov Dis Clin Pract* 2018; 5(2): 183–190.

Marmol S, M Feldman, C Singer, J Margolesky. Amantadine revisited: a contender for initial treatment in Parkinson's disease? *CNS Drugs* 2021; 35(11): 1141–1152.

Rascol O, M Fabbri, W Poewe. Amantadine in the treatment of Parkinson's disease and other movement disorders. *Lancet Neurol* 2021; 20(12): 1048–1056.

Thomas A, L Bonanni, F Gambi, A Di Iorio, M Onofrj. Pathological gambling in Parkinson disease is reduced by amantadine. *Ann Neurol* 2010; 68(3): 400–404.

References

Aarsland D, L Batzu, GM Halliday, GJ Geurtsen, C Ballard, K Ray Chaudhuri, D Weintraub. Parkinson disease-associated cognitive impairment. *Nature Rev Dis Primers* 2021; 7(1): 47.

AHFS Drug information. Bethesda: American Society of Health-System Pharmacists (2012). Accessed via www.medicinescomplete .com on 29 December 2022.

Amantadine. In: Brayfield A (Ed), *Martindale: The Complete Drug Reference*. London: The Royal Pharmaceutical Society of Great Britain. Accessed online via www.medicinescomplete.com on 31 October 2021.

Amantadine. In: DRUGDEX® System (electronic version). Truven Health Analytics, Greenwood Village, Colorado, USA. Accessed via www.micromedexsolutions.com on 31 October 2021.

Chang C, K Ramphul. Amantadine. StatPearls. Treasure Island (FL): StatPearls Publishing. Copyright © 2022, StatPearls Publishing LLC; 2022.

da Silva-Júnior, FP, P Braga-Neto, F Sueli Monte, VM de Bruin. Amantadine reduces the duration of levodopa-induced dyskinesia: a randomized, double-blind, placebo-controlled study. *Parkinsonism Relat Disord* 2005; 11(7): 449–452.

Giladi N, TA Treves, ES Simon, H Shabtai, Y Orlov, B Kandinov, D Paleacu, AD Korczyn. Freezing of gait in patients with advanced Parkinson's disease. *J Neural Transm (Vienna)* 2001; 108(1): 53–61.

Isaacson, SH, S Fahn, R Pahwa, CM Tanner, AJ Espay, C Trenkwalder, CH Adler, R Patni, R Johnson Parkinson's patients with dyskinesia switched from immediate release amantadine to open-label ADS-5102. *Mov Disord Clin Pract* 2018; 5(2): 183–190.

Joint Formulary Committee. British National Formulary (online). London: BMJ Group and Pharmaceutical Press. Accessed via www .medicinescomplete.com on 29 December 2022.

REFERENCES

Lechin F, B van der Dijs, B Pardey-Maldonado, JE Rivera, S Baez, ME Lechin. Effects of amantadine on circulating neurotransmitters in healthy subjects. *J Neural Transm (Vienna)* 2010; 117(3): 293–299.

Malkani RC Zadikoff, O Melen, A Videnovic, E Borushko, T Simuni. Amantadine for freezing of gait in patients with Parkinson disease. *Clin Neuropharmacol* 2012; 35(6): 266–268.

Metman LV, P Del Dotto, K LePoole, S Konitsiotis, J Fang, TN Chase. Amantadine for levodopa-induced dyskinesias: a 1-year follow-up study. *Arch Neurol* 1999; 56(11): 1383–1386.

Moresco RM, MA Volonte, C Messa, et al. New perspectives on neuro-chemical effects of amantadine in the brain of parkinsonian patients: a PET–[(11)C]raclopride study. *J Neural Transm (Vienna)* 2002; 109(10): 1265–1274.

Oertel WK Eggert, R Pahwa, CM Tanner, RA Hauser, C Trenkwalder, R Ehret, JP Azulay, S Isaacson, L Felt, MJ Stempien. Randomized, placebo-controlled trial of ADS-5102 (amantadine) extended-release capsules for levodopa-induced dyskinesia in Parkinson's disease (EASE LID 3). *Mov Disord* 2017; 32(12): 1701–1709.

Ory-Magne F, JC Corvol, JP Azulay, AM Bonnet, C Brefel-Courbon, P Damier, E Dellapina, A Destée, F Durif, M Galitzky, T Lebouvier, W Meissner, C Thalamas, F Tison, A Salis, A Sommet, F Viallet, M Vidailhet, O Rascol. Withdrawing amantadine in dyskinetic patients with Parkinson disease: the AMANDYSK trial. *Neurology* 2014; 82(4): 300–307.

Ossola B, N Schendzielorz, SH Chen, GS Bird, RK Tuominen, PT Männistö, JS Hong. Amantadine protects dopamine neurons by a dual action: reducing activation of microglia and inducing expression of GDNF in astroglia [corrected]. *Neuropharmacology* 2011; 61(4): 574–582.

Pahwa R, CM Tanner, RA Hauser, SH Isaacson, PA Nausieda, DD Truong, P Agarwal, KL Hull, KE Lyons, R Johnson, MJ Stempien. ADS-5102 (amantadine) extended-release capsules for levodopa-induced dyskinesia in Parkinson disease (EASE LID Study): a ran-domized clinical trial. *JAMA Neurol* 2017; 74(8): 941–949.

Rascol O, M Fabbri, W Poewe. Amantadine in the treatment of Par-kinson's disease and other movement disorders. *Lancet Neurol* 2021; 20(12): 1048–1056.

Rascol O, L Tönges, T deVries, M Jaros, A Quartel, D Jacobs. Immediate-release/extended-release amantadine (OS320) to treat Parkinson's disease with levodopa-induced dyskinesia: analysis of the randomized, controlled ALLAY-LID studies. *Parkinsonism Relat Disord* 2022; 96: 65–73.

Sanders WL. Creutzfeldt–Jakob disease treated with amantadine. *J Neu-rol Neurosurg Psychiatry* 1979; 42(10): 960–961.

Sawada H, T Oeda, S Kuno, M Nomoto, K Yamamoto, M Yamamoto, K Hisanaga, T Kawamura. Amantadine for dyskinesias in Parkinson's disease: a randomized controlled trial. *PLoS One* 2010; 5(12): e15298.

A

AMANTADINE

A

Snow BJ, L Macdonald, D McAuley, W Wallis. The effect of amantadine on levodopa-induced dyskinesias in Parkinson's disease: a double-blind, placebo-controlled study. *Clin Neuropharmacol* 2000; 23(2): 82–85.

Sommerauer C, P Rebernik, H Reither, C Nanoff, C Pifl. The noradrenaline transporter as site of action for the anti-Parkinson drug amantadine. *Neuropharmacology* 2012; 62(4): 1708–1716.

Summary of Product Characteristics – Amantadine hydrochloride 100 mg capsules. Electronic Medicines Compendium: Amantadine hydrochloride 100 mg capsules – summary of product characteristics (SmPC) – (emc). Accessed on 31 October 2021 via www.medicines .org.uk.

Tanner CM, R Pahwa, RA Hauser, WH Oertel, SH Isaacson, J Jankovic, R Johnson, D Chernick, J Hubble. EASE LID 2: a 2-year open-label trial of Gocovri (amantadine) extended release for dyskinesia in Parkinson's Disease. *J Parkinsons Dis* 2020; 10(2): 543–558.

Thomas A, L Bonanni, F Gambi, A Di Iorio, M Onofrj. Pathological gambling in Parkinson disease is reduced by amantadine. *Ann Neurol* 2010; 68(3): 400–404.

Verhagen Metman L, P Del Dotto, P van den Munckhof, J Fang, MM Mouradian, T Chase. Amantadine as treatment for dyskinesias and motor fluctuations in Parkinson's disease. *Neurology* 1998; 50(5): 1323–1326.

Weintraub D, M Sohr, MN Potenza, AD Siderowf, M Stacy, V Voon, J Whetteckey, GR Wunderlich, AE Lang. Amantadine use associated with impulse control disorders in Parkinson disease in cross-sectional study. *Ann Neurol* 2010; 68(6): 963–968.

Wolf E, K Seppi, R Katzenschlager, G Hochschorner, G Ransmayr, P Schwingenschuh, E Ott, I Kloiber, D Haubenberger, E Auff, W Poewe. Long-term antidyskinetic efficacy of amantadine in Parkinson's disease. *Mov Disord* 2010; 25(10): 1357–1363.

REFERENCES

AMITRIPTYLINE

*Amitriptyline doses reported in the literature and the following chapter refer to amitriptyline hydrochloride, unless stated otherwise.

Therapeutics

Chemical Name and Structure

Amitriptyline hydrochloride (3-(10,11-dihydro-5H-dibenzo[a,d]cycloheptene-5-ylidene)-N,N-dimethylpropan-1-amine; hydrochloride) has a molecular weight of 313.9 and a molecular formula of $C_{20}H_{23}N,HCl$. Amitriptyline is usually given as the hydrochloride and doses are expressed in terms of this salt. Amitriptyline hydrochloride 75 mg is equivalent to about 66.3 mg of the base.

Brand Names

- **Adepril** (*Italy*); **ADT** (*Portugal*); **Amderip** (*South Africa*); **Amineurin** (*Germany, South Africa*); **Amioxid** (Germany); **Amiptril** (*Argentina*); **Amirol** (*Cyprus, New Zealand*); **Amit** (*India*); **Amitec** (*Thailand*); **Amitone** (*India*); **Amitor** (*India*); **Amitrip** (*India*); **Amitryn** (*Thailand*); **Amrea** (*India*); **Amypres** (*India*); **Amytril** (*Brazil, Tunisia*); **Amyzol** (*Russian Federation*); **Anapsique** (*Mexico*); **Astilin** (*Ireland*).
- **Conmitrip** (*Thailand*); **Crypton** (*India*).
- **Deprelio** (*Spain*).
- **Elatrol** (*Israel*); **Elatrolet** (*Israel*); **Elavil** (*Canada, France, UK, USA*); **Eliwel** (*India, Russian Federation*); **Endep** (*Australia, Hong Kong*); **Entrip** (*Australia*).
- **Fiorda** (*Argentina*).
- **Gentrip** (*India*).
- **Kamitrin** (*India*).
- **Laroxyl** (*France, Italy, Turkey*); **Latilin** (*India*).
- **Maxivalet** (*Greece*); **Mitryp** (*India*).
- **Noriline** (*South Africa*).
- **Odep** (*India*).
- **Polytanol** (*Thailand*); **Protanol** (*Brazil*).
- **Qualitriptine** (*Hong Kong*).
- **Redomex** (*Belgium*).
- **Saroten** (*Australia, Austria, Denmark, Estonia, Germany, Greece, Russian Federation, South Africa, Sweden, Switzerland, Ukraine*); **Sarotena** (*India*); **Sarotex** (*Norway*); **Sinequan** (*Argentina*); **Stelminal** (*Germany, Greece*); **Syneudon** (*Germany*).
- **Teperin** (*Hungary*); **Thymontil** (*Greece*); **Trepiline** (*Hong Kong, South Africa*); **Trilin** (*Indonesia*); **Tripgen** (*Philippines*); **Tripsyl** (*Hong Kong*); **Tripsyline** (*Thailand*); **Tripta** (*Hong Kong, Malaysia, Singapore, Thailand*); **Triptizol** (*Italy, Spain*); **Triptyl** (*Finland*); **Triptyline** (*Thailand*); **Tripzol** (*Thailand*); **Tryptalgin** (*Argentina*);

Tryptanol (*Argentina, Brazil, Thailand, Venezuela*); **Tryptomer** (*India*); **Tryptizol** (*Spain*).
* **Veikirin** (*South Africa*).
In combination with other supplements:
* **Klotriptyl** (*Finland*); **Limbitrol** (*Brazil, Finland, South Africa*); **Minitran** (*Greece*); **Nobritol** (*Spain*); **Pertriptyl** (*Finland*).

Generics Available
* Yes.

Licensed Indications for Parkinson's Disease
* None.

Licensed Indications for Other Conditions
* Depression (FDA, EMA, EMC).
* Neuropathic pain, including post-herpetic neuralgia (EMA, EMC).
* Prophylactic treatment of migraine and chronic tension type headache (EMA, EMC).

Non-Licensed Use for Parkinson's Disease
* Depressive symptoms in Parkinson's disease.

Non-Licensed Use for Other Conditions
* Eating disorders.
* Intractable hiccup (anecdotal reports).
* Irritable bowel syndrome.

Ineffective
* Not reported.

Mechanism of Action
* The antidepressant properties of amitriptyline seem to be related to its inhibition of the reuptake of noradrenaline and serotonin at nerve terminals, leading to increased concentrations of these neurotransmitters in the synapse.
  * It inhibits the uptake of noradrenaline and serotonin equally well.
* It is believed to block sodium and potassium channels and NMDA receptors in the brain and the spinal cord, which is thought to mediate the pain-reducing effect.
* It also possesses varying affinity for muscarinic and histamine H1 receptors.

Efficacy Profile
* Amitriptyline has been characterized as 'possibly useful' in the management of depressive symptoms in Parkinson's disease patients, although there is 'insufficient evidence' of efficacy (MDS EBM Committee).

A

THERAPEUTICS

A

AMITRIPTYLINE

- According to an RCT comparing low-dose amitriptyline with low-dose fluoxetine in Parkinson's disease patients with depression for a follow-up period of 12 months, the former was found to be significantly effective in the management of depressive symptoms, although 15% of the enrolled patients had to end treatment due to side effects.
- A prospective single-blind randomized study comparing sertraline to low doses of amitriptyline in Parkinson's disease patients with depression showed that both drugs efficiently addressed depressive symptoms, although only sertraline was associated with a significant benefit on QoL.
- According to a recent systematic review and network meta-analysis in non- Parkinson's disease populations, amitriptyline is one of the most efficacious antidepressants in head-to-head studies, although less tolerable than others.
- Although the antidepressant effect of amitriptyline is expected after 2–4 weeks of therapy, adverse effects might appear earlier in treatment.

Pharmacokinetics

Absorption and Distribution
- Oral bioavailability: about 53%.
- Food co-ingestion: no food interactions have been reported.
- Tmax: 4 h (range 1–6 h).
- Time to steady state: within 1 week.
- Pharmacokinetics: a great variance is observed between individuals, which cannot be described by simple correlation.
- Protein binding: 95%.
- Volume of distribution: 16 ± 3 l/kg (after IV administration).

Metabolism
- Amitriptyline undergoes hepatic metabolism, mostly by CYP2C19 and CYP2D6 producing the active metabolite nortriptyline; the latter's metabolism is also clinically relevant.
- Amitriptyline is also metabolized by CYP3A4, CYP1A2 and CYP2C9.
- Amitriptyline metabolism is subject to genetic polymorphism (CYP450 isoenzymes).

Elimination
- Half-life for amitriptyline can range from 9 h to 25 h.
  - Half-life values can be significantly prolonged in overdosage.
- About 2% of an administered dose is excreted unchanged in urine and small amounts are found in faeces.
- Amitriptyline is mostly excreted in the form of metabolites.

Drug Interaction Profile

Pharmacokinetic Drug Interactions
- Effects by amitriptyline:
  - Amitriptyline might increase the levels of drugs that are metabolized by CYP2D6, such as *thioridazine, tramadol.*
- Effects on amitriptyline:
  - Strong (e.g. *bupropion, quinidine, fluoxetine, paroxetine*) and moderate CYP2D6 inhibitors (e.g. *duloxetine*) might increase amitriptyline serum levels.
  - Antifungals (e.g. *fluconazole, terbinafine*) might increase amitriptyline serum levels.
  - Inhibitors of other CYP350 isoenzymes, including *cimetidine, methylphenidate, ethanol, valproic acid* and calcium-channel blockers (e.g. *diltiazem, verapamil*), may increase plasma concentration of amitriptyline.
  - Oral contraceptives, *rifampicin, phenytoin, barbiturates,* and *carbamazepine* may lower plasma concentration of amitriptyline.

Pharmacodynamic Drug Interactions
- Co-medication with other serotonergic agents, including SSRIs/SNRIs, tricyclic antidepressants, opioids, *lithium, buspirone,* amphetamines, and triptans, can lead to a potentially life-threatening serotonin syndrome.
- Co-medication with neuroleptics or drugs causing electrolyte imbalance or increasing QT interval, such as Class IA and III anti-arrhythmics, antipsychotics (e.g. *haloperidol, phenothiazine derivatives*), tricyclic antidepressants, certain antimicrobial agents (e.g. *moxifloxacin, erythromycin*), certain antihistamines (e.g. *astemizole, mizolastine*), opiates, *pimozide, lithium,* and others, might lead to potentially fatal Torsade de Pointes arrhythmias and is considered a risk factor for sudden cardiac death.
- Co-medication with CNS depressants (e.g. benzodiazepines, most antipsychotics, antihistamines H1 antagonists, opioids) or alcohol might lead to synergistic sedative effects, including somnolence and dizziness.
- Co-administration with diuretics might increase the risk of hyponatremia or hypokalaemia (e.g. *furosemide*).

Adverse Effects

How Drug Causes Adverse Effects
- Although the activity of amitriptyline is mediated via a number of different neuronal receptors, its anticholinergic and antihistaminic effects are thought to be responsible for the most common adverse effects.
- If patients are poor CYP2D6 or CYP2C19 metabolizers, elevated serum levels of amitriptyline can occur with a higher risk of adverse effects.

A

ADVERSE EFFECTS

- A great percentage of amitriptyline adverse effects result from additive toxicity or from altered metabolism by other drugs.

Common Adverse Effects
- Very common (≥1/10):
  - Aggression, somnolence, tremor, dizziness, headache, drowsiness, dysarthria, accommodation disorder, palpitations, tachycardia, orthostatic hypotension, congested nose, dry mouth, constipation, nausea, increased perspiration, fatigue, feeling thirsty.
- Common (≥1/100 to <1/10):
  - Nervous/psychiatric: confusion, decreased libido, agitation, attention deficits, dysgeusia, paraesthesia, ataxia.
  - Eye/ear: mydriasis.
  - Cardiovascular: atrioventricular/bundle branch block, ECG abnormalities.
  - Renal/urinary: micturition disorders.
  - Reproductive: erectile dysfunction.
  - General: hyponatraemia.
- Uncommon (≥1/1,000 to <1/100):
  - Nervous/psychiatric: (hypo)mania, anxiety, insomnia, nightmares, convulsions.
  - Eye/ear: tinnitus, increased intraocular pressure.
  - Cardiovascular: collapse, aggravation of cardiac failure, hypertension.
  - Gastrointestinal: diarrhoea, vomiting, tongue oedema, hepatic impairment.
  - Skin: rash, urticaria, face oedema.
  - Renal/urinary: urinary retention.
  - Reproductive: galactorrhoea.

Life-Threatening or Dangerous Adverse Effects
- Rare (≥1/10,000 to <1/1,000):
  - Bone marrow suppression, agranulocytosis, leucopenia, eosinophilia, thrombocytopenia.
  - Delirium (especially in the elderly).
  - Acute glaucoma.
  - Arrhythmias.
  - Ileus paralytic.
- Very rare (<1/10,000):
  - Suicidal thoughts/behaviour.
  - Acute glaucoma.
  - Cardiomyopathy.
  - Alveolitis.
  - Ileus paralytic.

Rare and Not Life-Threatening Adverse Effects
- Decreased appetite.
- Hallucinations.

A

- Akathisia.
- Polyneuropathy.
- Salivary gland enlargement.
- Jaundice.
- Alopecia, photosensitivity reaction.
- Gynaecomastia.

Weight Change
- Weight increase is very common with amitriptyline use.
- Weight decrease is rare with amitriptyline use.

What to Do About Adverse Effects
- Before introducing amitriptyline, discuss common or life-threatening adverse effects with patients and/or caregivers, including symptoms that should be reported to the physician.
- Patients and their caregivers should be informed of the possibility of amitriptyline causing suicidal ideation/behaviour, especially in the early phase of treatment. If such signs/symptoms emerge, patients should urgently seek medical advice and be treated accordingly. Amitriptyline should be discontinued.
  - Due to suicidality risk, consider giving a limited quantity of amitriptyline to the patient.
- Patients and caregivers should be informed and be particularly vigilant for anticholinergic side effects of amitriptyline, including dry mouth, constipation, blurred vision, confusion, and seizures.
- Where a patient using amitriptyline reports bone pain, swelling, bruising, or point tenderness, the possibility of a subjacent bone fracture should be excluded.
- Tricyclic antidepressants might aggravate RBD in Parkinson's disease patients; consider removing amitriptyline before initiating treatment for RBD.
- Regular dental assessments are advised, as dry mouth is a common side effect of amitriptyline use.

Dosing and Use
Usual Dosage Range
- 10–150 mg.

Available Formulations
- Tablets: 10 mg, 25 mg, 50 mg, 75 mg, 100 mg, 150 mg.
- Oral solution: 10 mg/5 ml, 25 mg/5 ml, 50 mg/5 ml.

How to Dose
- Initial dose of 10–25 mg BID. If necessary, consider increasing the dose by 10–25 mg every 3–7 days (a minimum of every other day is

suggested) up to a maximum of 100–150 mg per day divided in two equal doses.

- A dosage of over 100 mg should only be administered on special occasions; extra caution is advised with higher dosage.
- Amitriptyline can also be administered as a single dose at night. The additional dose can be given late in the afternoon or in the evening.
- For those aged over 65 or those with cardiovascular disease an initial total dose of 10 mg is suggested; maximum total dose should not exceed 75–100 mg, either in one or two divided doses per day.
- Amitriptyline dose schedules should be carefully individualized; maintenance dose should be the lowest effective for the shortest possible duration.

Dosing Tips
- If amitriptyline therapy is effective, it should be used for a minimum of 6 months to ensure that the patient is free of symptoms and lower the risk of relapse.

How to Withdraw Drug
- Dosage tapering over a period of several weeks is necessary to lower the risk of withdrawal symptoms, especially in case of high dosage or a long treatment period (more than 8 weeks).
- A minimum of 4 weeks of tapering is suggested, depending on the initial dose and the duration of therapy (higher dosage and longer periods of treatment need longer tapering, which might be as long as 6 months).
- Withdrawal symptoms usually manifest as one of the following distinct syndromes:
  - Gastrointestinal disturbances and generalized symptoms, such as malaise, chills, headache, increased sweating, agitation, and anxiety.
  - Sleep impairment with insomnia, followed by vivid dreams.
  - Parkinsonism or akathisia.
  - Hypomania or mania.
- Cardiac arrhythmias might also be a consequence of abrupt discontinuation of amitriptyline.
- In case of severe or prolonged symptoms during dosage reduction or withdrawal, consider resuming the previously prescribed dose and follow a longer tapering period.
- Treating physicians need to be aware of the possibility of withdrawal symptoms to avoid misinterpretation of such symptoms as indications of relapse.

Overdose
- Amitriptyline overdose might present with mydriasis, tachycardia, urinary retention, dry mucous membranes, reduced bowel motility, fever, convulsions, alterations of level of consciousness, respiratory

A

depression, cardiac arrhythmias, hypotension, heart failure, cardio-genic shock, metabolic acidosis, hypokalaemia/hyponatraemia.
  • Broadening of the QRS complex (especially >0.16 s) is commonly analogous to the degree of amitriptyline toxicity following acute overdose.
• Ingestion of more than 750 mg of amitriptyline poses a higher risk for severe toxicity.
  • Simultaneous ingestion of alcohol or other psychotropic substances aggravates the effects of amitriptyline.
• Supportive measures, close monitoring, and maintenance of a clear airway with adequate ventilation are recommended. Continuous ECG monitoring for 3–5 days after overdose is advised.
• Consider activated charcoal (50 g) or gastric lavage if presenting within 1 h after amitriptyline ingestion.
• Avoid flumazenil administration in cases of benzodiazepine mixed overdose.
• Convulsions can be managed with diazepam; phenytoin should be avoided.
  • Diazepam can also be given orally or intravenously to sedate a patient in case of overdosage-related agitation.
• Consider rhabdomyolysis if the patient presents with persistent loss of consciousness.

Tests and Therapeutic Drug Monitoring
• Before initiation of amitriptyline therapy:
  • A baseline ECG should be performed to check for QT prolongation.
  • A metabolic panel should be performed, including electrolytes, renal and hepatic function.
• During amitriptyline therapy:
  • Patients should be regularly evaluated for worsening of depression, suicidality, behaviour changes or other common adverse effects, especially after introducing therapy or during dose modifications.
  • Consider regular ECG in geriatric patients.

Other Warnings/Precautions
• There is a black box warning for young adults (less than 24 years old) who take amitriptyline for depression and other psychiatric disorders concerning suicidal thinking and behaviour.
  • A slight increase in suicidal thinking has also been seen in those over 65 years old.
  • Patients with a history of suicide-related events are at higher risk and careful monitoring during treatment is required, especially early in therapy and following changes in dosage.
• Close monitoring is advised in patients with benign prostate hyper-plasia, urinary or GI retention, respiratory impairment, hepatic or renal impairment.

DOSING AND USE

- Caution is advised in patients with a history of epilepsy or brain tumour because amitriptyline might lower the seizure threshold, especially with concomitant use of neuroleptics.
- Caution is advised in patients with hyperthyroidism or those taking thyroid medication, as amitriptyline might precipitate cardiac arrhythmias.
- Caution is advised in patients with mania, bipolar disorder, or schizophrenia, as amitriptyline might aggravate psychosis.
- Close monitoring is recommended in patients with a history of bipolar disorder, as amitriptyline may trigger a manic episode.
  - Amitriptyline should be withdrawn in any patient entering a manic phase.
- Caution is advised in patients with diabetes mellitus, because amitriptyline might affect glycaemic control; insulin or other antidiabetic regimes may need to be modified accordingly.
- Close monitoring is advised in patients with frequent hypotensive episodes, including those with cardiovascular disease, hypovolemia, or simultaneous use of medication predisposing to hypotension or bradycardia.
- An angle-closure attack may be triggered in patients with high intraocular pressure or those at risk of angle closure glaucoma (e.g. anatomically narrow angles without a patent iridectomy).
- Amitriptyline may cause CNS depression, affecting the ability to drive or operate machinery.
  - Co-administration with CNS depressants or alcohol should be avoided.
- In case of co-administration with CYP2D6 inhibitors, dose adjustments of amitriptyline and monitoring of amitriptyline serum levels might be necessary.
- Clinically relevant interactions might be encountered with strong CYP3A4 inhibitors (e.g. *ketoconazole*, *itraconazole*, *ritonavir*); thus, caution is advised.
- Caution is advised in case of co-administration with diuretics that induce hypokalaemia.

Do Not Use (Contraindications)
- Known sensitivity to amitriptyline or to any of its excipients, including lactose.
  - Patients with rare hereditary problems of galactose intolerance, total lactase deficiency, or glucose–galactose malabsorption.
- During recovery after recent MI or in coronary artery insufficiency.
- Patients with any degree of heart block or cardiac rhythm disorders.
- In confirmed or suspected Brugada syndrome, as fatal cases have been reported.
- Co-administration with drugs that predispose to QT prolongation.
- Co-administration with MAOIs (including *selegiline* and *rasagiline*) or within 2 weeks after their discontinuation due to increased risk of

potentially fatal serotonin syndrome. MAOIs should not be administered for 1 week after amitriptyline discontinuation. The same applies for co-administration with *safinamide*.

- Co-administration with *linezolid* or *methylene blue* IV.
  - In case linezolid administration is necessary, amitriptyline should be immediately discontinued, and the patient should be monitored for CNS toxicity. Amitriptyline therapy can be resumed 24 h after last linezolid dose or after 2 weeks of monitoring, whichever applies first.
- Co-administration with *cisapride* and *fluvoxamine* is not recommended.
- Co-administration with sympathomimetic agents (e.g. *adrenaline*, *ephedrine*, *isoprenaline*, *noradrenaline*, *phenylephrine*, *phenylpropanolamine*), often included in anaesthetics and nasal decongestants, and adrenergic neuron blockers/centrally active antihypertensives (e.g. *clonidine*, *reserpine*).
- Co-medication with anticholinergic agents might enhance their effects and should be avoided.
- Co-administration with CYP2D6 substrates should be avoided due to increased risk of side effects (e.g. *thioridazine* – cardiotoxicity; *tramadol* – opioid toxicity).
- Cholinergic subtype of Parkinson's disease where use of anticholinergics can be hazardous owing to worsening cognitive function.

Special Populations

Renal Impairment
- No dosage modifications are suggested for patients with renal impairment.

Hepatic Impairment
- Dosage modification and careful monitoring might be necessary in case of hepatic impairment; measurement of amitriptyline plasma levels is suggested, if applicable.
- Amitriptyline use is not recommended in severe liver disease.

Elderly
- A reduced metabolism of amitriptyline leads to longer half-life values and lower clearance rates in the elderly.
- A lower initial and total dose, with up titration over a longer period, is generally suggested for the elderly.
- Elderly patients are more susceptible to adverse events, including orthostatic hypotension.

Pregnancy
- Category C (FDA): use with caution if benefits outweigh risks.
- Amitriptyline use is generally not recommended in pregnancy.
- Neonates exposed to amitriptyline late in the third trimester might develop withdrawal symptoms, such as irritability, hypertonia, tremor, irregular breathing, weak suckling, and anticholinergic symptoms.

A

Breastfeeding
- Amitriptyline is excreted in human milk in low concentrations.
- A risk to the nursing child cannot be excluded; thus, amitriptyline use is not recommended during breastfeeding.

Costs
NHS indicative price accessed 4 December 2022:
- 10 mg tablets, 28 tabs: £0.21–£0.68.
- 25 mg tablets, 28 tabs: £0.61–£0.93.
- 50 mg tablets, 28 tabs: £0.55–£1.03.
- 10 mg/5 ml oral solution, 150 ml: £116.00–£136.47.
- 25 mg/5 ml oral solution, 150 ml: £15.70–£18.00.
- 50 mg/5 ml oral solution, 150 ml: £17.20–£24.00.

The Overall Place of Amitriptyline in the Treatment of Parkinson's disease

Amitriptyline is a tricyclic antidepressant and a non-selective mono-amine reuptake inhibitor, which can be effectively used for the treatment of moderate to severe depression in Parkinson's disease. Its use in Parkinson's disease is mostly based on the experience from the general population, rather than on focused studies in the Parkinson's disease population. In head-to-head studies, amitriptyline was found to be one of the most effective antidepressants in the treatment of major depression, although it has also been associated with a high dropout rate due to tolerability issues. Amitriptyline therapy requires great vigilance for adverse effects and careful evaluation of patients for co-morbidities and simultaneous medications for drug-to-drug interactions, which are common and significantly increase the risk for serious complications, especially among elderly patients. The anticholinergic adverse events, which are characteristic for all tricyclic antidepressants, render their use particularly problematic among Parkinson's disease patients owing to concerns about worsening of cognition, aggravation of gut motility, and orthostatic hypotension, which might lead to falls. All of the above make amitriptyline an unpopular option for the management of Parkinson's disease-related depressive symptoms in routine clinical practice, although it can be useful in younger patients with intact cognition and relevant co-morbidities (e.g. migraine, neuropathic pain), particularly when other antidepressants fail to produce results. Moreover, it can be helpful in a subgroup of Parkinson's disease patients suffering from drooling or nocturia. Finally, clinicians are much more experienced with its use and pharmacological profile and can take advantage of its sedative properties in depression cases with co-morbid agitation or anxiety.

A

Potential Advantages
- Amitriptyline might be helpful in depressive patients with co-morbid chronic pain.
- Amitriptyline might be helpful in Parkinson's disease patients with drooling or those with sleep impairment when administered at night.
- Compared to SSRIs, tricyclic antidepressants have an inherent advantage in improving sleep.
- It can be given as a single dose to improve patients' adherence.
- Low cost.
- According to a recent study, amitriptyline has been associated with a lower risk of incident pneumonia among Parkinson's disease patients.

Potential Disadvantages
- Administration of tricyclic antidepressants to Parkinson's disease patients might precipitate or worsen psychosis, sedation, somnolence, cognitive impairment, or delirium, especially in those with impaired cognition.
- Amitriptyline is one of the most sedating tricyclic antidepressants.
- A long list of drug-to-drug interactions accompanies amitriptyline administration.
- Among all antidepressants, tricyclic antidepressants and citalopram at elevated doses bear the greatest risk for QT prolongation, especially for those over 60 years old; thus, regular ECG monitoring is required.
- In a number of countries amitriptyline might only be available in combination with other supplements (combined formulations, usually with an antipsychotic agent), which inhibits its use in Parkinson's disease patients.

CLINICAL BOX

Clinical Box
A 42-year-old woman, who was recently diagnosed with Parkinson's disease, presented at the Neurology Department Outpatient Clinic for her regular follow-up assessment. The patient mentioned low mood and frequent episodes of crying with impaired sleep; these symptoms were constant during the day and were not related to non-motor fluctuations associated with Parkinson's disease. She also mentioned an aggravation of daily frontal headaches during the past few months, which she has tried treating with common analgesics, which were ineffective. The patient was taking pramipexole 2.1 mg OD and the rest of her medical history was unremarkable. A diagnosis of moderate depression and chronic daily headache accompanying Parkinson's disease was made, and the patient was given the option of receiving amitriptyline, both as an antidepressant and a preventive therapy for headache, in order to address both conditions. No contraindications were found and a low dose of amitriptyline 25 mg OD before bedtime was prescribed with a good response of her symptoms and without any significant adverse events.

Suggested Reading

Antonini A, S Tesei, A Zecchinelli, P Barone, D De Gaspari, M Canesi, G Sacilotto, N Meucci, C Mariani, G Pezzoli. Randomized study of sertraline and low-dose amitriptyline in patients with Parkinson's disease and depression: effect on quality of life. *Mov Disord* 2006; 21(8): 1119–1122.

Cipriani A, TA Furukawa, G Salanti, A Chaimani, LZ Atkinson, Y Ogawa, S Leucht, HG Ruhe, EH Turner, JPT Higgins, M Egger, N Takeshima, Y Hayasaka, H Imai, K Shinohara, A Tajika, JPA Ioannidis, JR Geddes. Comparative efficacy and acceptability of 21 antidepressant drugs for the acute treatment of adults with major depressive disorder: a systematic review and network meta-analysis. *Lancet* 2018; 391(10128): 1357–1366.

Serrano-Dueñas M. [A comparison between low doses of amitriptyline and low doses of fluoxetin used in the control of depression in patients suffering from Parkinson's disease]. *Rev Neurol* 2002; 35(11): 1010–1014 [in Spanish].

References

AHFS Drug Information, 2012. Bethesda: American Society of Health-System Pharmacists. Accessed on 4 December 2022 via www.medicinescomplete.com.

Amitriptyline. In: DRUGDEX® System (electronic version). Truven Health Analytics, Greenwood Village, Colorado, USA. Accessed on 4 December 2022 via www.micromedexsolutions.com.

Amitriptyline. In: Brayfield A (Ed.), *Martindale: The Complete Drug Reference*. London: The Royal Pharmaceutical Society of Great Britain. Accessed on 4 December 2022 via www.medicinescomplete.com.

Greten S, JI Müller-Funogea, F Wegner, GU Höglinger, N Simon, U Junius-Walker, S Gerbel, O Krause, M Klietz. Drug safety profiles in geriatric patients with Parkinson's disease using the FORTA (Fit fOR The Aged) classification: results from a mono-centric retrospective analysis. *J Neural Transm (Vienna)* 2021; 128(1): 49–60.

Joint Formulary Committee. British National Formulary (online). London: BMJ Group and Pharmaceutical Press. Accessed on 4 December 2022 via www.medicinescomplete.com.

Kuo WY, KH Huang, YH Kuan, YC Chang, TH Tsai, CY Lee. Antidepressants usage and risk of pneumonia among elderly patients with the Parkinson's disease: a population-based case–control study. *Front Med (Lausanne)* 2022; 9: 740182.

Lee MY, S Hong, N Kim, KS Shin, SJ Kang. Tricyclic antidepressants amitriptyline and desipramine induced neurotoxicity associated with Parkinson's disease. *Mol Cells* 2015; 38(8): 734–740.

Paumier KL, CE Sortwell, L Madhavan, B Terpstra, BF Daley, TJ Collier. Tricyclic antidepressant treatment evokes regional changes in neurotrophic factors over time within the intact and degenerating nigrostriatal system. *Exp Neurol* 2015; 266: 11–21.

Summary of Product Characteristics – Amitriptyline 10 mg film-coated tablets. Brown and Burk UK Ltd. Electronic Medicines Compendium: Amitriptyline 10 mg film-coated tablets – summary of product characteristics (SmPC) – (emc). Accessed on 4 December 2022 via www.medicines.org.uk.

A

REFERENCES

APOMORPHINE HYDROCHLORIDE SUBCUTANEOUS INFUSION

APOMORPHINE HYDROCHLORIDE SUBCUTANEOUS

Therapeutics

Chemical Name and Structure

Apomorphine hydrochloride (6aβ-aporphine-10,11-diol hydrochloride hemihydrate; (R)-10,11-dihydroxy-6a-aporphine hydrochloride hemihydrate; (6aR)-5,6,6a,7-tetrahydro-6-methyl-4H-dibenzo[de,g] quinoline-10,11-diol hydrochloride hemihydrate) has a molecular weight of 303.8 and a molecular formula of $C_{17}H_{18}ClNO_2$.

Brand Names
* **Apofin** (*Italy*); **APO-go** (*Austria, Chile, Denmark, Finland, Greece, Hong Kong, Ireland, Israel, Netherlands, Portugal, Spain, Sweden, Switzerland, Thailand, Turkey, UK*); **Apokinon** (*Argentina, France*); **Apokyn** (*Japan, USA*); **Apomine** (*Australia, New Zealand*); **Apowok** (*Australia*).
* **Britaject** (*Norway*).
* **Dacepton** (*Austria, Czech Republic, Denmark, Finland, Netherlands, Norway, Poland, Portugal, Spain, Sweden, UK*); **Dopacepton** (*France*); **Dopamor** (*Turkey*).
* **Epamor** (*Turkey*).
* **Li Ke Ji** (*China*).
* **Movapo** (*Australia, Canada, New Zealand*).
* **Pargicyl** (*Turkey*).

Generics Available
* No.

Licensed Indications for Parkinson's Disease
* Motor fluctuations (usually levodopa–induced) inadequately controlled by oral dopaminergic agents (FDA, EMA, EMC).
* Patients with good response to apomorphine SC injections, but whose overall control remains unsatisfactory using intermittent injections, or patients who might require frequent injections (>10/day), may be initiated on or transferred to continuous SC infusion (FDA, EMA, EMC).

Licensed Indications for Other Conditions
* None.

Non-Licensed Use for Parkinson's Disease
* Non-motor fluctuations (cognitive, autonomic, and sensory) inadequately controlled by oral dopaminergic agents.
* Sleep dysfunction (motor off at night, nocturnal akinesia, nocturia, early morning off, periodic limb movements) inadequately controlled by oral dopaminergic agents (night-time infusion).

A

Non-Licensed Use for Other Conditions
• None.

Ineffective
• Not reported.

Mechanism of Action
• Apomorphine is a non-ergot-derivative dopamine receptor agonist, which is structurally and pharmacologically related to dopamine.
• It is a broad-spectrum dopamine agonist, acting on both D1-like (D1 and D5) and D2-like (D2, D3, D4) receptors, with a higher affinity for the latter.
  ○ In vitro studies have demonstrated different increasing affinity for D1, D5, D2, and D3 receptors, with the greatest affinity observed for D4 receptors.
• It has a moderate affinity to α-adrenergic (α1D, α2B, α2C) receptors.
• It has little or no affinity for serotonergic (5-HT1A, 5-HT2A, 5-HT2B, 5-HT2C) receptors, β1- or β2-adrenergic receptors, or histamine H1 receptors.

Efficacy Profile
• The goal of treatment is to reduce frequency and severity of OFF episodes and improve ON periods without troublesome dyskinesias.
• Apomorphine has been characterized as 'likely efficacious' and 'possibly useful' for the treatment of motor fluctuations in Parkinson's disease (MDS EBM Committee).
• Onset of action is rapid, usually within 10–20 min (it is the fastest acting dopaminergic therapy currently available).

PHARMACOKINETICS

Pharmacokinetics
Absorption and Distribution
• Bioavailability: 100%; well-absorbed after SC injection.
• Time to maximum concentration: 10–60 min.
• Time to steady state: not documented.
• Pharmacokinetic: possibly dose-dependent, but linear between 2 mg and 8 mg via SC administration through abdominal wall.
• Protein binding: 90% bound to plasma proteins.
• Volume of distribution: 218 l (123–404 l).

Metabolism
• Apomorphine is extensively metabolized in the liver mainly by conjugation with glucuronic acid or sulphate (major metabolite: apomorphine sulphate).
• It is also demethylated to norapomorphine.
• Cytochrome P-450 (CYP) enzymes play a minor role.

A

APOMORPHINE HYDROCHLORIDE SUBCUTANEOUS

Elimination
- Mean elimination half-life is about 40 min.
- It is mostly excreted in the urine, mainly as metabolites.

Drug Interaction Profile
Pharmacokinetic Drug Interactions
- Pharmacokinetic interactions with drugs affecting or metabolized by hepatic microsomal enzymes are unlikely.

Pharmacodynamic Drug Interactions
- Co-administration with antihypertensives may lead to enhanced hypotensive effect.
- Co-administration with 5HT3-receptor antagonists (e.g. *alosetron, dolasetron, granisetron, ondansetron, palonosetron*) may lead to increased hypotensive effects.
- Co-administration with nitrates may lead to enhanced hypotensive effect.
- Co-medication with drugs causing electrolyte imbalance or increasing QT interval, such as Class IA and III anti-arrhythmics, antipsychotics (e.g. *haloperidol, phenothiazine derivatives, pimozide*), tricyclic antidepressants, certain antimicrobial agents (e.g. *moxifloxacin, erythromycin*), certain antihistamines (e.g. *astemizole, mizolastine*), and others may lead to potentially fatal Torsade de Pointes arrhythmias and is considered a risk factor for sudden cardiac death.
- Co-administration with dopamine antagonists (e.g. *metoclopramide,* antipsychotics) may reduce the therapeutic effect of apomorphine.
- Co-administration with CNS depressants (e.g. *alcohol*) may lead to enhanced sedative and hypotensive effects.

Adverse Effects
How Drug Causes Adverse Effects
- Mainly (but not only) by increasing dopaminergic activity.

Common Adverse Effects
- Very common (≥1/10):
  - Hallucinations (although troublesome hallucinations are less common in clinical practice), injection site reactions (e.g. SC nodules, induration, erythema, tenderness, panniculitis, irritation, itching, bruising, pain).
- Common (≥1/100 to <1/10):
  - Neuropsychiatric: transient mild confusion, transient sedation, somnolence, dizziness, light-headedness, intrusive hallucinations.
  - Respiratory: yawning (considered proof of effect of apomorphine on CNS during challenge test).

- GI: nausea, vomiting (usually if domperidone is omitted and therefore domperidone is recommended in safe doses).
- Uncommon (≥1/1,000 to <1/100):
  - Neuropsychiatric: dyskinesias, sudden sleep onset episodes (likely in susceptible individuals with serotonergic subtype of Parkinson's disease).
  - Cardiovascular: postural hypotension (usually transient because tachyphylaxis develops).
  - Skin: injection site necrosis/ulceration (especially in those with fragile skin such as type 1 diabetes).
  - Other: positive Coomb's tests.

Life-Threatening or Dangerous Adverse Effects
- Uncommon (≥1/1,000 to <1/100):
  - Haemolytic anaemia, thrombocytopenia.
  - ICDs.
- Rare (≥1/10,000 to <1/1,000):
  - DDS.
  - Eosinophilia.
  - Allergic reactions, including anaphylaxis and bronchospasm.
- Unknown frequency:
  - Syncope.
  - QT-interval prolongation, angina, MI, cardia arrhythmia/arrest, and/or sudden death

Rare and Not Life-Threatening Adverse Effects
- Unknown frequency:
  - Aggression, agitation.
  - Headache.
  - Peripheral oedema.
  - Increased salivation and perspiration.
  - Paradoxical akinetic response.
  - Priapism.

Weight Change
- Not reported.

What to Do About Adverse Effects
- Discuss common adverse effects with patients or caregivers before starting medication, including symptoms that should be reported to the physician.
- In case of troublesome adverse effects, consider withdrawing therapy with concomitant increase in dosing of levodopa or other dopaminergic agents.
- Transient sedation may develop at the start of apomorphine therapy, which usually resolves over the first few weeks of therapy.

A

ADVERSE EFFECTS

APOMORPHINE HYDROCHLORIDE SUBCUTANEOUS

Dosing and Use

Challenge Test Prior to Initiation
Usually started after an apomorphine challenge test, which is done:
• Domperidone pre-treatment (optional).
• Ideally fasting state.
• Provoked off period (overnight drug dopaminergic therapy withdrawal).
• ECG (rule out QT interval abnormality).
• Initiate apomorphine starting at 1 mg SC with observation for 45 min and increase dose up to 7 mg (or more in selected cases) and assess motor and non-motor response for positive test.

Usual Dosage Range
• 1–4 mg/h during waking hours.

Available Formulations
• Solution for infusion in pre-filled syringe: 5 mg/ml.

How to Dose
• Start infusion at a rate of 1 mg/h; then daily increase according to individual response.
  • Increases should not exceed 0.5 mg at intervals of not less than 4 h.
• Intermittent bolus boosts can be administered as necessary and according to physician's instructions.
• A 24-h infusion scheme is not recommended, unless there is severe sleep dysfunction.
  • A washout period of at least 4 h is needed.
• Total daily dose should not exceed 100 mg.

Dosing Tips
• Anti-emetic prophylaxis is advisable; patient should be instructed to receive domperidone or trimethobenzamide hydrochloride 3 days before apomorphine initiation.
• Once apomorphine treatment is established, anti-emetic therapy may be gradually reduced and discontinued in some patients.
• Alternate injection sites on daily basis (abdomen, thigh, or upper arm); good skin hygiene is vital.
• A concomitant and progressive reduction of other dopamine agonists and levodopa daily dose if possible is suggested.

How to Withdraw Drug
• Progressive and slow dose reduction is recommended to reduce risk of dopaminergic withdrawal syndrome.

Overdose
• Signs and symptoms of overdose include persistent vomiting, respiratory depression, bradycardia, hypotension, and coma; death may occur.

A

- Empirical treatment: opioid antagonist, such as *naloxone*, for excessive vomiting, central nervous system and respiratory depression may be considered in severe cases.

Tests and Therapeutic Drug Monitoring
- Before apomorphine therapy:
  - Screen for QT-prolongation, especially if concomitant domperidone use.
  - In case of concomitant use with levodopa, screen for haemolytic anaemia and thrombocytopenia.
- During apomorphine therapy:
  - Patients receiving apomorphine with levodopa should be screened for haemolytic anaemia and thrombocytopenia every 6 months.
  - Periodic monitoring of hepatic, renal, haematopoietic, and cardiovascular function is advisable.
  - In case of concomitant use of domperidone, regular ECG assessments and monitoring of electrolytes are recommended.

Other Warnings / Precautions
- Careful patient selection is advisable (apomorphine is not recommended in patients with severe symptomatic orthostatic hypotension, severe excessive daytime sleepiness with history of sudden onset of sleep, troublesome psychosis, or intrusive ICDs).
- IV administration is contraindicated due to possible serious adverse effects (e.g. thrombosis).
- Use with caution in patients susceptible to nausea/vomiting or when vomiting is likely to pose a risk.
- Use with caution in patients with known cardiovascular/cerebrovascular disease due to potential hypotensive effects.
- Use with caution in patients with pulmonary or endocrine disease.
- Concomitant use with sublingual nitroglycerin may lead to greater decreases in blood pressure, so patients are advised to lie down before and after taking sublingual nitroglycerin.
- Caution is advised while driving or operating hazardous machines during apomorphine treatment, as it predisposes to daytime somnolence or sudden sleep episodes.

Do Not Use (Contraindications)
- Hypersensitivity to apomorphine or any ingredient in the formulation (e.g. sodium metabisulphite).
- Patients with respiratory depression, psychotic diseases, dementia, or hepatic insufficiency.
- Concomitant use of 5-HT3 receptor antagonists (e.g. *alosetron, dolasetron, granisetron, ondansetron, palonosetron*) or central dopamine receptors (e.g. *metoclopramide*).
- Co-administration with alcohol.

DOSING AND USE

APOMORPHINE HYDROCHLORIDE SUBCUTANEOUS

Special Populations

Renal Impairment
- Close monitoring is advised in case of renal impairment.
- Apomorphine should not be used in patients with severe renal impairment.

Hepatic Impairment
- Not recommended in case of hepatic impairment.

Elderly
- Use with caution because of higher risk of confusion, hallucinations, serious adverse events, falls, cardiovascular events, respiratory disorders, and gastrointestinal events.

Pregnancy
- Apomorphine should not be used during pregnancy unless necessary.
- There is no experience of apomorphine usage in pregnant women.
- No teratogenic effects have been found in animal studies; however, doses given to rats which are toxic to the mother can lead to failure to breathe in the newborn.

Breastfeeding
- Apomorphine use is not recommended during breastfeeding.
- It is not known whether apomorphine is excreted in human milk.

Costs
NHS indicative price accessed 5 December 2022:
- APO-go PFS 50 mg/10 ml solution for injection pre-filled syringes (Britannia Pharmaceuticals Ltd) – five pre-filled syringes £73.11.
- Dacepton 100 mg/20 ml solution for infusion vials (Ever Pharma) – five vials £145.00.

The Overall Place of Apomorphine SC infusion in the Treatment of Parkinson's Disease
Apomorphine infusion is an excellent therapeutic option with results comparable to levodopa infusion and DBS for the treatment of motor and non-motor fluctuations (urinary urgency, pain, depression, and anxiety), which are inadequately controlled by oral or transdermal dopaminergic agents. Patients with good response to apomorphine SC injections but whose overall control remains unsatisfactory using intermittent injections, or patients who might require frequent injections (>10/day), may be initiated on or transferred to continuous SC infusion. It is commonly used as a bridge therapy between oral

A

dopaminergic agents and other device-aided therapies (levodopa–carbidopa/levodopa–carbidopa–entacapone intestinal infusion or DBS). Apomorphine infusion can also be successfully used for a range of sleep disorders such as nocturnal akinesia and early morning off periods as a nocturnal infusion with lower dose (1–4 mg/h).

Clinical Box
A 60-year-old, left-handed man with a 9-year history of Parkinson's disease was assessed at the Movement Disorders Outpatient Clinic for his regular follow-up appointment. His current medication regimen consisted of apomorphine SC injection 3 mg 10 times daily (as rescue for recurring off periods), levodopa–benserazide 100 m/25 mg 5 times daily, levodopa–carbidopa CR 200 mg/55 mg at night-time, and rotigotine transdermal patch 4 mg/24 h. He was initiated on apomorphine SC injection for the management of his troublesome, unpredictable, motor and non-motor fluctuations (off related local pain, severe anxiety, and anhedonia) one year ago with good response and without side effects. He mentioned his motor and non-motor fluctuations have increased in frequency and severity. A switch to apomorphine subcutaneous infusion was suggested, which led to optimal fluctuation control at an infusion rate of 2 mg/h for 16 h and resolution of non-motor phenomena. Anti-emetic prophylaxis and ECG monitoring was not needed, as the gentleman was already on apomorphine SC injections, which were optimally tolerated.

Suggested Reading

Carbone F, A Djamshidian, K Seppi, W Poewe. Apomorphine for Parkinson's disease: efficacy and safety of current and new formulations. *CNS Drugs* 2019; 33(9): 905–918. doi: 10.1007/s40263-019-00661-z. PMID: 31473980; PMCID: PMC6776563.

Katzenschlager R, W Poewe, O Rascol, C Trenkwalder, G Deuschl, KR Chaudhuri, T Henriksen, T van Laar, K Spivey, S Vel, H Staines, A Lees. Apomorphine subcutaneous infusion in patients with Parkinson's disease with persistent motor fluctuations (TOLEDO): a multicentre, double-blind, randomised, placebo-controlled trial. *Lancet Neurol* 2018; 17(9): 749–759. doi: 10.1016/S1474-4422(18)30239-4. Epub 2018 Jul 25. PMID: 30055903.

Titova N, KR Chaudhuri. Apomorphine therapy in Parkinson's and future directions. *Parkinsonism Relat Disord* 2016; 33(Suppl 1): S56–S60. doi: 10.1016/j.parkreldis.2016.11.013. Epub 2016 Nov 30. PMID: 27913125.

SUGGESTED READING

References

AHFS Drug information 2012. Bethesda: American Society of Health-System Pharmacists. Accessed on 5 December 2022 via www.medicinescomplete.com.

Apomorphine. In: Brayfield A (Ed.), *Martindale: The Complete Drug Reference*. London: The Royal Pharmaceutical Society of Great Britain. Accessed on 5 December 2022 via www.medicinescomplete.com.

Apomorphine. In: DRUGDEX® System (electronic version). Truven Health Analytics, Greenwood Village, Colorado, USA. Accessed on 5 December 2022 via www.micromedexsolutions.com.

Auffret M, S Drapier, M Vérin. Pharmacological insights into the use of apomorphine in Parkinson's disease: clinical relevance. *Clin Drug Investig* 2018; 38(4): 287–312.

Chaudhuri KR, V Leta. Apomorphine infusion for improving sleep in Parkinson's disease. *Lancet Neurol* 2022; 21(5): 395–398.

Chaudhuri KR, A Todorova, MJ Nirenberg, M Parry, A Martin, P Martinez-Martin, A Rizos, T Henriksen, W Jost, A Storch, G Ebersbach, H Reichmann, P Odin, A Antonini. A pilot prospective, multicenter observational study of dopamine agonist withdrawal syndrome in Parkinson's disease. *Mov Disord Clin Pract* 2015; 2(2): 170–174.

Dafsari HS, P Martinez-Martin, A Rizos, M Trost, MG dos Santos Ghilardi, P Reddy, A Sauerbier, JN Petry-Schmelzer, M Kramberger, RWK Borgemeester, MT Barbe, K Ashkan, M Silverdale, J Evans, P Odin, ET Fonoff, GR Fink, T Henriksen, G Ebersbach, ... K Ray Chaudhuri ; EUROPAR and the International Parkinson and Movement Disorders Society Non-Motor Parkinson's Disease Study Group. EuroInf 2: subthalamic stimulation, apomorphine, and levodopa infusion in Parkinson's disease. *Mov Disord* 2019; 34: 353–365.

Jenkins JR, JMS Pearce. Paradoxical akinetic response to apomorphine in parkinsonism. *J Neurol Neurosurg Psychiatry* 1992; 55: 414–415.

Joint Formulary Committee. British National Formulary (online). London: BMJ Group and Pharmaceutical Press. Accessed on 29 December 2022 via www.medicinescomplete.com.

Marras C, KR Chaudhuri, N Titova, TA Mestre. Therapy of Parkinson's disease subtypes. *Neurotherapeutics* 2020; 17(4): 1366–1377.

Martinez-Martin P, P Reddy, A Antonini, T Henriksen, R Katzenschlager, P Odin, A Todorova, Y Naidu, S Tluk, C Chandiramani, A Martin, KR Chaudhuri. Chronic subcutaneous infusion therapy with apomorphine in advanced Parkinson's disease compared to conventional therapy: a real life study of non motor effect. *J Parkinsons Dis* 2011; 1(2): 197–203.

Stocchi F, MF De Pandis, FA Delfino, T Anselmo, D Frangillo. Transient atrial fibrillation after subcutaneous apomorphine bolus. *Mov Disord* 1996; 11: 584–585.

Summary of Product Characteristics – APO-go PFS 5 mg/ml solution for infusion in pre-filled syringe. Britannia Pharmaceuticals Limited. Electronic Medicines Compendium: APO-go PFS 5 mg/ml solution for infusion in pre-filled syringe – summary of product characteristics (SmPC) – (emc). Accessed on 5 December 2022 via www.medicines.org.uk.

A

REFERENCES

APOMORPHINE HYDROCHLORIDE SUBCUTANEOUS INJECTION

Therapeutics

Chemical Name and Structure

Apomorphine hydrochloride (6aβ–aporphine-10,11-diol hydrochloride hemihydrate; (*R*)-10,11-dihydroxy-6*a*-aporphine hydrochloride hemihydrate; (6aR)-5,6,6*a*,7-tetrahydro-6-methyl-4H-dibenzo[de,g] quinoline-10,11-diol hydrochloride hemihydrate) has a molecular weight of 303.8 and a molecular formula of $C_{17}H_{18}ClNO_2$.

Brand Names

- **Apofin** (*Italy*); **APO-go** (*Austria, Chile, Denmark, Finland, Greece, Hong Kong, Ireland, Israel, Netherlands, Portugal, Spain, Sweden, Switzerland, Thailand, Turkey, UK*); **Apokinon** (*Argentina, France*); **Apokyn** (*Japan, USA*); **Apomine** (*Australia, New Zealand*); **Apowok** (*Australia*).
- **Britaject** (*Norway*).
- **Dacepton** (*Austria, Czech Republic, Denmark, Finland, Netherlands, Norway, Poland, Portugal, Spain, Sweden, UK*); **Dopacepton** (*France*); **Dopamor** (*Turkey*).
- **Epamor** (*Turkey*).
- **Li Ke Ji** (*China*).
- **Movapo** (*Australia, Canada, New Zealand*).
- **Pargicyl** (*Turkey*).

Generics Available

- No.

Licensed Indications for Parkinson's Disease

- Motor fluctuations inadequately controlled by oral dopaminergic agents (FDA, EMA, EMC).

Licensed Indications for Other Conditions

- None.

Non-Licensed Use for Parkinson's Disease

- Non-motor fluctuations inadequately controlled by oral dopaminergic agents.
- Open-label studies have shown a benefit of SC apomorphine on erectile dysfunction in PD patients.

Non-Licensed Use for Other Conditions

- In homoeopathic medicines for emetic properties.
- Erectile dysfunction.
- Vegetative state (orphan).
- Acute myeloid leukaemia (orphan).
- Amyotrophic lateral sclerosis (orphan).

A

Ineffective
- Not reported.

Mechanism of Action
- Apomorphine is a non-ergot-derivative dopamine receptor agonist, which is structurally and pharmacologically related to dopamine.
- It is a broad-spectrum dopamine agonist, acting on both D1-like (D1 and D5) and D2-like (D2, D3, D4) receptors, with a higher affinity for the latter.
  - In vitro studies have demonstrated different increasing affinity for D1, D5, D2, and D3 receptors, with the greatest affinity observed for D4 receptors.
- It has a moderate affinity to α-adrenergic (α1D, α2B, α2C) receptors.
- It has little or no affinity for serotonergic (5-HT1A, 5-HT2A, 5-HT2B, 5-HT2C) receptors, β1- or β2-adrenergic receptors, or histamine H1 receptors.

Efficacy Profile
- The goal of treatment is to reduce frequency and severity of OFF episodes.
- Apomorphine has been characterized as 'likely efficacious' and 'clinically useful' for the treatment of motor fluctuations in PD (MDS EBM Committee).
- Onset of action is rapid, usually within 10–20 min, but has a short duration of action (about 60 min).

PHARMACOKINETICS

Pharmacokinetics
Absorption and Distribution
- Bioavailability: 100%; well absorbed after SC injection.
- Time to maximum concentration: 10–60 min.
- Time to steady state: not documented.
- Pharmacokinetic: possibly dose-dependent, but linear between 2 mg and 8 mg via SC administration through abdominal wall.
- Protein binding: 90% bound to plasma proteins.
- Volume of distribution: 218 l (123–404 l).

Metabolism
- Apomorphine is extensively metabolized in the liver mainly by conjugation with glucuronic acid or sulphate (major metabolite: apomorphine sulphate).
- It is also demethylated to norapomorphine.
- Cytochrome P-450 (CYP) enzymes play a minor role.

Elimination
- Mean elimination half-life is about 40 min.
- It is mostly excreted in the urine, mainly as metabolites.

HYDROCHLORIDE SUBCUTANEOUS INJECTION

Drug Interaction Profile

Pharmacokinetic Drug Interactions
- Pharmacokinetic interactions with drugs affecting or metabolized by hepatic microsomal enzymes are unlikely.

Pharmacodynamic Drug Interactions
- Co-administration with antihypertensives may lead to enhanced hypotensive effect.
- Co-administration with 5HT3-receptor antagonists (e.g. *alosetron, dolasetron, granisetron, ondansetron, palonosetron*) may lead to increased hypotensive effects.
- Co-administration with nitrates may lead to enhanced hypotensive effect.
- Co-medication with drugs causing electrolyte imbalance or increasing QT interval, such as Class IA and III anti-arrhythmics, antipsychotics (e.g. *haloperidol, phenothiazine derivatives, pimozide*), tricyclic antidepressants, certain antimicrobial agents (e.g. *moxifloxacin, erythromycin*), certain antihistamines (e.g. *astemizole, mizolastine*), and others may lead to potentially fatal Torsade de Pointes arrhythmias and is considered a risk factor for sudden cardiac death.
- Co-administration with dopamine antagonists (e.g. *metoclopramide,* antipsychotics) may reduce the therapeutic effect of apomorphine.
- Co-administration with CNS depressants (e.g. *alcohol*) may lead to enhanced sedative and hypotensive effects.

Adverse Effects

How Drug Causes Adverse Effects
- Mainly (but not only) by increasing dopaminergic activity.

Common Adverse Effects
- Very common (≥1/10):
  ○ Hallucinations (although troublesome hallucinations are less common in clinical practice), injection site reactions (e.g. SC nodules, induration, erythema, tenderness, panniculitis, irritation, itching, bruising, pain).
- Common (≥1/100 to <1/10):
  ○ Neuropsychiatric: transient mild confusion, transient sedation, somnolence, dizziness, light-headedness, intrusive hallucinations.
  ○ Respiratory: yawning (considered proof of effect of apomorphine on CNS during challenge test).
  ○ GI: nausea, vomiting (usually if domperidone is omitted and therefore domperidone is recommended in safe doses).
- Uncommon (≥1/1,000 to <1/100):
  ○ Neuropsychiatric: dyskinesias, sudden sleep onset episodes (likely in susceptible individuals with serotonergic subtype of PD).

- ◦ Cardiovascular: postural hypotension (usually transient because tachyphylaxis develops).
- ◦ Skin: injection site necrosis/ulceration (especially in those with fragile skin such as type 1 diabetes).
- ◦ Other: positive Coomb's tests.

Life-Threatening or Dangerous Adverse Effects
- Uncommon (≥1/1,000 to <1/100):
  - Haemolytic anaemia, thrombocytopenia.
  - ICDs.
- Rare (≥1/10,000 to <1/1,000):
  - DDS.
  - Eosinophilia.
  - Allergic reactions, including anaphylaxis and bronchospasm.
- Unknown frequency:
  - Syncope.
  - QT-interval prolongation, angina, MI, cardia arrhythmia/arrest, and/or sudden death

Rare and Not Life-Threatening Adverse Effects
- Unknown frequency:
  - ◦ Aggression, agitation.
  - ◦ Headache.
  - ◦ Peripheral oedema.
  - ◦ Increased salivation and perspiration.
  - ◦ Paradoxical akinetic response.
  - ◦ Priapism.

Weight Change
- Not reported.

What to Do About Adverse Effects
- Discuss common adverse effects with patients or caregivers before starting medication, including symptoms that should be reported to the physician.
- In case of troublesome adverse effects, consider withdrawing therapy with concomitant increase in dosing of levodopa or other dopaminergic agents.
- Transient sedation may develop at the start of apomorphine therapy, which usually resolves over the first few weeks of therapy.

Dosing and Use
Usual Dosage Range
- 3–30 mg daily, given as 1–10 injections.
- At least a 2-h interval between injections.

A

HYDROCHLORIDE SUBCUTANEOUS INJECTION

Available Formulations
- Solution for injection (pre-filled pen): 10 mg/ml.

How to Dose
- Introduction of apomorphine should be done in a medical setting where blood pressure and pulse can be monitored (20 min before administration, baseline, 20 min after administration, 40 min after administration and 60 min after administration).
- The appropriate dose for each patient is established by incremental dosing schedules (see figure 1). The following schedule might be suggested: Start with a dose of 1 mg given subcutaneously during an 'OFF' period and then observe motor response over 30 min. If no response, or response is inadequate, then a second dose of 2 mg may be used and the same observation period undertaken. This can then be repeated at 40-min intervals with escalation of dose only if the previous dose is well tolerated and produces a suboptimal response.

Patient in off state (withholding antiparkinsonian therapy overnight)

Task	Time (min)
Baseline motor and LSBP assessment	−15
Administer 1 mg s/c	0
Motor and LSBP reassessment	15
Administer 3 mg s/c*	30
Motor and LSBP reassessment	45
Administer 5 mg*	60
Motor and LSBP reassessment	75
Administer 6 mg s/c*	105
Motor and LSBP reassessment	120
Administer 7 mg*	150
Motor and LSBP reassessment	165

Check ECG and blood tests before challenge test
On completion, reintroduce anti-Parkinson's medications as per prescription

*Dose escalation only if previous dose well tolerated and suboptimal response

---

Figure 1 Suggested apomorphine challenge test.

Dosing Tips
- Anti-emetic prophylaxis is advisable; patient should be instructed to receive domperidone or trimethobenzamide hydrochloride 3 days before apomorphine initiation.
- Once apomorphine treatment is established, anti-emetic therapy may be gradually reduced and discontinued in some patients.
- Alternate injection sites on daily basis (abdomen, thigh, or upper arm); good skin hygiene is necessary.

A

How to Withdraw Drug
- Progressive and slow dose reduction is recommended to reduce risk of dopaminergic withdrawal syndrome.

Overdose
- Signs and symptoms of overdose include persistent vomiting, respiratory depression, bradycardia, hypotension, and coma; death may occur.
- Empirical treatment: opioid antagonist, such as *naloxone*, for excessive vomiting, central nervous system and respiratory depression may be considered in severe cases.

Tests and Therapeutic Drug Monitoring
- Before apomorphine therapy:
  - Screen for QT-prolongation, especially if concomitant domperidone use.
  - In case of concomitant use with levodopa, screen for haemolytic anaemia and thrombocytopenia.
- During apomorphine therapy:
  - Patients receiving apomorphine with levodopa should be screened for haemolytic anaemia and thrombocytopenia every 6 months.
  - Periodic monitoring of hepatic, renal, haematopoietic, and cardiovascular function is advisable.
  - In case of concomitant use of domperidone, regular ECG assessments and monitoring of electrolytes are recommended.

Other Warnings/Precautions
- Careful patient selection is advisable (apomorphine is not recommended in patients with symptomatic orthostatic hypotension, excessive daytime sleepiness, troublesome psychosis, or ICDs).
- IV administration is not recommended due to possible serious adverse effects (e.g. thrombosis).
- Use with caution in patients susceptible to nausea/vomiting or when vomiting is likely to pose a risk.
- Use with caution in patients with known cardiovascular/cerebrovascular disease due to potential hypotensive effects.
- Use with caution in patients with pulmonary or endocrine disease.
- Concomitant use with sublingual nitroglycerin may lead to greater decreases in blood pressure, so patients are advised to lie down before and after taking sublingual nitroglycerin.
- Caution is advised while driving or operating hazardous machines during apomorphine treatment, as it predisposes to daytime somnolence or sudden sleep episodes.

Do Not Use (Contraindications)
- Hypersensitivity to apomorphine or any ingredient in the formulation (e.g. sodium metabisulphite).

DOSING AND USE

45

- Patients with respiratory depression, dementia, psychotic diseases, or hepatic insufficiency.
- Concomitant use of 5-HT3 receptor antagonists (e.g. *alosetron, dolasetron, granisetron, ondansetron, palonosetron*) or central dopamine receptors (e.g. *metoclopramide*).
- Co-administration with alcohol.

Special Populations
Renal Impairment
- In patients with mild or moderate renal impairment, the recommended initial test dose and subsequent starting dose is 0.1 ml (1 mg).
- Apomorphine should not be used in patients with severe renal impairment.

Hepatic Impairment
- Not recommended in case of hepatic impairment.

Elderly
- Use with caution because of higher risk of confusion, hallucinations, serious adverse events, falls, cardiovascular events, respiratory disorders, and gastrointestinal events.

Pregnancy
- Apomorphine should not be used during pregnancy unless necessary.
- There is no experience of apomorphine usage in pregnant women.
- No teratogenic effects have been found in animal studies; however, doses given to rats, which are toxic to the mother, can lead to failure to breathe in the newborn.

Breastfeeding
- Apomorphine use is not recommended during breast-feeding.
- It is not known whether apomorphine is excreted in human milk.

Costs
NHS indicative price accessed 5 December 2022:
- APO-go 50 mg/5 ml solution for injection ampoules (Britannia Pharmaceuticals Ltd) – 5 amps £73.11.
- APO-go PEN 30 mg/3 ml solution for injection (Britannia Pharmaceuticals Ltd) – 5 pens £123.91.
- Dacepton 30 mg/3 ml solution for injection cartridges (Ever Pharma Ltd) – 5 cartridges £123.00.

A

The Overall Place of Apomorphine Subcutaneous Injections in the Treatment of Parkinson's Disease

Apomorphine constitutes a useful therapeutic option for the treatment of unpredictable OFF episodes, requiring prompt resolution (rescue medicine), the treatment of delayed ON or dose failure, and the treatment of early-morning OFF. If more than six daily injections are required, a switch to apomorphine SC infusion is recommended.

Clinical Box

A 54-year-old, right-handed woman with an 8-year history of PD started to experience unpredictable motor and non-motor fluctuations. She had no relevant co-morbidities. Her current medication regime consisted of levodopa–carbidopa 25/100 mg QID; levodopa–carbidopa CR 25/200 mg at night-time; opicapone 50 mg OD, and rotigotine 6 mg/24 h. No history of orthostatic hypotension, excessive daytime sleepiness, psychosis, or ICDs was mentioned. She was fully active and independent in her activities of daily living. She worked as a professional saxophonist. Her main concern was the onset of an OFF episode before getting on the stage. She was initiated on anti-emetic prophylaxis (domperidone 10 mg TDS) and apomorphine SC injections (optimal dose 3 mg/injection) with beneficial effect; the former was discontinued after 3 weeks.

Suggested Reading

Carbone F, A Djamshidian, K Seppi, W Poewe. Apomorphine for Parkinson's disease: efficacy and safety of current and new formulations. *CNS Drugs* 2019; 33(9): 905–918. doi: 10.1007/s40263-019-00661-z. PMID: 31473980; PMCID: PMC6776563.

Titova N, KR Chaudhuri. Apomorphine therapy in Parkinson's and future directions. *Parkinsonism Relat Disord* 2016; 33(Suppl 1): S56–S60. doi: 10.1016/j.parkreldis.2016.11.013. Epub 2016 Nov 30. PMID: 27913125.

References

AHFS Drug information, 2012. Bethesda: American Society of Health-System Pharmacists. Accessed on 5 December 2022 via www.medicinescomplete.com.

Apomorphine. In: DRUGDEX® System (electronic version). Truven Health Analytics, Greenwood Village, Colorado, USA. Accessed on 5 December 2022 via www.micromedexsolutions.com.

Apomorphine. In: Brayfield A (Ed.), *Martindale: The Complete Drug Reference*. London: The Royal Pharmaceutical Society of Great Britain. Accessed on 5 December 2022 via www.medicinescomplete.com.

REFERENCES

A

HYDROCHLORIDE SUBCUTANEOUS INJECTION

Auffret M, S Drapier, M Vérin. Pharmacological insights into the use of apomorphine in Parkinson's disease: clinical relevance. *Clin Drug Investig* 2018; 38(4): 287–312.

Chaudhuri KR, A Todorova, MJ Nirenberg, M Parry, A Martin, P Martinez-Martin, A Rizos, T Henriksen, W Jost, A Storch, G Ebersbach, H Reichmann, P Odin, A Antonini. A pilot prospective, multicenter observational study of dopamine agonist withdrawal syndrome in Parkinson's disease. *Mov Disord Clin Pract* 2015; 2(2): 170–174. doi: 10.1002/mdc3.12141. PMID: 30713891; PMCID: PMC6353371.

Jenkins JR, JMS Pearce. Paradoxical akinetic response to apomorphine in parkinsonism. *J Neurol Neurosurg Psychiatry* 1992; 55: 414–415.

Joint Formulary Committee. British National Formulary (online). London: BMJ Group and Pharmaceutical Press. Accessed on 5 December 2022 via www.medicinescomplete.com.

O'Sullivan JD, AJ Hughes. Apomorphine-induced penile erections in Parkinson's disease. *Mov Disord* 1998; 13(3): 536–539.

Stocchi F, MF De Pandis, FA Delfino, T Anselmo, D Frangillo. Transient atrial fibrillation after subcutaneous apomorphine bolus. *Mov Disord* 1996; 11: 584–585.

Summary of Product Characteristics – APO-go pen 10 mg/ml solution for injection. Britannia Pharmaceuticals Limited. Electronic Medicines Compendium: APO-go Pen 10mg/ml Solution for Injection – Summary of Product Characteristics (SmPC) – (emc). Accessed on 5 December 2022 via www.medicines.org.uk.

APOMORPHINE HYDROCHLORIDE SUBLINGUAL FILM

Therapeutics

Chemical Name and Structure

Apomorphine hydrochloride (6aβ-aporphine-10,11-diol hydrochloride hemihydrate; (R)-10,11-dihydroxy-6a-aporphine hydrochloride hemihydrate; (6aR)-5,6,6a,7-tetrahydro-6-methyl-4H-dibenzo[de,g] quinoline-10,11-diol hydrochloride hemihydrate) has a molecular weight of 303.8 and a molecular formula of $C_{17}H_{18}ClNO_2$.

Brand Names
- **Ixense** (*Thailand*).
- **Kynmobi** (*USA*).
- **Taluvian** (*Greece*).
- **Uprima** (*Greece, Thailand*).

Generics Available
- No.

Licensed Indications for Parkinson's Disease
- Motor fluctuations inadequately controlled by oral dopaminergic agents (FDA).

Licensed Indications for Other Conditions
- None.

Non-Licensed Use for Parkinson's Disease
- Non-motor fluctuations inadequately controlled by oral dopaminergic agents.

Non-Licensed Use for Other Conditions
- Erectile dysfunction.

Ineffective
- Not reported.

Mechanism of Action
- Apomorphine is a non-ergot-derivative dopamine receptor agonist, which is structurally and pharmacologically related to dopamine.
- It is a broad-spectrum dopamine agonist, acting on both D1-like (D1 and D5) and D2-like (D2, D3, D4) receptors, with a higher affinity for the latter.
  - In vitro studies have demonstrated different increasing affinity for D1, D5, D2, and D3 receptors, with the greatest affinity observed for D4 receptors.
- It has a moderate affinity to α-adrenergic (α1D, α2B, α2C) receptors.

A

APOMORPHINE HYDROCHLORIDE SUBLINGUAL

- It has little or no affinity for serotonergic (5-HT1A, 5-HT2A, 5-HT2B, 5-HT2C) receptors, β1- or β2-adrenergic receptors, or histamine H1 receptors.

Efficacy Profile
- The goal of treatment is resolution of OFF episodes.
- If multiple daily intakes are needed (more than five per day), switching to apomorphine SC infusion is advisable.

Pharmacokinetics
Absorption and Distribution
- Bioavailability: 17–18%.
- Food co-ingestion: no interactions reported.
- Tmax: 30–60 min.
- Time to steady state: not documented.
- Pharmacokinetic: less than dose-proportional increases in exposure over a dose range of 10–35 mg following single administration.
- Protein binding: 90% bound to plasma proteins.
- Volume of distribution: 3,630–3,650 l.

Metabolism
- Apomorphine is extensively metabolized in the liver mainly by conjugation with glucuronic acid or sulphate (major metabolite: apomorphine sulphate).
- It is also demethylated to norapomorphine.
- Cytochrome P-450 (CYP) enzymes play a minor role.

Elimination
- Mean elimination half-life is about 1.7 h.
- It is mostly excreted in the urine, mainly as metabolites.

Drug Interaction Profile
Pharmacokinetic Drug Interactions
- Pharmacokinetic interactions with drugs affecting or metabolized by hepatic microsomal enzymes are unlikely.

Pharmacodynamic Drug Interactions
- Co-administration with antihypertensives may lead to enhanced hypotensive effect.
- Co-administration with 5HT3-receptor antagonists (e.g. *alosetron, dolasetron, granisetron, ondansetron, palonosetron*) may lead to increased hypotensive effects.
- Co-administration with nitrates may lead to enhanced hypotensive effect.

THE MOVEMENT DISORDERS PRESCRIBER'S GUIDE TO PARKINSON'S DISEASE

A

- Co-medication with drugs causing electrolyte imbalance or increasing QT interval, such as Class IA and III anti-arrhythmics, antipsychotics (e.g. *haloperidol, phenothiazine derivatives, pimozide*), tricyclic antidepressants, certain antimicrobial agents (e.g. *moxifloxacin, erythromycin*), certain antihistamines (e.g. *astemizole, mizolastine*), and others may lead to potentially fatal Torsade de Pointes arrhythmias and is considered a risk factor for sudden cardiac death.
- Co-administration with dopamine antagonists (e.g. *metoclopramide*, antipsychotics) may reduce the therapeutic effect of apomorphine.
- Co-administration with CNS depressants (e.g. *alcohol*) may lead to enhanced sedative and hypotensive effects.

Adverse Effects

How Drug Causes Adverse Effects
- Mainly (but not only) by increasing dopaminergic activity.

Common Adverse Effects
- Very common (≥1/10):
  - Hallucinations (although troublesome hallucinations are less common in clinical practice), nausea, oral/pharyngeal soft tissue swelling/pain/paraesthesia, somnolence, dizziness.
- Common (≥1/100 to <1/10):
  - Neuropsychiatric: transient mild confusion, transient sedation, somnolence, dizziness, light-headedness, intrusive hallucinations.
  - Cardiovascular: syncope, hypotension.
  - Respiratory: yawning (considered proof of effect of apomorphine on CNS during challenge test), rhinorrhoea.
  - GI: vomiting (usually if domperidone is omitted and therefore domperidone is recommended in safe doses), oral mucosa erythema, oral ulceration and stomatitis, dry mouth, laceration.
  - Other: fatigue, hypersensitivity, falls, hyperhidrosis.
- Uncommon (≥1/1,000 to <1/100):
  - Neuropsychiatric: dyskinesias, sudden sleep onset episodes (likely in susceptible individuals with serotonergic subtype of Parkinson's disease).
  - Respiratory: respiratory difficulties.
  - Other: positive Coomb's tests.

Life-Threatening or Dangerous Adverse Effects
- Uncommon (≥1/1,000 to <1/100):
  - Haemolytic anaemia
  - Thrombocytopenia
- Rare (≥1/10,000 to <1/1,000):
  - Eosinophilia.
  - Allergic reactions, including anaphylaxis and bronchospasm.
  - ICDs, DDS.

ADVERSE EFFECTS

- Unknown frequency:
  - Dyspnoea.
  - QT-interval prolongation, angina, MI, cardiac arrhythmia/arrest, and/or sudden death.

Rare and Not Life-Threatening Adverse Effects
- Unknown frequency:
  - Aggression, agitation.
  - Peripheral oedema.
  - Increased salivation and perspiration.
  - Paradoxical akinetic response.
  - Priapism.

Weight Change
- Not reported.

What to Do About Adverse Effects
- Discuss common adverse effects with patients or caregivers before starting medication, including symptoms that should be reported to the physician.
- In case of troublesome adverse effects, consider withdrawing therapy with concomitant increase in dosing of levodopa or other dopaminergic agents.
- Transient sedation may develop at the start of apomorphine therapy, which usually resolves over the first few weeks of therapy.

Dosing and Use
Usual Dosage Range
- 10–50 mg; the maximum single dose is 30 mg.

Available Formulations
- Sublingual film: 10 mg, 15 mg, 20 mg, 25 mg, 30 mg.

How to Dose
- Sublingual apomorphine is administered on demand when the patient feels it is needed in order to address an OFF episode.
- Before introducing sublingual apomorphine, instruct patients not to take their regular morning dose of levodopa/DDI or any other anti-parkinsonian medications and to take their last levodopa/DDI dose no later than midnight the night before.
- An initial dose of 10 mg is suggested; the patient should not exceed five doses per day.
- An interval of at least 2 h should exist between each dose.
- If a single dose is ineffective for a particular OFF episode, a second dose should not be given for that OFF episode.

A

- In case of an insufficient response after an initial dose of 10 mg:
  - Resume patient's usual anti-parkinsonian medications and up-titrate with apomorphine within 3 days.
  - Increase dosage by 5-mg increments and assess response.
  - Continue titration in a similar manner under physician supervision, until an effective and tolerable dose is achieved.
- Appropriate dose is established by incremental dosing schedules.

Dosing Tips
- Anti-emetic prophylaxis is advisable; patient should be instructed to receive domperidone or trimethobenzamide hydrochloride 3 days before apomorphine initiation.
- Once apomorphine treatment is established, anti-emetic therapy may be gradually reduced and discontinued in some patients.
- Drinking water is recommended before using the film. Patients should be instructed to place the film under the tongue and wait for at least 3 min without swallowing in order to allow the film to dissolve.

How to Withdraw Drug
- Progressive and slow dose reduction is recommended to reduce risk of dopaminergic withdrawal syndrome.

Overdose
- Signs and symptoms of overdose include persistent vomiting, respiratory depression, bradycardia, hypotension, and coma; death may occur.
- Empirical treatment: opioid antagonist, such as *naloxone*, for excessive vomiting, central nervous system and respiratory depression may be considered in severe cases.

Tests and Therapeutic Drug Monitoring
- Before apomorphine therapy:
  - Screen for QT-prolongation, especially if concomitant domperidone use.
  - In case of concomitant use with levodopa, screen for haemolytic anaemia and thrombocytopenia.
- During apomorphine therapy:
  - Patients receiving apomorphine with levodopa should be screened for haemolytic anaemia and thrombocytopenia every 6 months.
  - Periodic monitoring of hepatic, renal, haematopoietic, and cardiovascular function is advisable.
  - In case of concomitant use of domperidone, regular ECG assessments and monitoring of electrolytes are recommended.

DOSING AND USE

Other Warnings / Precautions
- Careful patient selection is advisable (apomorphine is not recommended in patients with symptomatic orthostatic hypotension, excessive daytime sleepiness, troublesome psychosis, or ICDs).
- Use with caution in patients susceptible to nausea/vomiting or when vomiting is likely to pose a risk.
- Use with caution in patients with known cardiovascular/cerebrovascular disease due to potential hypotensive effects.
- Use with caution in patients with pulmonary or endocrine disease.
- Concomitant use with sublingual nitroglycerin may lead to greater decreases in blood pressure, so patients are advised to lie down before and after taking sublingual nitroglycerin.
- Caution is advised while driving or operating hazardous machines during apomorphine treatment, as it predisposes to daytime somnolence or sudden sleep episodes.

Do Not Use (Contraindications)
- Hypersensitivity to apomorphine or any ingredient in the formulation (e.g. sodium metabisulphite).
- Patients with respiratory or CNS depression, dementia, psychotic diseases, or hepatic insufficiency.
- Concomitant use of 5-HT3 receptor antagonists (e.g. *alosetron, dolasetron, granisetron, ondansetron, palonosetron*) or central dopamine receptors (e.g. *metoclopramide*).
- Co-administration with alcohol.

Special Populations
Renal Impairment
- In patients with mild or moderate renal impairment: no dose adjustment is necessary; dose titration should be done under medical supervision.
- CrCl<30 ml/min: not recommended.

Hepatic Impairment
- Mild-to-moderate impairment: use with caution.
- Not recommended in case of severe hepatic impairment.

Elderly
- Use with caution because of higher risk of confusion, hallucinations, serious adverse events, falls, cardiovascular events, respiratory disorders, and gastrointestinal events.

Pregnancy
- Apomorphine should not be used during pregnancy unless necessary.
- There is no experience of apomorphine usage in pregnant women.

- No teratogenic effects have been found in animal studies; however, doses given to rats which are toxic to the mother can lead to failure to breathe in the newborn.

Breastfeeding
- Apomorphine use is not recommended during breastfeeding.
- It is not known whether apomorphine is excreted in human milk.

Costs
Not available in the UK.

The Overall Place of Apomorphine Sublingual Film in the Treatment of Parkinson's Disease

Sublingual preparations of apomorphine are useful for the treatment of OFF episodes (rescue medicine) in Parkinson's disease. If frequent daily intakes (>5 daily) are required, switching to apomorphine subcutaneous infusion is suggested.

Clinical Box

A 67-year-old, right-handed woman with an 8-year history of Parkinson's disease duration started to experience unpredictable motor and non-motor fluctuations. Current and past medical history included diabetes mellitus type II. Her current medication regime consisted of levodopa–carbidopa–entacapone 100/25/200 mg 5 times daily, levodopa–carbidopa CR200/50 mg at night-time, ropirinole MR 8 mg in the morning, and metformin 500 mg twice daily. No history of orthostatic hypotension, excessive daytime sleepiness, psychosis, or impulse control disorder was reported. She was fully active and independent in her activities of daily living. She was initiated on anti-emetic prophylaxis and apomorphine sublingual film (optimal dose 25 mg/film – usually 3 times daily) with beneficial effect; the former was discontinued after 4 weeks.

Suggested Reading

Carbone F, A Djamshidian, K Seppi, W Poewe. Apomorphine for Parkinson's disease: efficacy and safety of current and new formulations. *CNS Drugs* 2019; 33(9): 905–918. doi: 10.1007/s40263-019-00661-z. PMID: 31473980; PMCID: PMC6776563.

Olanow CW, SA Factor, AJ Espay, RA Hauser, HA Shill, S Isaacson, R Pahwa, M Leinonen, P Bhargava, K Sciarappa, B Navia, D Blum ;

CTH-300 Study investigators. Apomorphine sublingual film for off episodes in Parkinson's disease: a randomised, double-blind, placebo-controlled phase 3 study. *Lancet Neurol* 2020; 19(2): 135–144. doi: 10.1016/S1474-4422(19)30396-5. Epub 2019 Dec 7. PMID: 31818699.

Titova N, KR Chaudhuri. Apomorphine therapy in Parkinson's and future directions. *Parkinsonism Relat Disord* 2016; 33(Suppl 1): S56–S60. doi: 10.1016/j.parkreldis.2016.11.013. Epub 2016 Nov 30. PMID: 27913125.

References

Apomorphine. In: Brayfield A (Ed.), *Martindale: The Complete Drug Reference*. London: The Royal Pharmaceutical Society of Great Britain. Accessed on 5 December 2022 via www.medicinescomplete.com.

Apomorphine. In: DRUGDEX® System (electronic version). Truven Health Analytics, Greenwood Village, Colorado, USA. Accessed on 5 December 2022 via www.micromedexsolutions.com.

Chaudhuri KR, Todorova A, Nirenberg MJ, Parry M, Martin A, Martinez-Martin P, Rizos A, Henriksen T, Jost W, Storch A, Ebersbach G, Reichmann H, Odin P, Antonini A. A Pilot Prospective, Multicenter Observational Study of Dopamine Agonist Withdrawal Syndrome in Parkinson's Disease. Mov Disord Clin Pract. 2015 Mar 16;2(2):170–174. doi:10.1002/mdc3.12141.PMID:30713891; PMCID:PMC6353371.

Jenkins JR, JMS Pearce. Paradoxical akinetic response to apomorphine in parkinsonism. *J Neurol Neurosurg Psychiatry* 1992; 55: 414–415.

Stocchi F, MF De Pandis, FA Delfino, T Anselmo, D Frangillo. Transient atrial fibrillation after subcutaneous apomorphine bolus. *Mov Disord* 1996; 11: 584–585.

THE MOVEMENT DISORDERS PRESCRIBER'S GUIDE TO PARKINSON'S DISEASE

BOTULINUM TOXIN

B

Therapeutics

Chemical Name and Structure

Botulinum toxins are potent neurotoxins produced by *Clostridium botulinum*. Two of the seven available biological serotypes of botulinum toxin are used in clinical practice, those being serotypes A and B. They are proteins comprising a heavy chain and a light chain. The two chains link via a disulphide bond.

- IncobotulinumtoxinA is the only botulinum product that consists solely of the active neurotoxin.

Brand Names

- **Alluzience** (*France, Sweden, Switzerland*); **Antipar** (*Mexico*); **Azzalure** (*Austria, Belgium, Denmark, Finland, France, Germany, Ireland, Netherlands, Norway, Poland, Portugal, Spain, Sweden, Switzerland, UK*).
- **Bocouture** (*Austria, Belgium, Czech Republic, Finland, France, Germany, Greece, Netherlands, Poland, Portugal, Spain, Sweden, Switzerland, UK*); **Botox** (*Argentina, Australia, Austria, Belgium, Brazil, Canada, Chile, China, Czech Republic, Denmark, Finland, France, Germany, Greece, Hong Kong, New Zealand, Norway, Philippines, Poland, Portugal, Russian Federation, Singapore, South Africa, Spain, Sweden, Switzerland, Thailand, Turkey, UK, Ukraine, USA, Venezuela*); **Botulax** (*Russian Federation, Thailand*); **Botulift** (*Brazil*); **BTXA** (*Hong Kong*).
- **Dysport** (*Argentina, Australia, Austria, Belgium, Brazil, Canada, Czech Republic, Denmark, Finland, France, Germany, Greece, Hong Kong, Hungary, Ireland, Israel, Italy, Malaysia, Mexico, Netherlands, New Zealand, Norway, Philippines, Poland, Portugal, Russian Federation, Singapore, South Africa, Spain, Sweden, Switzerland, Thailand, Turkey, UK, Ukraine, USA*).
- **Jeuveau** (*USA*).
- **Lantox** (*Russian Federation*); **Lanzox** (*Indonesia*); **Letybo** (*UK*).
- **Myobloc** (*USA*).
- **Nabota** (*Philippines, Thailand*); **NerBloc** (*Japan*); **NeuroBloc** (*Austria, Czech Republic, Denmark, Finland, Greece, Hungary, Ireland, Italy, Netherlands, Norway, Poland, Portugal, Spain*); **Nuceiva** (*Canada, Netherlands, Poland*).
- **Prosigne** (*Brazil*).
- **Reage** (*Chile*); **Relatox** (*Russian Federation*).
- **Siax** (*Hong Kong*).
- **Vistabel** (*Belgium, Czech Republic, Denmark, Finland, France, Germany, Greece, Hungary, Ireland, Netherlands, Norway, Poland, Portugal, Spain, Sweden, Switzerland*); **Vistabex** (*Italy*).
- **Xeomeen** (*Belgium, Mexico*); **Xeomin** (*Australia, Austria, Brazil, Canada, Czech Republic, Denmark, Finland, France, Germany, Hong Kong, Hungary, Ireland, Israel, Italy, Netherlands, New Zealand, Norway,*

B

Philippines, Poland, Portugal, Russian Federation, Singapore, Spain, Sweden, Switzerland, UK, USA).
• **Zentox** *(Thailand).*

Generics Available
• No.

Licensed Indications for Parkinson's Disease
• None.

Licensed Indications for Other Conditions
• Blepharospasm and strabismus associated with dystonia (FDA, EMC).
• Primary axillary hyperhidrosis (FDA, EMC).
• Cervical dystonia (FDA, EMC).
• Hemifacial spasm (EMC).
• Focal spasticity (FDA, EMA, EMC).
• Chronic migraine (FDA, EMA, EMC).
• Neurogenic detrusor over activity (FDA, EMC).
• Overactive bladder (FDA, EMC).
• Chronic sialorrhoea (IncobotulinumtoxinA, RimabotulinumtoxinB) (FDA)
• Cosmetic use (FDA, EMC).

Non-Licensed Use for Parkinson's Disease
• Sialorrhoea.
• Drug-resistant tremor in poor candidates for advanced therapies (OnabotulinumtoxinA, AbobotulinumtoxinA).

Non-Licensed Use for Other Conditions
• Tics.
• Tardive dyskinesia.
• Oromandibular dystonia.

Ineffective
• Restless leg syndrome, levodopa-induced dyskinesia and freezing of gait in Parkinson's disease.
• Generalized significant perspiration.

Mechanism of Action
• Botulinum toxin blocks calcium-ion-mediated release of ACh from presynaptic cholinergic nerve terminals, resulting in lower ACh concentration and reduced endplate potential at the neuromuscular junction. This leads to weakness (or even paralysis) of locally affected muscles through chemical denervation; this effect persists until new nerve terminals form, usually within 2–4 months.

B

- Botulinum toxin also disrupts neurotransmission at ganglionic nerve terminals of the autonomic nervous system.
  - ACh is the neurotransmitter at the parasympathetic junction in the salivary glands and direct injection of botulinum toxin into the salivary glands inhibits ACh release leading to lower saliva production.

Efficacy Profile
- Both botulinum toxins A and B have been characterized as 'efficacious' and 'clinically useful' for the management of drooling in Parkinson's disease, if administered by well-trained injectors with specialized monitoring techniques, including ultrasound guidance (MDS EBM Committee).
- From the available botulinum preparations, only IncobotulinumtoxinA and RimabotulinumtoxinB are approved as a first-line therapy for chronic sialorrhoea treatment (irrespective of Parkinson's disease) based on evidence from high-quality studies.
  - Although OnabotulinumtoxinA is the most widely used botulinum product with the largest number of indications, only some small studies are available to confirm its efficacy on sialorrhoea. The same applies to AbobotulinumtoxinA.
- The effect of botulinum toxin on Parkinson's disease-related drooling becomes apparent 1 week after injection with maximum improvement observed at 4 weeks; this effect is expected to be sustained for 15–19 weeks.
- Four open-label studies and one RCT have reported a beneficial effect of botulinum toxin on Parkinson's disease-related tremor, although this indication is limited by a significant risk of subsequent muscle weakness.
- The effect of botulinum toxin on tremor was shown to last for about 29 months on average with moderate to significant improvement reported by more than 80% of patients.
- Currently available studies suggest a potential benefit of botulinum toxin injections on Pisa syndrome in expert centres.
- There are also reports of botulinum toxin use for other symptoms of Parkinson's disease:
  - Dystonia-related pain in Parkinson's disease, especially of the foot (dystonic plantar flexion).
  - Anterocollis, when it is a result of dystonic activation of the ventral musculature and not of weak neck extensors (dropped head).
  - Overactive bladder (detrusor hyperreflexia).
  - Constipation (botulinum toxin into the puborectalis muscle to decrease outflow resistance).
  - OFF-related limb dystonia with pain.
- Fluctuations in clinical response to botulinum toxin injection might be a result of different vial reconstitution procedures, injection intervals, site of injection, and potency values of the product.

THERAPEUTICS

B

Pharmacokinetics

Absorption and Distribution
* ★Classical studies on the pharmacokinetics of the toxin have not been performed due to the extreme toxicity of botulinum toxin type A.
* Bioavailability: minimal levels are found in the general circulation after injection.

Metabolism
* Botulinum toxin is probably metabolized by proteases and the products are believed to be recycled through normal metabolic pathways.

Elimination
* The effect of IM injection typically reverses within 12 weeks as nerve terminals sprout and reconnect with the endplates.
* Studies suggest that botulinum toxin A has the longest half-life.

Drug Interaction Profile

Pharmacokinetic Drug Interactions
* Not reported.

Pharmacodynamic Drug Interactions
* Co-medication of botulinum toxin and aminoglycosides or other agents interfering with neuromuscular transmission (e.g. curare-like compounds, *magnesium sulphate*, *quinidine*) might potentiate the effects of the toxin.
* Co-medication of botulinum toxin and anticholinergic agents may potentiate systemic anticholinergic effects.
* Co-medication of botulinum toxin and muscle relaxants may predispose to excessive weakness.

Adverse Effects

How Drug Causes Adverse Effects
* Adverse effects may be related to the drug, injection technique, or both.
* Administration of separate botulinum toxin products concomitantly or earlier than suggested might aggravate the toxin effects.
* Exaggerated muscle weakness may appear even with therapeutic doses, although the extent of muscle weakness correlates directly with the amount of toxin injected.
  * Weakness begins to appear 2–4 days after injections, while total paralysis occurs within 10 days.
  * Actively contracting muscles may internalize the toxin faster.
* Serious adverse events, including fatal outcomes, have been reported when using botulinum toxin outside approved indications; these complications do not appear to be related to the distant spread of toxins, but rather to the injection site and/or adjacent structures.

Common Adverse Effects
- The most commonly reported adverse effect when administering botulinum toxin for drooling is dry mouth.
- Other reported adverse effects of intraglandular injection of botulinum toxin are peripheral oedema, breath odour, coated tongue, musculoskeletal stiffness, trismus, dysgeusia, dysphagia, dental hygiene-related issues.
- Digit weakness or decreased grip strength may develop when administering botulinum toxin to treat hand tremor.
- Procedure-related side effects, including localized infection, pain, inflammation, paraesthesia, hypoesthesia, tenderness, swelling, erythema, and/or bleeding/bruising/haematoma.
  - Needle-related pain and/or anxiety may lead to vasovagal responses, such as hypotension and syncope.
- Systemic spread of botulinum toxin beyond local sites of injection can occur, leading to muscular weakness in non-contiguous anatomic structures or other effects resembling botulism.
- Systemic autonomic or anticholinergic effects are more common with rimabotulinumtoxin B compared to onabotulinumtoxinA.

Life-Threatening or Dangerous Adverse Effects
- Rare ($\geq 1/10,000$ to $<1/1,000$):
  - Hypersensitivity reactions.
  - Aspiration.
- Very rare ($<1/10,000$):
  - Immune-mediated brachial plexopathy/neuritis.
- Unknown frequency:
  - Atrial fibrillation or other arrhythmias, MI.
  - New onset or recurrent seizures.
  - Botulism-like syndrome.

Rare and Not Life-Threatening Adverse Effects
- Fever and flu syndrome.

Weight Change
- According to animal studies (rats, monkeys), repeated botulinum toxin injections might lead to a transient decrease in body weight.

What to Do About Adverse Effects
- Before introducing botulinum toxin, discuss common or life-threatening adverse effects with patients and/or caregivers, including symptoms that should be reported to the physician.
- In case of speech impairment, swallowing difficulties, breathing problems, or other possible systemic effects (e.g. urinary incontinence, blurred vision) patients and/or caregivers should be instructed to seek immediate medical care.
- Before therapy initiation, patients should be asked if they have received any botulinum toxin preparation within the last 4 months.
- Patients should be aware that adverse effects might develop even if previous botulinum toxin injections were well-tolerated.

B

BOTULINUM TOXIN

Dosing and Use

Available Formulations
- There are four approved preparations currently on the market:
  - OnabotulinumtoxinA (Botox): 50 units/vial, 100 units/vial, 200 units/vial.
  - AbobotulinumtoxinA (Dysport): 300 units/vial, 500 units/vial.
  - IncobotulinumtoxinA (Xeomin): 50 units/vial, 100 units/vial.
  - RimabotulinumtoxinB (Myobloc/NeuroBloc): 2,500 units/vial, 5000 units/vial, 10,000 units/vial.
- All preparations are packaged and distributed in powder form and need to be diluted in saline before administration.

How to Dose
- For the management of sialorrhoea:
  - IncobotulinumtoxinA: total dose of 100 units (60% parotid gland, 40% submandibular gland).
  - RimabotulinumtoxinB: doses of 500–1,500 units per parotid gland and 250 units per submandibular gland (total dose of 1,500–3,500 units).
- The different botulinum toxin products are not interchangeable.
- Ultrasound-guided injections in the parotid and submandibular glands have been suggested as a first-line therapy for drooling, particularly in patients who cannot be prescribed anticholinergic medications due to increased risk of confusion, cognitive issues, or psychosis.
  - Ultrasound-guided approaches target for the maximum gland thickness.
- In the anatomical approach of localization of the salivary glands, injectors use known landmarks and positioning based on published recommendations.
  - For parotid gland: locate the midpoint between the tragus and the angle of the mandible; injection is delivered 1 cm anterior to this point.
  - For submandibular gland: locate the midpoint between the angle of the mandible and the tip of the chin; injection is delivered one finger breadth medially to the inferior surface of the mandible.

Dosing Tips
- A lower initial dose is suggested if botulinum toxin is administered for the first time in treatment naïve patients; the lowest effective dose should be maintained.
- Intraglandular injection of botulinum toxin should only be administered by well-trained physicians with access to specialized monitoring techniques in accordance with national guidelines.
- When treating patients for more than one indication, the maximum cumulative botulinum toxin dose should not exceed 400 units in 3 months.

B

- Single-dose vials can be used within 24 h after reconstitution; any remaining solution should be discarded afterwards.
- Caution is required with dilution, as it may cause spread to unwanted regions and yield suboptimal results.
- When botulinum toxin is administered to treat tremor, forearm flexors and extensors are the typical muscles to target, with priority given to the former due to a higher possibility of causing weakness to the latter.

How to Withdraw Drug
- Non applicable.

Overdose
- Higher botulinum toxin doses may result in local or distant, generalized and profound neuromuscular paralysis and botulism-like syndrome (100–700 units for onabotulinumtoxinA).
- Overdose symptoms do not differ between different botulinum toxin formulations.
- No cases of botulinum toxin ingestion have been described.
- In case of a suspected over dosage, the patient should be monitored closely for several weeks (even if asymptomatic) in order to detect progressive signs and symptoms or muscular weakness, such as ptosis, diplopia, dysphagia, dysarthria, generalized weakness, or respiratory failure.
- Supportive measures, close monitoring, and maintenance of a clear airway with adequate ventilation are recommended, especially if the musculature of the oropharynx and oesophagus has been affected, because it might lead to aspiration.
  - In case of respiratory muscle weakness, intubation and assisted respiration may be required.
- A botulism antitoxin is available, which cannot reverse any botulinum toxin-induced muscle weakness already evident at the time of antitoxin administration, but may stabilize the deficits.
- Recovery after botulinum toxin overdose might take weeks or even months (re-innervation of the paralysed muscle).

Tests and Therapeutic Drug Monitoring
- Not reported.

Other Warnings / Precautions
- The recommended dosages and frequencies of administration of each botulinum toxin formulation should not be exceeded to reduce the risk for overdose, exaggerated muscle weakness, distant spread of toxin, and the formation of serum neutralizing antibodies.
  - Neutralizing antibodies may reduce the effectiveness of botulinum toxin therapy; higher doses or earlier administrations should be

DOSING AND USE

B

avoided. When appropriate, the lowest effective dose at the longest clinically indicated interval is suggested to decrease the possibility of antibody formation.

- Uncontrolled studies suggest that patients might continue to respond to botulinum toxin therapy despite the presence of neutralizing antibodies.
- If a patient becomes unresponsive to a serotype preparation, the presence of neutralizing antibodies should be suspected, even if they are not detected, and a trial with another serotype could be attempted.

  Incobotulinumtoxin A is the only botulinum product that has not been associated with the production of neutralizing antibodies.

- There is a black box warning for the possibility of botulinum toxin effects spreading from the area of injection to produce systemic symptoms similar to botulism, including asthenia, generalized muscle weakness, diplopia, blurred vision, ptosis, dysphagia, dysphonia, dysarthria, urinary incontinence, and breathing difficulties.
  - These symptoms might develop hours to weeks after injection (typically within the first few days) and are usually transient (rarely they last several months).
  - Swallowing and breathing difficulties might be life-threatening.
  - Adults with predisposing underlying conditions (e.g. neuromuscular disorders, peripheral motor neuropathic diseases) are at higher risk for the above symptoms.
- Extra caution is advised when botulinum toxin is administered in patients with compromised respiratory function.
- Patients with pre-existing cardiovascular disease are at increased risk of adverse events involving the cardiovascular system, such as arrhythmia and MI.
- Extra caution is advised for patients with a history of dysphagia and aspiration.
- Caution is advised in patients with a history of epilepsy or other conditions predisposing to seizures, as new-onset or recurrent seizures have been reported with botulinum toxin administration.
- Caution is advised when administering botulinum toxin in patients with inflammation at the proposed site of injection or excessive weakness/atrophy of the target muscle.
- Caution is advised when administering botulinum toxin in patients with thrombocytopenia or bleeding disorders or where co-administered with anticoagulant therapy.
- Botulinum toxin formulations contain human albumin, which carries an extremely low risk for transmissions of viruses and variant Creutzfeldt–Jacob disease; despite this warning, no such cases have been described up to now in other albumin-containing licensed products.
- Caution is advised if co-administered with aminoglycosides or other products affecting the neuromuscular transmission due to additive effects.

B

- Caution is advised if co-administered with anticholinergic drugs due to additive effects.
- Botulinum toxin might cause asthenia, muscle weakness, somnolence, dizziness and visual impairment, affecting the ability to drive or operate dangerous machinery.

Do Not Use (Contraindications)
- Hypersensitivity to botulinum toxin or any of its excipients.
- Known neuromuscular disease or disease of the neuromuscular junction.
- Infection at the proposed injection site.
- Keloidal scarring.

Special Populations
Renal Impairment
- No dose adjustments needed.

Hepatic Impairment
- No dose adjustments needed.

Elderly
- No dosage modification is suggested for the elderly; however, the lowest therapeutic dose should be used.

Pregnancy
- Available data on the use of botulinum toxin during pregnancy are not adequate.
- Animal studies have revealed adverse effects of botulinum toxin on fetal growth at clinically relevant doses.
- Botulinum toxin use is not recommended during pregnancy and in women of childbearing potential not using contraception.

Breastfeeding
- It is not known whether botulinum toxin is excreted in human milk and its effect on nursing infants is not established.
- Botulinum toxin cannot be recommended during breastfeeding.

Costs
NHS indicative price accessed on 12 December 2022:
- Botulinum toxin type A:
  - Azzalure 125-unit powder for solution for injection (Galderma (UK) Ltd) 2 × vials £126.00.
  - Bocouture 50-unit powder for solution for injection (Merz Pharma UK Ltd) £72.00, 100-unit injection £229.90.

COSTS

B

BOTULINUM TOXIN

- Botox 50-unit power for solution for injection (AbbVie Ltd) £77.50, 100-unit injection £138.20, 200-unit injection £276.40.
- Dysport 300-unit powder for injection vials (Ipsen Ltd) £92.40, 2 × 500-unit injection £308.00.
- Letybo 50-unit powder for solution for injection (Croma-Pharma GmbH) £65.00.
- Xeomin 50-unit powder for solution for injection (Merz Pharma UK Ltd) £72.00, 100-unit injection £129.90, 200-unit injection £259.80.
- Botulinum toxin type B: no longer available in the UK.

The Overall Place of Botulinum Toxin in the Treatment of Parkinson's Disease

Botulinum toxin is a protein produced by *Clostridium botulinum*, which blocks ACh release at the neuromuscular junction, leading to muscle weakness or paralysis. There are seven available serotypes of botulinum neurotoxin; however, only two of them, A and B, are currently used in a clinical setting. Botulinum toxin has several well-established licensed indications, some of which can also be encountered in the context of Parkinson's disease, such as cervical dystonia and blepharospasm. Moreover, numerous high-quality studies have demonstrated a robust efficacy of botulinum toxin (both type A and B) on chronic sialorrhoea (licensed indication in the USA), including Parkinson's disease-related troublesome drooling. Indeed, botulinum toxin constitutes an efficient alternative to anticholinergic medications, which are associated with frequent and troublesome adverse effects in the elderly or cognitively impaired patients.

For other Parkinson's disease-related symptoms, where therapeutic options are often limited, there is some evidence that botulinum toxin might be useful; for example, in dystonic pain often encountered in patients with advanced-stage Parkinson's disease. The use of botulinum toxin might also be considered in cases of detrusor hyperactivity, if standard pharmacological treatments are not effective. Furthermore, it would be a reasonable option in drug-refractory tremor of the upper limb, especially in patients who are poor candidates for device-aided therapies. Finally, botulinum toxin injections into the external anal sphincter may be considered in selected cases of resistant and severe constipation caused by pelvic floor dyssynergia.

In general, botulinum toxin efficacy is largely dependent on dose, dose interval, injection site selection and the injector's experience. Therefore, personalized injection patterns are commonly used. It should also be noted that kinematic-based injections seem promising, as they were found to yield similar outcomes to expert injectors. Botulinum toxin is generally considered well-tolerated (doses of 1,500–4,000 units) with

B

currently available extension studies of repeated dosing exhibiting a sustained efficacy for up to 64 (sialorrhoea) or 96 weeks (tremor).

Potential Advantages
- Botulinum toxin is beneficial on a variety of symptoms.
- It is generally well tolerated in the long term.
- Any potential adverse events are expected to be transient in nature.
- It can be used in elderly and/or cognitively impaired patients.
- Botulinum toxin is more cost-effective than antimuscarinic agents in the management of overactive bladder in adults.

Potential Disadvantages
- Botulinum toxin injections can only be administered by experienced, well-trained clinicians with access to specialized administration techniques.
- Botulinum toxin therapy is an invasive procedure, requiring re-administration every few months.

Clinical Box
A 78-year-old man with an 8-year history of Parkinson's disease and moderate cognitive impairment, presented at the Movements Disorders Outpatient Clinic with his wife for his regular follow-up appointment. Apart from a mild deterioration of his motor performance, the patient's wife mentioned excessive drooling, which was socially isolating. The patient was receiving levodopa–carbidopa 200 mg/50 mg QID, transdermal rivastigmine patch of 9.5 mg/24 h, and quetiapine 25 mg OD. Due to the patient's age and existing cognitive impairment, management of sialorrhoea with anticholinergic agents was not considered a safe option and a personalized scheme of botulinum toxin injections into the parotid and submandibular glands was implemented with good effects.

Suggested Reading
Chinnapongse R, K Gullo, P Nemeth, Y Zhang, L Griggs. Safety and efficacy of botulinum toxin type B for treatment of sialorrhea in Parkinson's disease: a prospective double-blind trial. *Mov Disord* 2012; 27(2): 219–226.
Isaacson SH, W Ondo, CE Jackson, RM Trosch, E Molho, F Pagan, M Lew, K Dashtipour, T Clinch, AJ Espay. Safety and efficacy of rima-botulinumtoxinB for treatment of sialorrhea in adults: a randomized clinical trial. *JAMA Neurol* 2020; 77(4): 461–469.
Jost WH. Use of botulinum neurotoxin in Parkinson's disease: a critical appraisal. *Toxins (Basel)* 2021; 13(2): 87.

SUGGESTED READING

Jost WH, A Friedman, O Michel, C Oehlwein, J Slawek, A Bogucki, S Ochudlo, M Banach, F Pagan, B Flatau-Baqué, J Csikós, CJ Cairney, A Blitzer. SIAXI: placebo-controlled, randomized, double-blind study of incobotulinumtoxinA for sialorrhea. *Neurology* 2019; 92(17): e1982–e1991.

Ondo WG, C Hunter, W Moore. A double-blind placebo-controlled trial of botulinum toxin B for sialorrhea in Parkinson's disease. *Neurology* 2004; 62(1): 37–40.

References

Abusrair AH, W Elsekaily, S Bohlega. Tremor in Parkinson's disease: from pathophysiology to advanced therapies. *Tremor Other Hyperkinet Mov (NY)* 2022; 12: 29.

AHFS Drug information, 2012. Bethesda: American Society of Health-System Pharmacists. Accessed on 22 December 2022 via www.medicinescomplete.com.

Botulinum toxin. In: Brayfield A (Ed.), *Martindale: The Complete Drug Reference.* London: The Royal Pharmaceutical Society of Great Britain. Accessed on 22 December 2022 via www.medicinescomplete .com.

Hajebrahimi S, CR Chapple, F Pashazadeh, H Salehi-Pourmehr. Management of neurogenic bladder in patients with Parkinson's disease: a systematic review. *Neurourol Urodyn* 2019; 38(1): 31–62.

Huang P, YY Li, JE Park, P Huang, Q Xiao, Y Wang, S Chen, SD Chen, J Liu, YW Wu. Effects of onabotulinum toxin A on gait in Parkinson's disease patients with foot dystonia. *Can J Neurol Sci* 2022; 49(1): 123–128.

Isaacson J, S Patel, Y Torres-Yaghi, F Pagán. Sialorrhea in Parkinson's disease. *Toxins (Basel)* 2020; 12(11): 691.

Joint Formulary Committee. British National Formulary (online). London: BMJ Group and Pharmaceutical Press. Accessed on 22 December 2022 via www.medicinescomplete.com.

Jost WH, A Friedman, O Michel, C Oehlwein, J Slawek, A Bogucki, S Ochudlo, M Banach, F Pagan, B Flatau-Baqué, U Dorsch, J Csikós, A Blitzer. Long-term incobotulinumtoxinA treatment for chronic sialorrhea: efficacy and safety over 64 weeks. *Parkinsonism Relat Disord* 2020; 70: 23–30.

Knüpfer SC, SA Schneider, MM Averhoff, CM Naumann, G Deuschl, KP Jünemann, MF Hamann. Preserved micturition after intradetrusor onabotulinumtoxinA injection for treatment of neurogenic bladder dysfunction in Parkinson's disease. *BMC Urol* 2016; 16(1): 55.

Lagalla G, M Millevolte, M Capecci, L Provinciali, MG Ceravolo. Long-lasting benefits of botulinum toxin type B in Parkinson's disease-related drooling. *J Neurol* 2009; 256(4): 563–567.

B

Mittal SO, D Machado, D Richardson, D Dubey, B Jabbari. Botulinum toxin in Parkinson disease tremor: a randomized, double-blind, placebo-controlled study with a customized injection approach. *Mayo Clin Proc* 2017; 92(9): 1359–1367.

Rukavina K, V Leta, C Sportelli, Y Buhidma, S Duty, M Malcangio, K Ray Chaudhuri. Pain in Parkinson's disease: new concepts in pathogenesis and treatment. *Curr Opin Neurol* 2019; 32(4): 579–588.

Samotus O, J Lee, M Jog. Long-term tremor therapy for Parkinson and essential tremor with sensor-guided botulinum toxin type A injections. *PLoS One* 2017; 12(6): e0178670.

Samotus O, Y Mahdi, M Jog. Real-world longitudinal experience of botulinum toxin therapy for Parkinson and essential tremor. *Toxins (Basel)* 2022; 14(8): 557.

Shabir H, S Hashemi, M Al-Rufayie, T Adelowo, U Riaz, U Ullah, B Alam, M Anwar, L de Preux. Cost–utility analysis of oxybutynin vs. onabotulinumtoxinA (Botox) in the treatment of overactive bladder syndrome. *Int J Environ Res Public Health* 2021; 18(16): 8743.

Tassorelli C, R De Icco, E Alfonsi, M Bartolo, M Serrao, M Avenali, I De Paoli, C Conte, NG Pozzi, P Bramanti, G Nappi, G Sandrini. Botulinum toxin type A potentiates the effect of neuromotor rehabilitation of Pisa syndrome in Parkinson disease: a placebo controlled study. *Parkinsonism Relat Disord* 2014; 20(11): 1140–1144.

Vurture G, B Peyronnet, A Feigin, MC Biagioni, R Gilbert, N Rosenblum, S Frucht, A Di Rocco, VW Nitti, BM Brucker. Outcomes of intradetrusor onabotulinum toxin A injection in patients with Parkinson's disease. *Neurourol Urodyn* 2018; 37(8): 2669–2677.

REFERENCES

C CITALOPRAM

Therapeutics

Chemical Name and Structure

Citalopram (1-[3-(dimethylamino)propyl]-1-(4-fluorophenyl)-3H-2-benzofuran-5-carbonitrile) is a fine white to off-white powder with a molecular weight of 324.4 and an empirical formula of $C_{20}H_{21}FN_2O$. Citalopram 20 mg is equivalent to 24.99 mg citalopram hydrobromide.

Brand Names

- **A-Depress-Therapy** (*Greece*); **Acelopram** (*Greece*); **Actipram** (*Chile, Venezuela*); **Acti-Lift** (*South Africa*); **Adco-Talomil** (*South Africa*); **Adeprenal** (*Cyprus, Greece*); **Alcytam** (*Brazil*); **Alepram** (*Greece*); **Apo-Cital** (*Czech Republic*); **Arpolax** (*Hong Kong*); **As-Cilog** (*Turkey*); **Aurex** (*Poland*); **Auropram** (*Hong Kong*).
- **Belmazol** (*Greece*); **Bivien** (*Greece*).
- **C-Pram** (*India*); **C-Talo** (*India*); **Celepram** (*Australia, Brazil, New Zealand*); **Celepra** (*India*); **Celexa** (*Canada, USA*); **Celica** (*Australia, India*); **Celius** (*Greece*); **Celopram** (*Tunisia*); **Cibrom** (*Mexico*); **Cilate** (*South Africa*); **Cilift** (*South Africa*); **Cilodral** (*Cyprus*); **Cilopress** (*Greece*); **Cilopram** (*South Africa*); **Cilopress** (*Greece*); **Cimal** (*Chile*); **Cinapen** (*Greece*); **Ciprager** (*Ireland*); **Cipram** (*Hong Kong, Malaysia, Singapore, Turkey*); **Cipramil** (*Australia, Belgium, Brazil, Chile, China, Denmark, Estonia, Germany*, Ireland, *Israel, Netherlands, New Zealand, Norway, Poland, Russian Federation, South Africa, Sweden, UK, Ukraine*); **Cipraned** (*Greece*); **Ciprotan** (*Ireland*); **Ciral** (*Estonia, Lithuania*); **Citabax** (*Poland*); **Citadep** (*India*); **Citaforin** (*Brazil*); **Citagen** (*Hungary*); **Citagran** (*Brazil*); **Cital** (*Poland*); **Citalec** (*Czech Republic, Estonia*); **Citalgert** (*Greece*); **Citalift** (*Russian Federation*); **Citalo** (*Australia*); **Citaloc** (*Hong Kong*); **Citalogen** (*South Africa*); **Citalohexal** (*South Africa*); **Citalomine** (*India*); **Citalon** (*Germany, Russian Federation*); **Citalop** (*India*); **Citalorin** (*Russian Federation*); **Citalostad** (*Austria*); **Citalvir** (*Spain*); **Citapram** (*Hungary*); **Citara** (*India, Turkey*); **Cita Sandoz** (*Ukraine*); **Citaxin** (*Poland*); **Citexam** (*Turkey*); **Citol** (*Russian Federation, Turkey*); **Citola** (*India*); **Citolap** (*Turkey*); **Citalgert** (*Greece*); **Citaloprol** (*Greece*); **Citolixin** (*Turkey*); **Citopram** (*India*); **Citox** (*Mexico*); **Citpram** (*New Zealand*); **Citrex** (*Turkey*); **Citrol** (*Ireland*); **Citronil** (*Poland*); **Citta** (*Argentina, Brazil*); **Claropram** (*Switzerland*); **Copsam** (*Turkey*); **CTP** (*Canada*); **Cytop** (*India*).
- **Decilop** (*Greece*); **Denyl** (*Brazil*); **Depramil** (*South Africa*); **Depretal** (*Greece*); **Duo Fo** (*China*).
- **Ecloram** (*Greece*); **Elopram** (*Italy*); **Erlicon** (*Greece*); **Eslopram** (*Turkey*); **Etapiam** (*Greece*); **Europram** (*Hong Kong*); **Exenadil** (*Greece*).
- **Feliximir** (*Italy*); **Feliz** (*India, Philippines*); **Frimaind** (*Italy*).
- **Galopran** (*Greece*).

C

- **Humorap** (*Argentina, Russian Federation*).
- **Kaidor** (*Italy*); **Kylipram** (*Greece*).
- **Laira** (*Turkey*); **Lenepal** (*Argentina*); **Levixe** (*Brazil*); **Locitafer** (*Greece*); **Lopracil** (*Greece*); **Lopradep** (*Argentina*); **Lopram** (*India*); **Lopraxer** (*Greece, Hong Kong*); **Loptar** (*Greece*).
- **Madam** (*India*); **Mai Ke Wei** (*China*); **Malicon** (*Greece*); **Marpram** (*Italy*); **Maxapran** (*Brazil*).
- **Norecsero** (*Mexico*); **Nevdep** (*India*); **Nevropram** (*Greece*); **Nypram** (*Brazil*).
- **Opra** (*Russian Federation*); **Oropram** (*Poland*).
- **Palocit** (*India*); **Percitale** (*Italy*); **Pralotam** (*Greece*); **Pram** (*Austria, Czech Republic, Estonia, Lithuania, Poland, Russian Federation, Ukraine*); **Pramcil** (*Chile*); **Pramital** (*Greece*); **Prefucet** (*Greece*); **Prepram** (*Mexico*); **Pricital** (*Greece*); **Prisdal** (*Spain*); **Procimax** (*Brazil*); **Psiconor** (*Argentina*).
- **Ran-Citalo** (*Canada*); **Recita** (*South Africa, Ukraine*); **Recital** (*Israel*); **Relaxol** (*Turkey*); **Remicital** (*Mexico*); **Renevil** (*Greece*); **Return** (*Italy*); **Ricap** (*Italy*); **Ropramin** (*Cyprus, Greece*).
- **Sedopram** (*Russian Federation*); **Selon** (*Greece, Hong Kong*); **Sepram** (*Finland*); **Seproc** (*Greece*); **Seran** (*South Africa*); **Seregra** (*Spain*); **Seretover** (*Greece*); **Seropram** (*Argentina, Austria, Cyprus, Czech Republic, France, Greece, Hungary, Italy, Mexico, Spain, Switzerland, Venezuela*); **Seror** (*Greece*); **Setronil** (*Chile*); **Siloam** (*Greece*); **Sintab** (*Turkey*); **Sintopram** (*Italy*); **Siozam** (*Russian Federation*); **Sitaleau** (*Greece*); **Sotovon** (*Greece*).
- **Talam** (*Australia, Hong Kong*); **Taloped** (*Venezuela*); **Talopram** (*Greece*); **Talosin** (*Greece*); **Tasonade** (*Greece*); **Tazen** (*Philippines*); **Te Lin Na** (*China*); **Trolam** (*Venezuela*).
- **Unstress** (*Greece*).
- **Varom** (*Greece*); **Verisan** (*Italy*); **Verus** (*Greece*); **Vesema** (*Greece*); **Vodelax** (*Turkey*).
- **Wang You** (*China*).
- **Xadorek** (*Greece*).
- **Yi Tai Na** (*China*); **YiTeAn** (*China*).
- **Zanipram** (*Greece*); **Zeclicid** (*Greece*); **Zentius** (*Argentina, Chile, Ecuador*); **Zinetron** (*Mexico*); **Zoxipan** (*Brazil*).

Generics Available
- Yes.

Licensed Indications for Parkinson's Disease
- None.

Licensed Indications for Other Conditions
- Depression/major depressive disorder (FDA, EMA, EMC).
  - Initial and maintenance phase to avert potential relapse.
- Panic disorders with or without agoraphobia (EMA, EMC).

THERAPEUTICS

C

CITALOPRAM

Non-Licensed Use for Parkinson's Disease
• Depression and anxiety in Parkinson's disease.

Non-Licensed Use for Other Conditions
• Alcoholism.
• Binge-eating disorder.
• Generalized anxiety disorder, panic disorder.
• Obsessive-compulsive disorder.
• Hot flashes.
• Premenstrual dysphoric syndrome.
• Headache.

Ineffective
• Not reported.

Mechanism of Action
• A potent inhibitor of serotonin reuptake in presynaptic neurones, classified as an SSRI.
• Little or no affinity is reported for dopamine (D1 and D2), α-adrenergic (α1, α2, and β), histamine H1, muscarine cholinergic, GABA, benzodiazepine, and opioid receptors.

Efficacy Profile
• According to the MDS EBM Committee, citalopram has been characterized as 'clinically useful' for the treatment of depression and anxiety symptoms in Parkinson's disease.
• The antidepressant effect of citalopram takes 1–4 weeks to appear, while the full response is expected after 8–12 weeks from therapy initiation.
• Similarly to other antidepressants and MAOIs, citalopram suppresses REM sleep and amplifies deep slow-wave sleep. This activity is thought to be a predictor of the antidepressant effect.
• Citalopram does not disturb intellectual function or psychomotor performance and has no sedative effects, even when combined with alcohol.
• There is preliminary evidence of citalopram efficacy on Parkinson's disease-related psychosis and behavioural impulsivity/response inhibition in the absence of ICD in a subset of Parkinson's disease patients.

Pharmacokinetics
Absorption and Distribution
• (Oral) bioavailability: 80%.
• Food co-ingestion: no effect on citalopram bioavailability.
• Tmax: 1–6 h (average of 4 h).
• Time to steady state: 1–2 weeks.
• Pharmacokinetics: linear.

C

- Protein binding: <80%.
- Volume of distribution: 12.3 l/kg.

Metabolism
- Citalopram undergoes hepatic metabolism, mostly by CYP2C19 (~38%), CYP3A4 (~31%), and CYP2D6 (~31%), producing metabolites (also SSRIs) with potency and selectivity that are lower compared to the parent drug.
  - Because the biotransformation of citalopram is mediated by numerous P450 isoenzymes rather than one, its inhibition through drug interactions is less likely in clinical practice.

Elimination
- Half-life for citalopram is 24–48 h.
- Citalopram is excreted predominantly via the liver (85%) with the remainder via the kidneys (15%).
  - About 12% of an administered dose is excreted unchanged in the urine and about 10% in the faeces.

Drug Interaction Profile
Pharmacokinetic Drug Interactions
- Effects by citalopram:
  - Citalopram may increase the levels of drugs that are mainly metabolized by CYP2D6 (e.g. *desipramine, nortriptyline, risperidone, haloperidol, flecainide, metoprolol*).
- Effects on citalopram:
  - *Cimetidine* causes a moderate increase in citalopram levels.

Pharmacodynamic Drug Interactions
- Co-medication with other serotonergic agents, including SSRIs/ SNRIs, tricyclic antidepressants, opioids, lithium, buspirone, amphetamines, MAOIs, and triptans, can lead to potentially life-threatening serotonin syndrome.
- Co-medication with agents affecting platelet function, including antiplatelets (e.g. *aspirin*), anticoagulants (e.g. *warfarin*), and NSAIDs, increases the risk of bleeding events, including life-threatening haemorrhage.
- Co-administration with diuretics might increase the risk of hyponatraemia.
- Co-medication with drugs causing electrolyte imbalance or increasing QT interval, such as Class IA and III anti-arrhythmics, antipsychotics (e.g. *haloperidol, phenothiazine derivatives, pimozide*), tricyclic antidepressants, certain antimicrobial agents (e.g. *moxifloxacin, erythromycin*), certain antihistamines (e.g. *astemizole, mizolastine*), and others may lead to potentially fatal Torsade de Pointes arrhythmias and is considered a risk factor for sudden cardiac death.
- Co-medication with opioids aggravates the antinociceptive effect of commonly used opioid analgesics.

C

Adverse Effects

How Drug Causes Adverse Effects
- The activity of citalopram is thought to be mediated through inhibition of serotonin reuptake in the presynaptic neurons, leading to fewer anticholinergic side effects than tricyclic antidepressants.

Common Adverse Effects
- Very common (≥1/10):
  - Dry mouth, nausea, somnolence, insomnia, increased perspiration, headache, asthenia.
- Common (≥1/100 to <1/10):
  - Nervous/psychiatric: tremor, anxiety, agitation, decreased libido, yawning, confusion, migraine, paraesthesia, abnormal dreams, dizziness, amnesia, attention impairment.
  - Eye/ear: tinnitus.
  - Cardiovascular: orthostatic hypotension, tachycardia, palpitations.
  - Respiratory: rhinitis, upper respiratory infections, cough.
  - Gastrointestinal: diarrhoea, constipation, dyspepsia, vomiting, abdominal pain, flatulence, sialorrhoea.
  - Skin: pruritus, rash.
  - Renal/urinary: polyuria.
  - Reproductive: erectile dysfunction/impotence, abnormal orgasm (female), dysmenorrhoea, amenorrhoea.
  - Other: fatigue, apathy, anorexia, arthralgia/myalgia, weight change.
- Uncommon (≥1/1,000 to <1/100):
  - Nervous/psychiatric: aggression, depersonalization, hallucinations, mania, increased libido, syncope.
  - Eye/ear: mydriasis.
  - Cardiovascular: bradycardia.
  - Skin: urticaria, alopecia, rash, purpura, photosensitivity reaction.
  - Urinary: urinary retention.
  - Reproductive: menorrhagia.
  - Other: increased appetite, oedema.

Life-Threatening or Dangerous Adverse Effects
- Rare (≥1/10,000 to <1/1,000):
  - Serotonin syndrome.
  - Hyponatraemia (probably due to SIADH).
  - Seizures.
  - Hepatitis
- Unknown frequency:
  - QT prolongation
  - Thrombocytopenia
  - Anaphylactic reaction

Rare and Not Life-Threatening Adverse Effects
- Dyskinesia, movement disorder.
- Taste disturbance.

- Visual disturbance.
- Panic attack, bruxism, restlessness, suicidal ideation/behaviour.
- Orthostatic hypotension.
- Coughing.
- Priapism and/or galactorrhoea in men.
- Pyrexia, malaise.

Weight Change
- Both increases and decreases in body weight have been reported as side effects of citalopram therapy.

What to Do About Adverse Effects
- Before introducing citalopram, discuss common or life-threatening adverse effects with patients and/or caregivers, including symptoms that should be reported to the physician.
- Patients and their caregivers should be informed about the possibility of citalopram causing suicidal ideation/behaviour, especially in the early phase of recovery. If such signs/symptoms emerge, patients should urgently seek for medical advice and be treated accordingly. Citalopram should be discontinued.
  - Due to suicidality risk, consider giving only a limited number of citalopram tablets on initiation.
- Some patients may report a paradoxical escalation of their anxiety symptoms at the initial phase of treatment with antidepressants. Although this reaction typically improves within 2 weeks, a low starting dose of citalopram is advised.
- If a serotonin syndrome is suspected (e.g. mental-status changes, autonomic instability, neuromuscular abnormalities, gastrointestinal symptoms), close monitoring and discontinuation of citalopram or other interacting agents is necessary.
- Treatment with citalopram should be discontinued if a patient presents with seizures or a manic episode.
- In the case of arrhythmia, citalopram should be withdrawn, and the patient should undergo an ECG.
- Before treatment initiation, patients (both male and female) should be informed about the possibility of citalopram causing sexual dysfunction, as patients may not spontaneously report it.
  - In case of sexual dysfunction, a detailed history should be obtained to exclude other causes, including subjacent psychiatric disorders.
  - Sexual dysfunction might persist despite treatment discontinuation.
  - In male patients, SSRI use may lead to ejaculatory delay or failure, decreased libido, and erectile dysfunction. In female patients, it may lead to decreased libido and delayed or absent orgasm.
- Where a patient using citalopram reports bone pain, the possibility of a subjacent bone fracture should be excluded.
- SSRIs might aggravate RBD in Parkinson's disease patients; consider removing citalopram before initiating treatment for RBD.

Dosing and Use

Usual Dosage Range
• 10–40 mg per day.

Available Formulations
• Tablets: 10 mg, 20 mg, 40 mg.
• Oral solution: 10 mg/5 ml.

How to Dose
• Initial dose of 10 mg OD is suggested; may be increased to 20 mg OD.
• Dosage should be reviewed within 3–4 weeks of therapy initiation; if an insufficient response is detected, consider increasing the dose up to a maximum of 40 mg/day (see notes below for patients over 60).
  • The lowest effective dose should be maintained.
• Dosage increases can be applied at a minimum of 1-week intervals.
  • Clinical evaluation is advised before any dosage increase due to dose-related side effects.

Dosing Tips
• Citalopram is administered as a single dose at the same time each day, preferably in the morning to avoid undue somnolence problems.
• Citalopram oral solution can be mixed with water.
• If citalopram therapy is effective, it should be used for a minimum of 6 months to ensure that the patient is free of symptoms and to lower the risk of relapse.

How to Withdraw Drug
• Dosage tapering is necessary to lower the risk of withdrawal symptoms.
• Citalopram dosage should be gradually decreased at intervals of 1–2 weeks.
• Withdrawal symptoms might include dizziness, sensory disturbances, sleep impairment, agitation/anxiety, nausea/vomiting, tremor, confusion, sweating, headache, diarrhoea, palpitations, emotional instability, irritability, and visual disturbances.
• Withdrawal symptoms typically appear during the first few days after citalopram discontinuation, are mild to moderate in intensity and usually subside spontaneously within 2 weeks.
• In case of severe or prolonged symptoms during dosage reduction or withdrawal, consider resuming the previously prescribed dose and follow a longer tapering period.

Overdose
• Citalopram overdose is usually encountered in combination with alcohol or other medicinal products and might be fatal.
• Overdose might present with nausea/vomiting, sweating, tremor, agitation, mydriasis, hyperventilation, seizures, QT prolongation,

CITALOPRAM

C

C

bradycardia/tachycardia, hypotension/hypertension, hyperpyrexia, serotonin syndrome, rhabdomyolysis, alteration in level of consciousness and cardiac arrythmias/arrest.
- There is no specific antidote for citalopram overdosage.
- Supportive measures, close monitoring and maintenance of a clear airway with adequate ventilation are recommended.
- Activated charcoal can be helpful if administered soon after ingestion. An osmotically working laxative (e.g. sodium sulphate) and gastric lavage may also be of use.
- In the case of frequent or prolonged seizures, consider IV diazepam administration.

Tests and Therapeutic Drug Monitoring
- Before initiation of citalopram therapy:
  - A baseline ECG should be performed to check for QT prolongation.
  - A metabolic panel should be performed, including electrolytes, renal and hepatic function.
- During citalopram therapy:
  - Regular ECG monitoring is necessary in patients over 60 years old when a citalopram dose of over 20 mg per day is prescribed or in cases of altered metabolism that might affect citalopram levels, such as liver impairment.
  - Patients should be regularly evaluated for worsening of depression, suicidality, behaviour changes, or other common adverse effects, especially after introducing therapy or during dose modifications.

Other Warnings/Precautions
- There is a black box warning for young adults (less than 24 years old) who take citalopram for depression and other psychiatric disorders concerning suicidal thinking and behaviour.
  - A slight increase in suicidal thinking has also been seen in the elderly (>65 years old) receiving citalopram.
  - Patients with a history of suicide-related events are at higher risk and careful monitoring during treatment is required, especially early in therapy and following changes in dosage.
- Close monitoring is recommended in patients with a history of bipolar disorder, as citalopram may trigger a manic episode.
  - Citalopram should be withdrawn in any patient entering a manic phase.
- Close monitoring is recommended in patients with a history of seizures or cardiovascular disease.
- Caution and careful monitoring is advised in patients at high risk of prolonged cardiac repolarization (e.g. co-medication with drugs increasing QT interval, patients with cardiovascular disease, family history of QT prolongation, congenital long QT syndrome, significant bradycardia, congestive heart failure, heart hypertrophy, recent acute myocardial infarction, hypokalaemia, or hypomagnesaemia),

DOSING AND USE

C

CITALOPRAM

especially in the elderly and those with hepatic impairment, as citalopram has been associated with dose-dependent QT prolongation. In
such cases, citalopram should better be avoided.

- An angle-closure attack may be triggered in patients with high
intraocular pressure or those at risk of angle closure glaucoma.
- Hyponatraemia and/or SIADH have been reported with citalopram
therapy, especially in dehydrated or volume-depleted patients.
- Because citalopram therapy can affect glycaemic control in diabetic
patients, insulin or other antidiabetic regimes might need to be modified accordingly.
- Citalopram might aggravate co-existent psychotic symptoms.
- Similarly to other SSRIs/SNRIs, citalopram use might predispose to
abnormal bleeding, especially in case of haemorrhagic diathesis or
co-administration with antiplatelets, anticoagulants, or NSAIDS.
- In case of co-administration with CYP2C19 inhibitors (e.g. *omeprazole, esomeprazole, fluconazole, ticlopidine*) or in patients who are known
to be poor CYP2C19 metabolizers, a maximum dose of 20 mg per
day should be prescribed.
- In case of co-administration with drugs that are mainly metabolized
by CYP2D6 dose modifications might be needed.
- In case of co-administration with *cimetidine* a dose modification might
be needed.

Do Not Use (Contraindications)
- Known sensitivity to citalopram or to any of its excipients.
- In patients with uncompensated heart failure.
- Co-administration with drugs that predispose to QT prolongation.
- Co-administration with MAOIs (including selegiline and rasagiline)
or within 2 weeks after their discontinuation due to increased risk of
potentially fatal serotonin syndrome. MAOIs should not be adminis-
tered for 1 week after citalopram discontinuation.
- Co-administration with linezolid or methylene blue IV.
  - In case linezolid administration is necessary, citalopram should be
  immediately discontinued, and the patient should be monitored for
  CNS toxicity. Citalopram therapy can be resumed 24 h after last
  linezolid dose or after 2 weeks of monitoring, whichever applies
  first.

Special Populations
Renal Impairment
- Mild to moderate impairment: no dose adjustments are needed.
- Severe impairment (CrCl<20 ml/min): not studied. Caution is
advised if citalopram use is deemed necessary.

C

Hepatic Impairment
- In case of mild or moderate hepatic impairment:
  - An initial dose of 10 mg per day is suggested for the first 2 weeks of treatment.
  - A maximum dose of 20 mg per day should not be exceeded.

Elderly
- Due to decreased rate of metabolism, which results in longer half-life and lower clearance, a dose of 20 mg per day should not be exceeded in patients over 60 years.

Pregnancy
- No major birth defects or miscarriages have been reported with citalopram use during pregnancy.
- Neonates exposed to SNRIs or SSRIs late in the third trimester might develop complications, requiring hospitalization, respiratory support, and tube feeding.
- There is conflicting evidence regarding use of SSRIs during pregnancy and an increased risk of persistent pulmonary hypertension in the newborn.
- Avoid abrupt withdrawal of citalopram during pregnancy.
- An increased risk for postpartum haemorrhage has been reported when pregnant women use SSRIs/SNRIs near delivery.
- Consider risk of untreated depression in case of discontinuation or change of treatment during pregnancy. Citalopram must only be used during pregnancy if the expected benefits outweigh any potential risks.

Breastfeeding
- Citalopram has been identified in human milk.
- Breastfed infants might develop irritability, weight loss, and abnormal sleep patterns.
- Health benefits of breastfeeding should be considered along with the mother's need for citalopram therapy along with any potential effects on the breastfed infant either from the drug or from the mother's underlying condition.

Costs
NHS indicative price accessed 4 December 2022:
- Cipramil 20 mg tablets (Lundbeck Ltd) – 28 tablets: £8.95.
- Cipramil 40 mg/ml drops (Lundbeck Ltd) – 28 tablets: £10.08.
- Citalopram 10 mg tablets – 28 tablets: £0.75–£12.36.
- Citalopram 20 mg tablets – 28 tablets: £0.92–£14.66.
- Citalopram 40 mg tablets – 28 tablets: £0.99–£16.47.
- Citalopram 40 mg/ml drops – 15ml: £7.07–£14.09.

COSTS

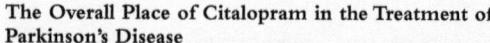

C

CITALOPRAM

The Overall Place of Citalopram in the Treatment of Parkinson's Disease

Citalopram is a well-established and widely used SSRI for the treatment of depression. Numerous RCTs have investigated the effect of SSRIs, including citalopram, in Parkinson's disease patients, usually reporting an amelioration in standardized depression scales, although complete resolution was uncommon. However, these results have been challenged in a thorough meta-analysis concluding that the pooled effect of SSRIs on depression in Parkinson's disease was not significant. Despite the fact that there are no robust data supporting the efficacy of citalopram in Parkinson's disease-related depressive symptoms, it is still considered a reasonable option in clinical practice due to the proven efficacy of SSRIs in depression beyond the context of Parkinson's disease. SSRIs are generally regarded as better tolerated compared to tricyclic antidepressants due to a lower rate of anticholinergic events or cardiac arrhythmias. Due to the better safety profile, SSRIs, including citalopram, are preferred as an initial choice in Parkinson's disease-related mild to moderate depression, especially in older patients or those with cognitive impairment. Although studies directly comparing citalopram to other antidepressants are limited, it was found to be more efficacious than paroxetine, but less than escitalopram. The latter sometimes replaces citalopram in routine clinical practice due to pharmacodynamic similarities, although it is not included in formal guidelines (MDS EBM Committee). High citalopram dosage (>20 mg/day) has been linked to a greater possibility of QT prolongation and, thus, regular ECG monitoring is deemed necessary in those over 60 years of age. Nevertheless, the reports on the extent of the potential citalopram cardiotoxicity are also conflicting.

Potential Advantages
- Citalopram is administered as a single dose, which improves adherence.
- Similarly to other SSRIs, citalopram might be useful in depressive patients with co-morbid anxiety.
- Compared to other antidepressants, SSRIs, including citalopram, might be the initial choice in older patients or those with co-morbidities and potential drug-to-drug interactions.
- According to data on Alzheimer's disease patients, citalopram might be useful in controlling agitation/irritability (not in acute settings) in cognitively impaired elderly patients when antipsychotics cannot be prescribed, even in the absence of depression.

Potential Disadvantages
- Delayed response to therapy.
- SSRI use has been associated with an aggravation of Parkinson's disease-related tremor in 1 in 20 patients, while worsening of parkinsonian features has also been reported. However, these results are conflicting.
- Among all antidepressants, tricyclic antidepressants and citalopram at elevated doses bear the greatest risk for QT prolongation, especially for those over 60 years of age; thus, regular ECG monitoring is required.

C

Clinical Box

A 55-year-old woman with a diagnosis of Parkinson's disease presented at the Neurology Department Outpatient Clinic for her regular follow-up appointment. The patient was receiving pramipexole 2.1 mg OD and levodopa/benserazide 100 mg/25 mg QID. The rest of her medical history included recent menopause with mild symptoms. After her assessment, the patient was found to be suffering from moderate depressive symptoms and anxiety. These symptoms were constant during the day and did not resemble the non-motor fluctuations associated with Parkinson's disease. A low dose of venlafaxine was initially prescribed; however, the patient developed troublesome gastrointestinal disturbances and was switched to a low dose of citalopram 10 mg OD in the morning. Due to lack of efficacy, and as the patient did not mention any side effects, the dose was increased to 20 mg OD after 4 weeks with a subsequent good response of her symptoms.

Suggested Reading

Devos D, K Dujardin, I Poirot, C Moreau, O Cottencin, P Thomas, A Destée, R Bordet, L Defebvre. Comparison of desipramine and citalopram treatments for depression in Parkinson's disease: a double-blind, randomized, placebo-controlled study. *Mov Disord* 2008; 23(6): 850–857.

Menza M, H Marin, K Kaufman, M Mark, M Lauritano. Citalopram treatment of depression in Parkinson's disease: the impact on anxiety, disability, and cognition. *J Neuropsychiatry Clin Neurosci* 2004; 16(3): 315–319.

Starkstein SE, S Brockman. Management of depression in Parkinson's disease: a systematic review. *Mov Disord Clin Pract* 2017; 4(4): 470–477.

Wermuth L, PS Sørensen, S Timm, B Christensen, NP Utzon, J Boas, E Dupont, E Hansen, I Magnussen, B Mikkelsen, J Worm-Petersen, L Lauritzen, L Bayer, P Bech. Depression in idiopathic Parkinson's disease treated with citalopram: a placebo-controlled trial. *Nordic J Psychiatry*, 1998; 52(2): 163–169.

REFERENCES

References

Aga VM. When and how to treat agitation in Alzheimer's disease dementia with citalopram and escitalopram. *Am J Geriatr Psychiatry* 2019; 27(10): 1099–1107.

AHFS Drug information 2012. Bethesda: American Society of Health-System Pharmacists. Accessed on 4 December 2022 via www.medicinescomplete.com.

Cipriani A, M Purgato, TA Furukawa, C Trespidi, G Imperadore, A Signoretti, R Churchill, N Watanabe, C Barbui. Citalopram versus other anti-depressive agents for depression. *Cochrane Database Syst Rev* 2012; 7(7): Cd006534.

C

Citalopram. In: Brayfield A (Ed.), *Martindale: The Complete Drug Reference*. London: The Royal Pharmaceutical Society of Great Britain. Accessed on 4 December 2022 via www.medicinescomplete.com.

Citalopram. In: DRUGDEX® System (electronic version). Truven Health Analytics, Greenwood Village, Colorado, USA. Accessed 4 December 2022 via www.micromedexsolutions.com.

Dell'Agnello G, R Ceravolo, A Nuti, G Bellini, A Piccinni, C D'Avino, L Dell'Osso, U Bonuccelli. SSRIs do not worsen Parkinson's disease: evidence from an open-label, prospective study. *Clin Neuropharmacol* 2001; 24(4): 221–227.

Joint Formulary Committee. British National Formulary (online). London: BMJ Group and Pharmaceutical Press. Accessed 4 December 2022 via www.medicinescomplete.com.

Montgomery S, T Hansen, S Kasper. Efficacy of escitalopram compared to citalopram: a meta-analysis. *Int J Neuropsychopharmacol* 2011; 14(2): 261–268.

Porsteinsson AP, LT Drye, BG Pollock, DP Devanand, C Frangakis, Z Ismail, C Marano, CL Meinert, JE Mintzer, CA Munro, G Pelton, PV Rabins, PB Rosenberg, LS Schneider, DM Shade, D Weintraub, J Yesavage, CG Lyketsos. Effect of citalopram on agitation in Alzheimer disease: the CitAD randomized clinical trial. *JAMA* 2014; 311(7): 682–691.

Rampello L, S Chiechio, R Raffaele, I Vecchio, F Nicoletti. The SSRI, citalopram, improves bradykinesia in patients with Parkinson's disease treated with L-dopa. *Clin Neuropharmacol* 2002; 25(1): 21–24.

Ryan M, CV Eatmon, JT Slevin. Drug treatment strategies for depression in Parkinson disease. *Expert Opin Pharmacother* 2019; 20(11): 1351–1363.

Sid-Otmane L, P Huot, M Panisset. Effect of antidepressants on psychotic symptoms in Parkinson disease: a review of case reports and case series. *Clin Neuropharmacol* 2020; 43(3): 61–65.

Summary of Product Characteristics – Cipramil 20 mg film-coated tablets. Lundbeck Limited. Electronic Medicines Compendium: Cipramil 20 mg film-coated tablets – Summary of Product Characteristics (SmPC) – (emc). Accessed on 4 December 2022 via www.medicines.org.uk.

Troeung L, SJ Egan, N Gasson. A meta-analysis of randomised placebo-controlled treatment trials for depression and anxiety in Parkinson's disease. *PLoS One* 2013; 8(11): e79510.

Ye Z, E Altena, C Nombela, CR Housden, H Maxwell, T Rittman, C Huddleston, CL Rae, R Regenthal, BJ Sahakian, RA Barker, TW Robbins, JB Rowe. Selective serotonin reuptake inhibition modulates response inhibition in Parkinson's disease. *Brain* 2014; 137(4): 1145–1155.

Zivin K, PN Pfeiffer, AS Bohnert, D Ganoczy, FC Blow, BK Nallamothu, HC Kales. Evaluation of the FDA warning against prescribing citalopram at doses exceeding 40 mg. *Am J Psychiatry* 2013; 170(6): 642–650.

CLONAZEPAM

C

Therapeutics

Chemical Name and Structure

Clonazepam (5-(2-chlorophenyl)-7-nitro-1,3-dihydro-1,4-benzodiazepin-2-one). It is an off-white to light yellow crystalline powder with a molecular weight of 315.71 and an empirical formula of $C_{15}H_{10}ClN_3O_3$.

Brand Names

- **Acepran** *(Chile)*; **Aklonil** *(Cyprus, Greece, Tunisia)*; **Alcona** *(India)*; **Anxrea** *(India)*.
- **Bejowa** *(Chile)*.
- **Clon** *(India)*; **Clonac** *(Venezuela)*; **Clonafit** *(India)*; **Clonagin** *(Argentina, Ecuador)*; **Clonam** *(South Africa)*; **Clonapam** *(Chile)*; **Clonapax** *(India)*; **Clonapik** *(India)*; **Clonotril** *(Thailand, Venezuela)*; **Clonatrac** *(India)*; **Clonax** *(Argentina)*; **Clonazen 2** *(Argentina)*; **Clonazepam** *(Greece)*; **Cloner** *(Argentina)*; **Clonetril** *(Brazil)*; **Clonex** *(Chile)*; **Clonopam** *(India)*; **Clonotril** *(Brazil, Cyprus, Greece, Hong Kong, Philippines, Singapore)*; **Clopam** *(Brazil, India)*; **Closed** *(India)*; **Clozanil** *(Chile)*; **Clozep** *(India)*; **Clozer** *(Mexico)*; **Convaclon** *(India)*; **Convolsil** *(Thailand)*; **Copam** *(India)*; **Coquan** *(Ecuador)*; **Crismol** *(Chile)*; **Czap** *(India)*.
- **Diocam** *(Argentina)*.
- **Edictum** *(Argentina)*; **Epcon** *(India)*; **Epitril** *(India)*; **Epizam** *(India)*.
- **Gabaclotec** *(Mexico)*.
- **Histrol** *(Ecuador)*.
- **Iktorivil** *(Sweden)*; **Incloz** *(India)*; **Induzepam** *(Argentina)*.
- **Jing Kang** *(China)*.
- **Kenoket** *(Mexico)*; **Klonopin** *(USA)*; **Kriadex** *(Ecuador, Mexico)*.
- **Landsen** *(Japan)*; **Leptic** *(Argentina)*; **Logen-MD** *(India)*; **Lonazep** *(India)*; **Lonin** *(India)*; **Lonna** *(India)*.
- **Melzap** *(India)*.
- **Neuryl** *(Argentina, Chile)*; **Norep** *(India)*.
- **Onz** *(India)*; **Ozepam** *(India)*.
- **Panazeclox** *(Mexico)*; **Panik** *(India)*; **Paxam** *(Australia, New Zealand)*; **Povanil** *(Thailand)*; **Prenarpil** *(Thailand)*.
- **Quazemic** *(Argentina)*.
- **Ravotril** *(Chile)*; **Ribocler** *(Argentina)*; **Riklona** *(Indonesia)*; **Riuclonaz** *(Argentina)*; **Rivatril** *(Finland)*; **Rivotril** *(Argentina, Australia, Austria, Belgium, Brazil, Canada, Czech Republic, Denmark, Ecuador, Estonia, France, Germany, Greece, Hong Kong, Hungary, Indonesia, Ireland, Italy, Japan, Lithuania, Malaysia, Mexico, Netherlands, New Zealand, Norway, Philippines, Portugal, Russian Federation, Singapore, South Africa, Spain, Switzerland, Turkey, Venezuela)*; **Ropsil** *(Chile)*.
- **Sedatril** *(Ecuador)*; **Solfidin** *(Argentina)*.
- **Uni Clonazepax** *(Brazil)*.

C

- **Valpax** (*Chile*, *Venezuela*).
- **Zilepam** (*Brazil*); **Zymanta** (*Mexico*).

Generics Available
- Yes.

Licensed Indications for Parkinson's Disease
- None.

Licensed Indications for Other Conditions
- Seizure disorders (broad spectrum) (FDA, EMA, EMC).
  - Status epilepticus (EMC), absence seizures (FDA, EMC), akinetic seizures (FDA), tonic seizures (EMC), tonic–clonic seizures (EMC), Lennox–Gastaut syndrome (FDA), myoclonic seizures (FDA, EMC), partial (focal) seizures with or without secondary generalization (EMC).
- Myoclonus and associated abnormal movements (EMC).
- Panic disorders (FDA).
  - Acute and short-term management (risk of rebound anxiety due to long $T_{1/2}$).

Non-Licensed Use for Parkinson's Disease
- REM sleep behavioural disorder and sleep onset insomnia in in Parkinson's disease.

Non-Licensed Use for Other Conditions
- Mania.
- RLS.
- Tardive dyskinesia.
- Idiopathic RBD.
- Spasticity (short-term relief).
- Tic disorders.

Ineffective
- Not a first-line therapy for any type of seizures.
- Sleep fragmentation.

Mechanism of Action
- Clonazepam is a positive allosteric modulator on GABA-A receptors, thus, enhancing the effects of the inhibitory neurotransmitter GABA and reduces the monosynaptic and polysynaptic reflexes. It also has some serotonergic activity and increases serotonin synthesis.
- It acts on the benzodiazepine binding sites of GABA-A receptors to provoke the inhibitory effect of GABA.
- Clonazepam has anticonvulsant and anxiolytic effects.
- It may have an effect on RBD through modulating either dreaming or complex motor behaviours at a supratentorial level and by prolonging non-REM sleep and reducing REM sleep duration.

C

Efficacy Profile
- Clonazepam may be an effective option for Parkinson's disease-related RBD and has been associated with RBD-linked nocturnal injury prevention, although the evidence is limited.
  - The average effective dose is 0.5 mg.
- A beneficial effect of clonazepam on periodic limb movements of sleep has also been reported.

Pharmacokinetics
Absorption and Distribution
- Oral bioavailability: about 90%.
- Food co-ingestion: absorption is unaffected by food consumption.
- Tmax: within 1–4 h after an oral dose.
- Time to steady state: 2–10 days.
- Pharmacokinetics: linear at therapeutic doses.
- Protein binding: about 85%.
- Volume of distribution: 1.5–3 l/kg.

Metabolism
- Clonazepam is metabolized in the liver by cytochrome P-450. CYP3A plays a major role in clonazepam reduction and oxidation.
- It mainly undergoes reduction of the 7-nitro group to the 7-amino derivative, which can be acetylated, hydroxylated, and glucuronidated, generating inactive metabolites, with the exception of 7-amino-clonazepam which retains some pharmacological activity.

Elimination
- The mean elimination half-life is 30 h (range of 17–56 h in healthy adults).
- Renal excretion: clonazepam is mostly excreted in the urine; less than 2% of an administered dose is excreted unchanged.

Drug Interaction Profile
Pharmacokinetic Drug Interactions
- Effects by clonazepam:
  - Clonazepam can increase *lithium* plasma levels.
- Effects on clonazepam:
  - Cytochrome P450 inducers (e.g. *phenytoin, carbamazepine, phenobarbital, rifampicin* antifungal agents) induce clonazepam metabolism, leading to 30% decrease in plasma clonazepam levels.
  - *Amiodarone, metoprolol, desmopressin, daptomycin, fluconazole, pantoprazole, folic acid* can increase clonazepam plasma levels.

CLONAZEPAM

Pharmacodynamic Drug Interactions
- Co-medication with CNS depressants (e.g. antidepressants, opiates, barbiturates, antipsychotics, anti-epileptics, MAO inhibitors, antihistamines, triptans, dopaminergic agents, *baclofen, sodium oxybate*) and alcohol might have additive sedative effects.

Adverse Effects
How Drug Causes Adverse Effects
- Same mechanism as for therapeutic effect.
- Long-term adaptation of benzodiazepine receptors may lead to dependence or tolerance and require withdrawal.

Common Adverse Effects
- Very common (≥1/10):
  - Somnolence.
- Common (≥1/100 to <1/10):
  - Nervous/psychiatric: abnormal coordination, slowed reaction, muscle weakness, ataxia, depression, dizziness, memory/concentration impairment, confusion, restlessness, nystagmus, hyperexcitability, nervousness.
  - Respiratory: upper respiratory infection, rhinitis, coughing.
  - GI: hypersalivation.
  - Other: fatigue.

Life-Threatening or Dangerous Adverse Effects
- Rare (≥1/10,000 to <1/1,000):
  - Respiratory depression.
  - Low platelet count.
- Unknown frequency:
  - Cardiac failure, including cardiac arrest.
  - Blood dyscrasias.

Rare and Not Life-Threatening Adverse Effects
- Headache.
- Nausea, gastrointestinal symptoms.
- Impotence, decreased libido.
- Urinary incontinence.
- Urticaria, pruritus, rash, transient hair loss, pigmentation changes, angioedema.
- Generalized fits.

Weight Change
- Weight loss or gain have been reported, although neither are common.

C

What to Do About Adverse Effects
- Before introducing clonazepam, discuss common or life-threatening adverse effects with patients and/or caregivers, including symptoms that should be reported to the physician.
- Patients and their caregivers should be informed of the possibility of clonazepam causing suicidal ideation/behaviour. If such signs/symptoms emerge, patients should urgently seek medical advice and be treated accordingly.
- Most adverse events are expected to subside spontaneously. If troublesome adverse events persist, consider tapering or withdrawing clonazepam.

Dosing and Use
Usual Dosage Range
- 0.25–1 mg in Parkinson's disease-related RBD.
  - Maximum dose of 2–4 mg in idiopathic RBD.

Available Formulations
- Oral solution: 0.5 mg/5 ml, 2 mg/5 ml.
- Tablets dispersible: 0.125 mg, 0.25 mg, 0.5 mg, 1 mg, 2 mg.
- Tablets: 0.5 mg, 1 mg, 2 mg.
- Liquid formulation: 1 mg/ml for dilution before IV injection.

How to Dose
- 0.25–0.5 mg OD 30 min prior to bedtime (RBD).
- May increase dose by 0.25–0.5 mg every 3–4 days if necessary, usually up to 0.5–1 mg/day; not to exceed 2 mg.

Dosing Tips
- Take with or without food.
- Patients on clonazepam should consider limiting caffeine intake.
- Suitable for administration via non-PVC nasogastric or PEG, as clonazepam is incompatible with polystyrene or PVC.
- In case of persistent RBD symptoms, co-medication with melatonin could be considered.

How to Withdraw Drug
- Even short-term use of clonazepam should be gradually discontinued.
- Withdrawal symptoms, especially after a lengthy period of clonazepam use or with high doses (usually >2 mg/day), might include tremor, sweating, agitation, sleep disturbances, anxiety, headaches, muscle pain, restlessness, confusion, irritability, and epileptic seizures (usually in those with an underlying epilepsy condition).
- Decrease the dose by 0.125–0.25 mg every 3 days until completely withdrawn.

DOSING AND USE

C

CLONAZEPAM

Overdose
- Overdose is rarely life-threatening if clonazepam is taken alone.
- Symptoms vary greatly depending on age, weight, and individual response and might include drowsiness, severe somnolence, muscle hypotonia, ataxia, dysarthria, nystagmus. In severe cases (e.g. elderly, pre-existent respiratory disorders), it might lead to coma, areflexia, apnoea, hypotension, and cardiorespiratory depression.
  - If patients are asymptomatic at 4 h, they are unlikely to become symptomatic later.
- Supportive measures and maintenance of a clear airway with adequate ventilation are recommended.
- Activated charcoal might be used to prevent further absorption, but in this case airway protection is necessary for drowsy patients. In case of mixed ingestion, gastric lavage may be more appropriate, but is not a routine measure.
- In severe cases of CNS depression, consider using the benzodiazepine antagonist flumazenil under closely monitored conditions. However, its use is strictly contraindicated in mixed overdose situations or as a 'diagnostic test', as it might precipitate seizures in patients with a medical history of epilepsy, especially if combined with drugs that lower the seizure threshold (e.g. tricyclic antidepressants).
- Haemodialysis might be useful.

Tests and Therapeutic Drug Monitoring
- During clonazepam therapy:
  - Periodic liver function tests and blood counts are recommended.

Other Warnings / Precautions
- Caution is advised when clonazepam is used in patients with excessive drooling (sialorrhoea), as it might increase salivation.
- Patients with a history of depression and/or suicide attempts should be closely monitored, as clonazepam predisposes to suicidal ideation and behaviour.
- Caution is advised in patients with cognitive impairment, as clonazepam might aggravate memory and cause confusion.
- Clonazepam should be used with extreme caution in patients with known respiratory diseases (e.g. COPD), especially in case of co-existent brain damage or co-medication with other agents that also depress respiration. A careful dose adjustment according to individual requirements is advised.
- Caution is advised in patients with sleep apnoea and the use of nasal CPAP should be strongly encouraged before starting therapy with clonazepam.
- Particular caution is advised in patients with spinal or cerebellar ataxia and those with porphyria.
- In case of loss or bereavement, psychological adjustment may be inhibited by benzodiazepines.

C

- Clonazepam may cause CNS depression and affect the ability to drive or operate machinery. Patients and caregivers should be properly informed before therapy initiation.

Do Not Use (Contraindications)
- Known sensitivity to benzodiazepines or hypersensitivity to the active substance or to any of its excipients, including lactose.
  - Patients with rare hereditary problems of galactose intolerance, total lactase deficiency, or glucose–galactose malabsorption.
- Acute pulmonary insufficiency or severe respiratory insufficiency or respiratory depression.
- Untreated sleep apnoea syndrome.
- Marked neuromuscular respiratory weakness, including myasthenia gravis.
- Patients in coma.
- Patients with a known addiction problem (pharmaceuticals, drugs, alcohol).
- Acute narrow-angle glaucoma.
- In patients who reported anterograde amnesia after benzodiazepine use.
- Co-administration with CNS depressants (e.g. anti-epileptics, opiates) or alcohol should be avoided, as it might lead to severe sedation and clinically significant respiratory and/or cardiovascular depression.
  - Black box warning for the concomitant use of benzodiazepines and opiates.

Special Populations
Renal Impairment
- No dose adjustment is required, although lower doses might be preferred.

Hepatic Impairment
- Lower doses might be preferred.
- Clonazepam is contraindicated in severe hepatic insufficiency.

Elderly
- Caution is advised and lower doses are preferred due to greater frequency of hepatic/renal/cardiac function impairment and due to polypharmacy.
- Paradoxical reactions, such as agitation, irritability, aggression, anxiety, nightmares, hallucinations, psychoses, are more likely to occur in the elderly.
- Clonazepam use in the elderly might predispose to falls.

C

CLONAZEPAM

Pregnancy
- Clonazepam is believed to cross the placental barrier and has harmful effects on pregnancy and the fetus/newborn.
- Clonazepam should not be used during pregnancy.

Breastfeeding
- Clonazepam has been found in maternal milk in small quantities.
- Women under clonazepam should not breastfeed.

Costs
NHS indicative price accessed 30 June 2022:
- 100 × 0.5 mg tablets: £34.34–£36.18
- 100 × 2 mg tablets: £37.24–£39.24
- 150 ml of 0.5 mg/5 ml oral solution: £69.50–£77.09
- 150 ml of 2 mg/5 ml oral solution: £90.30–£108.38
- 150 ml of 50 mg/5 ml oral solution: £140+VAT

The Overall Place of Clonazepam in the Treatment of Parkinson's Disease

Clonazepam is a long-acting benzodiazepine that has been used as a broad-spectrum anti-epileptic drug. In Parkinson's disease, low doses of clonazepam have been considered as a first-line therapeutic option in Parkinson's disease-related RBD (off-label indication and after sleep apnoea is excluded), although the evidence supporting this effect is rather limited and heterogeneous while large RCTs are lacking. Discontinuation of clonazepam may result in recurrence of RBD symptoms. Tapering or cessation of clonazepam might be followed by insomnia and reduced sleep quality. Side effects, including somnolence, cognitive impairment, and respiratory depression, along with tolerance and withdrawal issues, might arise, especially in higher doses, long-term treatment, and in individuals with respiratory disorders. Elderly and cognitively impaired patients are more prone to side effects.

Potential Advantages
- Rapid onset of action.
- Clonazepam has been associated with a decrease of sleep-related injury.

Potential Disadvantages
- Prolonged use of clonazepam may lead to dependence issues and withdrawal symptoms on cessation of use.
- Benzodiazepine use at therapeutic doses, including clonazepam, has been associated with anterograde amnesia and cognitive impairment.
- Clonazepam use has been associated with depression of the respiratory system, especially in the elderly and individuals with compromised respiratory function.

C

Clinical Box

A 45-year-old woman with a recent diagnosis of Parkinson's disease presented with symptoms of troublesome RBD, including intense motor behaviour which was irritating to her partner, vocalizations, and frequent falling out of bed, causing injury. Her current medication included a transdermal rotigotine patch of 8 mg/24 h OD. Her medical history included osteoporosis and well-controlled hypertension. She mentioned no respiratory problems. She was initially treated with a high dose of melatonin; however, symptoms persisted. A low dose of clonazepam 0.5 mg OD at bedtime was added with improvement in her symptoms and without any significant complications, although the patient was instructed to remain vigilant for potential side effects.

Suggested Reading

Jung Y, EK St Louis. Treatment of REM sleep behavior disorder. *Curr Treat Options Neurol* 2016; 18(11): 50.

St Louis EK, AR Boeve, BF Boeve. REM sleep behavior disorder in Parkinson's disease and other synucleinopathies. *Mov Disord* 2017; 32(5): 645–658.

References

AHFS Drug information, 2012. Bethesda: American Society of Health-System Pharmacists. Accessed on 30 June 2022 via www.medicinescomplete.com.

Brooks PL, JH Peever. Impaired GABA and glycine transmission triggers cardinal features of rapid eye movement sleep behavior disorder in mice. *J Neurosci* 2011; 31(19): 7111–7121.

Clonazepam. In:Brayfield A (Ed.), *Martindale: The Complete Drug Reference*. London: The Royal Pharmaceutical Society of Great Britain. Accessed on 30 June 2022 via www.medicinescomplete.com.

Joint Formulary Committee. British National Formulary (online). London: BMJ Group and Pharmaceutical Press. Accessed on 30 June 2022 via www.medicinescomplete.com.

Matar E, SJ McCarter, EK St Louis, SJG Lewis. Current concepts and controversies in the management of REM Sleep behavior disorder. *Neurotherapeutics* 2021; 18(1): 107–123.

REFERENCES

C

CLOZAPINE

Therapeutics

Chemical Name and Structure

Clozapine (3-chloro-6-(4-methylpiperazin-1-yl)-11H-benzo[*b*][1,4] benzodiazepine) has a molecular weight of 326.8 and an empirical formula of $C_{18}H_{19}ClN_4$.

Brand Names

- **Anzapine** (*Malaysia*); **Ayupil** (*Poland*); **Ayupine** (*Netherlands*); **Azaleprol** (*Russian Federation*); **Azaleptin** (*Russian Federation*); **Azaleptol** (*Ukraine*); **Azapin** (*Ukraine*).
- **Chrozap** (*India*); **Clomach** (*India*); **Cloment** (*South Africa*); **Clonex** (*Turkey*); **Clopaz** (*India*); **Clopaze** (*Thailand*); **Clopin** (*Switzerland*); **Clopine** (*Australia, Hong Kong, Malaysia, New Zealand*); **Clopixene** (*Philippines*); **Clopizam** (*Poland*); **Clopsine** (*Ecuador, Mexico*); **Cloril** (*Thailand*); **Clorilex** (*Indonesia*); **Closastene** (*Russian Federation*); **Clozamed** (*Thailand*); **Clozarem** (*Cyprus, Hong Kong, Malaysia*); **Clozaril** (*Australia, Canada, Hong Kong, Indonesia, Ireland, Japan, Malaysia, New Zealand, Singapore, South Africa, Spain, UK, USA*); **Clozasten** (*Russian Federation*); **Cozacin** (*India*).
- **Denzapine** (*Ireland, UK*); **Dicomex** (*Chile*).
- **FazaClo** (*USA*); **Froidir** (*Denmark, Finland, Sweden*).
- **Klozapol** (*Poland*).
- **Lanolept** (*Austria*); **Lapenex** (*Argentina*); **Leponex** (*Austria, Belgium, Brazil, Chile, Cyprus, Czech Republic, Denmark, Ecuador, Estonia, Finland, France, Germany, Greece, Hungary, Israel, Italy, Mexico, Netherlands, Norway, Philippines, Portugal, Russian Federation, Spain, Sweden, Switzerland, Tunisia, Turkey, Ukraine, Venezuela*); **Leydex** (*Ireland*); **Lodux** (*Chile*); **Lozap** (*Indonesia*); **Lozapin** (*India*); **Lozapine** (*Israel*); **Lozaril** (*India*); **Luften** (*Indonesia*).
- **Merbaril** (*Netherlands*).
- **Nemea** (*Spain*); **Nirva** (*Philippines*).
- **Okotico** (*Brazil*); **Ozapim** (*Portugal*).
- **Pinazan** (*Brazil*).
- **Refraxol** (*Ecuador*).
- **Sizopin** (*India, Philippines*); **Sizoril** (*Indonesia*); **Syclop** (*Philippines*); **Symcloza** (*Poland*).
- **Versacloz** (*Australia, New Zealand, USA*).
- **Xynaz** (*Brazil*).
- **Zapine** (*Malaysia*); **Zaponex** (*Netherlands, UK*); **Ziproc** (*Philippines*).

Generics Available

- Yes.

Licensed Indications for Parkinson's Disease

- Refractory psychosis in Parkinson's disease when other treatment strategies have failed (EMA, EMC).

Licensed Indications for Other Conditions
- Treatment-resistant schizophrenia (persistent or moderate delusions or hallucinations after failing two trials of antipsychotics) (FDA, EMA, EMC).
- Patients with schizophrenia or schizoaffective disorder and recurrent suicidal behaviour (FDA).

Non-Licensed Use for Parkinson's Disease
- Parkinson's disease-related resistant or refractory psychosis.
- Refractory tremor in Parkinson's disease.

Non-Licensed Use for Other Conditions
- Bipolar disorder.
- Schizophrenia with co-morbid depression.
- Major depressive disorder (preliminary evidence).
- Behavioural issues in patients with dementia, including Alzheimer's disease.

Ineffective
- Not reported.

Mechanism of Action
- Clozapine is an atypical antipsychotic, which acts as an antagonist at dopaminergic receptors, with high affinity for D4 receptors and weak blocking activity at D1, D2, D3, and D5 receptors, thus, causing fewer extrapyramidal symptoms than other antipsychotics.
- It is a partial 5-HT1A serotonergic agonist. It also acts at 5-HT1C, 5-HT2A/2C, and 5-HT3 serotonergic sites.
- It acts as an antagonist at M1, M2, M3, and M5 muscarinic, histamine, and α1 adrenergic receptors.
- Its metabolite, norclozapine, acts at M1 and M4 muscarinic receptors.

Efficacy Profile
- According to the MDS EBM Committee, clozapine is considered:
  - 'efficacious' and 'clinically useful' in the treatment of Parkinson's disease-related psychosis.
  - 'efficacious' and 'clinically useful' in the treatment of dyskinesias in Parkinson's disease.
- Two double-blind RCTs have found that a low clozapine dose (<50 mg/day) significantly improves Parkinson's disease-related psychosis without worsening of parkinsonian features; one of the studies suggested that a significant percentage of patients would relapse after therapy discontinuation.
- Results from three RCTs showed that clozapine and quetiapine were equally effective in Parkinson's disease-related psychosis. One study found a significant improvement of dyskinesias in both groups, one found a significant overall decrease in the UPDRS measurements of the clozapine group, and the other concluded that although there was a trend

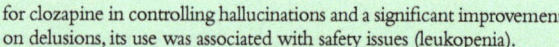

for clozapine in controlling hallucinations and a significant improvement on delusions, its use was associated with safety issues (leukopenia).
- The long-term benefit of clozapine on Parkinson's disease-related psychosis was confirmed for a minimum of 4 months in an open-label, extension study, although a high risk for morbidity and mortality was also found.
- A double-blind multi-centre RCT found that clozapine was beneficial for the management of LID in severe Parkinson's disease. This effect was confirmed in a small open-label study.
- There is evidence from two double-blind RCTs, an open-label extension study, a double-blind cross-over study, two retrospective studies, and a case series that clozapine can improve tremor in Parkinson's disease.

Pharmacokinetics
Absorption and Distribution
- Oral bioavailability: 50–60%.
- Food co-ingestion: no effect on the rate/extent of absorption.
- Tmax: 1–6 h.
- Pharmacokinetics: linear in doses ranging from 37.5 mg to 150 mg given twice daily.
- Protein binding: 97%.
- Volume of distribution: 6 l/kg.

Metabolism
- Clozapine is metabolized by hepatic P450 enzymes CYP1A2, CYP2D6, and CYP3A4. It undergoes N-demethylation, N-oxidation, 3′-carbon oxidation, epoxidation of chlorine-containing aromatic ring, substitution of chlorine by hydroxyl or thiomethyl groups, and sulphur oxidation.
- Its primary active metabolite is norclozapine.

Elimination
- Biphasic elimination with a mean terminal half-life of 12 h (9.1–17.4 h) in adults.
- About 50% of an administered dose is excreted as metabolites in urine and 30% in faeces. Only traces of unchanged drug are detected in the urine and faeces.

Drug Interaction Profile
Pharmacokinetic Drug Interactions
- Effects by clozapine:
  - It can increase levels of CYP2D6 substrates.
  - It can increase levels of highly protein bound drugs (e.g. *warfarin, digoxin*).

CLOZAPINE

C

- Effects on clozapine:
  - CYP450 inhibitors, especially CYP1A2 (e.g. *caffeine, fluvoxamine, perazine*) and less likely CYP2D6 (e.g. *fluoxetine, paroxetine, sertraline, hormonal contraceptives*) or CYP1A2 (e.g. *cimetidine, erythromycin,* protease inhibitors, azole antimycotics), can increase clozapine plasma levels and effects.
  - CYP450 inducers (e.g. *carbamazepine, phenytoin, rifampicin, omeprazole*) can decrease clozapine plasma levels and effects.
  - Sudden cessation of smoking might increase clozapine levels.

Pharmacodynamic Drug Interactions
- Co-medication with benzodiazepines or other psychotropic agents might lead to orthostatic hypotension with or without syncope, increasing the risk for circulatory collapse.
- Co-medication with CNS depressants (e.g. narcotics, antihistamines, benzodiazepines), drugs predisposing to bone marrow depression (e.g. *carbamazepine, chloramphenicol,* sulphonamides, *penicillamine,* long-acting depot injections of antipsychotics), drugs increasing QTc interval (e.g. Class IA and III anti-arrhythmics, antipsychotics, tricyclic antidepressants, certain antimicrobial agents, certain antihistamines) or causing electrolyte imbalance, and antihypertensives might have additive effects.
- Clozapine may compete with α-adrenergic agents (e.g. *epinephrine*) and reverse their pressor effects.
- Co-medication with *citalopram* may increase the risk of clozapine-induced adverse events.
- Co-medication with *lithium* may predispose to NMS.
- Co-medication with *valproic acid* may predispose to seizures.

Adverse Effects
How Drug Causes Adverse Effects
- Neutropenia/agranulocytosis are not considered dose-dependent, but an idiosyncratic (type B) immune-mediated reaction.
- Dopaminergic blocking activity, although weak, accounts for any potential extrapyramidal symptoms.
- Clozapine induces potent anticholinergic effects, which may result in CNS and peripheral anticholinergic adverse effects.
- Antimuscarinic properties of clozapine may cause confusion in cognitively impaired patients.
- Histamine receptor blockade accounts for sleep disturbance.

Common Adverse Effects
- Very common (≥1/10):
  - Drowsiness/sedation, dizziness, tachycardia, constipation, hypersalivation.

ADVERSE EFFECTS

C

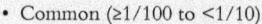

- Common (≥1/100 to <1/10):
  - Nervous/psychiatric: dysarthria, extrapyramidal symptoms, myoclonic jerks, akathisia, tremor, rigidity, headache, fatigue, seizures.
  - Cardiovascular: ECG changes, postural hypotension, hypertension, syncope.
  - Gastrointestinal: elevated liver enzymes.
  - Renal/urinary: urinary retention/incontinence.
  - Other: leukopenia/neutropenia, eosinophilia, leucocytosis, weight gain, blurred vision, benign hyperthermia, sweating impairment, temperature regulation disturbance, fever.
- Uncommon (≥1/1,000 to <1/100):
  - Falls (due to hypotension, somnolence, seizures, motor/sensory instability) leading to fractures or other injuries.

Life-Threatening or Dangerous Adverse Effects
- Common (≥1/100 to <1/10):
  - Seizures (dose-related risk) (black box warning).
  - Orthostatic hypotension, bradycardia, syncope, cardiac arrest (black box warning).
    - May occur even with the first dose and with dosage as low as 12.5 mg/day.
    - The risk is highest during the initial titration period, especially with rapid dose escalation.
- Uncommon (≥1/1,000 to <1/100):
  - Agranulocytosis/severe neutropenia (ANC <500/mm³), which can lead to serious infection and death (black box warning).
  - NMS.
- Rare (≥1/10,000 to <1/1,000):
  - Myocarditis, cardiomyopathy, mitral valve incompetence, especially during the first 2 months of therapy (black box warning).
  - Pericarditis/pericardial effusion.
  - Pulmonary embolism and DVT.
  - Hyperglycaemia or diabetes, which have very rarely been associated with oesophageal dysmotility, ketoacidosis, hyperosmolar coma, or death.
  - Confusion, delirium.
- Very rare (<1/10,000):
  - Hepatotoxicity, including hepatic failure, fulminant hepatic necrosis and hepatitis.
  - Intestinal obstruction, faecal impaction, paralytic ileus.
  - Thrombocytopenia, thrombocythemia.
  - Respiratory depression/arrest.

Rare and Not Life-Threatening Adverse Effects
- Anaemia.
- Hypercholesterolaemia, hypertriglyceridaemia.
- Agitation, restlessness.

CLOZAPINE

C

- Dysphagia.
- Skin reactions.
- Increased CPK.

Weight Change
- Similarly to other atypical antipsychotics, weight gain has been reported.

What to Do About Adverse Effects
- Before introducing clozapine, discuss common or life-threatening adverse effects with patients and/or caregivers, including symptoms that should be reported to the physician.
- Transient fever, especially during the first 3 weeks of clozapine therapy, has been considered benign and self-limiting. However, a potential infection, clozapine-induced neutropenia, or NMS should be excluded.
- Patients and caregivers should be advised to immediately report any symptoms consistent with severe neutropenia or infection, especially flu-like symptoms, and undergo a blood cell count. In the event of neutropenia or agranulocytosis:
  - WBC count 3,000–3,500/mm^3 or ANC 1,500–2,000/mm^3: clozapine can be continued with blood tests twice per week until values stabilize or increase.
  - WBC count <3,000/mm^3 or ANC<1,500/mm^3: clozapine should be discontinued immediately with daily blood tests until the abnormality is resolved. Concurrently, psychiatric monitoring is advised, while evaluations by a haematologist should take place at least twice per week.
  - Confirmation of the haematological values is recommended by performing two blood cell counts on two consecutive days, although clozapine should be discontinued after the first test.
- In case of eosinophilia with eosinophil count >3,000/mm^3, clozapine discontinuation is recommended; therapy can be re-initiated if values fall below 1,000/mm^3.
- If thrombocytopenia with a platelet count <50,000/mm occurs, clozapine discontinuation is recommended.
- If constipation occurs, ensure adequate hydration and supportive measures (e.g. laxatives); consultation with a gastroenterologist is suggested in more severe cases.
- If hyperglycaemia occurs, consider withdrawing clozapine; continuation of antidiabetic drugs might be needed despite clozapine cessation.
- Patients and caregivers should be advised to immediately report any symptoms or signs suggestive of hepatotoxicity (e.g. fatigue, malaise, anorexia, nausea, jaundice, bilirubinaemia, coagulopathy); if hepatitis or clinically relevant increased serum markers of hepatic function (more than 3 times the ULN) are present, consider withdrawing

C

clozapine; it can be re-initiated with close monitoring, if normal liver function is restored.
- If myocarditis or cardiomyopathy are suspected (e.g. persistent tachycardia at rest, palpitations, arrhythmias, chest pain, unexplained fatigue, dyspnoea, tachypnoea), clozapine therapy should be discontinued, and the patient should be referred for cardiac evaluation, including a 2D-echo Doppler examination to identify mitral valve incompetence.
  - It is common for non-specific flu-like symptoms (e.g. malaise, myalgia, pleuritic chest pain, low-grade fever) to precede more overt signs of cardiac failure.
- If seizures occur, the dose of clozapine should be reduced or the drug discontinued and, if necessary, anticonvulsant treatment should be introduced (not carbamazepine).
- If NMS occurs, clozapine should be immediately withdrawn, and appropriate medical treatment should be applied.
- If tardive dyskinesia appears, consider discontinuing clozapine therapy, which might lead to full or partial resolution of symptoms.
  - Longer therapy duration and higher doses of clozapine increase the risk for irreversible tardive dyskinesia.

Clozapine should be used by licensed physicians and with MDT backup and regular blood monitoring as per guidelines and including blood level monitoring in case of worsening falls, abnormal weight gain, excessive somnolence, worsening constipation. In addition, clozapine use must be supported by multidisciplinary monitoring of cardiac (including postural hypotension), weight, and bowel status.

Dosing and Use

Usual Dosage Range
- 6.25–50 mg; maximum dose of 150 mg.
  - The mean effective dose is usually 25–37.5 mg/day (significantly lower than dosage in schizophrenia).
  - The dose of 50 mg/day should only be exceeded in exceptional cases.

Available Formulations
In the USA and UK clozapine is only available through a restricted access programme due to the risk of neutropenia; patients must be registered, the prescriber must enrol and complete training, and pharmacies dispensing clozapine must be certified.
- Tablets: 25 mg, 50 mg, 100 mg, 200 mg.
- Oral tablet disintegrating: 12.5 mg, 25 mg, 100 mg, 150 mg, 200 mg.
- Oral suspension: 50 mg/ml.

How to Dose
- Initial dose of 12.5 mg/day, taken at bedtime; increase by 12.5 mg/day increments without exceeding an increase of 25 mg/day per week up to a maximum of 50 mg/day.

C

- A lower initial dose of 6.25 mg/day might be considered in cogni-tively impaired Parkinson's disease patients.
- In case a dose higher than 50 mg/day is needed, increase by 12.5 mg/day per week up to 100 mg/day.
- Cautious titration is recommended. The lowest effective dose and the shortest therapy duration necessary are suggested to limit the chances of potential side effects. Dosage must be adjusted individually.

Dosing Tips
- May be consumed with or without food.
- Modifications in clozapine dosage may be necessary in case of changes in coffee-drinking habits.
- The total daily dose should preferably be given as a single dose in the evening; alternatively in two divided doses.
- When complete remission of psychotic symptoms is achieved for at least 2 weeks, an increase in anti-parkinsonian medication can be considered, if applicable. If psychotic symptoms reappear, consider increasing clozapine dose up to a maximum of 100 mg/day, as needed.
- If clozapine therapy is interrupted for more than 48 h, an initiation scheme should be reapplied to minimize risk of hypotension, brady-cardia, and syncope.
- Lower doses may decrease the risk of sedation and metabolic syn-drome, although neutropenia remains an issue.
- It is generally advised that clozapine should not be used with other antipsychotics.
- Prescriptions should not be issued for periods longer than the interval between two blood cells counts.
- Avoid patients' immobilization due to risk of clozapine-induced thromboembolism.
- After clozapine discontinuation, consider not removing patients from the clozapine registry for a few months, even if symptoms have fully subsided (USA).

How to Withdraw Drug
- Rebound withdrawal effects may be reported following abrupt ces-sation of clozapine.
- If termination of therapy is not related to neutropenia, clozapine dose should be reduced gradually over a period of 1–2 weeks by steps of 12.5 mg/day.
- Blood monitoring should continue for at least 4 weeks after clozapine discontinuation, particularly in case of fever occurrence.
- If abrupt clozapine withdrawal is required for reasons not related to neutropenia, continue blood monitoring until ANC is ≥1,500/mm^3 (or ≥1,000/mm^3 in case of patients with benign ethnic neutropenia).
- All patients should be closely monitored during the withdrawal period for psychotic symptom recurrence and symptoms related to cholin-ergic rebound (e.g. sweating, headache, nausea, vomiting, diarrhoea).

DOSING AND USE

C

Overdose
- Mortality rate in clozapine overdose (usually doses above 2,000 mg) is about 12%, mostly due to cardiac failure or aspiration pneumonia.
- Overdose may present with drowsiness, lethargy, confusion, hallucinations, agitation, delirium, extrapyramidal symptoms, convulsions, hyperreflexia/areflexia; hypersalivation, mydriasis, blurred vision, thermolability; hypotension, tachycardia, arrhythmias, collapse; dyspnoea, respiratory depression, or failure.
- There is no specific antidote for clozapine overdose; supportive measures are recommended, continuous cardiac monitoring, respiration surveillance and monitoring of electrolytes and acid–base balance for at least 5 days due to delayed reactions.
  - Epinephrine use should be avoided ('reverse epinephrine' effect).
- Gastric lavage and/or activated charcoal administration within the first 6 h of ingestion is suggested. Peritoneal dialysis and haemodialysis are not recommended.

Tests and Therapeutic Drug Monitoring
- Before initiation of clozapine therapy (within 10 days):
  - Baseline ANC should be ≥1,500/mm³ for the general population and ≥1,000/mm³ for patients with documented benign ethnic neutropenia (FDA).
  - Baseline WBC count should be ≥3,500/mm³ and ANC ≥2,000/mm³ (EMA, EMC).
  - A baseline measurement of fasting glucose and lipids is recommended.
  - A baseline ECG should be performed.
  - Bowel function should be evaluated.
  - A fall risk assessment should be performed.
- During clozapine therapy:
  - WBC count with a differential count must be monitored at least weekly for the first 18 weeks of therapy and at least at 2-week intervals between 18 and 52 weeks of therapy. After 1 year of therapy with stable neutrophil counts, patients should be monitored at least every 4 weeks for as long as therapy continues (EMC).
    - If clozapine therapy is interrupted for more than 3 days and less than 4 weeks after the initial 18-week period, patients should continue with weekly blood tests for an additional 6 weeks.
    - If clozapine therapy is interrupted for more than 4 weeks, re-initiation of the standard monitoring scheme is necessary.
    - Without monitoring, mortality rate due to agranulocytosis is 0.3%.
  - Standing and supine blood pressure should be monitored during the first weeks of therapy in Parkinson's disease patients.
  - Periodic monitoring of blood lipids, fasting glucose, and weight is suggested.
  - Measuring natriuretic peptides levels may help detect early asymptomatic myocarditis.

CLOZAPINE

C

- Regular monitoring of blood glucose is suggested for patients at risk of hyperglycaemia and diabetes.
- Blood clozapine level monitoring is advised in specific situations (e.g. when a patient quits smoking or switches to e-cigarettes, when medications that interact with clozapine are used, in cases of serious infections).
- Regular liver function tests are advised in patients with stable pre-existing liver disorders.

Other Warnings / Precautions
- Caution is advised when using clozapine in patients with a history of:
  - Seizures or other factors predisposing to seizures (use lower possible dose).
  - Cardiovascular/cerebrovascular disease or conditions predisposing to hypotension.
  - Long QT syndrome or other conditions predisposing to QT prolongation (e.g. hypokalaemia, hypomagnesaemia, family history of QT prolongation).
  - Hyperglycaemia or diabetes.
- Due to potential anticholinergic effects, caution is advised when using clozapine in patients with narrow-angle glaucoma, prostatic hypertrophy, history of colonic disease or lower abdominal surgery, concomitant anticholinergic medications use (e.g. some antipsychotics, antidepressants, antiparkinsonian agents), or other relevant conditions (e.g. strenuous exercise, dehydration, heat exposure).
- If co-administered with strong CYP1A2 inhibitors, one-third of clozapine dose should be used. If co-administered with moderate or weak CYP1A2, CYP2D6, or CYP3A4 inhibitors, patients should be monitored for adverse effects; consider decreasing clozapine dose if needed.
- If co-administered with CYP2D6 substrates, lower doses of the latter may be necessary.
- If co-administered with moderate or weak CYP1A2 or CYP3A4 inducers, patients should be monitored for decreased effectiveness; consider increasing clozapine dose if needed.
- Caution is advised if co-administered with CNS depressants and substances with hypotensive or respiratory depressant effects.
- Close monitoring for side effects is advised if co-administered with *warfarin* and *digoxin*.
- Because clozapine may induce CNS depression, caution is advised for patients performing tasks that require mental alertness, like driving or operating machinery, especially during the initial weeks of therapy.

Do Not Use (Contraindications)
- Known sensitivity to the active substance or any of its excipients, including lactose monohydrate.
  - Patients with rare hereditary problems of galactose intolerance, total lactase deficiency, or glucose–galactose malabsorption.

DOSING AND USE

C

CLOZAPINE

- Patients with baseline WBC <3,500/mm³ or ANC <2,000/mm³ or patients who cannot adhere to regular blood monitoring.
- Clozapine should not be used in elderly patients with dementia-related psychosis, as its use has been associated with an increased risk of death due to cardiovascular or infectious causes (black box warning).
- History of toxic, idiosyncratic, or clozapine-induced granulocytopenia/agranulocytosis (unless induced by chemotherapy).
- Impaired bone marrow function.
- History of uncontrolled seizures.
- Circulatory collapse and/or CNS depression of any cause.
- Paralytic ileus.
- Severe cardiac disorders (e.g. myocarditis).
- Clozapine should not be re-initiated in patients with a history of clozapine-associated myocarditis or cardiomyopathy.
- Co-administration with:
  - CYP3A4 inducers; if co-administration is necessary, clozapine dose may need to be increased.
  - Drugs associated with bone marrow depression.
  - Long-acting depot antipsychotics, as they cannot be rapidly removed in case of severe adverse events (e.g. neutropenia).
  - Alcohol.

Special Populations
Renal Impairment
- Clozapine is contraindicated in severe renal disorders.

Hepatic Impairment
- Patients with hepatic impairment should receive clozapine with caution and regular monitoring of liver function. Dosage reduction might be necessary in severe cases. Clozapine is contraindicated in active liver disease, progressive liver disease, and hepatic failure.

Elderly
- For doses used in Parkinson's disease, no particular dose adjustments are recommended.
- Those over 60 are at increased risk of orthostatic hypotension and anticholinergic effects (e.g. urinary retention, constipation).

Pregnancy
- Caution is advised; adequate contraceptive measures must be ensured in women of childbearing potential.
- Animal studies have not found any direct or indirect harmful effects with respect to pregnancy; however, neonates exposed to clozapine during the third trimester are at risk of adverse reactions, including extrapyramidal and/or withdrawal symptoms, and newborns should be closely monitored.

C

Breastfeeding
- Clozapine is distributed in breast milk according to animal studies.
- Mothers on clozapine should not breastfeed.

Costs
NHS indicative price accessed 27 October 2022:
- Clozaril tablets (Viatris UK Healthcare Ltd) – 84 × 25 mg: £16.64; 84 × 100 mg: £66.53.
- Denzapine tablets (Britannia Pharmaceuticals Ltd) – 84 × 25 mg: £16.64; 100 × 50 mg: £39.60; 84 × 100 mg: £66.53; 100 × 200 mg: £158.40.
- Denzapine oral suspension (Britannia Pharmaceuticals Ltd) – 100 ml × 50 mg/ml: £53.50.
- Zaponex tablets (Leyden Delta B.V.) – 84 × 25 mg: £16.64; 84 × 100 mg: £66.53.
- Zaponex orodispersible tablets (Leyden Delta B.V.) – 28 × 12.5 mg: £2.77; 28 × 25 mg: £5.55; 28 × 50 mg: £11.09; 28 × 100 mg: £22.18; 28 × 200 mg: £44.35.

The Overall Place of Clozapine in the Treatment of Parkinson's Disease
Clozapine was the first agent studied for treatment of psychosis in Parkinson's disease, with abundant efficacy data from good-quality studies supporting its use. It has a proven efficacy in Parkinson's disease-related psychosis and can be used in patients who do not respond to treatment with *quetiapine* or *pimavanserin*. It is typically considered a first-line option for the treatment of Parkinson's disease-related psychosis, although it is not often not used this way in routine clinical practice due to the intensive blood cells count monitoring required as well as blood level monitoring (as indicated by clinical symptoms and patient frailty) and the range of side effects. Clozapine is not expected to significantly aggravate motor symptoms in Parkinson's disease, while it is efficacious in the management of dyskinesias and parkinsonian tremor. However, its use in this context is rare in clinical practice due to safety issues, with the only exception being intractable and bothersome tremor in patients not responsive to other therapies or not suitable for DBS. Granulocytopenia and agranulocytosis constitute an inherent risk in clozapine therapy, and seizures and cardiovascular effects have been labelled as 'black box warnings'. Although clozapine-induced leukopenia should not be a barrier in prescribing the drug in selected patients, as long as monitoring is maintained, a low adherence on clozapine has been found in the long term (8 years), mainly due to the inconvenience of regular blood testing. However, data suggest that clozapine continues to be effective and safe in the long term.

C

CLOZAPINE

Potential Advantages
- Clozapine efficacy on Parkinson's disease-related psychosis is based on strong evidence from good-quality studies.
- It has a relatively fast onset of action, ranging from a few days to 1 week.
- Clozapine has a lower risk of causing suicidal behaviour and tardive dyskinesias compared to other antipsychotic agents.
- Clozapine carries a lower risk of tardive dyskinesia compared to other antipsychotics.
- It has been associated with an improvement in cognition.

Potential Disadvantages
- Clozapine use has been associated with severe life-threatening adverse events.
- Stringent monitoring with blood tests is necessary throughout clozapine therapy, which might impair patients' adherence and is one of the main reasons for discontinuing therapy even when effective.
- Not an FDA-approved antipsychotic agent.

Clinical Box
A 68-year-old woman, with a 12-year history of Parkinson's disease, was referred to the Movement Disorders Outpatient Clinic due to troublesome visual hallucinations. Her current medication included levodopa/carbidopa 100 mg/25 mg QID and sertraline 50 mg OD. The rest of her medical history included hypercholesterolaemia and osteoporosis. Other causes of hallucinations were excluded, and the patient was initially prescribed quetiapine, because pimavanserin was not available in her country. Gradual increases of quetiapine dosage did not improve her symptoms. A decision for quetiapine cessation was made, and a low dose of clozapine 12.5 mg OD was introduced after a thorough discussion of the necessary blood test monitoring and the potential side effects. Symptoms resolved completely after a few days at a dose of 25 mg BD, while the patient also mentioned an improvement of her tremor. However, she complained about somnolence and dizziness during the day, which were addressed by administering the whole dose at bedtime.

Suggested Reading
Bonuccelli U, R Ceravolo, S Salvetti, C D'Avino, P Del Dotto, G Rossi, L Murri. Clozapine in Parkinson's disease tremor. Effects of acute and chronic administration. *Neurology* 1997; 49(6): 1587–1590.

Durif F, B Debilly, M Galitzky, D Morand, F Viallet, M Borg, S Thobois, E Brousolle, O Rascal. Clozapine improves dyskinesias in Parkinson disease: a double-blind, placebo-controlled study. *Neurology* 2004; 62(3): 381–388.

Gammon D, C Cheng, A Volkovinskaia, GB Baker, SM Dursun. Clozapine: why is it so uniquely effective in the treatment of a range of neuropsychiatric disorders? *Biomolecules* 2021; 11(7): 1030.

Parkinson Study Group. Low-dose clozapine for the treatment of drug-induced psychosis in Parkinson's disease. *N Engl J Med* 1999; 340(10): 757–763.

Pollak P, F Tison, O Rascol, A Destée, JJ Péré, JM Senard, F Durif, I Bourdeix. Clozapine in drug induced psychosis in Parkinson's disease: a randomised, placebo controlled study with open follow up. *J Neurol Neurosurg Psychiatry* 2004; 75(5): 689–695.

Yaw TK, SH Fox, AE Lang. Clozapine in parkinsonian rest tremor: a review of outcomes, adverse reactions, and possible mechanisms of action. *Mov Disord Clin Pract* 2016; 3(2): 116–124.

References

AHFS Drug information, 2012. Bethesda: American Society of Health-System Pharmacists. Accessed on 27 October 2022 via www.medicinescomplete.com.

Clonazepam. In: Brayfield A (Ed.), *Martindale: The Complete Drug Reference*. London: The Royal Pharmaceutical Society of Great Britain. Accessed on 27 October via www.medicinescomplete.com.

Clozapine. In: DRUGDEX® System (electronic version). Truven Health Analytics, Greenwood Village, Colorado, USA. Accessed on 11 March 2023 via www.micromedexsolutions.com.

Connolly BS, AE Lang. Pharmacological treatment of Parkinson disease: a review. *JAMA* 2014; 311(16): 1670–1683.

Divac N, R Stojanović, KS Vujović, B Medić, A Damjanović, M Postran. The efficacy and safety of antipsychotic medications in the treatment of psychosis in patients with Parkinson's disease. *Behav Neurol* 2016; 2016: 4938154.

Emre M, PJ Ford, B Bilgiç, EY Uç. Cognitive impairment and dementia in Parkinson's disease: practical issues and management. *Mov Disord* 2014; 29(5): 663–672.

Factor SA, JH Friedman, MC Lannon, D Oakes, K Bourgeois. Clozapine for the treatment of drug-induced psychosis in Parkinson's disease: results of the 12 week open label extension in the PSYCLOPS trial. *Mov Disord* 2001; 16(1): 135–139.

Fernandez HH, EM Donnelly, JH Friedman. Long-term outcome of clozapine use for psychosis in parkinsonian patients. *Mov Disord* 2004; 19(7): 831–833.

Fox SH. Non-dopaminergic treatments for motor control in Parkinson's disease. *Drugs* 2013; 73(13): 1405–1415.

Friedman JH, WC Koller, MC Lannon, K Busenbark, E Swanson-Hyland, D Smith. Benztropine versus clozapine for the treatment of tremor in Parkinson's disease. *Neurology* 1997; 48(4): 1077–1081.

C

C

CLOZAPINE

Hack N, SM Fayad, EH Monari, U Akber, A Hardwick, RL Rodriguez, IA Malaty, J Romrell, AAW Shukla, N McFarland, HE Ward, MS Okun. An eight-year clinic experience with clozapine use in a Parkinson's disease clinic setting. *PLoS One* 2014; 9(3): e91545.

Jann MW, SR Grimsley, EC Gray, WH Chang. Pharmacokinetics and pharmacodynamics of clozapine. *Clin Pharmacokinet* 1993; 24(2): 161–176.

Joint Formulary Committee. British National Formulary (online). London: BMJ Group and Pharmaceutical Press. Accessed on 27 October 2022 via www.medicinescomplete.com.

Klein C, J Gordon, L Pollak, JM Rabey. Clozapine in Parkinson's disease psychosis: 5-year follow-up review. *Clin Neuropharmacol* 2003; 26(1): 8–11.

Lee HB, JA Hanner, JK Yokley, B Appleby, L Hurowitz, CG Lyketsos. Clozapine for treatment-resistant agitation in dementia. *J Geriatr Psychiatry Neurol* 2007; 20(3): 178–182.

Merims D, M Balas, C Peretz, H Shabtai, N Giladi. Rater-blinded, prospective comparison: quetiapine versus clozapine for Parkinson's disease psychosis. *Clin Neuropharmacol* 2006; 29(6): 331–337.

Morgante L, A Epifanio, E Spina, M Zappia, AE Di Rosa, R Marconi, G Basile, G Di Raimondo, P La Spina, A Quattrone. Quetiapine and clozapine in parkinsonian patients with dopaminergic psychosis. *Clin Neuropharmacol* 2004; 27(4): 153–156.

Pierelli F, A Adipietro, G Soldati, F Fattapposta, G Pozzessere, C Scoppetta. Low dosage clozapine effects on L-dopa induced dyskinesias in parkinsonian patients. *Acta Neurol Scand* 1998; 97(5): 295–299.

Samudra N, N Patel, KB Womack, P Khemani, S Chitnis. Psychosis in Parkinson disease: a review of etiology, phenomenology, and management. *Drugs Aging* 2016; 33(12): 855–863.

Summary of Product Characteristics – Clozaril 25 mg tablets. Mylan. Electronic Medicines Compendium: Clozaril 25 mg Tablets – Summary of Product Characteristics (SmPC) – (emc). Accessed on 27 October 2022 via www.medicines.org.uk.

Teodorescu A, L Dima, P Ifteni, LM Rogozea. Clozapine for treatment-refractory behavioral disturbance in dementia. *Am J Ther* 2018; 25(3): e320–e325.

Trosch RM, JH Friedman, MC Lannon, R Pahwa, D Smith, LC Seeberger, CF O'Brien, PA LeWitt, WC Koller. Clozapine use in Parkinson's disease: a retrospective analysis of a large multicentered clinical experience. *Mov Disord* 1998; 13(3): 377–382.

Wang J, J-T Yu, H-F Wang, X-F Meng, C Wang, C-C Tan, L Tan. Pharmacological treatment of neuropsychiatric symptoms in Alzheimer's disease: a systematic review and meta-analysis. *J Neurol Neurosurg Psychiatry* 2015; 86(1): 101–109.

Wilby KJ, EG Johnson, HE Johnson, MHH Ensom. Evidence-based review of pharmacotherapy used for Parkinson's disease psychosis. *Ann Pharmacother* 2017; 51(8): 682–695.

DESIPRAMINE

D

Therapeutics

Chemical Name and Structure

Desipramine hydrochloride (3-(10,11-dihydro-5 H-dibenzo[*b,f*]azepin-5-yl)propyl(methyl)amine hydrochloride) is a dibenzazepine tricyclic antidepressant with a molecular weight of 302.8 and a molecular formula of $C_{18}H_{22}N_2$,HCl.

Brand Names
- **Deprexan** (*Israel*); **Desipram** (*Turkey*); **Distonal** (*Chile*).
- **Norpramin** (*USA*); **Nortimil** (*Italy*).

Generics Available
- Yes.

Licensed Indications for Parkinson's Disease
- None.

Licensed Indications for Other Conditions
- Depression (FDA).

Non-Licensed Use for Parkinson's Disease
- Depressive symptoms in Parkinson's disease.

Non-Licensed Use for Other Conditions
- Post-herpetic neuralgia.
- Neuropathic pain (limited evidence).
- Vulvodynia.
- Eating disorders.
- Difficult cases of attention deficit hyperactivity disorder.
- Cocaine dependence (individual studies).
- Irritable bowel syndrome.
- Overactive bladder.

Ineffective
- Not reported.

Mechanism of Action
- Desipramine is a monoamine reuptake inhibitor. It acts on presynaptic neuronal terminals to inhibit noradrenaline and serotonin reuptake leading to an acute increase in synaptic concentration (acute administration, before adaptive changes).
- Desipramine use is associated with a downregulation of beta-adrenergic and serotonergic receptor activity on chronic treatment (adaptive changes).
- Desipramine may also exhibit alpha-1 blocking, anti-histamine and anticholinergic activity.

D

Efficacy Profile
- Desipramine has been characterized as 'likely efficacious' and 'possibly useful' for the treatment of depressive symptoms in Parkinson's disease (MDS EBM Committee).
- A placebo-controlled study in Parkinson's disease has shown a beneficial effect of desipramine not only on depression, but also on fatigue, anxiety, and tremor.
- The therapeutic effect of desipramine is expected to start 2–5 days after the initiation of therapy, although its full therapeutic effect will only become apparent after 2–3 weeks.

Pharmacokinetics
Absorption and Distribution
- Oral bioavailability: about 40%.
- Food co-ingestion: no food interactions have been reported.
- Tmax: 4–6 h.
- Time to steady state: about 3 weeks.
- Pharmacokinetics: linear in the dose range 75–150 mg.
- Protein binding: up to 95%.
- Volume of distribution: 10–50 l/kg.

Metabolism
- Desipramine undergoes extensive hepatic metabolism, especially by CYP2D6 and to a lesser extent by CYP1A2, producing the active metabolite 2-hydroxydesipramine.

Elimination
- Half-life of desipramine ranges from 15 h to 24 h.
- Renal excretion: 70% of an administered dose is excreted in the urine.

Drug Interaction Profile
Pharmacokinetic Drug Interactions
- Effects by desipramine:
  - Desipramine will increase the levels and effects of *fentanyl, siponimod,* and others by affecting hepatic/intestinal CYP3A4 metabolism.
- Effects on desipramine:
  - *Amiodarone, bupropion, clarithromycin, diltiazem, duloxetine, fluconazole, haloperidol, quinidine, sertraline, venlafaxine, verapamil,* and other agents increase the levels and effects of desipramine by affecting hepatic/intestinal CYP450 isoenzymes.
  - *Phenytoin, rifabutin, rifampin,* and other agents decrease the levels and effects of desipramine by affecting hepatic/intestinal CYP450 isoenzymes.

DESIPRAMINE

D

Pharmacodynamic Drug Interactions
- Co-medication with other serotonergic agents, including SSRIs/SNRIs, tricyclic antidepressants, opioids, *lithium, buspirone,* amphetamines, and triptans, can lead to potentially life-threatening serotonin syndrome.
- Co-medication with drugs causing electrolyte imbalance or increasing QT interval, such as Class IA and III anti-arrhythmics, antipsychotics (e.g. *haloperidol, phenothiazine derivatives, pimozide*), tricyclic antidepressants, certain antimicrobial agents (e.g. *moxifloxacin, erythromycin*), certain antihistamines (e.g. *astemizole, mizolastine*), and others may lead to potentially fatal Torsade de Pointes arrhythmias and is considered a risk factor for sudden cardiac death.
- Co-medication with CNS depressants (e.g. benzodiazepines, most antipsychotics, antihistamines H1 antagonists, opioids) or alcohol might lead to synergistic sedative effects, including somnolence and dizziness.
- Co-medication with *guanethidine* or other compounds with similar activity may block their antihypertensive effects.

Adverse Effects
How Drug Causes Adverse Effects
- The activity of desipramine is mediated by a number of receptors mentioned above.

Common Adverse Effects
- Common ($\geq 1/100$ to $<1/10$):
  - Nervous/psychiatric: sedation, lethargy, agitation, anxiety, headache, insomnia.
  - Eye/ear: blurred vision.
  - Gastrointestinal: constipation, dry mouth, nausea, vomiting.
  - General: fatigue, weakness, sweating.
- Uncommon ($\geq 1/1,000$ to $<1/100$):
  - Nervous/psychiatric: confusion, dizziness, paraesthesia, extrapyramidal syndromes.
  - Eye/ear: tinnitus.
  - Cardiovascular: ECG changes, orthostatic hypotension, tachycardia.
  - Gastrointestinal: elevated liver enzymes.
  - Reproductive: sexual dysfunction.
  - Skin: rash.

Life-Threatening or Dangerous Adverse Effects
- Rare ($\geq 1/10,000$ to $<1/1,000$):
  - Seizures.
  - Agranulocytosis, eosinophilia, leukopenia, thrombocytopenia.
  - SIADH.

ADVERSE EFFECTS

D

- Unknown frequency:
  - Cardiac conduction defects, arrhythmia, tachycardia, stroke, acute myocardial infarction.
  - Acute liver injury.

Rare and Not Life-Threatening Adverse Effects
- Not reported.

Weight Change
- Anorexia and weight decrease are rarely reported.

What to Do About Adverse Effects
- Before introducing desipramine, discuss common or life-threatening adverse effects with patients and/or caregivers, including symptoms that should be reported to the physician.
- Patients and their caregivers should be informed about the possibility of desipramine causing suicidal ideation/behaviour, especially in the early phase of recovery. If such signs/symptoms emerge, patients should urgently seek for medical advice and be treated accordingly. Desipramine should be discontinued.
  - Due to suicidality risk, consider giving the patient only a small number of desipramine tablets.
- Patients and caregivers should be informed and be particularly vigilant for anticholinergic side effects of desipramine, including dry mouth, constipation, blurred vision, confusion, and seizures.

Dosing and Use
Usual Dosage Range
- 25–200 mg.

Available Formulations
- Tablets: 10 mg, 25 mg, 50 mg, 75 mg, 100 mg, 150 mg.

How to Dose
- An initial daily dose of 25–50 mg is suggested, which can be subsequently gradually increased (at a minimum of 1-week intervals) to 75–150 mg per day either as a single dose or divided in two doses with a 12-h interval according to tolerance and clinical response.
- A maximum of 300 mg per day can be used, but only for severe depression in hospitalized patients. Doses higher than 300 mg are not recommended.
- Desipramine dose regimens should be carefully individualized; maintenance dose should be the lowest effective for the shortest possible duration.

Dosing Tips
- At least one dose of desipramine should be given at night before bedtime to lower the possibility of daytime sleepiness. However, if a patient experiences insomnia, they could take the whole daily dose in the morning.
- Desipramine can be given in up to three divided doses a day.
- When depressive symptoms are controlled, the maintenance dose can be gradually reduced to the lowest possible level to sustain efficacy.

How to Withdraw Drug
- Desipramine should be gradually discontinued to reduce the possibility of withdrawal symptoms, especially in patients who received high doses for long periods of time.

Overdose
- Desipramine overdose may present as blurred vision, mydriasis, dry mouth, nausea/vomiting, constipation, urine retention, hypotension, tachycardia, arrhythmia, agitation, drowsiness, seizures, incoordination, rigidity/stiffness, serotonin syndrome, stupor, coma.
- Desipramine overdosage has an increased death rate compared to other tricyclic antidepressants.
- Supportive measures, close monitoring, serum alkalization and maintenance of a clear airway with adequate ventilation are recommended.
- The patient should be observed for a minimum of 6 h in case of unexplained syncope, shortness of breath, palpitations, or chest pain.
- Consider activated charcoal, if applied within 1 h after desipramine ingestion.
- Emesis is contraindicated.

Tests and Therapeutic Drug Monitoring
- Before initiation of desipramine therapy:
  - A baseline ECG should be performed to check for QT prolongation.
  - A metabolic panel should be performed, including electrolytes, renal and hepatic function.
- During desipramine therapy:
- Consider monitoring renal function and regular ECG in elderly patients.
  - Patients should be regularly evaluated for worsening of depression, suicidality, behaviour changes, or other common adverse effects, especially after introducing therapy or during dose modifications.

Other Warnings/Precautions
- There is a black box warning for young adults (less than 24 years old) who take desipramine for depression and other psychiatric disorders concerning suicidal thinking and behaviour.
  - Patients with a history of suicide-related events are at higher risk and careful monitoring during treatment is required, especially early in therapy and following changes in dosage.

D

DOSING AND USE

111

D

- Close monitoring is advised in patients with benign prostate hyperplasia, urinary or GI retention, respiratory impairment, hepatic or renal impairment.
- Caution is advised in patients with cardiovascular disease due to the cardiotoxicity potential of desipramine, especially in patients with a family history of sudden death, cardiac dysrhythmias, or conduction disturbances.
- Caution is advised in patients with a history of epilepsy or brain tumour because desipramine might lower the seizures threshold.
- Caution is advised in patients with hyperthyroidism or those taking thyroid medications, because desipramine might precipitate cardiac arrhythmias.
- An angle-closure attack may be triggered in patients with high intraocular pressure or those at risk of angle closure glaucoma (e.g. anatomically narrow angles without a patent iridectomy).
- Desipramine might cause CNS depression, affecting the ability to drive or operate dangerous machinery.
  - Co-administration with CNS depressants or alcohol should be avoided.

Do Not Use (Contraindications)
- Known sensitivity to desipramine or to any of the excipients.
- During recovery after recent MI.
- Desipramine is not indicated in patients with bipolar disorder, as it may trigger a manic episode.
  - Desipramine should be withdrawn in any patient entering a manic phase.
- Co-administration with MAOIs (including *selegiline* and *rasagiline*) or within 2 weeks after their discontinuation due to increased risk of potentially fatal serotonin syndrome. MAOIs should not be administered for 1 week after desipramine discontinuation. The same applies for co-administration with *safinamide*.
- Co-administration with linezolid or methylene blue IV.
  - In case linezolid administration is necessary, desipramine should be immediately discontinued, and the patient should be monitored for CNS toxicity. Desipramine therapy can be resumed 24 h after last linezolid dose or after 2 weeks of monitoring, whichever applies first.
- Co-medication with drugs causing QT prolongation.
- Co-medication with anticholinergic agents might enhance their effects and should be avoided.

Special Populations
Renal Impairment
- No dose adjustments are needed for eGFR 15–60 ml/min.
- In case of eGFR<15 ml/min or haemodialysis or peritoneal dialysis: an initial dose of 25 mg is suggested with extra caution in subsequent dosage increase.

Hepatic Impairment
• Patients with liver disease may require reduced doses.

Elderly
• Geriatric patients over 65 years old have not been sufficiently represented in desipramine studies.
• Regular follow-up and monitoring of renal function is advised for geriatric patients who use desipramine, because it is mainly excreted via the kidney and elderly patients are more likely to have decreased renal function.
• A lower total dosage of 25–100 mg per day is preferred; a maximum of 150 mg per day is suggested for severe depression and hospitalized patients.
• Desipramine use in the elderly has been associated with an increased risk of falls and confusion.

Pregnancy
• Safe use of desipramine during pregnancy has not been established and the results of animal studies have not been conclusive.
• Desipramine should only be given in pregnant women or women of childbearing potential if the expected benefits outweigh any potential risks.

Breastfeeding
• Limited data show that desipramine is detected in human milk in similar concentrations to maternal plasma.
• Safe use of desipramine during breastfeeding has not been established.
• Desipramine should only be given in nursing mothers if the expected benefits outweigh any potential risks for the patient and child.

Costs
• Not available in the UK.

The Overall Place of Desipramine in the Treatment of Parkinson's Disease
Desipramine is a tricyclic antidepressant, which has been typically used for the treatment of depression in Parkinson's disease, although it is not considered a first-line therapy option due to tolerability issues. In a head-to-head comparison with citalopram, desipramine showed a slightly more positive short-term effect on Parkinson's disease-related depression. However, it was concluded that desipramine had an increased rate of adverse effects compared to SSRIs and that this might outweigh the beneficial effect.

D

DESIPRAMINE

Potential Advantages
- Desipramine is one of the less-sedating tricyclic antidepressants and its antimuscarinic effects are mild.
- It can be given as a single dose to improve patients' adherence.
- Compared to SSRIs, tricyclic antidepressants have an inherent advantage in improving sleep.

Potential Disadvantages
- Administration of tricyclic antidepressants to Parkinson's disease patients might precipitate or worsen psychosis, sedation, somnolence, cognitive impairment, or delirium, especially in those with impaired cognition.
- A long list of drug-to-drug interactions accompanies desipramine administration.
- Among all antidepressants, tricyclic antidepressants and citalopram at elevated doses bear the greatest risk for QT prolongation, especially for those over 60 years old; thus, regular ECG monitoring is required.
- Desipramine use is not encouraged in elderly patients.
- Desipramine is not commercially available in numerous countries.

Clinical Box
A 50-year-old man with a diagnosis of Parkinson's disease presented at the Movement Disorders Outpatient Clinic for a follow-up appointment. The patient was recently diagnosed with moderate depression and had been offered trials with a number of antidepressant agents, including citalopram, venlafaxine, paroxetine and amitriptyline. He had discontinued all of these due to either lack of efficacy or tolerability issues. The patient was subsequently given the option of desipramine treatment. A low dose of desipramine 25 mg OD at night was suggested, which was gradually increased to 200 mg OD during the following days without any troublesome side effects.

Suggested Reading
Devos D, K Dujardin, I Poirot, C Moreau, O Cottencin, P Thomas, A Destée, R Bordet, L Defebvre. Comparison of desipramine and citalopram treatments for depression in Parkinson's disease: a double-blind, randomized, placebo-controlled study. *Mov Disord* 2008; 23(6): 850–857.

Laitinen L. Desipramine in treatment of Parkinson's disease. A placebo-controlled study. *Acta Neurol Scand* 1969; 45(1): 109–113.

D

References

Ciraulo DA, JG Barnhill, JH Jaffe. Clinical pharmacokinetics of imipramine and desipramine in alcoholics and normal volunteers. *Clin Pharmacol Ther* 1988; 43(5): 509–518.

Desipramine. In: Brayfield A (Ed.), *Martindale: The Complete Drug Reference*. London: The Royal Pharmaceutical Society of Great Britain. Accessed on 5 December 2022 via www.medicinescomplete.com.

Desipramine. In: DRUGDEX® System (electronic version). Truven Health Analytics, Greenwood Village, Colorado, USA. Accessed on 5 December 2022 via www.micromedexsolutions.com.

Hearn L, RA Moore, S Derry, PJ Wiffen, T Phillips. Desipramine for neuropathic pain in adults. *Cochrane Database Syst Rev* 2014; 2014(9): Cd011003.

Maan JS, A Rosani, A Saadabadi. Desipramine. In: StatPearls, 2022. StatPearls Publishing.

D

DOMPERIDONE

Therapeutics

Chemical Name and Structure

Domperidone (6-chloro-3-[1-[3-(2-oxo-3H-benzimidazol-1-yl)pro-pyl]piperidin-4-yl]-1H-benzimidazol-2-one) has a molecular weight of 425.9 and an empirical formula of $C_{22}H_{24}ClN_5O_2$. Each tablet contains domperidone maleate 10 mg, which is equivalent to 10 mg domperidone base.

Brand Names

- **Costi** (*Cyprus, Hong Kong*).
- **Domedon** (*Hong Kong*); **Domerid** (*Ireland*); **Domped** (*Brazil*); **Dompedon** (*Hong Kong*); **Dompenyl** (*Singapore*); **Dompeon** (*Hong Kong*); **Domper** (*Singapore*); **Domperan** (*Hong Kong*); **Domperix** (*Brazil*); **Dompgran** (*Brazil*); **Dompliv** (*Brazil*); **Dompyrex** (*Tunisia*); **Domstal** (*Lithuania*); **Doperan** (*Hong Kong*); **Dopidium** (*Tunisia*); **Doridone** (*Hong Kong, Singapore*); **Dosin** (*Hong Kong*).
- **Cilroton** (*Greece*); **Costi** (*Cyprus, Hong Kong*).
- **Eurotilium** (*Hong Kong*).
- **Feselin** (*Hong Kong*).
- **Gastrium** (*Singapore*); **Gastromotil** (*Hong Kong*); **Genolin** (*Hong Kong*).
- **Kalmivum** (*Tunisia*); **Kantuu** (*Hong Kong*).
- **Molax-M** (*Hong Kong*); **Molidon** (*Brazil*); **Monell** (*Hong Kong*); **Moridone** (*Singapore*); **Motilium** (*Australia, Austria, Brazil, Cyprus, France, Germany, Hong Kong, Ireland, Lithuania, Netherlands, New Zealand, Singapore, South Africa, Spain, UK*); **Motiridona** (*Brazil*).
- **Naupastad** (*Hong Kong*); **Nidolium** (*Hong Kong*).
- **Oroperidys** (*Estonia, Greece, Lithuania, Tunisia*).
- **Peptomet** (*Cyprus, Hong Kong, Singapore*); **Peridal** (*Brazil*); **Peridom** (*Hong Kong*); **Peridys** (*Tunisia*); **Perilium** (*Tunisia*); **Pesdon** (*Hong Kong*); **Piradium** (*Tunisia*).
- **Ridonex** (*Ireland*).
- **Synotilium** (*Hong Kong*).
- **Vicktilin** (*Hong Kong*); **Vicktilium** (*Hong Kong*); **Vocinium** (*Hong Kong*); **Vomi-Guard** (*South Africa*); **Vomicalm** (*Tunisia*); **Vomidon** (*South Africa*).

Generics Available

- Yes.

Licensed Indications for Parkinson's Disease

- None.

Licensed Indications for Other Conditions

- Relief of nausea/vomiting (EMA, EMC).
  - Particularly useful in diabetic gastropathy.

D

Non-Licensed Use for Parkinson's Disease
- Co-administration with apomorphine during the initial phase of apomorphine therapy to reduce the occurrence of nausea and/or vomiting.
- To treat excessive emesis in apomorphine overdose.
- Dopaminergic therapy-related symptoms of nausea/vomiting.
- Orthostatic hypotension in Parkinson's disease, mostly related to dopaminergic therapy.

Non-Licensed Use for Other Conditions
- Gastrointestinal pain in palliative care.
- Gastro-oesophageal reflux disease.

Ineffective
- Not reported.

Mechanism of Action
- Domperidone is a peripheral dopamine D-2 selective receptor antagonist with minor penetration through the blood–brain barrier.

Efficacy Profile
- Domperidone increases lower oesophageal pressure, improves antro-duodenal motility and accelerates gastric emptying, without any impact on gastric secretion.
- According to randomized studies, domperidone is efficacious in the management of GI and emetic effects of dopaminergic medications without affecting their therapeutic efficacy.
- Considering GI dysfunction in Parkinson's disease, including dopaminergic therapy-related anorexia, nausea, and vomiting, domperidone has been characterized as 'likely efficacious' and 'possibly useful' (MDS EBM Committee).
- There are numerous studies offering some evidence of the positive effect of domperidone on orthostatic hypotension in Parkinson's disease, even independently of the initiation of dopaminergic medication, although most evidence is related to combination with apomorphine therapy or other dopamine agonists.
  - One RCT has demonstrated a beneficial effect of domperidone on orthostatic hypotension in Parkinson's disease patients.
- Domperidone use in the treatment of orthostatic hypotension in Parkinson's disease has been labelled as 'investigational' with 'insufficient evidence' currently available (MDS EBM Committee).

Pharmacokinetics
Absorption and Distribution
- Oral bioavailability: about 15%.
- Food co-ingestion: domperidone should be taken 15–30 min before meals, otherwise absorption might be delayed.

D

- Tmax: approximately 1 h.
- Pharmacokinetics: linear in the therapeutic range.
- Protein binding: 91–93%.
- Volume of distribution: 5.7 l/kg.

Metabolism
- Domperidone undergoes an extensive first-pass metabolism in the gut wall and liver, mainly via CYP3A4 (N-dealkylation and aromatic hydroxylation) and to a lesser extent via CYP1A2 and CYP2E1 (aromatic hydroxylation).

Elimination
- Half-life ranges between 7 h and 9 h.
- About 31% and 66% of an administered dose is excreted (1% and 10% is unchanged) in the urine and faeces, respectively.

Drug Interaction Profile
Pharmacokinetic Drug Interactions
- Effects on domperidone:
  - Potent and moderate CYP3A4 inhibitors, including protease inhibitors, systemic azole antifungals, some macrolides (e.g. *erythromycin, clarithromycin*), *diltiazem, verapamil* and others, may increase plasma levels and effects of domperidone.
  - Grapefruit products might increase plasma levels of domperidone.
  - Co-administration of *cimetidine* and *sodium bicarbonate* may lower domperidone levels due to decreased oral bioavailability.

Pharmacodynamic Drug Interactions
- Co-medication with drugs causing electrolyte imbalance or increasing QT interval, such as Class IA and III anti-arrhythmics, antipsychotics (e.g. *haloperidol, phenothiazine derivatives, pimozide*), tricyclic antidepressants, certain antimicrobial agents (e.g. *moxifloxacin, erythromycin*), certain antihistamines (e.g. *astemizole, mizolastine*), and others may lead to potentially fatal Torsade de Pointes arrhythmias and is considered a risk factor for sudden cardiac death.

Adverse Effects
How Drug Causes Adverse Effects
- Domperidone is anticipated to act as a highly potent hERG/K_v11.1 channel blocker at therapeutic clinical doses, which is believed to be the mechanism mediating its arrhythmogenic potential.

Common Adverse Effects
- Common (≥1/100 to <1/10):
  - Dry mouth.

D

- Uncommon (≥1/1,000 to <1/100):
  - Nervous/psychiatric: loss of libido, anxiety, somnolence, headache.
  - Gastrointestinal: diarrhoea, impaired liver function tests.
  - Skin: rash, pruritus.
  - Reproductive: galactorrhoea, breast pain/tenderness, increased blood prolactin.

Life-Threatening or Dangerous Adverse Effects
- Very rare (<1/10,000):
  - QT prolongation, Torsades de Pointes.
- Unknown frequency:
  - Ventricular arrhythmias, sudden cardiac death.
  - Anaphylactic reaction/shock.
  - Convulsions.
  - Extrapyramidal disorders, including RLS.
  - Urticaria, angioedema.
  - Urinary retention.

Rare and Not Life-Threatening Adverse Effects
- Agitation, nervousness.
- Gynaecomastia, amenorrhoea.

Weight Change
- Not reported.

What to Do About Adverse Effects
- Before introducing domperidone, discuss common or life-threatening adverse effects with patients and/or caregivers, including symptoms that should be reported to the physician.
- Patients and caregivers should be thoroughly informed and be particularly vigilant for any signs or symptoms of new-onset arrhythmia during domperidone therapy (e.g. palpitations, dizziness/light-headedness, fatigue, fainting/near fainting, sweating) and report them to the treating physician.
  - In case of arrhythmia, domperidone therapy should be discontinued.

Dosing and Use
Usual Dosage Range
- 10–30 mg daily.

Available Formulations
- Tablets: 10 mg.
- Tablets orally disposable (OR): 10 mg.
- Suppository: 60 mg.
- Oral solution: 1 mg/1 ml.
- Sachets: 10 mg.

D

How to Dose
- The usual starting dose is 10 mg BID, which can be increased to 10 mg TID.
- A maximum total dose of 30 mg per day should not be exceeded, as it has been associated with serious ventricular arrhythmias or sudden cardiac death.
- Although there is a clear recommendation on the drug maximum dose allowed, prior to regulatory safety warnings higher doses of up to 150 mg per day have also been used in routine clinical practice, with schemes of 20 mg TID or 50 mg TID being commonly encountered.

Dosing Tips
- Domperidone therapy should not be prolonged for more than 1 week.
  - Although a clear cut-off point of 1 week is given by the manufacturer, domperidone therapy is often further prolonged in routine clinical practice when the drug is used to suppress drug-related symptoms of nausea and/or vomiting during the introduction of apomorphine, levodopa, or other dopamine agonists therapy.
    - This period is expected to be longer with acute subcutaneous injection of apomorphine compared to continuous subcutaneous infusion.
    - Careful cardiac monitoring is strongly recommended.
- The maintenance dose should be the lowest effective dose.
- It is suggested that each domperidone dose should be taken at a scheduled time.
- Suppository forms of domperidone might be useful in patients with vomiting who cannot receive oral formulations.

How to Withdraw Drug
- Abrupt domperidone discontinuation might lead to withdrawal symptoms, especially if patients have been treated with domperidone for long time periods or with high dosage.
- Withdrawal symptoms might include insomnia, anxiety, agitation, nausea, palpitations, tachycardia, cognitive problems, and depression.
- When patients receive domperidone during the introductory phase of levodopa or dopamine agonists and after their dose is established, the dose of domperidone can be decreased by 10 mg per day every week.
- In case of severe or prolonged symptoms during dosage reduction or withdrawal, consider resuming the previously prescribed dose and follow a longer tapering period.

Overdose
- Domperidone overdosage may present with agitation, somnolence, disorientation, altered consciousness, convulsions, and extrapyramidal reactions.
- There is no specific antidote to domperidone.

D

- Supportive measures, close monitoring with regular ECG assessments, and maintenance of a clear airway with adequate ventilation are recommended.
- Consider activated charcoal or gastric lavage, if applied close to domperidone ingestion.
- Anticholinergic and antiparkinsonian agents may be useful in the management of potential extrapyramidal symptoms.

Tests and Therapeutic Drug Monitoring
- Before initiation of domperidone therapy:
  - A baseline ECG should be performed to check for QT prolongation.
  - A metabolic panel should be performed, including electrolytes, renal and hepatic function.
    - Electrolyte disorders should be corrected before domperidone administration.
- During domperidone therapy:
  - Regular ECG assessments and monitoring of electrolytes are recommended.

Other Warnings/Precautions
- Caution is advised in patients with cardiovascular disease due to the risk of cardiotoxicity with domperidone, especially in patients with a predisposition to QT prolongation or a family history of long QT syndrome.
  - Caution is advised in patients with electrolyte imbalance (hypokalaemia, hyperkalaemia, hypomagnesaemia), as domperidone administration might lead to arrhythmias, potentially fatal Torsade de Pointes, and sudden cardiac death.
  - Domperidone use has been associated with a higher risk of ventricular tachycardia/sudden cardiac death in PD patients, especially for those with a history of cardiovascular disease. This risk was not significantly related to dose and duration of domperidone therapy.
- Caution is advised in patients with galactosaemia.
- Caution is advised in co-administration with the macrolides *azithromycin* and *roxithromycin* and with hypokalaemia-inducing drugs, for example *furosemide*.

Do Not Use (Contraindications)
- Known sensitivity to domperidone or any of its excipients, including lactose, sorbitol, and hydroxybenzoate.
  - Patients with hereditary problems of galactose intolerance, total lactase deficiency, glucose–galactose malabsorption, or fructose intolerance.
- Patients with cardiac conduction disorders, particularly long QT syndrome or Torsades de Pointes, those with underlying cardiac disease, including congestive heart failure and those with significant electrolyte impairment.
- Patients with GI haemorrhage/perforation or GI obstruction.

D

DOMPERIDONE

- Patients with a known prolactin-releasing pituitary tumour (prolactinoma).
- Co-administration with drugs that predispose to QT prolongation, such as Class IA (e.g. *hydroquinidine, quinidine*) and III anti-arrhythmics (e.g. *amiodarone, sotalol*), certain antipsychotics (e.g. *haloperidol, phenothiazine derivatives, pimozide*), tricyclic and other antidepressants (e.g. *citalopram, escitalopram*), certain antimicrobial, antifungal, and antimalarial agents (e.g. *moxifloxacin, erythromycin*), certain antihistamines (e.g. *astemizole, mizolastine*), and others, with the exception of *apomorphine*.
- Co-administration with potent and moderate CYP3A4 inhibitors.
- Patients should not consume grapefruit while on domperidone.

Special Populations
Renal Impairment
- When repeated domperidone doses are needed, a frequency reduction to 10 mg BID or OD is necessary depending on the level of impairment. A dose reduction might also be considered.
  - No dose adjustments are needed in case of a single administration.
- Regular assessments of renal function are needed in case of prolonged therapy.

Hepatic Impairment
- No dosage modification is necessary in mild hepatic impairment.
- Domperidone use is not recommended in moderate and severe hepatic impairment.

Elderly
- Caution is advised when domperidone is used in geriatric patients over 60 years, as it has been associated with an increased risk of serious ventricular arrhythmias or sudden cardiac death.

Pregnancy
- Data on domperidone use during pregnancy are scarce and any potential risks to humans have not been established.
- Domperidone can be used with caution during pregnancy only when the beneficial effect is expected to outweigh any potential risks.
- It is recommended that domperidone should be avoided during pregnancy, especially in the first trimester.

Breastfeeding
- Domperidone is excreted in human milk in low concentrations.
- Data on domperidone use during breast-feeding are scarce; no potential risks to humans have been identified, although they cannot be excluded.
- Potential benefits and risks from domperidone therapy or the mother's subjacent condition should be weighed before deciding if domperidone should be discontinued or the mother should abstain from breastfeeding.

D

Costs

NHS indicative price accessed 12 December 2022:

- Domperidone tablets – 30 × 10 mg tablets: £0.66–£2.17; 100 × 10 mg tablets: £1.90–£7.23.
- Motilium tablets (Zentiva Pharma UK Ltd) – 30 × 10 mg tablets: £2.71; 100 × 10 mg tablets: £9.04.
- Domperidone oral suspension – 200 ml × 1 mg/ml: £17.11–£24.85.

The Overall Place of Domperidone in the Treatment of Parkinson's Disease

Domperidone is a dopamine receptor antagonist with antiemetic effects. It acts on dopamine receptors in the periphery; there is no significant crossing of the blood–brain barrier. The most typical use of domperidone among Parkinson's disease patients is its co-administration with apomorphine when the latter is prescribed in a Parkinson's disease patient for the first time, but it can also be used in combination with levodopa or other dopamine agonists. Co-administration of domperidone with dopamine agonists or levodopa preparations has been recommended during their titration period to reduce the possibility of therapy failure due to adverse events. Patients will need to receive domperidone for a few days before the initiation of levodopa or dopamine agonists, particularly apomorphine, in order to reduce the risk of nausea, vomiting, or orthostatic hypotension. Domperidone therapy usually continues during the titration process of levodopa or dopamine agonists, which varies between individuals and may occasionally be prolonged beyond one week. Once the dose is established, domperidone can be gradually withdrawn. Domperidone dose should be the lowest effective and administered for the shortest time possible. Domperidone is generally well tolerated with a favourable safety profile; however, it has cardiotoxic potential, so extra caution is advised for elderly patients, those with a history of cardiac disease, and when used in high doses.

Potential Advantages

- Domperidone is considered a safe alternative to other antiemetics (e.g. *metoclopramide*) in Parkinson's disease, as it induces minimal CNS adverse effects, including extrapyramidal symptoms.

Potential Disadvantages

- Not approved for marketing by the FDA, although it is available from some compounding pharmacies in the USA.
- Domperidone cannot be used for long-term therapy.
- Extra caution is suggested in elderly patients and those with a history of cardiac disease.
- A long list of drug-to-drug interactions should be considered.
- A twofold increase of mortality risk has been found in Parkinson's disease patients who have used domperidone compared to those who have not, especially within the first month of therapy.

D

Clinical Box

A 55-year-old man presented at the Neurology Department for a scheduled admission to initiate apomorphine injection therapy due to early morning dystonic OFF phenomena. The patient had been instructed to take domperidone 10 mg TID for 3 days prior to apomorphine initiation. The patient's past medical history was unremarkable, and no contraindications were found either for domperidone or apomorphine. After a 5-day trial, a dose of apomorphine 4 mg once every morning was found effective for the patient and domperidone was reduced to 10 mg BID. The patient was discharged with instructions to continue domperidone 10 mg BID for 1 week and subsequently at 10 mg OD for another week before complete discontinuation of therapy. However, after domperidone cessation, symptoms of nausea emerged, and the patient was instructed to restart the medication at a dose of 10 mg OD. A longer withdrawal period of 2 weeks was suggested, after which the patient was able to successfully discontinue domperidone.

Suggested Reading

Jansen PA, RM Herings, MM Samson, PL De Vreede, LM Schuurmans-Daemen, A Hovestadt, HJ Verhaar, T Van Laar. Quick titration of pergolide in cotreatment with domperidone is safe and effective. *Clin Neuropharmacol* 2001; 24(3): 177–180.

Langdon N, PN Malcolm, JD Parkes. Comparison of levodopa with carbidopa, and levodopa with domperidone in Parkinson's disease. *Clin Neuropharmacol* 1986; 9(5): 440–447.

Quinn N, A Illas, F Lhermitte, Y Agid. Bromocriptine and domperidone in the treatment of Parkinson disease. *Neurology* 1981; 31(6): 662–667.

Schoffer KL, RD Henderson, K O'Maley, JD O'Sullivan. Nonpharmacological treatment, fludrocortisone, and domperidone for orthostatic hypotension in Parkinson's disease. *Mov Disord* 2007; 22(11): 1543–1549.

References

AHFS Drug information, 2012. Bethesda: American Society of Health-System Pharmacists. Accessed on 12 December 2022 via www.medicinescomplete.com.

Bacchi S, I Chim, P Kramer, RB Postuma. Domperidone for hypotension in Parkinson's disease: a systematic review. *J Parkinsons Dis* 2017; 7(4): 603–617.

Barone JA. Domperidone: a peripherally acting dopamine2-receptor antagonist. *Ann Pharmacother* 1999; 33(4): 429–440.

Domperidone, in Drugs and Lactation Database (LactMed). 2022, National Library of Medicine (US): Bethesda (MD).

D

Domperidone. In: Brayfield A (Ed.), *Martindale: The Complete Drug Reference*. London: The Royal Pharmaceutical Society of Great Britain. Accessed on 12 December 2022 via www.medicinescomplete.com.

Domperidone. In: DRUGDEX® System (electronic version). Truven Health Analytics, Greenwood Village, Colorado, USA. Accessed on 12 December 2022 via www.micromedexsolutions.com.

Joint Formulary Committee. British National Formulary (online). London: BMJ Group and Pharmaceutical Press. Accessed on 12 December 2022 via www.medicinescomplete.com.

Reddymasu SC, I Soykan, RW McCallum. Domperidone: review of pharmacology and clinical applications in gastroenterology. *Am J Gastroenterol* 2007; 102(9): 2036–2045.

Renoux C, S Dell'Aniello, P Khairy, C Marras, S Bugden, TC Turin, L Blais, H Tamim, C Evans, R Steele, C Dormuth, P Ernst. Ventricular tachyarrhythmia and sudden cardiac death with domperidone use in Parkinson's disease. *Br J Clin Pharmacol* 2016; 82(2): 461–472.

Rios Romenets S, Y Dauvilliers, V Cochen De Cock, B Carlander, S Bayard, C Galatas, C Wolfson, RB Postuma. Restless legs syndrome outside the blood–brain barrier – exacerbation by domperidone in Parkinson's disease. *Parkinsonism Relat Disord* 2013; 19(1): 92–94.

Simeonova M, F de Vries, S Pouwels, JHM Driessen, HGM Leufkens, SM Cadarette, AM Burden. Increased risk of all-cause mortality associated with domperidone use in Parkinson's patients: a population-based cohort study in the UK. *Br J Clin Pharmacol* 2018; 84(11): 2551–2561.

Song BG, YC Lee, YW Min, K Kim, H Lee, HJ Son, PL Rhee. Risk of domperidone induced severe ventricular arrhythmia. *Sci Rep* 2020; 10(1): 12158.

Summary of Product Characteristics – Motilium 10 mg film-coated tablets. Zentiva. Electronic Medicines Compendium: Motilium 10 mg film-coated tablets – summary of product characteristics (SmPC) – (emc). Accessed on 12 December 2022 via www.medicines.org.uk.

REFERENCES

D | DONEPEZIL

Therapeutics

Chemical Name and Structure

Donepezil hydrochloride ((±)-2,3-dihydro-5,6-dimethoxy-2-[[1-phenyl-methyl)-4-piperidinyl]methyl]-1H-inden-1-oneHClor(±)-2-[(1-benzyl-4-piperidyl)methyl]-5,6-dimethoxy-1-indanone hydrochloride). It is a white crystalline powder, soluble in water, with a molecular weight of 415.95 and an empirical formula of $C_{24}H_{29}NO_3.HCl$.

Brand Names

- **A Rui Si** (*China*); **Adlarity** (*USA*); **Adtreat** (*Greece*); **Aldomer** (*Indonesia*); **Aldonil** (*Greece*); **Alfimet** (*Argentina*); **Alizil** (*Portugal*); **Alkimus** (*Portugal*); **Almer** (*Ukraine*); **Alzamed** (*Turkey*); **Alzancer** (*Turkey*); **Alzdone** (*Poland*); **Alzedon** (*Hong Kong*); **Alzepezil** (*Poland*); **Alzepil** (*Hungary, Russian Federation, Turkey, Ukraine*); **Alzhemept** (*Hong Kong*); **Alzido** (*South Africa*); **Alzil** (*Czech Republic, Turkey*); **Alzim** (*Indonesia*); **Alzime** (*Thailand*); **Apo-Doperil** (*Poland*); **Arazil** (*Australia, Hong Kong*); **Aricep** (*India*); **Aricept** (*Australia, Austria, Belgium, Canada, China, Czech Republic, Denmark, Finland, France, Germany, Greece, Hong Kong, Hungary, Indonesia, Ireland, Israel, Italy, Japan, Malaysia, Norway, Philippines, Poland, Portugal, Russian Federation, Singapore, South Africa, Spain, Sweden, Switzerland, Thailand, Turkey, Ukraine, USA*); **Aridon** (*Australia*); **Arimentia** (*South Africa*); **Arimer** (*South Africa*); **Aripezil** (*Greece*); **Aripil** (*Ireland*); **Arizil** (*Malaysia, Philippines, Poland*); **Arypez** (*Turkey*); **Asenta** (*Israel*); **Aurobral** (*Argentina*).

- **Caricia** (*Greece*); **Cebrocal** (*Argentina*); **Cenipil** (*Greece*); **Cogiton** (*Poland*); **Cognezil** (*Poland*); **Covolos** (*Greece*); **Crialix** (*Argentina*); **Cristaclar** (*Argentina*); **Curlovon** (*South Africa*).

- **Daxolin** (*Chile*); **Demelan** (*Austria*); **Dement** (*Turkey*); **Dementis** (*Greece, Russian Federation*); **Depzil** (*India*); **Dezial** (*Greece*); **Dezira** (*Turkey*); **Divare** (*Greece, Turkey*); **Dobedipil** (*Poland*); **Doenza** (*Turkey, Ukraine*); **Donacept** (*Greece, Indonesia*); **Donasure** (*India*); **Donaz** (*India*); **Doncep** (*Turkey*); **Donebrain** (*Spain*); **Donecept** (*Hong Kong, Hungary, India, Ireland, Poland, South Africa, Thailand*); **Donecleus** (*Poland*); **Donectil** (*Hungary, Poland*); **Donefix** (*Turkey*); **Donegal** (*Greece*); **Donelet** (*Greece*); **DoneLiquid GeriaSan** (*Germany*); **Donemed** (*Poland*); **Donenerton** (*Poland*); **Donep** (*India*); **Donepes** (*Argentina*); **Donepesan** (*Poland*); **Donepestan** (*Poland*); **Donepex** (*Poland*); **Doneprion** (*Poland*); **Donept** (*Thailand*); **Donerin** (*South Africa*); **Donesan** (*Greece*); **Donestad** (*Hungary, Poland*); **Donester** (*Greece*); **Donesyn** (*Hungary, Ireland, Poland*); **Donethon** (*Poland*); **Donezel** (*Philippines*); **Donezil** (*Malaysia*); **Donila** (*Brazil*); **Donpethon** (*Czech Republic*); **Donpex** (*Argentina*); **Dopaben** (*Chile*); **Dospelin** (*Czech Republic, Greece*); **Dopezil** (*India, Philippines, Thailand*); **Dorent** (*India*); **Dozemo**

D

(*Thailand*); **Dozept** (*Ireland*); **Dozil** (*Hong Kong, Indonesia*); **Dozilax** (*Greece*); **Dozyl** (*Turkey*).
- **Endoclar** (*Argentina*); **Epez** (*Brazil*); **Eranz** (*Brazil, Venezuela*); **Evimal** (*Chile*); **Evocaz** (*Chile*).
- **Fang Qing** (*China*); **Fordesia** (*Indonesia*); **Fu Si Ke** (*China*); **Filosept** (*Greece*).
- **Gai Fei** (*China*).
- **Hania** (*Greece*).
- **Ideclar** (*Chile*).
- **Jia Qi** (*China*); **Jubezil** (*South Africa*).
- **Kognezil** (*Czech Republic*).
- **Labrea** (*Brazil*); **Landex** (*Czech Republic*); **Lirpan** (*Argentina*); **Lixben** (*Portugal, Spain*); **Lizidra** (*Italy*); **Lupracil** (*Argentina*).
- **Memac** (*Italy*); **Memkar** (*Turkey*); **Memoboost** (*Turkey*); **Memorit** (*Israel*); **Mensapex** (*Poland*); **Miltus** (*Greece*).
- **Navazil** (*Netherlands*); **Nepanizil** (*Greece*); **Nepecil** (*Venezuela*); **Nepezil** (*Greece*); **Nepizel** (*South Africa*); **Nepokare** (*Chile*); **Neurem** (*Turkey*); **Niritos** (*Greece*); **Nopez** (*Turkey*); **Nozil** (*India*); **Nuo Chong** (*China*).
- **Oldinot** (*Argentina*); **Onefin** (*Argentina*).
- **Palixid** (*Hungary*); **Pamigen** (*Poland*); **Penezil** (*Greece*); **Pezale** (*Greece*); **Peziled** (*Greece*); **Pezzil** (*Mexico*); **Promemore** (*Czech Republic*).
- **Rafazil** (*Greece*); **Rewind** (*Turkey*); **Ricordo** (*Poland*).
- **Sai Ling Si** (*China*); **Secca** (*Turkey*); **Senes** (*Brazil*); **Servonex** (*Philippines, Thailand*); **Si Bo Hai** (*China*); **Sulbenin** (*Greece*); **Sundonnez** (*Mexico*); **Symepezil** (*Poland*).
- **Tevapezil** (*Australia*); **Tonizep** (*Thailand*); **Torpezil** (*Philippines*).
- **Uxazen** (*Spain*).
- **Valpex** (*Argentina*); **Vastia** (*Hong Kong*); **Venaxen** (*Greece*).
- **Yasnal** (*Czech Republic, Poland, Russian Federation, Spain*); **Yasnoro** (*Italy*).
- **Zakalmer** (*Greece*); **Zamper** (*Venezuela*); **Zauton** (*Finland*); **Zepanalz** (*South Africa*); **Zhedon** (*Turkey*); **Ziledon** (*Brazil*); **Zilokline** (*Venezuela*); **Zinocept** (*Greece*); **Zopitel** (*Greece*).

Generics Available
- Yes.

Licensed Indications for Parkinson's Disease
- None.

Licensed Indications for Other Conditions
- Mild to severe dementia of the Alzheimer type (FDA, EMA, EMC).
- LBD (Japan).

THERAPEUTICS

D

DONEPEZIL

Non-Licensed Use for Parkinson's Disease
• Dementia associated with Parkinson's disease (FDA).

Non-Licensed Use for Other Conditions
• LBD.
• Traumatic brain injury.
• Vascular dementia.

Ineffective
• Mild cognitive impairment.
• Schizophrenia.
• MS-related cognitive impairment.
• Attention Deficit Hyperactivity Disorder.
• Post-Coronary Artery Bypass Graft surgery cognitive impairment.
• Down syndrome.
• CADASIL syndrome.

Mechanism of Action
• Donepezil is a reversible acetylcholinesterase inhibitor, which increases the availability of acetylcholine (ACh) in cholinergic synapses, thus enhancing cholinergic transmission.
    • Donepezil is highly selective for acetylcholinesterase with a much lower affinity for butyrylcholinesterase.
• Cholinesterase inhibitors, including donepezil, may reduce falls in Parkinson's disease because they affect gait and balance centres in the brain stem, which are believed to be cholinergic.
• Some non-cholinergic mechanisms have been reported:
    • It inhibits voltage-gated sodium currents reversibly and delays potassium currents, although no clinical effects have been linked to this mechanism.

Efficacy Profile
• Donepezil offers improvement of cognitive symptoms and improves global function in Parkinson's disease-related dementia.
    • At least one month of therapy is required in order to assess the clinical response to donepezil.
    • Individual response to donepezil cannot be predicted.
• According to the MDS EBM Committee, donepezil is considered:
    • 'Possibly useful' in the management of dementia in Parkinson's disease at a dose of 10 mg/day.
    • There are insufficient data to support the use of donepezil in improving gait and balance in Parkinson's disease; however, a reduction in the number of falls has been reported.
• Several high-quality studies with long follow-up periods (up to 96 weeks) have found that donepezil significantly improved cognitive performance in patients with Parkinson's disease or LBD.

D

- According to the results of a small study, donepezil may exert a beneficial effect on visual hallucinations in LDB patients, which is maintained for more than 6 months of therapy. An increased rate of relapse of visual hallucinations was also observed, which was effectively addressed with an increase in donepezil dosage. However, these findings were not confirmed in other studies.
- In Alzheimer's disease patients, the effects of donepezil were maintained in the long-term (up to 4.9 years) in open-label studies.

Pharmacokinetics

Absorption and Distribution
- Oral bioavailability: around 100%.
- Food co-ingestion: food does not affect donepezil absorption.
- Tmax: about 3–4 h after oral administration.
- Time to steady state: within 3 weeks of therapy initiation.
- Pharmacokinetics: linear at therapeutic dose range.
- Protein binding: about 95%.
- Volume of distribution: 12–16 l/kg.

Metabolism
- Donepezil is partially metabolized by cytochrome P450 to multiple metabolites, some of which have not been identified.
  - CYP3A4 isoenzymes and to a minor extent CYP2D6 are involved in donepezil metabolism.

Elimination
- Elimination half-life is 70 h.
- About 57% of an administered dose is excreted in the urine (17% as unchanged donepezil) and about 15% is found in the faeces, while 28% remained unrecovered.

Drug Interaction Profile

Pharmacokinetic Drug Interactions
- Effects on donepezil:
- CYP3A4 and CYP2D6 inhibitors (e.g. *ketoconazole, itraconazole, erythromycin, quinidine, fluoxetine*) can inhibit the metabolism of donepezil and increase its plasma levels and effects.
  - CYP3A4 and CYP2D6 inducers (e.g. *rifampicin, phenytoin, carbamazepine*) may decrease donepezil plasma concentrations and effects.

Pharmacodynamic Drug Interactions
- Co-medication with other cholinesterase blocking agents (e.g. *neostigmine, physostigmine*) may lead to synergistic effects.

D

DONEPEZIL

- Co-medication with beta-blockers (e.g. *carvedilol, metoprolol, atenolol, propranolol*) may increase the risk of bradycardia.
- Donepezil may prolong the effects of depolarizing neuromuscular blocking agents (e.g. *suxamethonium*).
- Co-medication with drugs causing electrolyte imbalance or increasing QT interval, such as Class IA and III anti-arrhythmics, antipsychotics (e.g. *haloperidol, phenothiazine derivatives, pimozide*), tricyclic antidepressants, certain antimicrobial agents (e.g. *moxifloxacin, erythromycin*), certain antihistamines (e.g. *astemizole, mizolastine*), and others may lead to potentially fatal Torsade de Pointes arrhythmias and is considered a risk factor for sudden cardiac death.

Adverse Effects

How Drug Causes Adverse Effects
- Most of the adverse effects are cholinergic in nature.

Common Adverse Effects
- Very common (≥1/10):
  ○ Diarrhoea, nausea, headache.
- Common (≥1/100 to <1/10):
  ○ Nervous/psychiatric: hallucinations, agitation, aggressive behaviour, abnormal dreams/nightmares, syncope, dizziness, insomnia, confusion.
  ○ Cardiovascular: hypertension.
  ○ Gastrointestinal: abdominal discomfort, vomiting.
  ○ Skin: rash, pruritus.
  ○ Urinary: urinary incontinence.
  ○ General: common cold, anorexia, muscle cramps, fatigue, pain, accidents.
- Uncommon (≥1/1,000 to <1/100):
  ○ Cardiovascular: bradycardia.
  ○ Gastrointestinal: gastrointestinal haemorrhage, gastric/duodenal ulcers.
  ○ General: CPK increase.

Life-Threatening or Dangerous Adverse Effects
- NMS.
- Sino-atrial/atrioventricular block.
- Generalized convulsions.
- Rhabdomyolysis.

Rare and Not Life-Threatening Adverse Effects
- Extrapyramidal symptoms.
- Hepatic impairment.
- Bladder outflow obstruction.

D

Weight Change
- Donepezil might cause weight loss.

What to Do About Adverse Effects
- Before introducing donepezil, discuss common or life-threatening adverse effects with patients and/or caregivers, including symptoms that should be reported to the treating physician.
- Donepezil should only be prescribed if a caregiver is available to regularly monitor drug intake and the occurrence of adverse effects for the patient.
- Patients and/or caregivers should be made aware that donepezil use might worsen parkinsonian symptoms (including tremor and dystonia) and to inform their treating physician if this occurs. This was not confirmed in patients with LBD or PDD.
- Patients and/or caregivers should be aware of the potential vagotonic effects of donepezil (e.g. bradycardia), as there might be synergistic effects with the antiparkinsonian drugs (e.g. orthostatic hypotension), which may lead to loss of consciousness.
- If troublesome or persistent adverse effects are present, considering lowering the dose of donepezil or completely withdrawing the drug.
- Caution is advised in patients with increased risk for rhabdomyolysis (e.g. predisposing medication). In case of increased levels of CPK or development of relevant symptoms, consider discontinuing donepezil therapy.
- If patients develop manifestations indicative of NMS or present with unexplained fever (even without any additional signs and symptoms suggestive of neuroleptic malignant-like syndrome), donepezil therapy should be discontinued.
- The ability of patients on donepezil to drive or operate machinery should be regularly monitored, not only because donepezil can cause fatigue, dizziness, and muscle cramps, but also due to the patients' background of dementia.

Dosing and Use

Usual Dosage Range
- Tablets or oral disintegrating tablet (ODT): 5–10 mg per day for Parkinson's disease–related dementia.

Available Formulations
- Tablet: 5 mg, 10 mg, 23 mg.
- Tablet, ODT: 5 mg, 10 mg.

How to Dose
- Initial dose of 5 mg OD at bedtime; may increase to 10 mg OD after 4–6 weeks, if needed.
  - The tablets' formulations are bioequivalent to the ODT formulations, so the same dosing principles apply.

DOSING AND USE

D

DONEPEZIL

Dosing Tips
- Donepezil is taken at bedtime, with or without food.
- ODT: dissolve on tongue and follow with water.
- Maintenance therapy can be continued for as long as there is therapeutic benefit.

How to Withdraw Drug
- Abrupt discontinuation of donepezil in patients with PDD and LBD has been associated with cognitive and behavioural decline; thus, a gradual withdrawal is suggested.
- A dose reduction at the next lower dose is suggested for 2 weeks before the dose is stopped completely.
- The recommended tapering schedule may be tailored according to circumstances. In case of severe adverse events, donepezil can be discontinued without tapering.

Overdose
- Overdosage with cholinesterase inhibitors, including donepezil, can lead to a cholinergic crisis, characterized by severe nausea, vomiting, salivation, sweating, bradycardia, hypotension, respiratory depression, collapse, and convulsions. Muscle weakness is also possible and might be fatal if respiratory muscles are involved.
- General supportive measures are suggested.
- It is unknown whether donepezil or its metabolites can be removed by haemodialysis, peritoneal dialysis, or haemofiltration.
- Anticholinergics, like *atropine*, might serve as antidote.
- Donepezil and/or its metabolites may persist in the body for more than 10 days.

Tests and Therapeutic Drug Monitoring
- An ECG should be performed before initiation of donepezil therapy to check for QT prolongation.
- An objective scoring of cognitive performance should take place during donepezil therapy.

Other Warnings/Precautions
- Donepezil can increase gastric acid secretion; thus, caution is advised for individuals at risk of gastric ulcer disease or gastrointestinal bleeding (e.g. co-medication with NSAIDs).
- Due to donepezil cholinomimetic actions, caution is advised in patients with pre-existing seizures disorders, urinary tract obstruction, cardiac conduction abnormalities, or respiratory disease, including COPD and asthma and those at risk of cardiac repolarization.
- Cholinesterase inhibitors, including donepezil, might enhance succinylcholine-type muscle relaxation during anaesthesia.
- Donepezil is metabolised by CYP450 enzymes, concomitant use with CYP450 inhibitors or inducers should be done with caution due to unknown magnitude of effects on drug concentrations.

D

Do Not Use (Contraindications)
- Known hypersensitivity to donepezil or its excipients, including lactose monohydrate.
  - Patients with rare hereditary problems of galactose intolerance, total lactase deficiency, or glucose–galactose malabsorption should not receive donepezil.
- Donepezil administration in patients at high risk of prolonged cardiac repolarization (e.g. co-medication with drugs increasing QT interval) should be avoided.

Special Populations
Renal Impairment
- Donepezil use has not been studied in renal impairment.
- Caution is recommended in case of renal impairment.

Hepatic Impairment
- Donepezil use has not been studied in hepatic impairment.
- Caution is recommended in case of hepatic impairment.

Elderly
- No dose adjustments are required.

Pregnancy
- Animal studies have not confirmed a teratogenic effect of donepezil, but have shown peri- and postnatal toxicity. Data on humans are insufficient.
- Donepezil should not be used during pregnancy.

Breastfeeding
- Donepezil is found in the milk of rats. Data on humans are insufficient.
- Women on donepezil should not breastfeed.

COSTS

Costs
NHS indicative price accessed 30 June 2022:
- Aricept: 28 × 5 mg tablets £59.85.
- Aricept 28 × 10 mg tablets £83.89.
- Generic: 28 × 5 mg tablets £0.73–£59.85.
- Generic: 28 × 10 mg tablets £0.91–£83.89.
- Aricept Evess: 28 × 5 mg orodispersible tablets £59.85.
- Aricept Evess 28 × 10 mg orodispersible tablets £83.89.
- Generic: 28 × 5 mg orodispersible tablets £15.30–£83.89.
- Generic: 28 × 10 mg orodispersible tablets £59.02–£71.31.
- 150 ml of 1 mg/ml oral solution £81.23.

D

The Overall Place of Donepezil in the Treatment of Parkinson's Disease

Donepezil is a highly specific and reversible acetylcholinesterase inhibitor, which, despite being typically used in Alzheimer's disease, also constitutes an off-label therapeutic option for other kinds of dementia, including LBD and PDD. It delays the progression of cognitive symptoms and improves global function in Parkinson's disease-related dementia, while it has been associated with a decreased risk of falls and a potential beneficial effect on Parkinson's disease-related hallucinations and psychosis. Compared to rivastigmine, there is less evidence to support its efficacy in Parkinson's disease-related dementia; however, it is believed to have a more benign safety profile. It is generally considered well-tolerated with the majority of side effects being mild, transient, and cholinergic in nature. Vigilance is required, though, especially from the patient's caregiver, to detect potential adverse events and inform the treating physician.

Potential Advantages
- The rapidly disintegrating formulation can assist patients with swallowing difficulties.
- Once daily administration of donepezil might improve patients' adherence.
- Donepezil has a broad spectrum of efficacy (mild to severe dementia) and a simple titration scheme.
- Donepezil is thought to have a more benign safety profile compared to rivastigmine.

Potential Disadvantages
- Donepezil use has been associated with cholinergic adverse effects and drug interaction, which might be an issue for elderly Parkinson's disease patients, as co-morbidities and polypharmacy in this group are frequent.

Clinical Box

An 80-year-old man with a 9-year history of Parkinson's disease presented at the Neurology Department Outpatient Clinic with his wife due to deteriorating memory problems. He also mentioned a few episodes of visual hallucinations (e.g. human figures, children), especially at dusk, which were not frightening to him and he acknowledged they were not real. His current medication included levodopa/benserazide 200 mg/50 mg QID and rasagiline 1 mg OD. The patient was relatively independent in his everyday life, experienced no particular motor fluctuations, and both he and his wife were satisfied with general performance and his current regimen. The rest of his medical history included well-controlled diabetes mellitus II and hypercholesterolaemia. During the assessment, mild-to-moderate cognitive impairment was detected.

D

The patient was scheduled for blood tests and a brain MRI scan, which came back with unremarkable findings. A diagnosis of Parkinson's disease-related dementia was considered possible. As the hallucinations were not particularly troublesome to the patient, changes to his current dopaminergic medications were not considered necessary. A decision to initiate an acetylcholinesterase inhibitor was made. The patient opted for the simplest possible dosing scheme, and therefore donepezil 5 mg OD at bedtime was prescribed. The patient and his caregiver were informed about potential side effects and given instructions to double the dose in 6 weeks.

Suggested Reading

Aarsland D, K Laake, JP Laron, C Janvin. Donepezil for cognitive impairment in Parkinson's disease: a randomised controlled study. *J Neurol Neurosurg Psychiatry* 2002; 72(6): 708–712.

Chung KA, BM Lobb, JG Nutt, FB Horak. Effects of a central cholinesterase inhibitor on reducing falls in Parkinson disease. *Neurology* 2010; 75(14): 1263–1269.

Dubois B, E Tolosa, R Katzenschlager, M Emre, AJ Lees, G Schumann, E Pourcher, J Gray, G Thomas, J Swartz, T Hsu, ML Moline. Donepezil in Parkinson's disease dementia: a randomized, double-blind efficacy and safety study. *Mov Disord* 2012; 27(10): 1230–1238.

Ravina B, M Putt, A Siderowf, JT Farrar, M Gillespie, A Crawley, HH Fernandez, MM Trieschmann, S Reichwein, T Simuni. Donepezil for dementia in Parkinson's disease: a randomised, double blind, placebo controlled, crossover study. *J Neurol Neurosurg Psychiatry* 2005; 76(7): 934–939.

Shigeta M, A Homma. Donepezil for Alzheimer's disease: pharmacodynamic, pharmacokinetic, and clinical profiles. *CNS Drug Rev* 2001; 7(4): 353–368.

References

AHFS Drug information 2012. Bethesda: American Society of Health-System Pharmacists. Accessed on 30 June 2022 via www.medicinescomplete.com.

Allen NE, CG Canning, LRS Almeida, BR Bloem, SHJ Keus, N Löfgren, A Niewboer, GSAF Verheyden, TP Yamato, C Sherrington. Interventions for preventing falls in Parkinson's disease. *Cochrane Database Syst Rev* 2022; 6(6): CD011574.

Bergman J, V Lerner. Successful use of donepezil for the treatment of psychotic symptoms in patients with Parkinson's disease. *Clin Neuropharmacol* 2002; 25(2): 107–110.

Burns A, S Gauthier, C Perdomo. Efficacy and safety of donepezil over 3 years: an open-label, multicentre study in patients with Alzheimer's disease. *Int J Geriatr Psychiatry* 2007; 22(8): 806–812.

D

Donepezil. In: Brayfield A (Ed.), *Martindale: The Complete Drug Reference*. London: The Royal Pharmaceutical Society of Great Britain. Accessed on 30 June 2022 via www.medicinescomplete.com.

Donepezil. In: DRUGDEX® System (electronic version). Truven Health Analytics, Greenwood Village, Colorado, USA. Accessed on 30 June 2022 via http://www.micromedexsolutions.com.

Joint Formulary Committee. British National Formulary (online). London: BMJ Group and Pharmaceutical Press. Accessed on 30 June 2022 via www.medicinescomplete.com.

Leroi I, J Brandt, SG Reich, CG Lyketsos, S Grill, R Thompson, L Marsh. Randomized placebo-controlled trial of donepezil in cognitive impairment in Parkinson's disease. *Int J Geriatr Psychiatry* 2004; 19(1): 1–8.

Minett TS, A Thomas, LM Wilkinson, SL Daniel, J Sanders, J Richardson, E Littlewood, P Myint, J Newby, IG McKeith. What happens when donepezil is suddenly withdrawn? An open label trial in dementia with Lewy bodies and Parkinson's disease with dementia. *Int J Geriatr Psychiatry* 2003; 18(11): 988–993.

Mueller C, AP Rajkumar, YM Wan, L Velayudhan, D Ffytche, KR Chaudhuri, D Aarsland. Assessment and management of neuropsychiatric symptoms in Parkinson's disease. *CNS Drugs* 2018; 32(7): 621–635.

Rogers SL, RS Doody, RD Pratt, JR Ieni. Long-term efficacy and safety of donepezil in the treatment of Alzheimer's disease: final analysis of a US multicentre open-label study. *Eur Neuropsychopharmacol* 2000; 10(3): 195–203.

Rolinski M, C Fox, I Maidment, R McShane ; Cochrane Dementia and Cognitive Improvement Group. Cholinesterase inhibitors for dementia with Lewy bodies, Parkinson's disease dementia and cognitive impairment in Parkinson's disease. *Cochrane Database Syst Rev* 2012; 2012(3): CD006504.

Sawada H, T Oeda, M Kohsaka, A Umemura, S Tomita, K Park, K Mizoguchi, H Matsuo, K Hasegawa, H Fujimura, H Sugiyama, M Nakamura, S Kikuchi, K Yamamoto, T Fukuda, S Ito, M Goto, K Kiyohara, T Kawamura. Early use of donepezil against psychosis and cognitive decline in Parkinson's disease: a randomised controlled trial for 2 years. *J Neurol Neurosurg Psychiatry* 2018; 89(12): 1332–1340.

Sobow T. Parkinson's disease-related visual hallucinations unresponsive to atypical antipsychotics treated with cholinesterase inhibitors: a case series. *Neurol Neurochir Pol* 2007; 41(3): 276–279.

Summary of Product Characteristics – Aricept tablets 10 mg. Eisai Ltd. Electronic Medicines Compendium: Aricept tablets 10 mg – summary of product characteristics (SmPC) – (emc). Accessed on 30 June 2022 via www.medicines.org.uk.

Ukai K, H Fujishiro, S Iritani, N Ozaki. Long-term efficacy of donepezil for relapse of visual hallucinations in patients with dementia with Lewy bodies. *Psychogeriatrics* 2015; 15(2): 133–137.

DONEPEZIL

DROXIDOPA

D

Therapeutics

Chemical Name and Structure
Droxidopa ((–)-threo-3-(3,4-dihydroxyphenyl)-L-serine) is an odourless, tasteless, white to off-white crystalline powder, which is slightly soluble to water. It has a molecular weight of 213.2 and a molecular formula of $C_9H_{11}NO_5$.

Brand Names
• **Dops** (*Japan*).
• **Northera** (*USA*).

Generics Available
• Yes.

Licensed Indications for Parkinson's Disease
• Neurogenic orthostatic hypotension in Parkinson's disease (FDA).

Licensed Indications for Other Conditions
• Neurogenic orthostatic hypotension in patients with primary autonomic failure, dopamine beta-hydroxylase deficiency, and non-diabetic autonomic neuropathy (FDA).

Non-Licensed Use for Parkinson's Disease
• Orthostatic hypotension in Parkinson's disease.

Non-Licensed Use for Other Conditions
• None.

Ineffective
• Fatigue in the context of parkinsonism (NCT03446807).

Mechanism of Action
• Droxidopa is a synthetic amino-acid analogue, which acts as a prodrug to the neurotransmitter noradrenaline. After absorption, droxidopa is converted to noradrenaline by the enzyme dopa-decarboxylase, which is ubiquitously distributed in human tissues.
• Droxidopa is believed to exert its pharmacological effect through its conversion to noradrenaline.
  • Noradrenaline increases blood pressure through peripheral arterial and venous vasoconstriction.
  • Peak droxidopa and noradrenaline plasma concentrations coincide with the increase in blood pressure.
• In contrast to noradrenaline, droxidopa may cross the blood–brain barrier.

THERAPEUTICS

D

Efficacy Profile
- Droxidopa has been characterized as 'efficacious' and 'possibly useful' in the treatment of orthostatic hypotension in Parkinson's disease, but only for short-term use (1 week).
  - There is insufficient evidence to conclude efficacy in the long term; thus, prolonged use of droxidopa in Parkinson's disease patients is not recommended.
- The effect of droxidopa on orthostatic hypotension in Parkinson's disease was examined in one RCT with an 8-week follow-up period, which was preceded by a titration period of up to 2 weeks. A statistically significant change was only found for the first week of therapy with droxidopa compared to placebo.
- In multi-centre clinical trials, droxidopa was found to have a positive effect on orthostatic hypotension-related dizziness, vision disturbance, weakness, and fatigue, while the patients' ability to stand or walk was enhanced.
- In Japan, there have been earlier reports of droxidopa in the management of FoG in Parkinson's disease patients with conflicting results. More recent reports have published some encouraging results on levodopa-resistant FoG co-administered with a COMT inhibitor (entacapone) to prevent droxidopa peripheral metabolism. A Chinese group has reported a beneficial effect of droxidopa on overall mobility, including tremor and stiffness and activities of daily living in moderate-to-severe Parkinson's disease. No such effects have been reported from other countries.

Pharmacokinetics
Absorption and Distribution
- Oral bioavailability: about 90%.
- Food co-ingestion: high-fat meals may affect droxidopa absorption, resulting in lower plasma concentration and longer Tmax (~2 h).
- Tmax: 1–4 h.
- Pharmacokinetics: droxidopa and noradrenaline levels decrease mono- and multi-exponentially, respectively.
  - Despite the short half-life of noradrenaline (1–2 min), its levels remain elevated due to gradual conversion from droxidopa, which is apparently taken up by neuronal and non-neuronal tissues.
- Protein binding: 75% (100 ng/ml), 26% (10000 ng/ml).
- Volume of distribution: 200 l.

Metabolism
- Droxidopa metabolism is mediated by the catecholamine pathway:
  - COMT converts droxidopa to methoxylated dihydroxyphenylserine (3-OM-DOPS),
  - DOPA decarboxylase converts droxidopa to noradrenaline, and
  - DOPS aldolase converts droxidopa to protocatechualdehyde.

- Apart from noradrenaline, the role of droxidopa metabolites in its clinical effects is not clear.
- Droxidopa is not metabolized by CYP450.

Elimination
- Half-life of droxidopa is 2–3 h.
- Renal excretion: 75% of an administered dose is excreted in urine within 24 h of oral dosing.

Drug Interaction Profile
Pharmacokinetic Drug Interactions
- Effects on droxidopa:
  - Co-medication with aromatic amino-acid decarboxylase inhibitors (e.g. *carbidopa*, *benserazide*) may lead to lower levels of droxidopa due to peripheral inhibition of the enzyme dopa-decarboxylase, which converts droxidopa to norepinephrine.

Pharmacodynamic Drug Interactions
- Co-medication with triptans (e.g. *sumatriptan*), sympathomimetic agents (e.g. *phenylephrine*, *pseudoephedrine*), non-selective MAOIs, SNRIs, and caffeine may potentiate the pressor effects of droxidopa.
- Co-medication with neuroleptics may cause NMS.

Adverse Effects
How Drug Causes Adverse Effects
- Droxidopa mainly causes adverse effects through adrenergic activity.

Common Adverse Effects
- Very common (≥1/10):
  - Headache (mostly in long-term use), falls, syncope, urinary tract infections.
- Common (≥1/100 to <1/10):
  - Neuropsychiatric: dizziness.
  - Cardiovascular: (supine) hypertension.
  - GI: nausea.

Life-Threatening or Dangerous Adverse Effects
- Unknown frequency:
  - Hypersensitivity reactions, such as anaphylaxis, angioedema, bronchospasm, urticaria and rash.
  - Pancreatitis.
  - Delirium.
  - Cerebrovascular events.
  - Neuroleptic malignant-like syndrome.

D

Rare and Not Life-Threatening Adverse Effects
• Abdominal pain, vomiting, diarrhoea.
• Fatigue.
• Psychosis, hallucinations, agitation, memory disorder.
• Blurred vision.

Weight Change
• Not reported.

What to Do About Adverse Effects
• Before introducing droxidopa therapy, discuss common or life-threatening adverse effects with patients and/or caregivers, including symptoms that should be reported to the physician.
• Patients can be instructed to elevate the head of their bed at least 30–45° at night when sleeping in order to lower the risk for supine hypertension. If supine hypertension occurs despite this manoeuvre, reconsider dose reduction or cessation of droxidopa.
• In case of hypersensitivity reaction, droxidopa therapy should be discontinued and appropriate treatment should be applied.
• Droxidopa may trigger an uncommon but fatal symptom complex, similar to neuroleptic malignant-like syndrome, which may present with fever or hyperthermia, muscle rigidity, involuntary movements, altered consciousness, and mental status changes. In order to lower this risk, close monitoring is advised when droxidopa dose modifications are introduced, particularly in patients receiving neuroleptics.

Dosing and Use
Usual Dosage Range
• 300–1,800 mg.

Available Formulations
• Capsules: 100 mg, 200 mg, 300 mg.

How to Dose
• An initial dose of droxidopa 100 mg TID is suggested; titrate in increments of 100 mg TID every 1–2 days according to symptomatic response; a maximum dose of 600 mg TID (total dose of 1,800 mg per day) is recommended.
• Continued benefit of droxidopa should be reassessed periodically during therapy.

Dosing Tips
• The first dose should be received upon rising in the morning, the second at midday and the third late in the afternoon at least 3 h before bedtime to lower the risk of supine hypertension.
• Droxidopa should be given at the same times every day.

D

- In case of advanced patients who are ambulatory only for a few hours in the morning, consider administering a single droxidopa dose in the morning.
- Depending on patients' needs, higher droxidopa doses may be needed in the morning compared to the afternoon or evening; droxidopa scheme can be tailored accordingly.
- Droxidopa should be received consistently with or without food.
- Droxidopa therapy duration in Parkinson's disease should not exceed 2 weeks of titration plus 1 week of maintenance therapy.

How to Withdraw Drug
- Droxidopa can be abruptly discontinued in case of adverse events.

Overdose
- Reported cases of droxidopa overdosage presented with hypertension-related complications, such as intracranial haemorrhage.
- There is no known antidote for droxidopa overdose.
- If high blood pressure is measured after droxidopa overdose, consider cessation of droxidopa, close monitoring, supportive measures, and symptomatic therapy.

Tests and Therapeutic Drug Monitoring
- Before initiation of droxidopa therapy:
  - Supine, sitting, and 3-min standing blood pressure should be measured.
- During droxidopa therapy:
  - Supine, sitting, and 3-min standing blood pressure should be regularly monitored, especially in dosage increases. Night measurements should also be included.

Other Warnings/Precautions
- Droxidopa has a black box warning for causing supine hypertension, which, if left untreated, can predispose to cardiovascular events, particularly strokes.
- Special consideration should be given before starting droxidopa therapy in patients with ischaemic heart disease, arrhythmias, or congestive heart failure, as the sympathomimetic properties of droxidopa may aggravate these conditions.
- Close monitoring is advised in case of co-administration with triptans, sympathomimetics, SNRIs, and caffeine due to additive sympathetic effects, including an increased risk for supine hypertension.
  - The same applies in case of co-administration with *fludrocortisone* or *midodrine*.
- In case of co-administration with an aromatic L-amino acid decarboxylase inhibitor (such as carbidopa or benserazide), higher doses of droxidopa (within the defined usual dosage range) may be needed.

DOSING AND USE

D

DROXIDOPA

• Co-administration with non-selective MAOIs and *linezolid* may result in increased blood pressure.
• No side effects have been observed with the co-administration of droxidopa with selective MAO-B inhibitors, including *rasagiline* or *selegiline*.

Do Not Use (Contraindications)
• Known sensitivity to droxidopa or to any of the excipients, including FD+C Yellow No. 5 (tartrazine).

Special Populations
Renal Impairment
• Mild to moderate impairment (GFR > 30 ml/min): no dosage modifications needed.
• Severe impairment (GFR < 30 ml/min): no data available; caution is advised.

Hepatic Impairment
• Not reported.

Elderly
• No differences reported.

Pregnancy
• No data are available on the effects of droxidopa in pregnant women or the fetus.
• Droxidopa use is generally not recommended in pregnancy.

Breastfeeding
• No data are available on the effects of droxidopa on breastfeeding infants or on milk production.
• A risk to the nursing child cannot be excluded; thus, droxidopa use is not recommended during breastfeeding.

Costs
• Not available in the UK for comparison.

The Overall Place of Droxidopa in the Treatment of Parkinson's Disease
Droxidopa is a precursor/prodrug of noradrenaline with conversion mediated by the ubiquitous enzyme dopa-decarboxylase. Droxidopa exerts its beneficial effects in Parkinson's disease by elevating noradrenaline levels. It was initially approved in Japan in 1989 for the treatment

D

of neurogenic orthostatic hypotension associated with various disorders, including Parkinson's disease. Early applications of droxidopa included management of freezing phenomena and dysarthria in Parkinson's disease patients, but also of levodopa-resistant gait apraxia in parkinsonian patients, including those with a post-mortem neuropathological diagnosis of PSP. In 2014, droxidopa was approved by the FDA for the short-term treatment of neurogenic orthostatic hypotension (no more than 2 weeks of therapy) based on high-quality studies, including one RCT which focused on Parkinson's disease-related orthostatic hypotension, although the results were not always favourable for droxidopa.

Orthostatic hypotension is a particularly troublesome non-motor symptom in Parkinson's disease and specifically in the noradrenergic subtype of Parkinson's disease, which can limit daily activities and result in falls, but also affect the therapeutic options for the management of motor symptoms. Droxidopa levels may be mildly affected (lower concentration) by the co-administration of a peripheral decarboxylase inhibitor (such as carbidopa or benserazide). Furthermore, COMT inhibitors may decrease the metabolism of droxidopa by O-methylation resulting in enhanced activity.

Short regimens of droxidopa administration are generally well tolerated. It is worth noting, however, that droxidopa use might result in comparable increases in standing and supine blood pressure. Thus, treating physicians should be vigilant in noting potential supine hypertension. Open-label studies have demonstrated a sustained effect of droxidopa on orthostatic hypotension without significant supine hypertension or other major safety issues; however, longer high-quality studies are still required to verify these findings.

Potential Advantages
• Unlike noradrenaline, it can be administered orally.

Potential Disadvantages
• It is only available in Japan and the USA.
• Droxidopa is only effective in the short term.
• Its use is associated with a significant risk of supine hypertension.

CLINICAL BOX

Clinical Box
A 70-year-old man with a 7-year history of Parkinson's disease was referred to the Movement Disorders Outpatient Clinic by his GP. The patient was on levodopa/carbidopa 100 mg/25 mg TID and rotigotine patch 4 mg/24 h. For the past 6 months the patient reported symptoms of dizziness upon standing and fatigue. His GP made a diagnosis of orthostatic hypotension after regular measurements of blood pressure in the supine and standing position. He was initially instructed to follow non-pharmacological interventions (increased fluids and salt intake), but without success. Rotigotine was subsequently gradually withdrawn and

D

replaced by an extra dose of levodopa/carbidopa (levodopa/carbidopa 100 mg/25 mg QID) to avoid compromising his motor performance. Due to persistent symptoms, which did not correlate with levodopa administration timing, he was prescribed fludrocortisone and then midodrine, which were effective for a short while, but he had repeated faints related to orthostatic syncope. The patient was subsequently started on droxidopa 100 mg TID and was instructed to increase the dose by 100 mg every 1–2 days until alleviation of symptoms or the maximum dose of 600 mg TID was reached. Thorough instructions were given to avoid the development of supine hypertension (elevation of bed head). The patient reported that symptoms resolved at a droxidopa dose of 200 mg TID.

Suggested Reading

Elgebaly A, B Abdelazeim, O Mattar, M Gadelkarim, R Salah, A Negida. Meta-analysis of the safety and efficacy of droxidopa for neurogenic orthostatic hypotension. *Clin Auton Res* 2016; 26(3): 171–180.

Hauser RA, S Isaacson, JP Lisk, LA Hewitt, G Rowse. Droxidopa for the short-term treatment of symptomatic neurogenic orthostatic hypotension in Parkinson's disease (nOH306B). *Mov Disord* 2015; 30(5): 646–554.

Kaufmann H, R Freeman, I Biaggioni, P Low, S Pedder, A Hewitt, C Mathias. Treatment of neurogenic orthostatic hypotension with droxidopa: results from a multi-center, double-blind, randomized, placebo-controlled, parallel group, induction design study (PL02.001). *Neurology* 2012; 78(1 Supplement): PL02.001.

Zhao S, R Cheng, J Zheng, Q Li, J Wang, W Fan, L Zhang, Y Zhang, H Li, S Liu. A randomized, double-blind, controlled trial of add-on therapy in moderate-to-severe Parkinson's disease. *Parkinsonism Relat Disord* 2015; 21(10): 1214–1218.

References

AHFS Drug information, 2012. Bethesda: American Society of Health-System Pharmacists. Accessed on 12 December 2022 via www.medicinescomplete.com.

Biaggioni I, R Freeman, CJ Mathias, P Low, LA Hewitt, H Kaufmann. Randomized withdrawal study of patients with symptomatic neurogenic orthostatic hypotension responsive to droxidopa. *Hypertension* 2015; 65(1): 101–107.

Droxidopa. In: Brayfield A (Ed.), *Martindale: The Complete Drug Reference*. London: The Royal Pharmaceutical Society of Great Britain. Accessed on 12 December via www.medicinescomplete.com.

Droxidopa. In: DRUGDEX® System (electronic version). Truven Health Analytics, Greenwood Village, Colorado, USA. Accessed on 12 December via www.micromedexsolutions.com.

D

Fukada K, T Endo, M Yokoe, T Hamasaki, T Hazama, S Sakoda. L-threo-3,4-dihydroxyphenylserine (L-DOPS) co-administered with entacapone improves freezing of gait in Parkinson's disease. *Med Hypotheses* 2013; 80(2): 209–212.

Isaacson S, S Vernino, A Ziemann, GJ Rowse, U Kalu, WB White. Long-term safety of droxidopa in patients with symptomatic neurogenic orthostatic hypotension. *J Am Soc Hypertens* 2016; 10(10): 755–762.

Kaufmann H, L Norcliffe-Kaufmann, JA Palma. Droxidopa in neurogenic orthostatic hypotension. *Expert Rev Cardiovasc Ther* 2015; 13(8): 875–991.

Matsuo H, H Takashima, M Kishikawa, I Kinoshita, M Mori, M Tsujihata, S Nagataki. Pure akinesia: an atypical manifestation of progressive supranuclear palsy. *J Neurol Neurosurg Psychiatry* 1991; 54(5): 397–400.

Ogawa N, M Yamamoto, H Takayama. L-threo-3, 4-dihydroxyphenyl-serine treatment of Parkinson's disease. *J Med* 1985; 16(5–6): 525–534.

Ray Chaudhuri K, V Leta, K Bannister, DJ Brooks, P Svenningsson. The noradrenergic subtype of Parkinson disease: from animal models to clinical practice. *Nat Rev Neurol* 2023; 19: 333–345.

Tohgi H, T Abe, S Takahashi. The effects of L-threo-3,4-dihydroxyphe-nylserine on the total norepinephrine and dopamine concentrations in the cerebrospinal fluid and freezing gait in parkinsonian patients. *J Neural Transm Park Dis Dement Sect* 1993: 5(1): 27–34.

Yoshida M, S Noguchi, S. Kuramoto. L-threo-3,4-dihydroxyphenylser-ine treatment for gait apraxia in parkinsonian patients. *Kurume Med J* 1989; 36(2): 67–74.

REFERENCES

ENTACAPONE

Therapeutics

Chemical Name and Structure

Entacapone ((*E*)-2-cyano-3-(3,4-dihydroxy-5-nitrophenyl)-*N*,*N*-diethyl-2-propenamide) has a molecular weight of 305.29 and a molecular formula of $C_{14}H_{15}N_3O_5$.

Brand Names
* **Adcapone** (*India*).
* **Comtan** (*Argentina, Australia, Austria, Belgium, Brazil, Canada, China, Cyprus, Czech Republic, Estonia, Finland,* France, *Germany, Greece, Hong Kong, Hungary, Indonesia, Ireland, Israel, Italy, Japan, Malaysia, Mexico, Netherlands, New Zealand, Philippines, Poland, Portugal, Singapore, South Africa, Spain, Switzerland, Thailand, Tunisia, Turkey, Ukraine, USA, Venezuela*); **Comtess** (*Czech Republic, Denmark, Estonia, Finland, Greece, Ireland, Lithuania, Netherlands, Norway, Poland, Portugal, Sweden, UK*).
* **Encapia** (*Cyprus, Estonia, Netherlands*); **Enkobist** (*South Africa*); **Enpon** (*Hong Kong*); **Entacom** (*India*); **Entapone** (*New Zealand*); **Entarkin** (*Brazil*).
* **Medapia** (*Lithuania, Spain*).

Generics Available
* Yes.

Licensed Indications for Parkinson's Disease
* Adjunctive treatment to standard preparations of levodopa/benserazide or levodopa/carbidopa and for end-of-dose motor fluctuations that cannot be stabilized on those combinations (FDA, EMA, EMC).

Licensed Indications for Other Conditions
* None.

Non-Licensed Use for Parkinson's Disease
* Adjunctive treatment to standard preparations of levodopa/benserazide or levodopa/carbidopa and end-of-dose non-motor fluctuations.

Non-Licensed Use for Other Conditions
* None.

Ineffective
* Ineffective in patients not receiving levodopa therapy at the same time as each entacapone dose.

Mechanism of Action
* Selective and reversible, peripherally acting, COMT inhibitor, designed for concomitant administration with levodopa preparations.

E

- It decreases the peripheral metabolism of levodopa to 3–O–methyldopa (3-OMD) by inhibiting COMT. This action leads to higher and more sustained plasma levodopa concentrations, while prolonging the clinical response to levodopa.
- In clinical practice, the addition of entacapone is expected to prolong the response of each levodopa dose by about 30–60 min, offering the patient 1–2 h of extra ON time a day.
- Entacapone does not cross the blood–brain barrier.

Efficacy Profile
- Entacapone is efficacious whether combined with standard or controlled-release levodopa preparations.
- Entacapone has been characterized as 'non-efficacious' and 'not useful' for symptomatic adjunct therapy in early or stable Parkinson's disease patients and to prevent/delay motor fluctuations.
- Entacapone has been characterized as 'efficacious' and 'clinically useful' for the treatment of motor fluctuations in Parkinson's disease.
- Numerous RCTs have found that entacapone can substantially increase ON time by 1–2 h (with a concomitant decrease in OFF time). Entacapone use has also been associated with a reduction of total levodopa dose in Parkinson's disease patients with motor fluctuations.
- Entacapone exhibits a good long-term safety profile and a sustained beneficial effect in Parkinson's disease patients with motor fluctuations according to results from a 3-year open-label extension study (NOMECOMT study group).
- Open-label study indicates motor benefit during sleep and improvement of Parkinson's Disease Sleep Scale (PDSS) scores with the use of nocturnal entacapone.

Pharmacokinetics
Absorption and Distribution
- Oral bioavailability: 35%.
- Food co-ingestion: neither delays nor reduces the rate of absorption.
- Tmax: 1 h.
- Pharmacokinetic: linear.
- Protein binding: 98% bound to plasma proteins (mainly albumin).
- Volume of distribution: 20 l.

Metabolism
- Entacapone undergoes hepatic glucuronidation.
- Data from in-vitro studies indicate that entacapone inhibits CYP2C9.

Elimination
- Elimination half-life of entacapone ranges between 1.6 h and 3.4 h.
- It is mainly by non-renal metabolic routes with up to 90% found in faeces, while 10% is excreted in the urine.
- Only traces of entacapone are found unchanged in the urine.

PHARMACOKINETICS

Drug Interaction Profile

Pharmacokinetic Drug Interactions
- Effects caused by entacapone:
  - Entacapone may increase levels and effects of drugs metabolized by COMT, such as inotropes, vasopressors, SSRIs, and SNRIs.
  - Potential pharmacokinetic interactions with drugs metabolized by CYP2C9, for example *warfarin*.
- Effects on entacapone:
  - Drugs interfering with biliary excretion, glucuronidation, and intestinal β-glucuronidase (e.g. *cholestyramine*, *probenecid*, some anti-infectives [e.g. *ampicillin*, *chloramphenicol*, *erythromycin*, *rifampicin*]) may decrease levels and effects of entacapone.

Pharmacodynamic Drug Interactions
- Potential pharmacodynamic interaction with non-selective MAOIs (e.g. *phenelzine*, *tranylcypromine*) due to entacapone inhibiting catecholamine metabolism.

Adverse Effects

How Drug Causes Adverse Effects
- Mainly (but not only) by increasing dopaminergic activity.
- Slow metabolizers may be more susceptible to COMT-inhibitor induced hepatotoxicity.

Common Adverse Effects
- Very common (≥1/10):
  - Urine discolouration (reddish-brown), dyskinesia, nausea.
- Common (≥1/100 to <1/10):
  - Neuropsychiatric: insomnia, hallucinations, confusion, paranoia, aggravated parkinsonism, dizziness, dystonia, hyperkinesia.
  - Cardiovascular: ischaemic heart disease events apart from MI (e.g. angina pectoris).
  - GI: diarrhoea, abdominal pain, dry mouth, constipation, vomiting.
  - Other: fatigue, perspiration, falls.
- Uncommon (≥1/1,000 to <1/100):
  - Cardiovascular: MI.

Life-Threatening or Dangerous Adverse Effects
- Very rare (<0.01%):
  - Severe rhabdomyolysis.
  - NMS.
- Unknown frequency:
  - Colitis.

Rare and Not Life-Threatening Adverse Effects
- Rare (>0.01% and <1%):
  - Agitation.
  - Abnormal hepatic function tests.
  - Erythematous/maculopapular rash.
- Very rare (<1/10,000):
  - Anorexia.
  - Urticaria.
- Unknown frequency:
  - Skin, hair, beard, and nail discolorations.
  - Cholestatic hepatitis.
- In association with levodopa (with unknown frequency):
  - Excessive daytime somnolence/sudden sleep onset episodes.
  - ICDs.

Weight Change
- Weight decreases have been reported.

What to Do About Adverse Effects
- Discuss common adverse effects with patients or caregivers before starting medication, including symptoms that should be reported to the physician.
- Patients and caregivers should be made aware of the possibility of entacapone in association with levodopa causing ICDs. A review of treatment is recommended if such symptoms develop.
- If troublesome adverse effects occur, consider withdrawing therapy with a concomitant increase in levodopa dosing or alternative levodopa-sparing strategies.
- Dopaminergic adverse reactions may be prominent after introducing entacapone, thus, dose adjustments of levodopa or other dopaminergic medications may be needed within the first days/weeks of therapy to address those.
  - Consider reducing levodopa daily dose by about 10–30% (usually greater decreases are necessary when using entacapone in combination with levodopa/benserazide), by either reducing each dose or overall frequency to prevent or address adverse events.
- If prolonged or persistent diarrhoea occurs, entacapone should be discontinued and the possibility of colitis should be excluded.
- General medical evaluation, including hepatic function tests, is recommended for those who develop progressive anorexia, asthenia, and weight loss within a short time of initiating treatment with entacapone.

E

ADVERSE EFFECTS

E

ENTACAPONE

Dosing and Use

Usual Dosage Range
- 300–1,000 mg (up to 2,000 mg).

Available Formulations
- Tablets: 200 mg.
- Also available as combination tablets with levodopa/carbidopa.

How to Dose
- Entacapone should be given at the same time as each dose of levodopa/DDI.

Dosing Tips
- Entacapone can be taken before meals.

How to Withdraw Drug
- Entacapone should be withdrawn gradually, and consideration should be given to increasing levodopa dose as required.
- Isolated cases of NMS have been reported following abrupt discontinuation of entacapone.

Overdose
- Signs and symptoms of overdose include confusion, decreased activity, somnolence, hypotonia, skin discoloration, and urticaria.
- Management of entacapone overdose is symptomatic.

Tests and Therapeutic Drug Monitoring
- Hepatic function should be assessed before entacapone initiation.

Other Warnings / Precautions
- Caution is advised in patients with known orthostatic hypotension, as entacapone may aggravate this condition.
- Caution is recommended in prescribing entacapone in patients with ischaemic heart disease.
- Biliary excretion is the principal route of entacapone elimination, so caution is advised in patients with biliary obstruction.
- Close monitoring is advised if co-administered with COMT substrates, as it may result in changes of the heart rate/rhythm and blood pressure.
- Close monitoring is advised if co-administered with *warfarin*, as increases of INR values of up to 20% have been reported.
- Close monitoring is advised if co-administered with selective MAOIs.
  - If co-administered with *selegiline*, a selective MAO-B inhibitor, the daily dose of *selegiline* should not exceed 10 mg.
- Entacapone and iron preparations should be taken at least 2–3 h apart, as entacapone may form chelates with iron in the GI tract.

E

- Caution is advised with driving or operating hazardous machinery in case of entacapone-induced dizziness, orthostatic hypotension, excessive day-time sleepiness, or sudden onset sleep, until effects have stopped recurring.

Do Not Use (Contraindications)
- Hypersensitivity to entacapone, or to peanut or soya or to any excipients in the formulation, including sucrose.
  ○ Patients with rare hereditary problems of fructose intolerance, glucose–galactose malabsorption, or sucrase–isomaltase insufficiency.
- Hepatic impairment.
- Phaeochromocytoma.
- Concomitant use of non-selective MAOIs (MAO-A and MAO-B).
- Concomitant use of a selective MAO-A inhibitor plus a selective MAO-B inhibitor.
- Previous history of NMS and/or non-traumatic rhabdomyolysis.

Special Populations
Renal Impairment
- Dosage adjustments are not necessary in renal impairment.
- Consider increasing dosage intervals in patients receiving dialysis.

Hepatic Impairment
- Entacapone is contraindicated in case of hepatic impairment.

Elderly
- No special warnings or precautions are advised for the elderly.

Pregnancy
- There are no data on therapeutic use of entacapone during pregnancy in humans.
- No overt teratogenic or primary fetotoxic effects have been noted in animal studies.
- Entacapone should not be used during pregnancy.

Breastfeeding
- According to animal studies, entacapone is excreted in breast milk.
- No data on human studies are available.
- Women are advised not to breastfeed during treatment with entacapone.

Costs
NHS indicative price accessed 16 April 2021:
- Comtess (Orion Pharma UK Ltd) – 30 × 200 mg tablets: £17.24; 100 × 200 mg tablets: £57.45.
- Generic formulations – 30 × 200 mg tablets: between £5.03 and £16.35; 100 × 200 mg tablets: £16.01–£54.58.

COSTS

E

ENTACAPONE

The Overall Place of Entacapone in the Treatment of Parkinson's Disease

Entacapone is the most common COMT inhibitor encountered in routine clinical practice. It is used as an adjunct to levodopa preparations (either as a combined preparation or separate tablet) to increase levodopa bioavailability, independent of other concomitant dopaminergic medication. Various high-quality studies have demonstrated that entacapone reduces end-of-dose fluctuations in Parkinson's disease patients, especially OFF time, and is associated with lower total levodopa dose. Entacapone needs to be given with each dose of levodopa/DDI, as the half-life of entacapone is similar to that of levodopa. If ineffective or only partially effective, entacapone can be replaced with another COMT inhibitor (tolcapone/opicapone) or combined with a MAO-B inhibitor or a dopamine agonist. Entacapone is a relatively safe drug that can be used for long time periods without serious side effects. Common adverse events, like dyskinesias, are due to increased dopaminergic activity, which can be mitigated to some degree by reduction in levodopa daily dosage.

Potential Advantages
- Entacapone is considered a safe drug after many years of experience in clinical practice.
- Entacapone can be safely co-administered with dopamine agonists, including SC apomorphine.

Potential Disadvantages
- Entacapone needs to be administered with every levodopa dose, which usually leads to multiple doses throughout the day and may negatively affect patients' adherence, particularly advanced Parkinson's disease patients who follow complicated regimens.
- Entacapone may commonly cause urine discoloration and diarrhoea.

Clinical Box

A 75-year-old man with a 5-year history of Parkinson's disease reported motor and non-motor (anxiety and pain) wearing off phenomena. His current medications were levodopa–carbidopa 100/25 mg QID and rasagiline 1 mg OD. His past and current medical history consisted of a mild renal failure. Entacapone 200 mg QID was prescribed. The patient developed discoloration of urine and mild–moderate generalized dyskinesia. The latter was addressed by reducing the levodopa–carbidopa daily dose from 100/25 mg QID to TID and decreasing entacapone daily intake from 200 mg QID to TID.

E

Suggested Reading

Li J, Z Lou, X Liu, Y Sun, J Chen. Efficacy and safety of adjuvant treatment with entacapone in advanced Parkinson's disease with motor fluctuation: a systematic meta-analysis. *Eur Neurol* 2017; 78(3–4): 143–153.

Müller T. Entacapone. *Expert Opin Drug Metab Toxicol* 2010; 6(8): 983–993.

Schrag A. Entacapone in the treatment of Parkinson's disease. *Lancet Neurol* 2005; 4(6): 366–370.

References

AHFS Drug information, 2012. Bethesda: American Society of Health-System Pharmacists. Accessed on 17 June 2021 via www.medicinescomplete.com.

Brooks DJ, H. Sagar. Entacapone is beneficial in both fluctuating and non-fluctuating patients with Parkinson's disease: a randomised, placebo controlled, double blind, six month study. *J Neurol Neurosurg Psychiatry* 2003; 74(8): 1071–1079.

Brusa L, A Bassi, G Lunardi, E Fedele, A Peppe, A Stefani, P Pasqualetti, P Stanzione, M Pierantozzi. Delayed administration may improve entacapone effects in parkinsonian patients non-responding to the drug. *Eur J Neurol* 2004; 11(9): 593–606.

Entacapone. In: Brayfield A (Ed.), *Martindale: The Complete Drug Reference*. London: The Royal Pharmaceutical Society of Great Britain. Accessed on 17 June 2022 via www.medicinescomplete.com.

Entacapone. In: DRUGDEX® System (electronic version). Truven Health Analytics, Greenwood Village, Colorado, USA. Accessed on 3 March 2023 via www.micromedexsolutions.com.

Joint Formulary Committee. British National Formulary (online). London: BMJ Group and Pharmaceutical Press. Accessed on 17 June 2022 via www.medicinescomplete.com.

Larsen JP, J Worm-Petersen, A Sidén, A Gordin, K Reinikainen, M Leinonen. The tolerability and efficacy of entacapone over 3 years in patients with Parkinson's disease. *Eur J Neurol* 2003; 10(2): 137–146.

Olanow CW, K Kieburtz, M Stern, R Watts, JW Langston, M Guarnieri, J Hubble. Double-blind, placebo-controlled study of entacapone in levodopa-treated patients with stable Parkinson disease. *Arch Neurol* 2004; 61(10): 1563–1568.

Parkinson Study Group. Entacapone improves motor fluctuations in levodopa-treated Parkinson's disease patients. *Ann Neurol* 1997; 42(5): 747–755.

Poewe WH, G Deuschl, A Gordin, ER Kultalahti, M Leinonen. Efficacy and safety of entacapone in Parkinson's disease patients with suboptimal levodopa response: a 6-month randomized placebo-controlled double-blind study in Germany and Austria (Celomen study). *Acta Neurol Scand* 2002; 105(4): 245–255.

REFERENCES

E

Rinne UK, JP Larsen, A Siden, J Worm-Petersen. Entacapone enhances the response to levodopa in parkinsonian patients with motor fluctuations. Nomecomt Study Group. *Neurology* 1998; 51(5): 1309–1314.

Summary of product characteristics – Comtess 200 mg film-coated tablets. Orion Pharma (UK) Ltd. Electronic Medicines Compendium: Comtess 200 mg film-coated tablets – Summary of product characteristics (SmPC) – (emc). Accessed on 3 March 2023 via www.medicines.org.uk.

ENTACAPONE

FLUDROCORTISONE

F

Therapeutics

Chemical Name and Structure

Fludrocortisone acetate (9α-fluoro-11β,17α,21-trihydroxypregn-4-ene-3,10-dione 21-acetate) is a synthetic adrenal steroid. It has a molecular weight of 422.5 and a molecular formula of $C_{23}H_{31}FO_6$.

Brand Names

- **Astonin** (*Austria, Estonia, Hungary, Spain, Turkey*); **Astonin H** (*Austria, Germany*).
- **Cortineff** (*Cyprus, Estonia, Greece, Lithuania, Poland, Russian Federation, Ukraine*).
- **Floricot** (*India*); **Florinef** (*Australia, Canada, Chile, Denmark, Estonia, Finland, Greece, Hong Kong, Japan, Malaysia, Mexico, Netherlands, New Zealand, Singapore, South Africa, Sweden, Switzerland, Thailand, UK, USA*); **Florinefe** (*Brazil*); **Flucortac** (*France*); **Fludrace** (*Netherlands*).
- **Lonikan** (*Argentina*).

Generics Available

- Yes.

Licensed Indications for Parkinson's Disease

- None.

Licensed Indications for Other Conditions

- Primary and secondary adrenocortical insufficiency in Addison disease (FDA, EMA, EMC).
- Salt-losing forms of adrenogenital syndrome (FDA, EMA, EMC).

Non-Licensed Use for Parkinson's Disease

- Orthostatic hypotension in Parkinson's disease.

Non-Licensed Use for Other Conditions

- Severe orthostatic hypotension.
- Iatrogenic hyperkalaemia.
- Hyponatraemia.
- As an adjunct therapy to septic shock in patients with adrenal insufficiency.

Ineffective

- Neurogenic orthostatic hypotension.

Mechanism of Action

- Fludrocortisone is a potent mineralocorticoid with high glucocorticoid activity.

THERAPEUTICS

F

- It increases blood volume and improves the ability of blood vessels to respond to changes in position. This effect is believed to be mediated by the binding of fludrocortisone to the aldosterone receptor, which promotes sodium and water retention in the distal tubule of the kidney, while increasing urinary excretion of potassium and hydrogen ions.
- Fludrocortisone also increases norepinephrine release and sensitizes vascular adrenergic receptors.
  - Chronic fludrocortisone use may result in a persistent blood pressure-raising effect through increased peripheral vascular resistance.
- Similarly to other corticosteroids, fludrocortisone exhibits anti-inflammatory and immunosuppressive properties.

Efficacy Profile
- Fludrocortisone has been labelled as 'possibly useful' in the treatment of Parkinson's disease-related orthostatic hypotension, although there is 'insufficient' evidence to support its efficacy (MDS EBM Committee).
- There are two published RCTs, which compare the efficacy of fludrocortisone with pyridostigmine or domperidone for the management of orthostatic hypotension in Parkinson's disease patients; both of them found a statistically significant positive effect of fludrocortisone on blood pressure management without significant safety issues. However, both were small studies with a short follow-up period.

Pharmacokinetics
Absorption and Distribution
- Oral bioavailability: 100%.
- Food co-ingestion: no food interactions have been reported.
- Tmax: less than 1.7 h.
- Protein binding: about 70–80% (mainly to globulin fractions).

Metabolism
- Fludrocortisone undergoes hepatic metabolism, likely via the CYP3A family, but not fully elucidated.

Elimination
- The plasma half-life of fludrocortisone is 3.5 h, but it has a more biological half-life of 18–36 h.
- Approximately 80% of an administered dose is found in urine with the remaining being excreted via the faecal or biliary route. Similar to other steroids, excretion into the bile is balanced by reabsorption in the intestine with a percentage of the drug found in faeces.

FLUDROCORTISONE

F

Drug Interaction Profile
Pharmacokinetic Drug Interactions
- Effects by fludrocortisone:
  - Levels and effects of serum *isoniazid* and *salicylate* may be decreased.
- Effects on fludrocortisone:
  - Oestrogens, including oral contraceptives, and *ketoconazole* may increase levels and effects of corticosteroids.
  - Hepatic enzyme inducers (e.g. barbiturates, *carbamazepine*, *phenytoin*, *rifabutin*, *rifampicin*) may decrease levels and effects of fludrocortisone.

Pharmacodynamic Drug Interactions
- Co-medication with *amphotericin B*, *furosemide* or other potassium-depleting agents may aggravate hypokalaemia.
- Co-medication with oral anticoagulants may potentiate or decrease anticoagulant action.
- Co-medication with *cyclosporin* may lead to increased toxicity of the latter.
- Co-medication with *digoxin* may lead to digitalis toxicity.
- Co-medication with fluoroquinolones (e.g. *ciprofloxacin*, *levofloxacin*, *moxifloxacin*, *norfloxacin*) may increase the risk for tendon rupture.
- Co-medication with *droxidopa* or *midodrine* may increase the risk for supine hypertension.
- Fludrocortisone may decrease or increase the neuromuscular blocking action.
- Similarly to other corticosteroids, fludrocortisone may increase the frequency and severity of NSAIDs-associated GI bleeding and ulceration.

ADVERSE EFFECTS

Adverse Effects
How Drug Causes Adverse Effects
- Fludrocortisone may cause adverse effects due to:
  - Suppression of the hypothalamic–pituitary–adrenal axis.
  - Anti-inflammatory and immunosuppressive effects.
  - Sodium and fluid retention, potassium loss, and calcium excretion.
  - Hypersensitivity reactions.
- Side effects relate to the drug potency, dosage, timing of administration, and treatment duration.

Common Adverse Effects
- Very common (≥1/10):
  - Metabolism and nutrition: hypokalaemia.
  - Cardiac: cardiac failure congestive, hypertension.
- Common (≥1/100 to <1/10):
  - Nervous system: headache.
  - Musculoskeletal: muscular weakness.
  - General: oedema, swelling.

F

FLUDROCORTISONE

- Uncommon (≥1/1,000 to <1/100):
  - Metabolism and nutrition: hypokalaemic alkalosis, decreased appetite.
  - Psychiatric: delusional perception, illusion, hallucination
  - Nervous system: seizure, epilepsy, syncope, loss of consciousness, dysgeusia.
  - Cardiac: cardiomegaly.
  - Gastrointestinal: diarrhoea.
  - Musculoskeletal: muscle atrophy.
  - Investigations: blood potassium decreased.
- When used at recommended doses the glucocorticoid side effects are not usually present; however, some adverse events have been spontaneous reported in patients taking fludrocortisone overdose:
  - Anti-inflammatory: increased susceptibility to infections, opportunistic infections, recurrence of latent tuberculosis.
  - Electrolyte/fluid disturbances: oedema, congestive heart failure, hypertension, cardiac arrhythmias, ECG changes.
  - Musculoskeletal: muscle weakness, fatigue, steroid myopathy, loss of muscle mass, osteoporosis, avascular osteonecrosis, vertebral compression fractures, delaying healing of fractures, aseptic necrosis of femoral and humeral heads, pathological fractures of long bones and spontaneous fractures, tendon rupture.
  - Gastrointestinal: dyspepsia, peptic ulcer, pancreatitis, abdominal distension and ulcerative esophagitis, candidiasis.
  - Hypersensitivity: angioedema, rash, pruritus, and urticaria.
  - Dermatologic: thin fragile skin, petechiae/ecchymoses, facial erythema, increased sweating, purpura, hirsutism, striae, acneiform eruptions, lupus erythematosus-like lesions, suppressed reactions to skin tests.
  - Neuropsychiatric: psychological dependence, sleep problems/insomnia, irritability, anxiety, behavioural disturbances, convulsions, pseudo-tumour cerebri, vertigo, headache, neuritis, or paraesthesias.
    - Affective disorders (depression, euphoria, labile mood, suicidal ideation).
    - Psychotic reactions (mania, delusions, hallucinations, psychosis aggravation).
    - Cognitive dysfunction (confusion, amnesia).
  - Endocrine/metabolic: menstrual irregularities/amenorrhoea, Cushingoid state, decreased carbohydrate tolerance, latent diabetes mellitus, increased appetite.
  - Ophthalmic: posterior subcapsular cataracts, glaucoma, exophthalmos, papilledema, corneal or scleral thinning, blurred vision.
  - Others: necrotizing angiitis, thrombophlebitis, leucocytosis, syncope.

Life-Threatening or Dangerous Adverse Effects
- Thromboembolic events, arrhythmias.
- Congestive heart failure.
- Steroid-myopathy.

F

- GI perforation/haemorrhage, pancreatitis.
- Anaphylactoid reactions.
- Severe psychosis.
- Epilepsy.

Weight Change
- Fludrocortisone therapy may lead to increased weight.
- Weight loss may occur during therapy discontinuation.

What to Do About Adverse Effects
- Before introducing fludrocortisone therapy, discuss common or life-threatening adverse effects with patients and/or caregivers, including symptoms that should be reported to the physician.
  - Corticosteroid-related adverse effects are usually reversible on cessation of therapy.
- Fludrocortisone is a potent mineralocorticoid, its dosage and salt intake should be carefully monitored during fludrocortisone therapy to avoid potential side effects, such as hypertension, oedema, or weight gain.
  - Patients can be instructed to elevate the head of their bed at least 30–45° at night when sleeping in order to lower the risk for supine hypertension.
- Patients and their caregivers should be informed about the possibility of fludrocortisone causing severe psychiatric adverse reactions, with those receiving higher doses being at greater risk.
  - If worrying psychological symptoms occur, particularly depressed mood or suspected suicidal ideation, medical advice should be sought.
  - These reactions typically respond to dose reduction or complete fludrocortisone withdrawal, although focused treatment may be necessary.
  - Psychiatric disturbances may also appear during or immediately after dose tapering or discontinuation.
- If the patient reports any visual disturbances (e.g. blurred vision), a referral to an ophthalmologist should be considered to exclude diagnoses of corticosteroid-induced conditions, such as cataract, glaucoma, or rare diseases like central serous chorioretinopathy.
- A worsening of existent or occurrence of latent diabetes mellitus may occur, necessitating higher dosage of antidiabetic medication, including insulin.
  - Extra caution is advised in case of corticosteroids dosage modifications or discontinuation of therapy.
- If a patient develops back pain during prolonged fludrocortisone therapy, osteoporosis should be excluded.
- Unvaccinated patients on fludrocortisone should seek medical advice if they are exposed to chickenpox, shingles, or measles.
  - If patients who are not immune are receiving systemic corticosteroids or have received them during the past 3 months are exposed to

ADVERSE EFFECTS

F

FLUDROCORTISONE

chickenpox, passive immunization with varicella zoster immuno-globulin may be needed. Corticosteroids discontinuation is not suggested.
- If non-immune patients are exposed to measles, prophylaxis with normal immunoglobulin may be needed.
- Glucocorticoid side effects may be mitigated by fludrocortisone dose reduction.
- Undesirable effects may be minimized using the lowest effective dose for the shortest period.

Dosing and Use

Usual Dosage Range
- 0.1–0.3 mg.

Available Formulations
- Tablets: 0.1 mg.
- Oral solution: 1 mg/ml.
- Ointment: 1 mg/g.

How to Dose
- Initial dose of 0.05 mg or 0.1 mg OD in combination with high salt diet and adequate fluid intake; may be increased by 0.1 mg per week; maximum total dose of 1 mg/day.

Dosing Tips
- Doses higher than 0.3 mg per day have not shown any significant benefit and have been associated with adverse events.
- Fludrocortisone tablets can be taken with food or milk to avoid stomach upset.

How to Withdraw Drug
- Prolonged therapy with corticosteroids, including fludrocortisone, is expected to cause adrenal cortical atrophy, which may persist for years after therapy discontinuation. It is, therefore, suggested that fludrocortisone therapy withdrawal should always be gradual to minimize the risk of acute adrenal insufficiency.
- Withdrawal syndrome may present with fever, myalgia, arthralgia, rhinitis, conjunctivitis, painful itchy skin nodules, and/or weight loss.
- Fludrocortisone withdrawal period may last for weeks or even months depending on the duration and dosage of therapy.

Overdose
- In case of consumption of a single large dose of fludrocortisone, the patient should be instructed to receive plenty of water and decrease dietary sodium intake.
- Careful monitoring of serum electrolytes is also needed.
- Administration of potassium chloride may be considered.

F

Tests and Therapeutic Drug Monitoring
- During fludrocortisone therapy:
  - Periodic assessment of blood glucose and serum electrolyte levels (especially sodium and potassium) is advised in prolonged therapy.
  - Periodic assessments of body weight and blood pressure (standing and supine) are advised in prolonged therapy.

Other Warnings/Precautions
- Caution is advised when administering fludrocortisone in patients with diabetes mellitus, hypertension, congestive heart failure, glaucoma, electrolyte abnormalities, sodium and water retention, infections, immunizations, ocular herpes simplex, myasthenia gravis, peptic ulcer disease (active or past), psychosis (acute or past, especially if steroid-induced), affective disorders (active or past or in their first-degree relatives), recent intestinal anastomoses, diverticulitis, thrombophlebitis, exanthematous disease, metastatic carcinoma, osteoporosis (especially in post-menopausal females), acute glomerulonephritis, chronic nephritis, previous steroid myopathyz or epilepsy.
- Fludrocortisone may cause electrolyte imbalance with sodium and fluid retention, which might result in oedemas, hypertension and congestive heart failure in susceptible individuals, and potassium loss, which might result in ECG changes and cardiac arrhythmias.
- Patients receiving fludrocortisone are expected to show an increased susceptibility to infections, including opportunistic infections; infections can have atypical presentations or be particularly severe, such as septicaemia or tuberculosis, which may be masked and only recognized at an advanced stage.
- Fludrocortisone therapy may delay wound healing.
- Patients on fludrocortisone or other corticosteroids should be warned to avoid exposure to people infected with measles, shingles, or chickenpox if they are unvaccinated, as these illnesses might be fatal in immunosuppressed individuals.
- Patients with positive tuberculin test should be monitored, as dormant tuberculosis may be reactivated.
- Prolonged use of fludrocortisone or other corticosteroids may lead to increased intra-ocular pressure, glaucoma, or cataracts.
- Hyper- and hypothyroidism may lead to lower and higher levels of adrenocorticoids, including fludrocortisone; fludrocortisone dosage should be re-examined whenever changes in thyroid status occur.
- Prolonged use of fludrocortisone or other corticosteroids has been associated with the development of Kaposi sarcoma.
- Female patients should be informed about potential menstrual irregularities.
- Fludrocortisone has been classified as possibly porphyrinogenic (Norwegian Porphyria Centre (NAPOS), Porphyria Centre Sweden).
- Caution is advised in co-administration with potassium-depleting agents (e.g. *amphotericin B*) due to potential additive effects of hypokalaemia.

DOSING AND USE

161

F

FLUDROCORTISONE

- Caution is advised in co-administration with anticholinesterases due to opposing action.
- Close monitoring is recommended in co-administration with oral anticoagulants and digitalis glycosides.
- If the patient receives fludrocortisone, CYP3A inhibitors should only be administered if expected benefits outweigh potential risks; close monitoring is recommended.
- Discontinuation of fludrocortisone therapy during high-dose salicylate therapy may lead to salicylate toxicity.

Do Not Use (Contraindications)
- Known sensitivity to fludrocortisone or to any of the excipients, including lactose.
  - Patients with rare hereditary problems of galactose intolerance, total lactase deficiency, or glucose-galactose malabsorption.
- Systemic fungal or other infections, unless specific anti-infective therapy is employed.
- Administration of live virus vaccines is contraindicated in patients receiving corticosteroid therapy in short-term schemes (<2 weeks), in low-to-moderate dosage, as long-term alternate-day therapy with short-acting preparations, or as replacement therapy, as their antibody response will be reduced.

Special Populations
Renal Impairment
- Caution is advised in case of renal impairment.

Hepatic Impairment
- Caution is advised in case of hepatic impairment.

Elderly
- No particular dose modifications are suggested.
- Supine hypertension as an adverse reaction to fludrocortisone use is more common among the elderly.

Pregnancy
- Corticosteroids use during pregnancy may be associated with an increased risk of cleft palate and intra-uterine growth retardation. Hypoadrenalism of the neonate has also been reported.
- Pregnancy category C: use with caution if benefits outweigh risks.

Breastfeeding
- It is not known whether fludrocortisone is excreted in human milk.
- Use with caution during lactation.

Costs
NHS indicative prices accessed 18 December 2022:
- Fludrocortisone 0.1 mg tablets – 30 × 0.1 mg tablets: £10.09–£17.10.

The Overall Place of Fludrocortisone in the Treatment of Parkinson's Disease

Fludrocortisone acetate is a synthetic adrenocortical steroid with profound corticoid activity, associated with fluid and sodium retention, leading to an increase in plasma volume, and sensitivity of α-adrenoreceptors. It is believed to exert its blood pressure-increasing effect through expansion of the circulating volume. This mechanism of action differentiates it from other medication used for the treatment of orthostatic hypotension; it is not expected to be efficacious in orthostatic hypotension due to volume loss (e.g. patients with chronic diarrhoea, inadequate fluid intake due to dysphagia, concomitant use of diuretics) if fluids are not adequately replenished. Although it has been extensively prescribed 'off-label' in routine clinical practice for the management of orthostatic hypotension, including Parkinson's disease patients, only scarce data are available to support its use. Two high-quality studies have demonstrated its efficacy on the management of orthostatic hypotension in Parkinson's disease patients; however, one of them noted that despite recording higher values of blood pressure after fludrocortisone therapy, patients' symptoms did not improve, thus suggesting that fludrocortisone effects might not be clinically relevant. Current evidence on the safety profile of fludrocortisone is uncertain, although the aforementioned studies have not revealed any significant adverse events. Among others, fludrocortisone use has been associated with a risk for supine hypertension, a condition that is often hard to recognize. Finally, its use may be limited by the sequelae of excessive fluid retention in vulnerable patients, such as peripheral oedema and congestive heart failure; thus, fludrocortisone should not be used in patients who cannot tolerate fluid retention.

Potential Advantages
- Fludrocortisone mechanism of action is differentiated by short-acting pressor agents (e.g. *droxidopa*, *midodrine*), whose action is mediated by adrenergic effects resulting in increased peripheral vascular resistance.

Potential Disadvantages
- Fludrocortisone is only efficient in the short term.
- Its use is associated with a significant risk for supine hypertension.

F

Clinical Box

A 62-year-old woman with a 7-year history of Parkinson's disease was referred to the Movement Disorders Outpatient Clinic by her GP due to marked episodes of light-headedness upon standing during the past 3 months. A diagnosis of orthostatic hypotension was made; non-pharmacological measures of increased salt and fluid intake were initially applied without success. The patient was on levodopa/carbidopa/entacapone 150 mg/37.5 mg/200 mg QID for the past 6 months and was satisfied with her motor performance. A dose of fludrocortisone 0.1 mg OD was prescribed, which was subsequently increased to 0.2 mg OD with significant improvement of her symptoms.

Suggested Reading

Schoffer KL, RD Henderson, K O'Maley, JD O'Sullivan. Nonpharmacological treatment, fludrocortisone, and domperidone for orthostatic hypotension in Parkinson's disease. *Mov Disord* 2007; 22(11): 1543–1549.

Schreglmann SR, F Büchele, M Sommerauer, L Epprecht, G Kägi, S Hägele-Link, O Götze, L Zimmerli, D Waldvogel, CR Baumann. Pyridostigmine bromide versus fludrocortisone in the treatment of orthostatic hypotension in Parkinson's disease – a randomized controlled trial. *Eur J Neurol* 2017; 24(4): 545–551.

Veazie S, K Peterson, Y Ansari, KA Chung, CH Gibbons, SR Raj, M Helfand. Fludrocortisone for orthostatic hypotension. *Cochrane Database Syst Rev* 2021; 5(5): CD012868.

References

AHFS Drug information, 2012. Bethesda: American Society of Health-System Pharmacists. Accessed on 18 December 2022 via www.medicinescomplete.com.

Fludrocortisone. In: Brayfield A (Ed.), *Martindale: The Complete Drug Reference*. London: The Royal Pharmaceutical Society of Great Britain. Accessed on 18 December 2022 via www.medicinescomplete.com.

Fludrocortisone. In: DRUGDEX® System (electronic version). Truven Health Analytics, Greenwood Village, Colorado, USA. Accessed on 18 December 2022 via www.micromedexsolutions.com.

Joint Formulary Committee. British National Formulary (online). London: BMJ Group and Pharmaceutical Press. Accessed on 18 December 2022 via www.medicinescomplete.com.

Summary of product characteristics – fludrocortisone acetate 0.1 mg tablets. Mylan. Electronic Medicines Compendium: Fludrocortisone Acetate 0.1 mg Tablets – Summary of Product Characteristics (SmPC) – (emc). Accessed on 18 December 2022 via www.medicines.org.uk.

GLYCOPYRROLATE

G

Therapeutics

Chemical Name and Structure

Glycopyrronium bromide (3-(α-cyclopentylmandeloyloxy)-1,1-dimethylpyrrolidinium bromide) has a molecular weight of 398.3 and a molecular formula of $C_{19}H_{28}BrNO_3$.

Brand Names
- **Assicco** (*UK*).
- **Cuvposa** (*Canada, USA*).
- **Dartisla** (*USA*).
- **Enurev** (*Greece, Netherlands, Poland, Spain*).
- **Glycate** (*USA*); **Glyco-P** (*India, Thailand*); **Glyprolate** (*India*); **Glyrx-PF** (*USA*).
- **Lycolate** (*India*).
- **Panthero** (*Turkey*).
- **Robinul** (*Australia, Austria, Belgium, Denmark, Finland, Germany, Greece, New Zealand, Norway, South Africa, Sweden, UK, USA*).
- **Sebraler** (*Turkey*); **Seebri** (*Argentina, Australia, Austria, Belgium, Brazil, Canada, Chile, China, Czech Republic, Denmark, Finland, France, Germany, Greece, Hong Kong, Hungary, Indonesia, Ireland, Israel, Japan, Malaysia, Netherlands, New Zealand, Norway, Poland, Portugal,* Russian Federation, *Singapore, Spain, Sweden, Switzerland, Thailand, Turkey, Ukraine, UK, Venezuela*); **Sialanar** (*Denmark, Finland, Germany,* Ireland, *Netherlands, Norway, Poland, Sweden, UK*).
- **Tovanor** (*Greece, Netherlands, Poland, Portugal, Spain*).
- **Ultibro** (*Venezuela*).

Generics Available
- Yes.

Licensed Indications for Parkinson's Disease
- None.

Licensed Indications for Other Conditions
- Severe sialorrhoea in children (>3 years) and adolescents (EMC) with neurological disorders (oral solution) (EMA, EMC).
- Perioperative reduction of saliva and tracheobronchial/pharyngeal secretions or intraoperative reduction of cholinergic effects (injectable solution) (FDA, EMA, EMC).
- Neuromuscular blockade reversal (injectable solution) (FDA, EMA, EMC).
- Adjunct to treatment of peptic ulcer (injectable solution) (FDA).
- Chronic obstructive pulmonary disease (inhalant formulation) (EMA).

THERAPEUTICS

GLYCOPYRROLATE

Non-Licensed Use for Parkinson's Disease
- Sialorrhoea.
- Glycopyrrolate therapy is recommended for short-term intermittent use.

Non-Licensed Use for Other Conditions
- Sialorrhoea.
- Frey syndrome (orphan drug).

Ineffective
- Not reported.

Mechanism of Action
- Glycopyrrolate is a potent, competitive inhibitor of the muscarinic cholinergic receptors. It blocks acetylcholine's action on structures innervated by post-ganglionic cholinergic nerves and on smooth muscles (attenuation of parasympathetic activity).
  - Peripheral cholinergic receptors are located on the autonomic effector cells of smooth muscle, cardiac muscle, the sinoatrial node, the atrioventricular node, exocrine glands, and in the autonomic ganglia (limited numbers).
- Glycopyrrolate's actions include lowering of the volume and free acidity of gastric secretions, plus the decrease of excessive pharyngeal/ tracheal/bronchial secretions.
- The highly polar quaternary ammonium group of glycopyrronium bromide inhibits penetration of lipid membranes, including the blood–brain barrier.

Efficacy Profile
- Glycopyrrolate has been characterized as 'efficacious' and 'possibly useful' for the short-term treatment of sialorrhoea in Parkinson's disease.
- Two double-blind RCTs have shown the efficacy of glycopyrrolate on Parkinson's disease-related drooling both in the short (4 weeks) and long term (12 weeks).
- High-quality studies have demonstrated the efficacy of glycopyrrolate 2 mg OD on clozapine-related nocturnal sialorrhoea.
- There have been case reports of nebulized glycopyrrolate as an effective treatment for drooling in non-Parkinson's disease patients with swallowing difficulties for short time periods.
- Glycopyrrolate duration is 8–12 h.

Pharmacokinetics

Absorption and Distribution (Oral Formulations)
- Oral bioavailability: very low.
- Food co-ingestion: high-fat food decreases oral bioavailability.
- Tmax: about 3 h.
- Pharmacokinetics: non-linear.
- Protein binding: 38%–41%.
- Volume of distribution: 0.64±0.29 l/kg in adults.

Metabolism
- Multiple CYP450 isoenzymes are involved in the oxidative biotransformation of glycopyrrolate.
- Members of the cholinesterase family are also involved in glycopyrrolate hydrolysis.

Elimination
- Half-life of oral solution ranges between 2.5 h and 4 h (highly variable).
- Glycopyrrolate is excreted mostly unchanged in urine and to a lesser extent in faeces via biliary elimination.

Drug Interaction Profile

Pharmacokinetic Drug Interactions
- Effects by glycopyrrolate:
  - Glycopyrrolate might increase levels and effects of *atenolol, digoxin,* and *metformin* by unknown mechanisms.
  - Glycopyrrolate may decrease the absorption of *levodopa.*

Pharmacodynamic Drug Interactions
- Co-medication with *botulinum toxin* products might lead to synergistic effects.
- Co-medication with neuroleptics (e.g. *aripiprazole, chlorpromazine, clozapine, haloperidol, quetiapine, risperidone*), tricyclic antidepressants, antihistamines, MAOIs, *amantadine, atropine, buprenorphine,* and other anticholinergic agents might lead to additive anticholinergic effects, including hyperthermia.
- Co-medication with cholinesterase inhibitors (e.g. *donepezil*) might lead to unclear results due to opposing activity in the cholinergic system.
- Co-medication with *domperidone* or *metoclopramide* has opposing effects on gastrointestinal activity.
- Co-medication with nitrates might lead to decreased effects of the latter, as dry mouth might inhibit nitrates from dissolving under the tongue.
- Co-medication with *metformin* may potentiate the effects of the latter.

Adverse Effects

How Drug Causes Adverse Effects
- The anticholinergic activity of glycopyrrolate is responsible for the most common adverse effects.
- Glycopyrrolate reduces GI motility and may result in delayed gastric emptying, constipation, and intestinal pseudo-obstruction. It may also trigger or aggravate paralytic ileus and toxic megacolon.
  - This risk is further increased if co-administered with anticholinergic agents or other drugs decreasing GI peristalsis.
- Caution in cholinergic subtype of Parkinson's disease.

Common Adverse Effects (Oral Formulations)
- Common (≥1/100 to <1/10):
  - Neuropsychiatric: mood disturbances.
  - Respiratory: pneumonia.
  - Renal/urinary: urinary retention.
  - GI: abdominal pain.
  - Other: pyrexia.
- Uncommon (≥1/1,000 to <1/100):
  - Nervous/psychiatric: seizures, insomnia.
  - Eye/ear: nystagmus.
  - GI: pseudo-obstruction, GI mobility disorder, oesophageal candidiasis, breath odour.
  - Urinary: urinary urgency.
  - Other: allergic reactions, hives, dehydration, thirst.

Life-Threatening or Dangerous Adverse Effects
- Unknown frequency:
  - Angle-closure glaucoma.
  - Angioedema.
  - Transient bradycardia.

Rare and Not Life-Threatening Adverse Effects
- Headache.
- Somnolence, drowsiness, dizziness.
- Mydriasis, blurred vision, photophobia, dry eyes.
- Epistaxis.
- Rash, dry skin, sweat inhibition.

Weight Change
- Not reported.

What to Do About Adverse Effects
- Before introducing glycopyrrolate, discuss common or life-threatening adverse effects with patients and/or caregivers, including symptoms that should be reported to the physician, such as constipation, diarrhoea, urinary retention, pneumonia, pyrexia, allergic reaction, changes in behaviour.

G

- Patients and their caregivers should be informed about the possibility of glycopyrrolate increasing intra-ocular pressure; if the patient experiences any symptoms of acute angle-closure glaucoma, such as sudden eye pain or headache, blurred vision, nausea/vomiting, marked conjunctival injection and dilated pupils, glycopyrrolate should be discontinued and the patient should urgently seek medical care.
  - Co-administration of anticholinergics and corticosteroids may lead to increased intra-ocular pressure.
- Therapy should be discontinued if troublesome anticholinergic symptoms appear, including cognitive or visual impairment.
- If incomplete mechanical intestinal obstruction or occurrence of diarrhoea occurs, especially in patients who have an ileostomy or colostomy, glycopyrrolate should be discontinued.

Dosing and Use

Usual Dosage Range
- Oral formulations: 3–4.5 mg.

Available Formulations
- Tablets: 1 mg, 1.5 mg, 2 mg.
- Tablets, orally disintegrating tablets (ODT): 1.7 mg.
- Oral solution: 1 mg/5ml.
- Injectable solution: 0.2 mg/ml.
- Capsules (inhalation powder): 50µg (44 µg/dose).

How to Dose
- Oral formulations: 1 mg BID or TID; not to exceed 4.5 mg/day.

Dosing Tips
- Oral formulations of glycopyrrolate should be administered 1 h before or 2 h after meals.
- ODT formulations should not be used if a lower dosage of another oral glycopyrrolate product may be administered.

How to Withdraw Drug
- No special instructions are given.

Overdose
- Glycopyrrolate overdose is expected to manifest with peripheral rather than central symptoms, including muscular weakness and possible paralysis, along with anticholinergic effects (e.g. mydriasis, dry mouth).
- Supportive measures, close monitoring and maintenance of a clear airway with adequate ventilation are recommended.
  - Pressor amines (e.g. *norepinephrine, metaraminol*) and respiratory stimulants (e.g. *doxapram hydrochloride*) can be applied to combat hypotension and respiratory depression, respectively.

DOSING AND USE

- Consider gastric lavage, cathartics and/or enemas to further reduce glycopyrrolate absorption.
- A quaternary ammonium anticholinesterase, such as neostigmine, could be administered to block peripheral anticholinergic effects.

Tests and Therapeutic Drug Monitoring
- Not reported.

Other Warnings/Precautions
- Caution is advised when administered in patients with concomitant conditions, which are aggravated by potential anticholinergic side reactions, such as autonomic neuropathy, pre-existing constipation, and hiatal hernia with reflux oesophagitis.
- Because glycopyrrolate may increase heart rate and might precipitate arrhythmias, caution is advised when administered in patients with hyperthyroidism, hypertension, or cardiovascular disease.
- Patients should be advised to avoid exposure to hot/very warm environmental temperatures, as glycopyrrolate reduces perspiration and might lead to fever and heat stroke, particularly in older patients.
- Glycopyrrolate might impair mental abilities and cause blurred vision; thus, the ability to drive or operate dangerous machinery may be affected.
- Close monitoring is advised if co-administered with *botulinum toxin*, *amantadine*, neuroleptics, tricyclic antidepressants, or other anticholinergic agents; concomitant use is not recommended.
- Consider a dose reduction of *metformin* if co-administered with glycopyrrolate.
- Close monitoring is advised in patients receiving inhalation anaesthesia.

Do Not Use (Contraindications)
- Known sensitivity to glycopyrrolate or to any of the excipients, such as sorbitol.
- Rare hereditary problems of fructose intolerance.
- Angle-closure glaucoma.
- Obstructive uropathies, including prostatic enlargement.
- Urinary retention.
- Obstructive diseases of the GI tract.
- GI motility disorders (e.g. achalasia, paralytic ileus).
- Bleeding GI ulcer.
- Active inflammatory or infectious colitis (risk of toxic megacolon).
- History of or current toxic megacolon.
- Myasthenia gravis.
- Co-administration with potassium chloride solid oral dose products.

Special Populations

Renal Impairment
- Caution is advised, as glycopyrrolate is primarily excreted by the kidney.
- Glycopyrrolate may cause urinary retention and further aggravate existing renal impairment; consider dose reduction in case of renal impairment.
- Glycopyrrolate therapy is contraindicated in severe renal impairment (eGFR < 30 ml/min/1.73 m²), including patients on dialysis.

Hepatic Impairment
- Regular monitoring is recommended.
- No specific dosage adjustments are suggested; consider dose reduction in case of hepatic impairment.

Elderly
- Glycopyrrolate use is not encouraged in the elderly, as it might cause anticholinergic side effects specifically in the cholinergic subtype and indirect consequences, including urinary retention, bowel obstruction, heat prostration, arrhythmias, delirium, falls, or fractures.
- It is particularly contraindicated in selected geriatric patients with underlying medical conditions.
- No specific dosage modifications are suggested.
- ODT formulations are not recommended in the elderly.

Pregnancy
- Although there are no reports of drug-associated adverse maternal or fetal outcomes, glycopyrrolate use is contraindicated during pregnancy.
- Women of childbearing potential are advised to use contraception during glycopyrrolate therapy.
- No adverse effects have been observed in animal studies at non-maternally toxic doses.

Breastfeeding
- Glycopyrrolate is contraindicated during breastfeeding.
- Due to the anticholinergic activity, glycopyrrolate may suppress lactation.
- There are no reports of drug-associated adverse effects on breastfed infants.

Costs

NHS indicative price on 18 December 2022:
- Assico Tablets (Morningside Healthcare) – 30 × 1 mg tablets: £79.00; 30 × 2 mg tablets: £123.00.
- Glycopyrronium bromide tablets 30 × 1 mg tablets: £180.00–£265.58; 30 × 2 mg tablets: £198.00–£292.63.

G

- Sialanar 320 micrograms/ml oral solution (Proveca Ltd) – 60 ml bottle: £76.80; 250 ml bottle: £320.00.
- Glycopyrronium bromide 1 mg/5 ml oral solution – 150 ml bottle: £91.00–£134.82.

The Overall Place of Glycopyrrolate in the Treatment of Parkinson's Disease

Glycopyrrolate is a competitive muscarinic inhibitor with well-established indications in a number of conditions and multiple potential administration routes. Two double-blind, randomized controlled studies have shown the efficacy of oral formulations on Parkinson's disease-related sialorrhoea, both in the short (4 weeks) and long term (12 weeks). The possibility of oral administration of glycopyrrolate is an important advantage compared to *botulinum toxin*, which is a first-line therapy in Parkinson's disease-related sialorrhoea. Despite being an anticholinergic agent with a long list of potential side effects and pharmacological interactions, glycopyrrolate crosses the blood–brain barrier only poorly. It therefore has a more favourable tolerability profile with fewer central adverse events, including neuropsychiatric effects and cognitive impairment, which is particularly important for the predominantly elderly Parkinson's disease population. Indeed, no serious complications have been found in studies of glycopyrrolate use in Parkinson's disease patients. However, these were small studies and well-acknowledged safety concerns over the drug cannot be ignored. Therefore, in order to weigh risks and benefits, glycopyrrolate therapy should only be introduced in severe cases of sialorrhoea.

Potential Advantages
- Due to a quaternary ammonium structure, glycopyrrolate crosses the blood–brain barrier to a limited degree; thus, it is expected to demonstrate minimal central side effects, such as neuropsychiatric effects and cognitive impairment.
- Glycopyrrolate can be taken via PEG.

Potential Disadvantages
- There are no long-term safety data beyond 24 weeks of therapy; thus, treatment duration should be kept as brief as possible. If therapy is repeated intermittently, close monitoring is advised.
- Anticholinergic effects are the most common reason for glycopyrrolate discontinuation.

G

Clinical Box
A 72-year-old woman with a 10-year history of Parkinson's disease presented to the Neurology Department Outpatient Clinics for her regular follow-up assessment. Among other symptoms, she complained of severe drooling, which made her socially isolated and worsened depression. An initial suggestion of botulinum toxin injections was made; however, the patient rejected it, as she would have to travel to another specialized medical centre a long distance from her home to receive treatment. An alternative choice of glycopyrrolate 1 mg BID was given and accepted. Symptom improvement was observed 14 days after therapy initiation with an increase in frequency of administration to 1 mg TID.

Suggested Reading

Arbouw ME, KL Movig, M Koopmann, PJ Poels, HJ Guchelaar, TC Egberts, C Neef, JP van Vugt. Glycopyrrolate for sialorrhea in Parkinson disease: a randomized, double-blind, crossover trial. *Neurology* 2010; 74(15): 1203–1207.

Man WH, JC Colen-de Koning, PF Schulte, W Cahn, IM van Haelst, HJ Doodeman, TC Egberts, ER Heerdink, I Wilting. The effect of glycopyrrolate on nocturnal sialorrhea in patients using clozapine: a randomized, crossover, double-blind, placebo-controlled trial. *J Clin Psychopharmacol* 2017; 37(2): 155–161.

Mestre TA, E Freitas, A Basndwah, MR Lopez, LM de Oliveira, DM Al-Shorafat, T Zhang, JP Lui, D Grimes, SH Fox. Glycopyrrolate improves disability from sialorrhea in Parkinson's disease: a 12-week controlled trial. *Mov Disord* 2020; 35(12): 2319–2323.

References

AHFS Drug information, 2012. Bethesda: American Society of Health–System Pharmacists. Accessed on 18 December 2022 via www.medicinescomplete.com.

Glycopyrronium. In: Brayfield A (Ed.), *Martindale: The Complete Drug Reference*. London: The Royal Pharmaceutical Society of Great Britain. Accessed on 18 December 2022 via www.medicinescomplete.com.

Glycopyrronium. In: DRUGDEX® System (electronic version). Truven Health Analytics, Greenwood Village, Colorado, USA. Accessed on 18 December 2022 via www.micromedexsolutions.com.

Joint Formulary Committee. British National Formulary (online). London: BMJ Group and Pharmaceutical Press. Accessed on 18 December 2022 via www.medicinescomplete.com.

Lee ZI, KJ Yu, DH Lee, SK Hong, SB Woo, JM Kim, D Park. The effect of nebulized glycopyrrolate on posterior drooling in patients with brain injury: two cases of different brain lesions. *Am J Phys Med Rehabil* 2017; 96(8): e155–e158.

Plunkett C. Sialorrhoea treated with inhaled glycopyrronium. *BMJ Support Palliat Care* 2021; 11(4): 406–407.

Summary of product characteristics – glycopyrronium bromide 1 mg tablets. Dawa Ltd. Electronic Medicines Compendium: glycopyrronium bromide 1 mg tablets – summary of product characteristics (SmPC) – (emc). Accessed on 18 December 2022 via www.medicines.org.uk.

GLYCOPYRROLATE

ISTRADEFYLLINE

Therapeutics
Chemical Name and Structure
Istradefylline (8-[(1E)-2-(3,4-dimethoxyphenyl)ethenyl]-1,3-dethyl-7-methyl-3,7-dihydro-1H-purine-2,6-dione) is a xanthine derivative with a molecular weight of 384.4 and an empirical formula of $C_{20}H_{24}N_4O_4$.

Brand Names
• **Nourianz** (*USA*); **Nouriast** (*Japan*).

Generics Available
• No.

Licensed Indications for Parkinson's Disease
• As an adjunct therapy to levodopa formulations in Parkinson's disease patients experiencing OFF episodes (FDA).

Licensed Indications for Other Conditions
• None.

Non-Licensed Use for Parkinson's Disease
• None.

Non-Licensed Use for Other Conditions
• None.

Ineffective
• Symptomatic monotherapy in Parkinson's disease.

Mechanism of Action
• Istradefylline is a selective adenosine A2A receptor antagonist.

Efficacy Profile
• Istradefylline has been characterized as 'likely efficacious' and 'possibly useful' for the treatment of motor fluctuations in Parkinson's disease. More specifically, istradefylline has been associated with a clinically significant decrease in OFF time.
• Patients on istradefylline have exhibited a sustained positive response without any tolerability issues over a 52-week period.
• Although there was some evidence that the higher 40 mg dosage of istradefylline had a greater benefit compared to the lower 20 mg dose, a dose–response association was not clearly demonstrated.
• The effect of istradefylline in reducing OFF time seems to be similar to that of other currently available adjunctive therapies.
• According to preliminary reports, istradefylline might have a potential to improve neuropsychiatric aspects of Parkinson's disease, including mood disorders, apathy, cognitive impairment, and somnolence.

ISTRADEFYLLINE

Pharmacokinetics

Absorption and Distribution
- (Oral) bioavailability: not reported.
- Food co-ingestion: no food interactions have been reported.
- Tmax: 4 h.
- Time to steady state: within 1 week.
- Pharmacokinetics: dose-proportional in the range 20–80 mg.
- Protein binding: approximately 98%.
- Volume of distribution: 557 l.

Metabolism
- Istradefylline undergoes hepatic metabolism and is mainly metabolized by CYP3A4 and CYP1A1.
- It is metabolized to a lesser extent by CYP1A2, CYP2B6, CYP2C8, CYP2C9, CYP2C18, and CYP2D6.
- Six metabolites of istradefylline have been detected in human plasma.

Elimination
- Half-life of istradefylline is about 83 h.
- About 39% of an administered dose is excreted in urine and 48% is found in faeces.
  - Unchanged istradefylline is not detected in urine.

Drug Interaction Profile

Pharmacokinetic Drug Interactions
- Istradefylline is both a weak CYP3A4 inhibitor and inducer.
- It is also a weak inhibitor for P-glycoprotein, breast cancer resistance protein (BCRP), organic cation transporter (OAT)P1B1, OATP1B3, OAT1, OCT2, multidrug and toxin extrusion protein (MATE)1 and MATE2-K.
- Effects by istradefylline:
  - Istradefylline, especially in higher dosage, may increase the levels and effects of CYP3A4 substrates (e.g. *alprazolam, amiodarone, amlodipine, apixaban, aripiprazole, atorvastatin, calcitriol, carbamazepine, chloroquine, citalopram, clarithromycin, clonazepam, diazepam, eletriptan, escitalopram, estradiol, haloperidol, mirtazapine, omeprazole, quetiapine, rivaroxaban, sildenafil, tramadol, venlafaxine, verapamil*).
  - Istradefylline, especially in higher dosage, may increase the levels and effects of sensitive P-glycoprotein substrates (e.g. some statins, *amitriptyline, apixaban, carvedilol, cimetidine, ciprofloxacin, clarithromycin, dabigatran, digoxin, dihydroergotamine, eletriptan, hydrocortisone, prednisone, verapamil*).
- Effects on istradefylline:
  - Strong CYP3A4 inducers (e.g. *carbamazepine, fosphenytoin, phenytoin, primidone, rifabutin, rifampin*) may decrease the levels and effects of istradefylline.

- CYP3A4 inhibitors (e.g. *chloramphenicol*) may increase the levels and effects of istradefylline.
- Grapefruit increases the levels and effects of istradefylline through affecting CYP3A4 metabolism.

Pharmacodynamic Drug Interactions
- Not reported.

Adverse Effects

How Drug Causes Adverse Effects
- The activity of istradefylline is mediated by adenosine A2A receptor antagonism.

Common Adverse Effects
- Very common (≥1/10):
  - Dyskinesia.
- Common (≥1/100 to <1/10):
  - Nervous/psychiatric: dizziness, hallucinations, insomnia, abnormal thinking/behaviour.
  - Respiratory: upper respiratory tract inflammation.
  - GI: constipation, nausea, diarrhoea.
  - Skin: rash.
  - Other: decreased appetite, increased blood glucose, increased blood urea, increased alkaline phosphatase.
- Uncommon (≥1/1,000 to <1/100):
  - Nervous/psychiatric: impulse control disorder.

Life-Threatening or Dangerous Adverse Effects
- Not reported.

Rare and Not Life-Threatening Adverse Effects
- Not reported.

Weight Change
- Rare reports of anorexia and weight decrease.

What to Do About Adverse Effects
- Before introducing istradefylline, discuss common adverse effects with patients and/or caregivers, including symptoms that should be reported to the physician.
- On a regular basis, monitor for ICDs, hallucinations, or psychotic-like behaviours with focused and direct questions to patients and caregivers, as patients might not acknowledge such symptoms as abnormal to report them.

ADVERSE EFFECTS

- Patients and their caregivers should be made aware about the possibility of istradefylline causing ICDs. A dose reduction or complete discontinuation of therapy should be considered.
- Istradefylline therapy may induce or worsen psychosis. If the patient develops hallucinations or psychotic behaviour consider dose reduction or complete discontinuation of istradefylline.

Dosing and Use

Usual Dosage Range
- 20–40 mg.

Available Formulations
- Tablets: 20 mg, 40 mg.

How to Dose
- Initial dose of 20 mg OD; may increase up to a maximum dose of 40 mg if needed.

Dosing Tips
- Not reported.

How to Withdraw Drug
- There is no need for gradual discontinuation of istradefylline.

Overdose
- No information is provided.

Tests and Therapeutic Drug Monitoring
- No particular monitoring is required.

Other Warnings / Precautions
- Istradefylline therapy may predispose patients to develop ICDs, including increased sexual urges, intense urges to gamble, spend money, binge or compulsive eating or other urges, with an inability to control them.
- Co-administration with levodopa may result in dyskinesias or worsen already existent dyskinesias. Most cases are of mild or moderate severity.
- If co-administered with CYP3A4 inhibitors a maximum daily dose of istradefylline 20 mg is recommended.
- Co-administration of istradefylline and CYP3A4 substrates is generally not encouraged. If co-administration cannot be avoided, consider a maximum daily dose of istradefylline 20 mg and a lower dose of the CYP3A4 substrate and close monitoring.
  - With some CYP3A4 substrates (e.g. *abametapir*) a minimum of 2 weeks interval is necessary before istradefylline therapy is started, while others should be completely avoided (e.g. *lonafarnib*).

ISTRADEFYLLINE

- If istradefylline is co-administered with sensitive P-glycoprotein substrates, a dose reduction of the latter is suggested.
- If the patient smokes more than 20 cigarettes per day (or equivalent tobacco dose), an istradefylline daily dose of 40 mg is suggested.

Do Not Use (Contraindications)
- Patients with a diagnosis of major psychiatric disorder.
- Co-administration with strong CYP3A4 inducers is not recommended.

Special Populations
Renal Impairment
- Mild, moderate or severe renal impairment (CrCl 15–89 ml/min): no dose adjustments are required.
- End-stage renal impairment or haemodialysis: not studied; istradefylline use is not advised.

Hepatic Impairment
- Mild impairment (Child–Pugh A): no dosage modification required.
- Moderate impairment (Child–Pugh B): a maximum dose of 20 mg and close monitoring is suggested.
- Severe impairment (Child–Pugh C): istradefylline use is not recommended.

Elderly
- Studies have shown no age-related differences in the pharmacokinetics of istradefylline and the patients' response to therapy.
- No dosage adjustments are necessary.

Pregnancy
- There are no data on istradefylline use during pregnancy in humans.
- Women of childbearing potential should be advised to use contraception during istradefylline therapy.
- A teratogenic potential of istradefylline was found in animal studies.

Breastfeeding
- There are no data concerning the presence of istradefylline in human milk or its effect on breastfed infants.
- In lactating rats, istradefylline was detected in milk at concentrations 10 times higher than in maternal plasma.
- Istradefylline is not recommended during breastfeeding. Potential benefits and risks from istradefylline therapy should be weighed before deciding if it should be discontinued or the mother should not breastfeed.

SPECIAL POPULATIONS

Costs
• Not available in the UK.

The Overall Place of Istradefylline in the Treatment of Parkinson's Disease

Istradefylline is a non-dopaminergic agent, which offers a novel mechanism of action in the treatment of Parkinson's disease. It is the only A2A antagonist currently available for the treatment of motor fluctuations in Parkinson's disease. It can only be used as an adjunctive therapy to levodopa formulations. Istradefylline offers a clinically meaningful decrease in OFF time in six high-quality studies (including a 12-month extension study). This effect was not confirmed in one high-quality study. Istradefylline has also been associated with an increase in ON time without troublesome dyskinesia; however, this effect was not so clearly detected in all clinical studies and it is not included in the drug's indications. Istradefylline has only been approved in Japan and the United States. The EMA has refused marketing authorization due to lack of sufficient evidence of its benefits in Parkinson's disease patients in phase III studies, particularly those involving European populations. Despite the conflicting reports, the overall efficacy of istradefylline, according to the MDS EBM Committee, seems to be positive. Istradefylline is generally considered well tolerated with minor adverse events, although more studies with longer follow-up periods are required.

Potential Advantages
• Istradefylline can be an alternative option for Parkinson's disease patients who cannot tolerate COMT inhibitors.
• Istradefylline is considered a safe option for elderly patients.
• Drug–drug interactions are limited.
• There are no major contraindications in istradefylline use.

Potential Disadvantages
• Not available in most countries, including Europe.
• Istradefylline is relatively expensive, which might be complicating for Medicare and private insurance coverage.

Clinical Box
An 80-year-old man with an 8-year-history of Parkinson's disease presented at the Movement Disorders Outpatient Clinic for his regular follow-up appointment. He reported motor end-of-dose phenomena and a significant increase in daily OFF time. His current medications were levodopa/carbidopa 100/25 mg QID and rasagiline 1 mg OD. His medical history consisted of a past stroke, hypertension, diabetes mellitus, and mild renal impairment for which he was receiving acetylsalicylic

acid 100 mg OD, olmesartan/hydrochlorothiazide 20/12.5 mg OD and metformin 850 mg BID. The patient was given the option of initiating either entacapone or istradefylline to decrease OFF time and he chose the latter because it was administered in a single daily dose. OFF time decreased, but the patient developed mild dyskinesia. As dyskinesia was not troublesome to the patient, no changes to the current regimen were made.

Suggested Reading

Hauser RA, JP Hubble, DD Truong. Randomized trial of the adenosine A(2A) receptor antagonist istradefylline in advanced PD. *Neurology* 2003; 61(3): 297–303.

Hauser RA, LM Shulman, JM Trugman, JW Roberts, A Mori, R Ballerini, NM Sussman. Study of istradefylline in patients with Parkinson's disease on levodopa with motor fluctuations. *Mov Disord* 2008; 23(15): 2177–2185.

Kondo T, Y Mizuno. A long-term study of istradefylline safety and efficacy in patients with Parkinson disease. *Clin Neuropharmacol* 2015; 38(2): 41–46.

LeWitt PA, M Guttman, JW Tetrud, PJ Tuite, A Mori, P Chaikin, NM Sussman. Adenosine A2A receptor antagonist istradefylline (KW-6002) reduces "off" time in Parkinson's disease: a double-blind, randomized, multicenter clinical trial (6002-US-005). *Ann Neurol* 2008; 63(3): 295–302.

Mizuno Y, T Kondo. Adenosine A2A receptor antagonist istradefylline reduces daily OFF time in Parkinson's disease. *Mov Disord* 2013; 28(8): 1138–1141.

Pourcher E, HH Fernandez, M Stacy, A Mori, R Ballerini, P Chaikin. Istradefylline for Parkinson's disease patients experiencing motor fluctuations: results of the KW-6002-US-018 study. Parkinsonism Relat Disord 2012; 18(2): 178–184.

Stacy M, D Silver, T Mendis, J Sutton, A Mori, P Chaikin, NM Sussman. A 12-week, placebo-controlled study (6002-US-006) of istradefylline in Parkinson disease. *Neurology* 2008; 70(23): 2233–2240.

References

AHFS Drug information, 2012. Bethesda: American Society of Health-System Pharmacists. Accessed on 4 December 2022 via www.medicinescomplete.com.

Istradefylline. In: Brayfield A (Ed.), *Martindale: The Complete Drug Reference*. London: The Royal Pharmaceutical Society of Great Britain. Accessed on 4 December 2022 via www.medicinescomplete.com.

Istradefylline. In: DRUGDEX® System (electronic version). Truven Health Analytics, Greenwood Village, Colorado, USA. Accessed on 4 December 2022 via www.micromedexsolutions.com.

REFERENCES

ISTRADEFYLLINE

Jenner P, A Mori, T Kanda. Can adenosine A_{2A} receptor antagonists be used to treat cognitive impairment, depression or excessive sleepiness in Parkinson's disease? *Parkinsonism Relat Disord*, 2020; 80: S28–S36.

Nagayama H, O Kano, H Murakami, K Ono, M Hamada, T Toda, R Sengoku, Y Shimo, N Hattori. Effect of istradefylline on mood disorders in Parkinson's disease. *J Neurol Sci* 2019; 396: 78–83.

LEVODOPA–BENSERAZIDE

L

Therapeutics

Chemical Name and Structure

Levodopa ((−)-3,4-dihydroxyphenyl)-L-alanine) has a molecular weight of 197.19 and a molecular formula of $C_9H_{11}NO_4$.

Benserazide hydrochloride ((*RS*)-2-amino-3-hydroxy-*N'*-(2,3,4-trihydroxybenzyl)propanehydrazide hydrochloride) has a molecular weight of 293.7 and a molecular formula of $C_{10}H_{16}ClN_3O_5$.

Brand Names
- **Benspar** (*India*); **Bopazir** (*Denmark*).
- **EC-Doparl** (*Japan*); **Ekson** (*Brazil*); **Eugenix** (*Indonesia*).
- **Leparson** (*Indonesia*); **Levazide** (*Indonesia*); **Levoben** (*Indonesia*); **Levopar** (*Indonesia*); **Levopar Plus** (*Israel, Thailand*).
- **Madopar** (*Argentina, Australia, Austria, China, Czech Republic, Denmark, Finland, Germany, Greece, Hong Kong, Ireland, Italy, Japan, Malaysia, Mexico, Netherlands, New Zealand, Norway, Philippines, Poland, Portugal, Russian Federation, Singapore, South Africa, Spain, Switzerland, Thailand, Turkey, UK, Ukraine, Venezuela*); **Madopar-F** (*India*); **Madopark** (*Sweden*); **Madozide** (*Chile*); **Melitase** (*Chile*); **Modopar** (*France*).
- **Neodopasol** (*Japan*).
- **Pardoz** (*Indonesia*); **Prolopa** (*Belgium, Brazil, Canada, Chile*).
- **Restex** (*Austria*).
- **Udopar-250** (*Thailand*).
- **Vopar** (*Thailand*).

Generics Available
- Yes.

Licensed Indications for Parkinson's Disease
- Symptomatic treatment of parkinsonism (EMA, EMC).

Licensed Indications for Other Conditions
- None.

Non-Licensed Use for Parkinson's Disease
- Dopamine-responsive non-motor symptoms.

Non-Licensed Use for Other Conditions
- Restless legs syndrome.
- Dopamine-responsive dystonia.

Ineffective
- Reduced or no response in atypical parkinsonism.

THERAPEUTICS

L

LEVODOPA–BENSERAZIDE

Mechanism of Action
- Levodopa crosses the blood–brain barrier and is converted to dopamine by dopa-decarboxylase, which then acts on dopamine receptors to reverse the dopamine deficiency occurring in Parkinson's disease.
- Benserazide hydrochloride is a peripheral DDI, which increases the amount of levodopa crossing the blood–brain barrier.

Efficacy Profile
- The goal of treatment is to control Parkinson's disease-related motor and non-motor symptoms.
- Onset of action may be rapid and usually within 30 min (more rapid with dispersible formulations).
- If ineffective/partially effective, the dose can be progressively increased, or it can be combined with a COMT inhibitor or a MAO-B inhibitor or a dopamine agonist.

Pharmacokinetics
Absorption and Distribution of Levodopa when Co-Administered with Benserazide
- Bioavailability: up to 98%; rapid absorption, mainly in the proximal small intestine.
- Food co-ingestion: peak levodopa plasma concentrations are approximately 30% lower, plus absorption is delayed when administered after a standard meal.
- Tmax: within 1 h.
- Pharmacokinetic: linear.
- Protein binding: none.
- Volume of distribution: 57 l.

Metabolism of Levodopa when Co-Administered with Benserazide
- Bacterial decarboxylation to dopamine in the intestinal lumen.
- O-methylation to 3-O-methyldopa by the ubiquitous enzyme COMT.
- Decarboxylation to dopamine in the brain and production of 3,4-dihydroxyphenylacetic acid by MAO-B enzyme.

Elimination of Levodopa when Co-Administered with Benserazide
- Levodopa and benserazide are both extensively metabolized.
- After 48 h, 0.17% is found in faeces, 0.28% is exhaled, and 78.4% in the urine.
- Less than 10% of levodopa is excreted unchanged in the urine.
- Elimination half-life of levodopa: 1.5 h.
- Benserazide is almost entirely eliminated by metabolism (metabolites mainly excreted in the urine (64%) and faeces (24%)).

Drug Interaction Profile
Pharmacokinetic Drug Interactions
- *Trihexyphenidyl* may reduce the rate, but not the extent, of levodopa/benserazide absorption. No impact on CR formulations.
- Antacids reduce the extent of levodopa absorption by approximately 32%.
- Ferrous sulphate decreases the maximum plasma concentration and the AUC of levodopa by 30–50%.
- *Metoclopramide* and *domperidone* increase the rate of levodopa absorption by stimulating gastric emptying.
- *Tolcapone* increases benserazide concentration.
- *Tryptophan* decreases levodopa concentration.
- COMT inhibitors and MAO-B inhibitors: reduced metabolism of levodopa and dopamine respectively.

Pharmacodynamic Drug Interactions
- Co-administration with dopamine-receptor blockers, *isoniazid*, *phenytoin*, and *papaverine* may lead to reduced levodopa effects.
- Co-administration with antihypertensives may enhance the antihypertensive properties of levodopa.
- Co-administration of sympathomimetics (e.g. *epinephrine*, *norepinephrine*, *isoproterenol*, or *amphetamine*) may enhance the sympathomimetic properties of levodopa.
- Co-administration with irreversible non-selective MAOIs or combination of MAO-B and MAO-A inhibitors increases the risk of hypertensive crisis.
- Co-administration with dopamine agonists may lead to enhanced dopaminergic effects.

Adverse Effects
How Drug Causes Adverse Effects
- Mainly (but not only) by increasing dopaminergic activity.

Common Adverse Effects
- Very common (≥1/10):
  - Anxiety, depression, insomnia, dyskinesias, orthostatic hypotension, nausea, constipation, falls.
- Common (≥1/100 to <1/10):
  - Neuropsychiatric: abnormal dreams, agitation, confusion, hallucinations, psychotic disorder, sleep attacks, sleep disorder, dizziness, dystonia, headache, hypoesthesia, paraesthesia, polyneuropathy, somnolence, tremor.
  - Cardiovascular: irregular heart rate, hypertension.
  - Respiratory: dyspnoea, oropharyngeal pain.
  - GI: abdominal distension, diarrhoea, dry mouth, dysgeusia, dyspepsia, dysphagia, flatulence, vomiting.

L

ADVERSE EFFECTS

- ∘ Skin: hyperhidrosis, peripheral oedema, pruritus, rash.
- ∘ Urinary/renal: urinary incontinence/retention.
- ∘ Other: anaemia, increased amino acid (methylmalonic acid) and homocysteine levels, vitamin B6/ B12 deficiency, syncope, muscle spasms, neck pain, fatigue, pain, asthenia, decreased appetite.
- Uncommon (≥1/1,000 to <1/100):
  - ∘ Neuropsychiatric: dementia, disorientation, euphoria, fear, increased libido, ataxia, gait disturbance.
  - ∘ Eye/ear: blepharospasm, diplopia.
  - ∘ Cardiovascular: palpitations, phlebitis, chest pain.
  - ∘ GI: salivary hypersecretion.
  - ∘ Skin: alopecia, erythema, urticaria.
  - ∘ Urinary/renal: chromaturia.
  - ∘ Other: dysphonia, malaise.

Life-Threatening or Dangerous Adverse Effects
- ICDs, DDS.
- Psychosis.
- Haemolytic anaemia, thrombocytopenia, leukopenia, agranulocytosis, and pancytopenia.
- Arrhythmia.

Rare and Not Life-Threatening Adverse Effects
- Decreased appetite.
- Ageusia/dysgeusia.
- Saliva/tongue/tooth/oral mucosa discolouration.
- Increased values of transaminases, alkaline phosphatase, γGT and/or blood urea.
- Pruritus, rash.

What to Do About Adverse Effects
- Discuss common adverse effects with patients or caregivers before starting medication, including symptoms that should be reported to the physician.
- Consider reducing daily dose if adverse effects are troublesome.
- Symptomatic treatment for specific adverse effects (i.e. nausea, orthostatic hypotension, dyskinesia) may be considered.
- If levodopa-induced nausea occurs, the patient can be instructed to take the medication after a meal; a temporary antiemetic therapy (e.g. *domperidone* 10 mg TID) could be considered.
  - It is important to manage GI dysfunction to improve intestinal absorption.

Dosing and Use
Usual Dosage Range
- 300–1,000 mg of levodopa.

L

Available Formulations
- ODT: 100 mg/25 mg.
- Tablets: 200 mg/50 mg.
- Capsules: 50 mg/12.5 mg, 100 mg/25 mg, 200 mg/50 mg.
- Capsules CR: 100 mg/25 mg.

How to Dose
- Start with a low dose of 50 mg/12.5 mg TID; progressively increase daily dose if necessary and tolerated.
- As an initial step, increase dose of each intake; when fluctuations occur, consider dividing the dosage into smaller, more frequent doses (spread the dose).

Dosing Tips
- Intake on an empty stomach is preferred in order to improve intestinal absorption.

How to Withdraw Drug
- A stepwise reduction of the daily dose of levodopa is recommended to lower the possibility of NMS.
- For patients on high doses (more than 1,000 mg of levodopa per day), a reduction of 50–100 mg per day is suggested. For patients receiving more than 500 mg of levodopa per day, a reduction of 25–50 mg per day is suggested. Finally, for patients on low doses (less than 500 mg of levodopa per day), a reduction of 25 mg every second or third day is suggested.
- Patients need to be closely monitored during the tapering off period and the reduction rate should be adjusted according to the clinical response of the patient or potential adverse events.
- The levodopa equivalence dosage of the antiparkinsonian drugs, which can be introduced to replace levodopa, can also be used.

Overdose
- Overdose symptoms are similar to levodopa/benserazide side effects in therapeutic doses, but they may be of greater severity.
- Overdosage may present with cardiovascular (e.g. cardiac arrhythmias), psychiatric (e.g. confusion and insomnia, psychosis), and/or GI (e.g. nausea and vomiting) symptoms and dyskinesia.
- Close monitoring of vital signs is advised; supportive measures should be applied if needed.

Tests and Therapeutic Drug Monitoring
- Periodical evaluation of hepatic, haemopoietic, renal, and cardiovascular function, including blood count, is recommended.
- Periodical dermatological review is suggested if there is a history of melanoma.
- Regular measurement of intraocular pressure is advised in patients with open-angle glaucoma.

DOSING AND USE

L

LEVODOPA–BENSERAZIDE

Other Warnings / Precautions
- Caution is advised in active psychiatric disease.
- Caution is advised if evidence of severe endocrine, renal, hepatic, peptic ulcer, pulmonary, or cardiovascular disease, particularly if the patient has a history of MI or arrhythmia.
- Caution is advised if the patient has a history of orthostatic hypotension, as levodopa/benserazide may aggravate this condition.
- Caution is advised in osteomalacia.
- Monitor regularly for: sleepiness (which might occur without preceding warning signs, even later in therapy, e.g. after 1 year), drowsiness, hypotension (especially during dosing escalation), ICDs, hallucinations or psychotic-like behaviours with focused and direct questions to patients and caregivers, as patients might not acknowledge such symptoms as abnormal to report them.
- If general anaesthetic is required, treatment should be discontinued as close to the surgery as possible; in the case of halothane, therapy should be discontinued for 12–48 h before surgical intervention.
- Caution is advised if there is concomitant use of antipsychotics, as a worsening of parkinsonian symptoms may be observed due to their dopamine-receptor blocking properties.
- Close cardiovascular surveillance is advised if there is concomitant use of sympathomimetics (e.g. epinephrine, norepinephrine, isoproterenol, or amphetamine); the dose of sympathomimetic agents may need to be reduced.
- When introducing an add-on therapy with a COMT inhibitor, a reduction of levodopa daily dose may be needed.
- If co-administered with an irreversible non-selective MAOIs or combination of MAO-B and MAO-A inhibitors, a 2-week washout is required to lower the risk for a hypertensive crisis.
- Levodopa may affect laboratory test results for catecholamines, ketone bodies, creatinine, uric acid, glycosuria, and Coombs' tests.
- Caution is advised while driving or operating hazardous machinery while initiating levodopa/benserazide or when increasing dosage.

Do Not Use (Contraindications)
- Known hypersensitivity to levodopa or benserazide or any of its excipients.
- Concomitant use of MAOIs.
- Decompensated endocrine disease (e.g. phaeochromocytoma, hyperthyroidism, Cushing syndrome), impaired renal or hepatic function, cardiac disorders (e.g. severe cardiac arrhythmias and cardiac failure).
- Closed-angle glaucoma.
- Age under 25 years old, as skeletal development may not be yet complete.

Special Populations
Renal Impairment
- No dose reduction is required in case of mild or moderate renal insufficiency.

Hepatic Impairment
- Safety and efficacy have not been evaluated in patients with hepatic impairment.

Elderly
- Use with caution, although it is generally well tolerated.

Pregnancy
- Levodopa/benserazide preparations are contraindicated during pregnancy.
- Women of childbearing potential should not receive the drug in the absence of adequate contraception; if pregnancy occurs, levodopa/benserazide must be discontinued.

Breastfeeding
- Levodopa/benserazide use is not recommended during breastfeeding, as occurrence of skeletal malformations in the infants cannot be excluded.

Costs
NHS indicative price (as per BNF) accessed 30 October 2022:
- Madopar dispersible tablets (Roche Products Ltd) – 50 mg/12.5 mg × 100 tablets: £5.90+VAT; 100 mg/25 mg × 100 tablets: £10.45+VAT.
- Madopar capsules (Roche Products Ltd) – 50 mg/12.5 mg × 100 capsules: £4.96 +VAT; 100 mg/25 mg × 100 capsules: £6.91 +VAT; 200 mg/50 mg × 100 capsules: £11.78 +VAT.
- Madopar CR capsules (Roche Products Ltd) – 100 mg/25 mg × 100 capsules: £12.77 +VAT.
- Co-beneldopa capsules (various generic products) – 12.5 mg/50 mg × 100 capsules: £4.10–£4.96 +VAT.

The Overall Place of Levodopa/Benserazide in the Treatment of Parkinson's Disease
Levodopa combined with a peripheral DDI is the gold standard treatment for Parkinson's disease. Treatment with levodopa/benserazide can be initiated at diagnosis or later in the course of the disease. The dispersible formulation can be particularly useful if a more rapid onset of action is required (early morning, delayed on, wearing off) or when patients present with difficulties swallowing capsules/tablets. Flask

L

LEVODOPA–BENSERAZIDE

therapy based on dispersible tablets has also been used to produce a more continuous drug delivery when device-aided therapies are not indicated. CR capsules are commonly used at night-time to provide a more prolonged dopaminergic effect while sleeping.

Clinical Box

A 70-year-old, right-handed man with a 3-year history of Parkinson's disease started to experience early morning OFF episodes characterized by troublesome rigidity, pain, and anxiety. He had a history of hypertension and hypercholesterolaemia. His current medication regime included levodopa/carbidopa tablet 100 mg/25 mg TID (at 7, 12, 18), atorvastatin 40 mg OD, and ramipril 2.5 mg OD. He was fully active and independent in his activities of daily living. Intake of levodopa/benserazide dispersible tablet 50 mg/12.5 mg in the morning (on top of his levodopa–carbidopa capsule 100 mg/25 mg at the same time) was started with a beneficial response.

Suggested Reading

Tambasco N, M Romoli, P Calabresi. Levodopa in Parkinson's disease: current status and future developments. *Curr Neuropharmacol* 2018; 16(8): 1239–1252. doi: 10.2174/1570159X15666170510143821. PMID: 28494719; PMCID: PMC6187751.

References

Co-beneldopa. In: Brayfield A (Ed.), *Martindale: The Complete Drug Reference*. London: The Royal Pharmaceutical Society of Great Britain. Accessed on 30 October 2022 via www.medicinescomplete.com.

Joint Formulary Committee. British National Formulary (online). London: BMJ Group and Pharmaceutical Press. Accessed on 30 October 2022 via www.medicinescomplete.com.

Koschel J, K Ray Chaudhuri, L Tönges, M Thiel, V Raeder, WH Jost. Implications of dopaminergic medication withdrawal in Parkinson's disease. *J Neural Transm (Vienna)* 2022; 129(9): 1169–1178.

Summary of product characteristics – Madopar 100 mg/25 mg hard capsules. Roche Products Ltd. Electronic Medicines Compendium: Madopar 100 mg/25 mg hard capsules – summary of product characteristics (SmPC) – (emc). Accessed on 30 October 2022 via www.medicines.org.uk.

LEVODOPA–CARBIDOPA

L

Therapeutics

Chemical Name and Structure

Levodopa (L-3,4-dihydroxyphenylalanine) has a molecular weight of 197.19 and a molecular formula of $C_9H_{11}NO_4$.

Carbidopa ((+)-2-(3,4-dihydroxybenzyl)-2-hydrazinopropionic acid monohydrate; (–)-L-α-hydrazino-3,4-dihydroxy-α-methylhydrocinnamic acid monohydrate) has a molecular weight of 226.23 and a molecular formula of $C_{10}H_{14}N_2O_4$.

Brand Names

- **Apo-Levocarb** (*Canada, Hong Kong, Malaysia*); **Atamet** (*USA*).
- **Carbidol** (*Brazil*); **Carbidel** (*Philippines*); **Carbilev** (*South Africa*); **Carcopa** (*Japan*); **Cardopar** (*Singapore*); **Cloisone** (*Mexico*); **Credanil** (*Greece, Singapore*); **Cronomet** (*Brazil*).
- **Dhivy** (*USA*); **Dopacol** (*Japan*); **Dopadex** (*Turkey*); **Dopamar** (*Poland*); **Dopicar** (*Israel*); **Duopa** (*USA*).
- **Flexilev** (*Denmark, Poland, Sweden*).
- **Grifoparkin** (*Chile*).
- **Half Sinemet** (*Greece, Ireland, UK*).
- **Isicom** (*Czech Republic, Germany*).
- **Kardopal** (*Finland*); **Kinson** (*Australia, New Zealand*).
- **Lavida** (*Philippines*); **LCD** (*India*); **Lebocar** (*Argentina*); **Lecardop** (*South Africa*); **Lecarge** (*Argentina*); **Leprinton** (*Japan*); **Levacin** (*Switzerland*); **Levocar** (*Austria, Sweden*); **Levocarb** (*Brazil*); **Levocarbhexal** (*Ukraine*); **Levodop** (*Germany*); **Levofamil** (*Chile*); **Levokom** (*Ukraine*); **Levomed** (*Hong Kong, Malaysia, Thailand*); **Levomet** (*Singapore, Thailand*); **Levopa-C** (*India*).
- **Menesit** (*Japan*).
- **Nacom** (*Germany*); **Nakom** (*Czech Republic, Russian Federation, Ukraine*); **Neocare** (*India*); **Neodopaston** (*Japan*).
- **Pardopa** (*Philippines*); **Parkidopa** (*Brazil*); **Parkimet** (*Philippines*); **Parkinel** (*Argentina*); **Parkiston** (*Japan*); **Parklen** (*Brazil*); **PMS-Levocarb** (*Canada*); **Prikap** (*Argentina*); **Pro-Levocarb** (*Canada*).
- **Racovel** (*Mexico*); **Rytary** (*USA*).
- **Sinedin** (*Philippines*); **Sinedopa** (*Malaysia*); **Sinepar** (*Czech Republic*); **Saniter Compuesto** (*Chile*); **Sinemet** (*Argentina, Australia, Austria, Brazil, Canada, Chile, China, Denmark, Finland, France, Greece, Hong Kong, Ireland, Israel, Italy, Malaysia, Mexico, Netherlands, New Zealand, Norway, Philippines, Portugal, Singapore, South Africa, Spain, Sweden, Switzerland, Thailand, Turkey, UK, USA, Venezuela*); **Sirio** (*Italy*); **Syndopa** (*India, Russian Federation, Thailand*).
- **Ternovag** (*Mexico*); **Tidomet** (*Philippines, Russian Federation, Singapore, Thailand*); **Tremonorm** (*Russian Federation*).
- **Xi Lai Mei** (*China*).
- **Zuades** (*Netherlands, Norway*).

L

Generics Available
- Yes.

Licensed Indications for Parkinson's Disease
- Symptomatic treatment of parkinsonism (FDA, EMA, EMC).

Licensed Indications for Other Conditions
- None.

Non-Licensed Use for Parkinson's Disease
- Dopamine-responsive non-motor symptoms.

Non-Licensed Use for Other Conditions
- RLS.
- Dopamine-responsive dystonia.

Ineffective
- Reduced or no response in atypical parkinsonism.

Mechanism of Action
- Levodopa crosses the blood–brain barrier, is converted to dopamine via the action of a dopa-decarboxylase and binds to dopamine receptors.
- Carbidopa hydrochloride is a peripheral DDI, which increases the amount of levodopa crossing the blood–brain barrier.

Efficacy Profile
- The goal of treatment is control of Parkinson's disease-related symptoms.
- Onset of action may be rapid and usually within 30 min.
- If ineffective/partially effective, dose can be progressively increased, or it can be combined with a COMT inhibitor, a MAO-B inhibitor, or a dopamine agonist.

Pharmacokinetics
Absorption and Distribution of Levodopa when Co-Administered with Carbidopa
- Bioavailability: up to 99%; rapid absorption, mainly in the proximal small intestine.
- Food co-ingestion: peak levodopa plasma concentrations are approximately 30% lower, and absorption is delayed when administered after a standard meal.
- Tmax: within 1 h.
- Pharmacokinetics: linear.
- Protein binding: none.
- Volume of distribution: 0.9–1.6 l/kg.

L

Metabolism of Levodopa when Co-Administered with Carbidopa
- Bacterial decarboxylation to dopamine in the intestinal lumen.
- O-methylation to 3-O-methyldopa by the ubiquitous enzyme COMT.
- Decarboxylation to dopamine in the brain and production of 3,4-dihydroxyphenylacetic acid by MAO-B enzyme.
- Main metabolic pathway for carbidopa: loss of the hydrazine functional group.

Elimination of Levodopa when Co-Administered with Carbidopa
- Levodopa and carbidopa are both extensively metabolized with less than 10% and 30%, respectively, excreted unchanged through the kidneys.
- Elimination half-life of levodopa: 1.5 h.

Drug Interaction Profile
Pharmacokinetic Drug Interactions
- Drugs inhibiting gastric emptying (e.g. anticholinergic, opioid analgesics) may reduce levodopa absorption.
- Drugs stimulating gastric emptying (e.g. *metoclopramide*, *domperidone*) may increase levodopa absorption.
- Antacids reduce the extent of levodopa absorption by approximately 32%.
- Ferrous sulphate decreases the maximum plasma concentration and the AUC of levodopa by 30–50%.
- *Tryptophan* decreases levodopa concentration.
- COMT inhibitors and MAO-B inhibitors: reduced metabolism of levodopa and dopamine, respectively.

Pharmacodynamic Drug Interactions
- Co-administration with dopamine-receptor blockers, *isoniazid*, *phenytoin*, and *papaverine* may lead to reduced levodopa effects.
- Co-administration with antihypertensives may enhance the antihypertensive properties of levodopa.
- Co-administration of sympathomimetics (e.g. *epinephrine*, *norepinephrine*, *isoproterenol*, or *amphetamine*) may enhance the sympathomimetic properties of levodopa.
- Co-administration with irreversible non-selective MAOIs or combination of MAO-B and MAO-A inhibitors increases the risk of hypertensive crisis.
- Co-administration with dopamine agonists may lead to enhanced dopaminergic effects.

DRUG INTERACTION PROFILE

L

LEVODOPA–CARBIDOPA

Adverse Effects

How Drug Causes Adverse Effects
- Mainly (but not only) by increasing dopaminergic activity.

Common Adverse Effects
- Very common (≥1/10):
  - anxiety, depression, insomnia, dyskinesias, orthostatic hypotension, nausea, constipation, falls.
- Common (≥1/100 to <1/10):
  - Neuropsychiatric: abnormal dreams, agitation, confusion, hallucinations, psychotic disorder, sleep attacks, sleep disorder, dizziness, dystonia, headache, hypoesthesia, paraesthesia, polyneuropathy, somnolence, tremor.
  - Cardiovascular: irregular heart rate, hypertension.
  - Respiratory: dyspnoea, oropharyngeal pain.
  - GI: abdominal distension, diarrhoea, dry mouth, dysgeusia, dyspepsia, dysphagia, flatulence, vomiting.
  - Skin: hyperhidrosis, peripheral oedema, pruritus, rash.
  - Urinary/renal: urinary incontinence/retention.
  - Other: anaemia, increased amino acid (methylmalonic acid) and homocysteine levels, vitamin B6/ B12 deficiency, syncope, muscle spasms, neck pain, fatigue, pain, asthenia, decreased appetite.
- Uncommon (≥1/1,000 to <1/100):
  - Neuropsychiatric: dementia, disorientation, euphoria, fear, increased libido, ataxia, gait disturbance.
  - Eye/ear: blepharospasm, diplopia.
  - Cardiovascular: palpitations, phlebitis, chest pain.
  - GI: salivary hypersecretion.
  - Skin: alopecia, erythema, urticaria.
  - Urinary/renal: chromaturia.
  - Other: dysphonia, malaise.

Life-Threatening or Dangerous Adverse Effects
- ICDs, DDS.
- Psychosis.
- Haemolytic anaemia, thrombocytopenia, leukopenia, agranulocytosis, and pancytopenia.
- Arrhythmia.
- GI bleeding, duodenal ulcer.
- NMS.
- Depression with or without suicidal ideation.
- Convulsions (causal relationship has not been established).

Rare and Not Life-Threatening Adverse Effects
- Increased values of transaminases, alkaline phosphatase, γGT, and/or blood urea.
- Alopecia, rash, flushing, increased sweating.

THE MOVEMENT DISORDERS PRESCRIBER'S GUIDE TO PARKINSON'S DISEASE

- Phlebitis.
- Dark saliva/sweat/urine.
- Diarrhoea, constipation, dyspepsia, dry mouth, bitter taste, sialorrhoea, dysphagia, bruxism, hiccups, abdominal pain, flatulence, burning sensation of the tongue.
- Dream abnormalities, agitation, confusion, numbness, muscle cramps, anxiety, euphoria.
- Increased libido.
- Oedema.
- Urinary retention/incontinence.
- Priapism.

What to Do About Adverse Effects
- Discuss common adverse effects with patients or caregivers before starting medication, including symptoms that should be reported to the physician.
- Consider reducing daily dose if adverse effects are troublesome.
- Symptomatic treatment for specific adverse effects (i.e. nausea, orthostatic hypotension, dyskinesia) may be considered.
- In case of levodopa-induced nausea, the patient can be instructed to take the medication after a meal; a temporary scheme of antiemetic therapy (e.g. *domperidone* 10 mg TID) could be considered.
  - It is important to manage GI dysfunction to improve intestinal absorption.
- Muscle twitching and blepharospasm may be interpreted as early signs of dyskinesias; consider a decrease in dosage.

Dosing and Use
Usual Dosage Range
- 300–1,000 mg of levodopa.

Available Formulations
- Tablets (levodopa/carbidopa): 50 mg/12.5 mg, 10 mg/100 mg, 25 mg/100 mg, 25 mg/250 mg.
- Prolonged-release tablets (levodopa/carbidopa): 100 mg/25 mg, 200 mg/50 mg.
- In the United States, carbidopa preparations (25-mg tablets) are also provided (not as a combined formulation with levodopa). They are only used in Parkinson's disease patients for whom the levodopa/carbidopa combined preparations provide less than adequate daily dosage of carbidopa or in patients whose dosage requirements necessitate separate titration of each entity (levodopa and carbidopa).

How to Dose
- Start with a low dose of 50 mg/12.5 mg TID; progressively increase daily dose if necessary and tolerated.

L

DOSING AND USE

L

- As an initial step, increase dose of each intake; when fluctuations occur, consider dividing the dosage into smaller, more frequent doses (spread the dose).

Dosing Tips
- Intake on an empty stomach is preferred in order to improve intestinal absorption.

How to Withdraw Drug
- A stepwise reduction of daily dose of levodopa is recommended to lower the possibility of NMS.
- For patients on high doses (more than 1,000 mg of levodopa per day), a reduction of 50–100 mg per day is suggested. For patients receiving more than 500 mg of levodopa per day, a reduction of 25–50 mg per day is suggested. Finally, for patients on low doses (less than 500 mg of levodopa per day), a reduction of 25 mg every second or third day is suggested.
- Patients need to be closely monitored during the tapering off period and the reduction rate should be adjusted according to the clinical response of the patient or potential adverse events.
- The levodopa equivalence dosage of the antiparkinsonian drugs, which can be introduced to replace levodopa, can also be used.

Overdose
- Overdose symptoms are similar to levodopa/carbidopa side effects in therapeutic doses, but they may be of greater severity.
- Overdosage may present with cardiovascular (e.g. cardiac arrhythmias), psychiatric (e.g. confusion and insomnia, psychosis), and/or gastrointestinal (e.g. nausea and vomiting) symptoms and dyskinesia.
- Close monitoring of vital signs is advised; supportive measures should be applied if needed.

Tests and Therapeutic Drug Monitoring
- Periodical evaluation of hepatic, haemopoietic, renal, and cardiovascular function, including blood count, is recommended.
- Periodical dermatological review is suggested in case of a melanoma history.
- Regular measurement of intraocular pressure is advised in patients with open-angle glaucoma.

Other Warnings / Precautions
- Caution is advised in active psychiatric disease.
- Caution is advised in severe endocrine, renal, hepatic, peptic ulcer, pulmonary, or cardiovascular disease, particularly if the patient has a history of MI or arrhythmia.
- Caution is advised if the patient has a history of orthostatic hypotension, as levodopa/carbidopa may aggravate this condition.

- Caution is advised in osteomalacia.
- On a regular basis, monitor for sleepiness (which might occur without preceding warning signs, even later in therapy, e.g. after 1 year), drowsiness, hypotension (especially during dosing escalation), ICDs, hallucinations, or psychotic-like behaviours with focused and direct questions to patients and caregivers, as patients might not acknowledge such symptoms as abnormal to report them.
- Caution is advised with concomitant use of antipsychotics, as a worsening of parkinsonian symptoms may be observed due to their dopamine-receptor blocking properties.
- Close cardiovascular surveillance is advised with concomitant use of sympathomimetics (e.g. epinephrine, norepinephrine, isoproterenol, or amphetamine); the dose of sympathomimetic agents may need to be reduced.
- When introducing an add-on therapy with a COMT inhibitor, a reduction of levodopa daily dose may be needed.
- In case of co-administration with irreversible non-selective MAOIs or combination of MAO-B and MAO-A inhibitors, a 2-week washout is required to lower the risk for a hypertensive crisis.
- Levodopa may affect laboratory test results for catecholamines, ketone bodies, creatinine, uric acid, glycosuria, and Coombs' tests.
- Caution is advised while driving or operating hazardous machines during initiating levodopa/carbidopa or when increasing dosage.

Do Not Use (Contraindications)
- Known hypersensitivity to levodopa or carbidopa or any of its excipients.
- Concomitant use of MAOIs.
- Decompensated endocrine disease (e.g. phaeochromocytoma, hyperthyroidism, Cushing syndrome), impaired renal or hepatic function, cardiac disorders (e.g. severe cardiac arrhythmias and cardiac failure).
- Closed-angle glaucoma.
- Age under 25 years old, as skeletal development may not yet be complete.

Special Populations
Renal Impairment
- No dose reduction is required in mild or moderate renal insufficiency.

Hepatic Impairment
- Safety and efficacy have not been evaluated in patients with hepatic impairment.

Elderly
- Use with caution, although it is generally well tolerated.

L

Pregnancy
- Unknown effect on humans.
- Levodopa and levodopa–carbidopa have been found to cause visceral and skeletal malformations in animal studies.
- Levodopa/carbidopa preparations are contraindicated during pregnancy.
- Women of childbearing potential should not receive the drug in the absence of adequate contraception; if pregnancy occurs, levodopa/carbidopa must be discontinued.

Breastfeeding
- Levodopa/carbidopa use is not recommended during breastfeeding.
- Whether carbidopa is excreted in human milk is unknown, although this possibility cannot be excluded.

Costs
NHS indicative price (as per BNF) accessed 1 November 2022:
- Sinemet tablets (Organon Pharma (UK) Ltd) – 90 × 12.5 mg/50 mg tablets £6.28; 100 × 10 mg/100 mg tablets £7.30; 100 × 25 mg/250 mg tablets: £18.29.
- Sinemet Plus tablets (Organon Pharma (UK) Ltd) – 100 × 25 mg/100 mg tablets: £12.88.
- Half Sinemet CR tablets (Organon Pharma (UK) Ltd) – 60 × 25 mg/100 mg tablets: £11.60.
- Sinemet CR tablets (Organon Pharma (UK) Ltd) – 60 × 50 mg/200 mg tablets: £11.60.
- Co-careldopa 12.5 mg/50 mg tablets – 90 tablets: £5.55–£19.31.
- Co-careldopa 10 mg/100 mg tablets – 100 tablets: £7.30–£14.00.
- Co-careldopa 25 mg/100 mg tablets – 100 tablets: £6.78–£13.50.
- Co-careldopa 25 mg/250 mg tablets – 100 tablets: £18.29–£35.42.
- Caramet 25 mg/100 mg CR tablets – 60 tablets: £11.47.
- Lecado 100 mg/25 mg modified-release tablets – 60 tablets: £9.86.
- Lecado 200 mg/50 mg modified-release tablets – 60 tablets: £9.86.

The Overall Place of Levodopa/Carbidopa in the Treatment of Parkinson's Disease
Levodopa combined with a peripheral DDI is the gold standard for the treatment of Parkinson's disease. Treatment with levodopa/carbidopa preparations can be initiated at diagnosis or later in the course of the disease. CR formulations are commonly used at night-time to ensure prolonged dopaminergic stimulation while sleeping.

L

REFERENCES

Clinical Box

A 77-year-old, right-handed man with a 2-year history of Parkinson's disease reported nocturnal akinesia, nocturia, and sleep maintenance insomnia. His current and past medical history consisted of asthma. His current medication regime included levodopa/carbidopa tablets 100 mg/25 mg TID (at 7, 12, 18), and salbutamol inhalers 1 puff when needed. He was retired, fully active, and independent in his activities of daily living. No side effects were reported. Intake of levodopa/carbidopa CR 100 mg/25 mg at night-time was suggested with a subsequent beneficial response.

Suggested Reading

Tambasco N, Romoli M, Calabresi P. Levodopa in Parkinson's disease: current status and future developments. *Curr Neuropharmacol.* 2018; 16(8): 1239–1252. doi: 10.2174/1570159X15666170510143821. PMID: 28494719; PMCID: PMC6187751.

References

AHFS Drug information, 2012. Bethesda: American Society of Health-System Pharmacists. Accessed on 1 November 2022 via www.medicinescomplete.com.

Carbidopa/levodopa. Brayfield A (Ed.), *Martindale: The Complete Drug Reference.* London: The Royal Pharmaceutical Society of Great Britain. Accessed on 1 November 2022 via www.medicinescomplete.com.

Carbidopa/levodopa. In: DRUGDEX® System (electronic version). Truven Health Analytics, Greenwood Village, Colorado, USA. Accessed on 1 November 2022 via www.micromedexsolutions.com.

Joint Formulary Committee. British National Formulary (online). London: BMJ Group and Pharmaceutical Press. Accessed on 1 November 2022 via www.medicinescomplete.com.

Koschel J, K Ray Chaudhuri, L Tönges, M Thiel, V Raeder, WH Jost. Implications of dopaminergic medication withdrawal in Parkinson's disease. *J Neural Transm (Vienna)* 2022; 129(9): 1169–1178.

Summary of product characteristics – Sinemet Plus 25 mg/100 mg tablets. Organon Pharma (UK) Ltd. Electronic Medicines Compendium: Sinemet Plus 25 mg/100 mg tablets – summary of product characteristics (SmPC) – (emc). Accessed on 1 November 2022 via www.medicines.org.uk.

LEVODOPA–CARBIDOPA INTESTINAL GEL

Therapeutics

Chemical Name and Structure

Levodopa (L-3,4–dihydroxyphenylalanine) has a molecular weight of 197.19 and a molecular formula of $C_9H_{11}NO_4$.

Carbidopa ((+)-2-(3,4–dihydroxybenzyl)-2-hydrazinopropionic acid monohydrate; (−)-L-α-hydrazino-3,4-dihydroxy-α-methylhydrocinnamic acid monohydrate) has a molecular weight of 226.23 and a molecular formula of $C_{10}H_{14}N_2O_4$.

Brand Names

- **Duodopa** (*Australia, Austria, Belgium, Canada, Cyprus, Czech Republic, Denmark, Estonia, Finland, France, Germany, Greece, Hungary,* Ireland, *Israel, Italy, Japan, Lithuania, Netherlands, New Zealand, Norway, Poland, Portugal, Romania, South Africa, Spain, Sweden, Switzerland, Thailand,* UK); **Duopa** (*USA*).

Generics Available
- No.

Licensed Indications for Parkinson's Disease
- Symptomatic treatment of advanced Parkinson's disease with severe motor fluctuations and/or dyskinesias refractory to oral treatment.

Licensed Indications for Other Conditions
- None.

Non-Licensed Use for Parkinson's Disease
- Non-motor fluctuations refractory to oral treatment.

Non-Licensed Use for Other Conditions
- None.

Ineffective
- Not reported.

Mechanism of Action
- Levodopa crosses the blood–brain barrier, is converted to dopamine via the action of a dopa-decarboxylase and that dopamine binds to dopamine receptors.
- Carbidopa hydrochloride is a peripheral DDI, which increases the amount of levodopa crossing the blood–brain barrier.

Efficacy Profile
- The goal of treatment is to control motor and non-motor fluctuations and/or troublesome dyskinesias.

L

- Onset of action is usually within 30 min of administration.
- Reduced fluctuations in levodopa plasma concentrations are associated with reduced fluctuations in treatment response.

Pharmacokinetics
- Administered via an inserted tube directly into the duodenum or upper jejunum and connected to a pump.

Absorption and Distribution of Levodopa–Carbidopa via Intestinal Gel
- Bioavailability: up to 99%; rapid absorption of levodopa, mainly in the proximal small intestine. Carbidopa is absorbed slightly.
- Food co-ingestion: peak levodopa plasma concentrations are reduced and absorption is delayed when administered after a standard meal.
- Tmax: 2.5 h.
- Pharmacokinetics: linear.
- Protein binding: levodopa 10–30%, carbidopa 36%.
- Volume of distribution: 0.9–1.6 l/kg.

Metabolism of Levodopa when Co-Administered with Carbidopa
- Bacterial decarboxylation to dopamine in the intestinal lumen.
- O-methylation to 3-O-methyldopa by the ubiquitous enzyme COMT.
- Decarboxylation to dopamine in the brain and production of 3,4-dihydroxyphenylacetic acid by MAO-B enzyme.
- Main metabolic pathway for carbidopa: loss of the hydrazine functional group.

Elimination of Levodopa when Co-Administered with Carbidopa
- Levodopa and carbidopa are both extensively metabolized with less than 10% and 30%, respectively, excreted unchanged through the kidneys.
- Elimination half-life of levodopa: 1.5 h.

Drug Interaction Profile
No interaction studies have been performed with levodopa–carbidopa intestinal gel. Find below known interactions from oral preparations of levodopa–carbidopa combinations.

Pharmacokinetic Drug Interactions
- Drugs inhibiting gastric emptying (e.g. anticholinergic, opioid analgesics) may reduce levodopa absorption.
- Drugs stimulating gastric emptying (e.g. *metoclopramide, domperidone*) may increase levodopa absorption.
- Antacids reduce the extent of levodopa absorption by approximately 32%.

DRUG INTERACTION PROFILE

- Ferrous sulphate decreases the maximum plasma concentration and the AUC of levodopa by 30–50%.
- *Tryptophan* decreases levodopa concentration.
- COMT inhibitors and MAO-B inhibitors: reduced metabolism of levodopa and dopamine, respectively.

Pharmacodynamic Drug Interactions
- Co-administration with dopamine-receptor blockers, *isoniazid*, *phenytoin*, and *papaverine* may lead to reduced levodopa effects.
- Co-administration with antihypertensives may enhance the antihypertensive properties of levodopa.
- Co-administration of sympathomimetics (e.g. *epinephrine*, *norepinephrine*, *isoproterenol*, or *amphetamine*) may enhance the sympathomimetic properties of levodopa.
- Co-administration with irreversible non-selective MAOIs or combination of MAO-B and MAO-A inhibitors increases the risk of hypertensive crisis.
- Co-administration with dopamine agonists may lead to enhanced dopaminergic effects.

Adverse Effects
How Drug Causes Adverse Effects
- Mainly (but not only) by increasing dopaminergic activity.
- Device-/procedure-related adverse effects (tube dislocation, tube occlusion, excessive granulation tissue, incision site erythema, infection, discharge, procedure-related pain) are also relevant.

Common Adverse Effects
Drug-related adverse effects:
- Very common (≥1/10):
  - Anxiety, depression, insomnia, dyskinesias, orthostatic hypotension, nausea, constipation, falls.
- Common (≥1/100 to <1/10):
  - Neuropsychiatric: abnormal dreams, agitation, confusion, hallucinations, psychotic disorder, sleep attacks, sleep disorder, dizziness, dystonia, headache, hypoesthesia, paraesthesia, polyneuropathy, somnolence, tremor.
  - Cardiovascular: irregular heart rate, hypertension.
  - Respiratory: dyspnoea, oropharyngeal pain.
  - GI: abdominal distension, diarrhoea, dry mouth, dysgeusia, dyspepsia, dysphagia, flatulence, vomiting.
  - Skin: hyperhidrosis, peripheral oedema, pruritus, rash.
  - Urinary/renal: urinary incontinence/retention.
  - Other: anaemia, increased amino acid (methylmalonic acid) and homocysteine levels, vitamin B6/B12 deficiency, syncope, muscle spasms, neck pain, fatigue, pain, asthenia, decreased appetite.

- Uncommon (≥1/1,000 to <1/100):
  - Neuropsychiatric: dementia, disorientation, euphoria, fear, increased libido, ataxia, gait disturbance.
  - Eye/ear: blepharospasm, diplopia.
  - Cardiovascular: palpitations, phlebitis, chest pain.
  - GI: salivary hypersecretion.
  - Skin: alopecia, erythema, urticaria.
  - Urinary/renal: chromaturia.
  - Other: dysphonia, malaise.

Device-/procedure-related adverse events:
- Very common (≥1/10):
  - Postoperative wound infection, abdominal pain, excessive granulation tissue, incision site erythema, post-procedural discharge.
- Common (≥1/100 to <1/10):
  - Incision site cellulitis, post-procedural infection, incision site pain.

Life-Threatening or Dangerous Adverse Effects
- Common (≥1/100 to <1/10):
  - ICDs.
  - Peritonitis, pneumo-peritoneum.
  - (Aspiration) pneumonia.
  - Device dislocation/occlusion.
  - Post-procedural ileus/haemorrhage.
- Uncommon (≥1/1,000 to <1/100):
  - Convulsions.
  - Angle-closure glaucoma, optic ischaemic neuropathy.
  - Leukopenia, thrombocytopenia.
  - Suicidal ideation/behaviour.
  - Postoperative abscess.
  - Bezoar.
  - GI obstruction.
  - Pancreatitis.
- Rare (≥1/10,000 to <1/1,000):
  - Malignant melanoma.
  - Sepsis.
- Unknown frequency:
  - Anaphylactic reactions.
  - DDS.
  - GI ischemia, GI perforation.
  - Guillain–Barré syndrome-like autoimmune polyradiculoneuropathy.
  - Buried bumper syndrome.

Rare and Not Life-Threatening Adverse Effects
- Abnormal thinking.
- Discoloration of saliva/sweat.
- Hiccups.
- Glossodynia.
- Priapism.

Weight Change
- Decreased weight is a very common complication of LCIG infusion.
- Increased weight is a common complication of LCIG infusion.

What to Do About Adverse Effects
- Discuss common adverse effects with patients or caregivers before starting medication, including symptoms that should be reported to the physician.
- Consider reducing daily dose if adverse effects are troublesome.
- Symptomatic treatment for specific adverse effects (i.e. nausea, orthostatic hypotension, dyskinesia) may be considered.
- If troublesome device-related adverse effects occur, consider switching to oral levodopa–carbidopa therapy.
- Constipation should be properly addressed and dietary advice should be given to patients to avoid the formation of LCIG-related bezoars (e.g. avoid fibre-rich foods, or have these foods chopped into small pieces before boiling them to soften them; they should be chewed thoroughly).

Dosing and Use
Available Formulations
- Duopa (carbidopa/levodopa): (4.63 mg/20 mg)/ml in a single-use cassette; each cassette contains ~100 ml.
- Duodopa (levodopa/carbidopa): (20 mg/5 mg)/ml in a single-use cassette; each cassette contains ~100 ml.

Usual Dosage Range
- Morning dose: 5–10 ml = 100–200 mg levodopa; maximum recommended morning dose is 15 ml (300 mg levodopa).
- Continuous maintenance dose: 2–6 ml/h (40–120 mg levodopa/h); maximum recommended daily dose is 200 ml (2,000 mg levodopa).
- Extra bolus doses: 0.5–2 ml (10–40 mg levodopa).

How to Dose
- The total daily dose is composed of three individually adjusted doses:
  ○ Morning bolus dose.
  ○ Continuous maintenance dose.
  ○ Extra bolus doses.
- Initial dose setting is based on patient's daily levodopa intake.
  ○ The morning dose is administered to rapidly achieve therapeutic dose levels (within 30 min). Consider administering the same size of previous levodopa morning intake plus the volume required to fill the tube (3 ml).
- Continuous maintenance dose is administered to maintain therapeutic dose levels during the day.

L

- ○ Continuous dose should be based on patient's daily levodopa intake (excluding the morning dose); it is initially reduced to 80% of the previous daily levodopa intake.
- ○ Consider an increase in continuous maintenance dose if more than 5 extra doses per day are needed.
- Treatment is usually limited to the patient's awake period.
- If ineffective/partially effective, dose can be progressively titrated up (also consider tube dislocation).
- Dose should be titrated gradually, based on clinical response:
  - ○ Dose adjustment by 0.1 ml (2 mg) increments for morning dose.
  - ○ Dose adjustment by 0.1 ml/h (2 mg/h) increments for continuous maintenance dose.

Dosing Tips
- Aim for monotherapy, if possible.
  - ○ To avoid dopamine agonist withdrawal symptoms, abrupt dopamine agonist discontinuation is not recommended.
- In case of a sudden deterioration in treatment response, consider duodenal/jejunal tube dislocation or occlusion; an abdomen X-ray is recommended.

How to Withdraw Drug
- Sudden significant reduction of levodopa equivalent daily dose should be avoided due to risk of NMS.
- A switch to oral levodopa equivalent daily dose is suggested; higher oral doses should be considered.

Overdose
- Overdose symptoms are similar to levodopa–carbidopa side effects in therapeutic doses, but they may be of greater severity.
- Overdosage may present with cardiovascular (e.g. cardiac arrhythmias), psychiatric (e.g. confusion and insomnia, psychosis), and/or GI (e.g. nausea and vomiting) symptoms and dyskinesia.
- Close monitoring of vital signs is advised; supportive measures should be applied if needed.
- Consider applying the lock function in the pump.

Tests and Therapeutic Drug Monitoring
- Periodic evaluation of the following parameters is recommended:
  - ○ Hepatic, haemopoietic, renal and cardiovascular function.
  - ○ Blood count, levels of vitamin B12, folate and homocysteine.
  - ○ Weight.
- Periodic inspection of the J-PEG site.
- Periodic clinical evaluation of peripheral nerve function.
- Periodic dermatological review is suggested in case of a melanoma history.
- Regular measurement of intra-ocular pressure is advised in patients with open-angle glaucoma.

DOSING AND USE

L

Other Warnings/Precautions
- The option of LCIG infusion should only be offered if the patient or their caregiver are able to manage the system safely.
- Caution is advised in case of active psychiatric disease.
- Caution is advised in case of severe endocrine, renal, hepatic, peptic ulcer, pulmonary, or cardiovascular disease, particularly if the patient has a history of MI or arrhythmia.
- Caution is advised if the patient has a history of orthostatic hypotension, as levodopa–carbidopa may aggravate this condition.
- Caution is advised in case of osteomalacia.
- Caution is advised in case of history of upper GI surgery, as difficulties may be encountered during performing gastrostomy/jejunostomy.
- On a regular basis, monitor for sleepiness (which might occur without preceding warning signs, even later in therapy), drowsiness, hypotension (especially during dose escalation), ICDs, hallucinations or psychotic-like behaviours with focused and direct questions to patients and caregivers, as patients might not acknowledge such symptoms as abnormal to report them.
- Caution is advised in case of concomitant use of antipsychotics, as a worsening of parkinsonian symptoms may be observed due to their dopamine-receptor blocking properties.
- Close cardiovascular surveillance is advised in case of concomitant use of sympathomimetics (e.g. epinephrine, norepinephrine, isoproterenol, or amphetamine); the dose of sympathomimetic agents may need to be reduced.
- When introducing an add-on therapy with a COMT inhibitor, a reduction of levodopa daily dose may be needed.
- In case of co-administration with irreversible non-selective MAOIs or combination of MAO-B and MAO-A inhibitors, a 2-week washout is required to lower the risk of precipitating a hypertensive crisis.
- Levodopa may affect laboratory test results for catecholamines, ketone bodies, creatinine, uric acid, glycosuria, and Coombs tests.
- Caution is advised while driving or operating hazardous machines when initiating LCIG or when increasing dosage.
- LCIG contains hydrazine, a degradation product of carbidopa, which can be genotoxic and possibly carcinogenic.

Do Not Use (Contraindications)
- Known hypersensitivity to levodopa or carbidopa or any of its excipients.
- Concomitant use of non-selective MAOIs and selective MAO type A inhibitors.
- Decompensated endocrine disease (e.g. phaeochromocytoma, hyperthyroidism, Cushing syndrome), impaired renal or hepatic function, cardiac disorders (e.g. severe cardiac arrhythmias and cardiac failure).
- Closed-angle glaucoma.
- Age of less than 25 years old, as skeletal development may not be complete.
- Known contraindications to undergoing an endoscopic procedure.

Special Populations

Renal Impairment
- No dose reduction is required in case of mild or moderate renal insufficiency.
- Close monitoring is recommended in case of severe renal impairment.

Hepatic Impairment
- No dose reduction is required in case of mild or moderate hepatic impairment.
- Close monitoring is recommended in case of severe hepatic impairment.

Elderly
- Use with caution, although it is generally well-tolerated.

Pregnancy
- Unknown effect on humans.
- Levodopa and levodopa–carbidopa have been found to cause visceral and skeletal malformations in animal studies.
- Levodopa–carbidopa preparations are contraindicated during pregnancy.

Breastfeeding
- Not recommended during breastfeeding.

Costs
NHS indicative price on 18 June 2023:
- Duodopa intestinal gel 100 ml cassette (AbbVie Ltd) – 7 cassettes: £539.00.

The Overall Place of LCIG infusion in the Treatment of Parkinson's Disease

LCIG infusion is a device-aided therapy available for the treatment of motor and non-motor complications refractory to oral treatment. It is the most effective levodopa-based therapy in Parkinson's disease with a strong footprint in motor and non-motor improvement as suggested by two global registry studies (GLORIA and Duoglobe) and the only therapy currently capable of maintaining advanced Parkinson's disease cases on monotherapy (COSMOS) study.

L

THE TREATMENT OF PARKINSON'S DISEASE

L

LEVODOPA–CARBIDOPA INTESTINAL GEL

Clinical Box

A 76-year-old right-handed man with an 11-year history of Parkinson's disease reported troublesome motor and non-motor complications, mainly characterized by peak-dose dyskinesias during ON and severe tremor, anxiety, depression, and hyperhidrosis during unpredictable OFF episodes. His current medication regime consisted of rasagiline 1 mg OD, levodopa–benserazide 100/25 mg one dispersible tablet in the morning, levodopa–benserazide 100/25 mg one tablet five times daily, levodopa–carbidopa 200/50 mg CR one tablet at night-time, and rotigotine transdermal patch 10 mg/24 h. COMT inhibitors and amantadine were previously tried but were discontinued due to tolerability issues. No symptoms of GI dysfunction were reported. Levodopa intake was on an empty stomach. The patient had mild non-troublesome ICDs (occasional and mild punding), and was independent in his activities of daily living. No relevant co-morbidities were reported. He lived with his partner. He was evaluated for device-aided therapies and considered eligible for LCIG infusion.

Example of initial dose setting prior to titration:

Previous levodopa morning dose: 100 mg.

Previous levodopa equivalent daily dose (excluding levodopa morning dose and rotigotine transdermal patch): 750 mg/day.

Morning dose: 100 mg.

Corresponds to a volume of 5 ml of 20 mg/ml gel.

Total morning dose: 5 ml + 3 ml (volume to fill the tube) = 8 ml.

Continuous maintenance dose: 750 mg/day.

Continuous maintenance dose reduced to 80%: 750 mg/day × 0.80 = 600 mg/day.

Intake per hour (calculated based on 16 h of administration per day): 600 mg/16 h = 38 mg/h.

Corresponding to an hourly flow rate of: 38 mg/h = 1.9 ml/h of 20 mg/ml gel.

Patient was initiated on LCIG infusion with the above-mentioned doses, extra bolus dose of 1 ml (20 mg), and continued treatment with rotigotine patch 10 mg/24 h.

Progressive up-titration enabled optimal control of his motor and non-motor fluctuations, as well as reduction of the rotigotine transdermal patch daily dose from 10 mg to 4 mg/24 h.

Suggested Reading

Leta V, HS Dafsari, A Sauerbier, V Metta, N Titova, L Timmermann, K Ashkan, M Samuel, E Pekkonen, P Odin, A Antonini, P Martinez-Martin, M Parry, DJ van Wamelen, K Ray Chaudhuri. Personalised advanced therapies in Parkinson's disease: the role of non-motor symptoms profile. *J Pers Med* 2021; 11(8): 773.

Titova N, K Ray Chaudhuri. Intrajejunal levodopa infusion therapy for Parkinson's disease: practical and pragmatic tips for successful maintenance of therapy. *Expert Rev Neurother* 2017; 17(6): 529–537.

L

References

AHFS Drug information, 2012. Bethesda: American Society of Health-System Pharmacists. Accessed on 12 November 2022 via www.medicinescomplete.com.

Antonini A, W Poewe, KR Chaudhuri, R Jech, B Pickut, Z Pirtošek, J Szasz, F Valldeoriola, C Winkler, L Bergmann, A Yegin, K Onuk, D Barch, P Odin; GLORIA study co-investigators. Levodopa-carbidopa intestinal gel in advanced Parkinson's: Final results of the GLORIA registry. *Parkinsonism Relat Disord* 2017; 45: 13–20.

Chaudhuri KR, N Kovács, FE Pontieri, J Aldred, P Bourgeois, TL Davis, E Cubo, M Anca-Herschkovitsch, R Iansek, MS Siddiqui, M Simu, L Bergmann, M Ballina, P Kukreja, O Ladhani, J Jia, DG Standaert. Levodopa carbidopa intestinal gel in advanced Parkinson's disease: DUOGLOBE final 3-year results. *J Parkinsons Dis* 2023; 13(5): 769–783.

Fasano A, T Gurevich, R Jech, N Kovács, P Svenningsson, J Szász, JC Parra, L Bergmann, A Johnson, O Sanchez-Soliño, Z Tang, L Vela-Desojo. Concomitant medication usage with levodopa-carbidopa intestinal gel: results from the COSMOS study. *Mov Disord* 2021; 36(8): 1853–1862.

Joint Formulary Committee. British National Formulary (online). London: BMJ Group and Pharmaceutical Press. Accessed on 12 November 2022 via www.medicinescomplete.com.

Levodopa. In: Brayfield A (Ed.), *Martindale: The Complete Drug Reference*. London: The Royal Pharmaceutical Society of Great Britain. Accessed on 12 November 2022 via www.medicinescomplete.com.

Levodopa. In: DRUGDEX® System (electronic version). Truven Health Analytics, Greenwood Village, Colorado, USA. Accessed on 12 November 2022 via www.micromedexsolutions.com.

Spanaki C, I Boura, A Avgoustaki, E Orfanoudaki, IA Giannopoulou, E Giakoumakis, G Chlouverakis, E Athanasakis, M Koulentaki. Buried bumper syndrome: a common complication of levodopa intestinal infusion for Parkinson disease. *Parkinsonism Relat Disord* 2021; 85: 59–62.

Summary of Product Characteristics – Duodopa intestinal gel. AbbVie Ltd. Electronic Medicines Compendium: Duodopa intestinal gel – summary of product characteristics (SmPC) – (emc). Accessed on 12 November 2022 via www.medicines.org.uk.

Ueno T, N Hanabata, A Katagai, R Okudera, A Arai, M Tomiyama. Phytobezoar associated with levodopa–carbidopa intestinal gel infusion in patients with Parkinson's disease: a case report and literature review. *Intern Med* 2021; 60(20): 3317–3320.

L

LEVODOPA–CARBIDOPA–ENTACAPONE INTESTINAL GEL

Therapeutics

Chemical Name and Structure

Levodopa (L-3,4–dihydroxyphenylalanine) has a molecular weight of 197.19 and a molecular formula of $C_9H_{11}NO_4$.

Carbidopa ((+)-2-(3,4-dihydroxybenzyl)-2-hydrazinopropionic acid monohydrate; (–)-L-α-hydrazino-3,4–dihydroxy-α-methylhydrocinnamic acid monohydrate) has a molecular weight of 226.23 and a molecular formula of $C_{10}H_{14}N_2O_4$.

Entacapone ((E)-2-cyano-3-(3,4-dihydroxy-5-nitrophenyl)-*N,N*-diethyl-2-propenamide) has a molecular weight of 305.29 and a molecular formula of $C_{14}H_{15}N_3O_5$.

Brand Names

• **Lecigon** (*Denmark, Finland, Netherlands, Sweden*).

Generics Available

• No.

Licensed Indications for Parkinson's Disease

• Symptomatic treatment of advanced Parkinson's disease with severe motor fluctuations and/or dyskinesia refractory to oral treatment.

Licensed Indications for Other Conditions

• None.

Non-Licensed Use for Parkinson's Disease

• Non-motor fluctuations refractory to oral treatment.

Non-Licensed Use for Other Conditions

• None.

Ineffective

• Not reported.

Mechanism of Action

• Levodopa crosses the blood–brain barrier, is converted to dopamine via the action of a dopa-decarboxylase and dopamine binds to dopamine receptors.
• Carbidopa hydrochloride is a peripheral DDI, which increases the amount of levodopa crossing the blood–brain barrier by inhibiting peripheral metabolism of levodopa.
• Entacapone is a selective and reversible, mainly peripherally acting, COMT inhibitor, designed for concomitant administration with levodopa preparations.

L

- Entacapone decreases the metabolism of levodopa to 3-O-methyldopa (3-OMD) by inhibiting COMT. This action leads to higher and more sustained plasma levodopa concentrations, increases levodopa availability to brain and prolongs the clinical response to levodopa.
- Entacapone and carbidopa do not cross the blood–brain barrier at usual therapeutic doses.

Efficacy Profile
- The goal of treatment is to control Parkinson's disease-related symptoms, including motor and non-motor fluctuations.
- Onset of action is usually within 30 min.

Pharmacokinetics
- See also pharmacokinetics of entacapone (see relevant chapter).
- Administered via an inserted tube directly into the duodenum or upper jejunum and connected to a pump.
- Substantial inter- and intra-individual variations in the absorption of levodopa, carbidopa, and entacapone, particularly concerning the maximum concentration reached in plasma.

Absorption and Distribution of Levodopa when Co-Administered with Carbidopa and Entacapone via Intestinal Gel
- Rapid absorption and attainment of therapeutic plasma levels.
- Food effect on levodopa–carbidopa–entacapone preparations has not been evaluated.
- Protein binding: levodopa 10–30%; carbidopa 36%; entacapone 98% over the concentration range of 0.4–50 μg/ml.
- Volume of distribution: 0.36–1.6 l/kg.

Metabolism of Levodopa when Co-Administered with Carbidopa and Entacapone
- Decarboxylation to dopamine in the brain and production of 3,4-dihydroxyphenylacetic acid by MAO-B enzyme.
- Main metabolic pathway for carbidopa: removal of the hydrazine moiety.
- Main metabolic pathway for entacapone: extensive first pass metabolism – isomerization to the *cis*-isomer (active metabolite).
- Bacterial decarboxylation of levodopa to dopamine in the intestinal lumen.

Elimination of Levodopa when Co-Administered with Carbidopa and Entacapone
- Levodopa is extensively metabolized and less than 10% is excreted unchanged through the kidneys.
- Elimination half-life: 1.7 h.

PHARMACOKINETICS

- Unchanged carbidopa accounts for 30% of the total urinary excretion.
- Entacapone and the *cis*-isomer eliminated in the urine as glucuronide conjugates. Only a very small amount is excreted unchanged in the urine.

Drug Interaction Profile

No interaction studies have been performed with levodopa–carbidopa–entacapone intestinal gel. Below are known interactions from combinations of oral levodopa/carbidopa and entacapone/levodopa/carbidopa.

Pharmacokinetic Drug Interactions
- Drugs inhibiting gastric emptying (e.g. anticholinergic, opioid analgesics) may reduce levodopa absorption.
- Drugs stimulating gastric emptying (e.g. *metoclopramide*, *domperidone*) may increase levodopa absorption.
- Antacids reduce the extent of levodopa absorption by approximately 32%.
- Ferrous sulphate decreases the maximum plasma concentration and the AUC of levodopa by 30–50%.
- *Tryptophan* decreases levodopa concentration.
- MAO-B inhibitors: reduced metabolism of dopamine.
- Entacapone may increase levels and effects of drugs metabolized by COMT, such as inotropes, vasopressors, SSRIs, and SNRIs.
- Potential pharmacokinetic interactions with drugs metabolized by CYP2C9, for example *warfarin*.
- Drugs interfering with biliary excretion, glucuronidation, and intestinal β-glucuronidase (e.g. *cholestyramine*, *probenecid*), some anti-infectives (e.g. *ampicillin*, *chloramphenicol*, *erythromycin*, *rifampin*) may decrease levels and effects of entacapone.

Pharmacodynamic Drug Interactions
- Co-administration with dopamine-receptor blockers, *isoniazid*, *phenytoin*, and *papaverine* may lead to reduced levodopa effects.
- Co-administration with antihypertensives may enhance the antihypertensive properties of levodopa.
- Co-administration of sympathomimetics (e.g. *epinephrine*, *norepinephrine*, *isoproterenol*, or *amphetamine*) may enhance the sympathomimetic properties of levodopa.
- Co-administration with irreversible non-selective MAOIs or combination of MAO-B and MAO-A inhibitors increases the risk of hypertensive crisis.
- Co-administration with dopamine agonists may lead to enhanced dopaminergic effects.

Adverse Effects

How Drug Causes Adverse Effects
- Mainly (but not only) by increasing dopaminergic activity.
- Device/procedure–related adverse effects (tube dislocation, tube occlusion, excessive granulation tissue, incision site erythema, infection, discharge, procedure–related pain) should also be considered.

Common Adverse Effects
- Very common (≥1/10):
  - Weight loss, anxiety, depression, insomnia, dyskinesia, orthostatic hypotension, nausea, constipation, diarrhoea, pain in muscles, muscoskeletal and connective tissue pain, abdominal pain, harmless reddish-brown discoloration of the urine (chromaturia).
- Common (≥1/100 to <1/10):
  - Blood disorders: anaemia.
  - Psychiatric: nightmares, agitations, confusion, hallucinations, ICD, sleep disorders.
  - Nervous system: dizziness, headache, somnolence, tremor.
  - Eye: blurred vision.
  - Gastrointestinal: dry mouth, abdominal distension, dyspepsia, vomiting.
  - Skin: rash, hyperhidrosis, pruritis.
  - General: fatigue, peripheral oedema.
  - Harmless reddish-brown discoloration of the urine.

Device-/Procedure-Related Adverse Events
- Very common (≥1/10):
  - Postoperative wound infection, abdominal pain, excessive granulation tissue, incision site erythema, post-procedural discharge.
- Common (≥1/100 to <1/10):
  - Incision site cellulitis, post-procedural infection, incision site pain.

Life-Threatening or Dangerous Adverse Effects
Usually uncommon or rare:
- ICDs, DDS.
- Severe psychosis
- Haemolytic anaemia, thrombocytopenia, leukopenia, agranulocytosis, pancytopenia.
- Severe rhabdomyolysis secondary to severe dyskinesia or NMS.
- GI haemorrhage.
- Angioedema.
- Bezoars.
- Post-procedure peritonitis/perforation.

Rare and Not Life-Threatening Adverse Effects
- Skin, hair, beard, and nail discolorations.
- Cholestatic hepatitis.

L

ADVERSE EFFECTS

L

LEVODOPA–CARBIDOPA–ENTACAPONE

Weight Change
Reduced appetite and weight decreases have been reported.

What to Do About Adverse Effects
- Discuss common adverse effects with patients or caregivers before starting medication, including symptoms that should be reported to the physician.
- Consider reducing daily dose if adverse effects are troublesome.
- Symptomatic treatment for specific adverse effects (i.e. nausea, orthostatic hypotension, and dyskinesia) may be considered.
- If troublesome adverse effects are clearly related to entacapone (e.g. diarrhoea), consider switching from levodopa/carbidopa/entacapone preparations to levodopa/carbidopa only and titrate dose.
- Constipation should be properly addressed, and dietary advice should be given to patients to avoid the formation of bezoars (e.g. avoid fibre-rich foods, or have these foods chopped into small pieces before boiling them to soften them; they should be chewed thoroughly).

Dosing and Use
Usual Dosage Range
- Morning dose: 5–10 ml = 100–200 mg levodopa; maximum recommended morning dose is 15 ml (300 mg levodopa).
- Continuous maintenance dose: 0.7–5.0 ml/h (15–100 mg levodopa/h); maximum recommended daily dose is 100 ml (2,000 mg levodopa).
- Extra bolus doses: less than 3 ml (less than 60 mg levodopa).

Available Formulations
- 1 ml contains 20 mg levodopa, 5 mg carbidopa monohydrate, and 20 mg entacapone.

How to Dose
- The total daily dose is composed of three individually adjusted doses:
  ○ Morning bolus dose.
  ○ Continuous maintenance dose (multiple daily options).
  ○ Extra bolus doses.
- Treatment is usually limited to the patient's awake period.
- Initial dose setting is based on patient's daily levodopa intake.
- The morning dose is administered to rapidly achieve therapeutic dose levels (within 30 min).
  ○ The same size of previous levodopa morning intake is suggested, plus the volume required to fill the tube (3 ml).
- The continuous maintenance dose is administered to maintain therapeutic dose levels.
  ○ The continuous dose should be based on the patient's daily levodopa intake (excluding the morning dose) and is initially reduced to 65% of the previous daily levodopa intake.

L

- ○ Consider 1:1 conversion, if transition from oral levodopa/carbidopa/entacapone to intestinal levodopa/carbidopa/entacapone.
- Consider an increase in continuous maintenance dose if more than five extra doses per day are needed.
- Doses should be titrated gradually, based on clinical response:
  - ○ Dose adjustments by 0.1 ml (2 mg levodopa) increments for morning dose.
  - ○ Dose adjustment by 0.1 ml/h (2 mg/h levodopa) increments for continuous maintenance dose.

Dosing Tips
- The effect of entacapone on levodopa is dose-dependent, meaning that larger dose reductions are expected in high-dose patients.
- Aim for monotherapy, if possible.
  - ○ To avoid dopamine agonist withdrawal symptoms, abrupt dopamine agonist discontinuation is not recommended.
- In case of sudden deterioration in treatment response, consider excluding a potential duodenal/jejunal tube dislocation or occlusion; an abdomen X-ray is recommended.

How to Withdraw Drug
- Sudden significant reduction of levodopa equivalent daily dose should be avoided due to risk of NMS.
- A switch to oral levodopa equivalent daily dose is suggested; higher oral doses should be considered.

Overdose
- Symptoms are similar to side effects in therapeutic doses, but more severe.
- Overdosage may present as agitation, confusion, coma, bradycardia, ventricular tachycardia, Cheyne–Stokes respiration, discolorations of skin, tongue, and conjunctiva, and chromaturia.
- Management of acute overdose is similar to acute overdose with levodopa/DDI only; close monitoring of vital signs is advised; supportive measures should be applied if needed.
- Consider applying the lock function in the pump.

Tests and Therapeutic Drug Monitoring
- Periodic evaluation of the following parameters is recommended:
  - ○ Hepatic, haemopoietic, renal, and cardiovascular function.
  - ○ Blood count, levels of vitamin B12, folate, and homocysteine.
  - ○ Weight.
- Periodic inspection of the J-PEG site.
- Periodic clinical evaluation of peripheral nerve function.
- Periodic dermatology review is suggested in case of a melanoma history.
- Regular measurement of intra-ocular pressure is advised in patients with open-angle glaucoma.

DOSING AND USE

215

Other Warnings / Precautions
- The option of levodopa/carbidopa/entacapone infusion should only be offered if the patient or their caregiver are able to handle the system.
- Caution is advised in cases of active psychiatric disease.
- Caution is advised in cases of severe endocrine, renal, hepatic, peptic ulcer, pulmonary, or cardiovascular disease, particularly if the patient has a history of MI or arrhythmia.
- Caution is advised if the patient has a history of orthostatic hypotension, as levodopa/carbidopa may aggravate this condition.
- Caution is advised in osteomalacia.
- Caution is advised if there is a case of history of upper GI surgery, as difficulties may be encountered during performing gastrostomy/jejunostomy.
- On a regular basis, monitor for sleepiness (which might occur without preceding warning signs, even later in therapy), drowsiness, hypotension (especially during dosing escalation), ICDs, hallucinations, or psychotic-like behaviours with focused and direct questions to patients and caregivers, as patients might not acknowledge such symptoms as abnormal to report them.
- Caution is advised if there is concomitant use of antipsychotics, as a worsening of parkinsonian symptoms may be observed due to their dopamine-receptor blocking properties.
- Close cardiovascular surveillance is advised if concomitant use of sympathomimetics (e.g. epinephrine, norepinephrine, isoproterenol, or amphetamine); the dose of sympathomimetic agents may need to be reduced.
- Levodopa may affect laboratory test results for catecholamines, ketone bodies, creatinine, uric acid, glycosuria, and Coombs' tests.
- Levodopa/carbidopa/entacapone infusion contains hydrazine, a degradation product of carbidopa, which can be genotoxic and possibly carcinogenic.
- Caution is advised while driving or operating hazardous machinery when initiating levodopa/carbidopa/entacapone or when increasing dosage.

Do Not Use (Contraindications)
- Known hypersensitivity or intolerance to levodopa, carbidopa, entacapone, or any other excipients.
- Concomitant use of MAOIs.
- Decompensated endocrine disease (e.g. phaeochromocytoma, hyperthyroidism, Cushing syndrome), impaired renal or hepatic function, cardiac disorders (e.g. severe cardiac arrhythmias and cardiac failure).
- Closed-angle glaucoma.
- Age less than 25 years old, as skeletal development may not be complete.
- Known contraindications to undergoing an endoscopic procedure.
- Severe hepatic impairment.
- Previous history of NMS and/or non-traumatic rhabdomyolysis.

L

Special Populations

Renal Impairment
- No dose reduction is required in case of mild or moderate renal insufficiency.
- Close monitoring is recommended in case of severe renal impairment.

Hepatic Impairment
- Dose reductions may be needed in case of mild or moderate hepatic impairment.
- Levodopa/carbidopa/entacapone preparations are contraindicated in case of severe hepatic impairment.

Elderly
- Use with caution; no dose adjustments are required.

Pregnancy
- Unknown effect on humans.
- Levodopa and levodopa/carbidopa have been found to cause visceral and skeletal malformations in animal studies. No overt entacapone-related teratogenic or primary fetotoxic effects have been noted in animal studies.
- Levodopa/carbidopa/entacapone preparations are contraindicated during pregnancy.

Breastfeeding
- Women are advised not to breastfeed during treatment with levodopa/carbidopa/entacapone.

Costs
- Not available in the UK for cost comparison.

The Overall Place of Levodopa/Carbidopa/Entacapone Intestinal Gel Infusion in the Treatment of Parkinson's Disease
Levodopa/carbidopa/entacapone intestinal gel infusion is a new device-aided therapy, available in some countries for the treatment of motor and non-motor complications of Parkinson's disease which are refractory to oral treatment. Post-marketing, registry-based data are needed for longer-term tolerability and safety-related information. There are currently no head-to-head comparisons in terms of global motor and non-motor effects, the latter being well established for intrajejunal levodopa/carbidopa infusion.

THE TREATMENT OF PARKINSON'S DISEASE

Clinical Box

A 72-year-old, right-handed man with a 9-year history of Parkinson's disease reported troublesome motor and non-motor complications, mainly characterized by peak-dose dyskinesia during ON and severe bradykinesia, pain, anxiety, and swallowing difficulties during unpredictable OFF episodes. His current medication regimen consisted of rasagiline 1 mg one tablet in the morning, levodopa/benserazide 100 mg/25 mg one dispersible tablet in the morning, levodopa/carbidopa 100 mg/25 mg one tablet five times daily, levodopa/carbidopa CR one tablet 200 mg/50 mg at night-time, rotigotine transdermal patch 12 mg/24 h, opicapone 50 mg one tablet in the evening, and amantadine 100 mg twice daily. No symptoms of GI dysfunction were reported. Levodopa intake was on an empty stomach. He had mild non-troublesome ICD (eating sweets at night), a mild cognitive impairment, and was independent in his activities of daily living; no relevant co-morbidities were reported. He lived with his partner. He was evaluated for device-aided therapies and considered eligible for levodopa intestinal gel infusion. He preferred levodopa–carbidopa–entacapone intestinal gel infusion given the smaller size of the pump.

Example of initial dose setting prior to titration:

Previous levodopa morning dose: 100 mg.

Previous levodopa equivalent daily dose (excluding levodopa morning dose and rotigotine transdermal patch): 1,275 mg/day.

Morning dose: 100 mg.

Corresponds to a volume of 5 ml of 20 mg/ml gel.

Total morning dose: 5 ml + 3 ml (volume to fill the tube) = 8 ml.

Continuous maintenance dose: 1,275 mg/day.

Continuous maintenance dose reduced to 65%: 1,275 mg/day × 0.65 = 829 mg/day.

Intake per hour (calculated based on 16 h of administration per day): 829 mg/16 h = 52 mg/h.

Corresponding to an hourly flow rate of: 52 mg/h = 2.6 ml/h of 20 mg/ml gel.

Patient was initiated on levodopa–carbidopa–entacapone intestinal gel infusion with the above-mentioned doses, extra bolus dose of 1 ml, and continued treatment with rotigotine patch 12 mg/24 h.

Progressive up-titration allowed an optimal control of his motor and non-motor fluctuations, as well as a reduction of the rotigotine transdermal patch daily dose from 12 mg to 6 mg/24 h.

L

Suggested Reading

Leta V, HS Dafsari, A Sauerbier, V Metta, N Titova, L Timmermann, K Ashkan, M Samuel, E Pekkonen, P Odin, A Antonini, P Martinez-Martin, M Parry, DJ van Wamelen, K Ray Chaudhuri. Personalised advanced therapies in Parkinson's disease: the role of non-motor symptoms profile. *J Pers Med* 2021; 11(8): 773.

Nyholm D, WH Jost. Levodopa–entacapone–carbidopa intestinal gel infusion in advanced Parkinson's disease: real-world experience and practical guidance. *Ther Adv Neurol Disord* 2022; 15: 17562864221108018.

References

Levodopa. In: Brayfield A (Ed.), *Martindale: The Complete Drug Reference*. London: The Royal Pharmaceutical Society of Great Britain. Accessed on 12 November 2022 via www.medicinescomplete.com.

LEVODOPA, INHALED

Therapeutics

Chemical Name and Structure

Levodopa ((2S)-2-amino-3-(3,4-dihydroxyphenyl)propanoic acid, 3,4-dihydroxy-L-phenylalanine) has a molecular weight of 197.19 and a molecular formula of $C_9H_{11}NO_4$.

Brand Names
• **Inbrija** (*USA*).

Generics Available
• No.

Licensed Indications for Parkinson's Disease
• Intermittent management of OFF episodes in Parkinson's disease patients already treated with levodopa/DDI preparations (FDA, EMA).

Licensed Indications for Other Conditions
• None.

Non-Licensed Use for Parkinson's Disease
• Not reported.

Non-Licensed Use for Other Conditions
• Anorexia nervosa, congestive heart failure, hypertension, orthostatic hypotension, phenylketonuria, post-anoxic myoclonus, psoriasis, restless legs syndrome, supranuclear paralysis, vitiligo.

Ineffective
• In patients not already taking levodopa/DDI preparations.

Mechanism of Action
• Levodopa is an amino acid precursor of dopamine, which is converted to dopamine by DOPA decarboxylase in the brain and then stimulates dopamine receptors compensating for the depletion of endogenous dopamine in Parkinson's disease.
• Levodopa can cross the blood–brain barrier.
• Inhaled levodopa enters the body through the lungs bypassing the GI system leading to a rapid onset of action.

Efficacy Profile
• In a double-blind, multi-centre RCT, inhaled levodopa enhanced motor performance in Parkinson's disease patients during in-clinic OFF periods without substantial safety issues.

L

- In a double-blind, randomized study with a two-way crossover design, administration of inhaled levodopa immediately after the first daily dose of levodopa–carbidopa was well tolerated for the management of early morning OFF episodes.
- A prospective, open-label, randomized controlled study showed that inhaled levodopa was safe and efficacious for up to 12 months of therapy as assessed by motor scores, OFF time, and patient-reported outcomes.
- Two phase 2 studies have confirmed the pulmonary safety and tolerability of inhaled levodopa among Parkinson's disease patients experiencing motor fluctuations.

Pharmacokinetics

Absorption and Distribution
- Bioavailability: about 70% compared to IR oral tablets.
- Food co-ingestion: no interactions reported.
- Tmax: 30 min.
- Time to steady state: not applicable.
- Pharmacokinetics: dose proportional pharmacokinetics from 13 mg to 122 mg.
- Protein binding: minimal.
- Volume of distribution: 168 l.

Metabolism
- Inhaled levodopa is extensively metabolized.
- O-methylation to 3-O-methyldopa by the ubiquitous enzyme COMT.
- Decarboxylation to dopamine in the brain and production of 3,4-dihydroxyphenylacetic acid by MAO-B.

Elimination
- In the presence of carbidopa, elimination half-life of inhaled levodopa following a single administration is 2.3 h.
- Levodopa and carbidopa are both extensively metabolized with less than 10% and 30%, respectively, excreted unchanged through the kidneys.

Drug Interaction Profile

Pharmacokinetic Drug Interactions
- Effects of inhaled levodopa:
  - Inhaled levodopa may increase levels and effects of *linezolid*.
- Effects on inhaled levodopa:
  - *Isoniazid* may decrease levels and effects of inhaled levodopa by altering its metabolism (DOPA-decarboxylase inhibition in the brain).
  - Iron salts can form chelates with levodopa and reduce its bioavailability.

DRUG INTERACTION PROFILE

Pharmacodynamic Drug Interactions
- Co-medication with non-selective or selective MAOIs (e.g. *phenelzine, isocarboxazid, tranylcypromine*) may lead to synergistic effects, including an increased risk for acute hypertensive episodes.
- Co-medication with selective MAO-B inhibitors (e.g. *rasagiline, safinamide*) may be associated with episodes of orthostatic hypotension.
- Co-medication with dopamine antagonists (e.g. *amisulpride, aripiprazole, chlorpromazine, clozapine, metoclopramide, olanzapine, pimavanserin, prochlorperazine, risperidone*) may lead to pharmacodynamic antagonism and alter the efficacy of both medications.

Adverse Effects
How Drug Causes Adverse Effects
- Mainly (but not only) by increasing dopaminergic activity.

Common Adverse Effects
- Very common (≥1/10):
  - Cough.
- Common (≥1/100 to <1/10):
  - Neuropsychiatric: dyskinesias, headache, insomnia.
  - Cardiovascular: orthostatic hypotension/decreased blood pressure.
  - Respiratory: upper respiratory tract infection, bronchitis/pneumonia, discoloured nasal discharge, throat irritation.
  - GI: discoloured sputum, nausea, vomiting, laceration, skin abrasion, oropharyngeal pain.
  - Other: falls, chest discomfort, increased bilirubin, reduced RBC count.

Life-Threatening or Dangerous Adverse Effects
- Unknown frequency:
  - Peptic ulcer, GI haemorrhage.
  - Atrial fibrillation.
- Reported with oral preparations:
  - ICDs, DDS.
  - NMS, rhabdomyolysis.
  - Malignant melanoma.
  - Anaemia, agranulocytosis, thrombocytopenia, leukopenia.
  - Allergic oedema.
  - Seizures.
  - Cardiac rhythm disorders.
  - Syncope, hot flush.
  - Angioedema.
  - Hypertension, thrombophlebitis.

Rare and Not Life-Threatening Adverse Effects
- Reported with oral preparations:
  - Confusion, hallucinations, depression, anxiety, abnormal dreams, agitation, disorientation, euphoria.
  - Increased libido.
  - Dystonia, paraesthesia, tremor.
  - Blurred vision, diplopia, mydriasis, blepharospasm.
  - Dyspnoea, dysphonia, hiccups.
  - Abdominal pain, constipation, diarrhoea, dry mouth, dysphagia, dyspepsia, glossodynia, flatulence, salivary hypersecretion.
  - Hyperhidrosis, rash, pruritus, alopecia, purpura, sweat discoloration.
  - Muscle spasms, trismus.
  - Urinary retention/incontinence, chromaturia.
  - Priapism.
  - Peripheral oedema, asthenia, fatigue, malaise, gait disturbance.
  - Increased liver function tests, increased blood glucose/creatinine/uric acid/urea, positive Coombs test.

Weight Change
- Decreased or increased weight have been reported with oral levodopa preparations.

What to Do About Adverse Effects
- Discuss common adverse effects with patients or caregivers before starting medication, including symptoms that should be reported to the physician.
- Coughing, the most common side effect of inhaled levodopa, is usually mild to moderate in intensity and appears within the first month after therapy initiation.
- On a regular basis, monitor for sleepiness (which might occur without preceding warning signs, even later in therapy, e.g. after 1 year), drowsiness, hypotension (especially during dose escalation), ICDs, hallucinations or psychotic-like behaviours with focused and direct questions to patients and caregivers, as patients might not acknowledge such symptoms as abnormal to report them.

Dosing and Use
Usual Dosage Range
- 84–420 mg.

Available Formulations
- Capsules, inhalation powder: 42 mg/capsule.
  - Each hard capsule contains 42 mg levodopa, but the delivered dose is 33 mg.
  - Capsules for oral inhalation only; used solely with the inhaler of the specific brand.

How to Dose
- Inhaled levodopa should be inhaled when an OFF episode starts to appear.
- Parkinson's disease patients should be on a stable levodopa/DDI regimen before being prescribed inhaled levodopa preparations. They should also be able to recognize the onset of their OFF symptoms and be able (them or their caregiver) to prepare the inhaler when required.
- A dose of 84 mg (2 capsules) should be inhaled orally via the supplied inhaler, as needed; a maximum of 5 doses per day is recommended.
- Patients should not take more than 2 capsules per OFF episode.

Dosing Tips
- The first capsule should be loaded into the inhaler and then the patient should breathe in; the used capsule should then be removed and a second capsule should be loaded with the patient repeating inhalation. The used capsule can be removed from the inhaler afterwards.
- Capsules should be removed from the package immediately before use; they should not be stored inside the inhaler.
- Intended effect will not be obtained if capsules are swallowed.

How to Withdraw Drug
- A progressive reduction of daily dose and close monitoring of the patient are recommended to lower the possibility of NMS, especially in patients receiving neuroleptics.

Overdose
- Inhaled levodopa overdose may appear if the patient uses multiple doses for the same OFF episode.
- Levodopa overdosage can present with cardiovascular disturbances, such as hypotension or tachycardia, and psychiatric problems.
- Close monitoring of vital signs is advised; supportive measures should be applied if needed.

Tests and Therapeutic Drug Monitoring
- Periodical evaluation of hepatic, haemopoietic, renal, and cardiovascular function, including blood count, is recommended.
- Periodical dermatological control is suggested in case of a melanoma history.
- Regular measurement of intra-ocular pressure is advised in patients with open-angle glaucoma.

Other Warnings/Precautions
- Caution is advised in cases of active psychiatric disease.
- Caution is advised if severe endocrine, renal, hepatic, peptic ulcer, pulmonary, or cardiovascular disease are present, particularly if the patient has a history of MI or arrhythmia.

L

- Caution is advised if the patient has a history of orthostatic hypotension, as levodopa may aggravate this condition.
- Caution is advised in osteomalacia.
- Levodopa inhaled may lead to an increase of intra-ocular pressure in patients with glaucoma.
- Caution is advised if co-administered with selective MAOIs due to additive effects and increased risk for an acute hypertensive episode or episodes of orthostatic hypotension.
- Caution is advised if co-administered with antihypertensives, as it may lead to reduced blood pressure; dose adjustments of antihypertensive agents may be needed.
- Caution is advised if co-administered with anticholinergic agents, although their combination may improve tremor, it may worsen involuntary motor disorders.
- Caution is advised if used concomitantly with antipsychotics, as a worsening of parkinsonian symptoms may be observed due to their dopamine-receptor blocking properties.
- Caution is advised while driving or operating hazardous machinery during initiation of inhaled levodopa therapy or when increasing dosage, as it may predispose to somnolence or sleep attacks without warning.
- Patients taking levodopa may exhibit increased levels of catecholamines and their metabolites in plasma and urine, suggesting pheochromocytoma (false-positive results).

Do Not Use (Contraindications)
- Known hypersensitivity to levodopa or any of its excipients.
- Patients with a history of asthma, COPD, or other chronic lung disease due to bronchospasm risk.
  - Interactions of levodopa inhaled with locally or systematically administered pulmonary medicinal products have not been investigated, as the former is contraindicated in chronic lung conditions.
- Impaired renal or hepatic function, cardiac disorders (e.g. severe cardiac arrhythmias and cardiac failure).
- Closed-angle glaucoma.
- Phaeochromocytoma.
- Age of less than 25 years old, as skeletal development may not be yet complete.
- A prior history of NMS and/or non-traumatic rhabdomyolysis.
- Co-administration with non-selective MAOIs is contraindicated; a washout period of at least 2 weeks is recommended.
  - Increased doses of orally administered selegiline (>10 mg/day tablet/capsule or >2.5 mg/day ODT) or transdermal selegiline exhibit non-selective MAOI activity.
- Co-administration with dopamine receptor antagonists should be avoided.
- *Clozapine* and *quetiapine* have been associated with a lower risk and their use may be considered with caution.

DOSING AND USE

L

Special Populations

Renal Impairment
- Close monitoring is recommended in severe renal impairment.

Hepatic Impairment
- Safety and efficacy have not been evaluated in patients with hepatic impairment.
- Close monitoring is recommended in severe hepatic impairment.

Elderly
- No dose adjustments are necessary for individuals over 65 years old.
- Limited data are available for patients over the age of 75.

Pregnancy
- Unknown effect on humans.
- Levodopa can cause visceral and skeletal malformations in animal studies.
- Levodopa preparations are contraindicated during pregnancy.

Breastfeeding
- Levodopa has been detected in human milk.
- Levodopa demonstrates a prolactin-lowering activity, which may interfere with lactation, although there are limited data on the effect of levodopa on milk production.
- Levodopa use is not recommended during breastfeeding.

Costs
- Not available in the UK for cost comparison.

The Overall Place of Levodopa Inhaled in the Treatment of Parkinson's Disease

Inhaled levodopa is a self-administered therapy recently approved for the intermittent treatment of OFF episodes in Parkinson's disease patients who are already on a stable regimen with levodopa/DDI preparations. Its mode of delivery offers an important advantage in bypassing the digestive system and accessing the bloodstream rapidly and effectively. It can be used as a rescue therapy for OFF periods. High-quality studies have confirmed the beneficial effect of inhaled levodopa on Parkinson's disease-related OFF episodes, without any significant adverse effects on long-term use. Inhaled levodopa can also be used for early morning OFF symptoms, although there is currently only preliminary data demonstrating a positive effect. However, concerns remain regarding the ability of patients to inhale during OFF periods, and to have enough manual dexterity to use the inhaler.

Potential Advantages
- Inhaled levodopa bypasses the GI tract; thus, fewer GI adverse events are expected.
- It has a rapid onset of action, which makes it suitable for the management of OFF episodes.
- In contrast to SC apomorphine, which can also be used for the same indication, it is a non-intrusive therapeutic option.

Potential Disadvantages
- As inhaled levodopa is a recently licensed medication, there is only limited experience of its use in routine clinical practice.
- It is not available globally.
- Patients need to be able to handle the device of the inhaler or have a capable caregiver who can do this for them.

Clinical Box

A 68-year-old man with a 9-year history of Parkinson's disease was assessed at the Movement Disorders Outpatient Clinics. He had experienced end-of-dose OFF phenomena over the past few months. He was accompanied by his wife. The patient was receiving levodopa/benserazide 200/50 mg five times per day, levodopa/benserazide PR 100/25 mg at night-time, rotigotine patch 8 mg/24 h and rasagiline 1 mg OD. OFF episodes (usually 2 per day) were predictably appearing about 30 min before the next levodopa dose was due, mostly in the afternoon, and included motor and non-motor symptoms. The rest of his medical history was unremarkable. The patient was prescribed inhaled levodopa and was instructed to administer a dose of 84 mg during the initiation phase of each OFF episode. The doses were to be at least 2 h apart and he could receive no more than 5 doses per day. Both he and his wife were also given instructions for the use of the inhaler. However, treatment was stopped because the patient found it difficult to inhale during an OFF episode.

Suggested Reading

Grosset DG, R Dhall, T Gurevich, J Kassubek, WH Poewe, O Rascol, M Rudzinska, J Cormier, A Sedkov, C Oh. Inhaled levodopa in Parkinson's disease patients with OFF periods: a randomized 12-month pulmonary safety study. *Parkinsonism Relat Disord* 2020; 71: 4–10.

Hauser RA, SH Isaacson, A Ellenbogen, BE Safirstein, DD Truong, SF Komjathy, DM Kegler-Ebo, P Zhao, C Oh. Orally inhaled levodopa (CVT-301) for early morning OFF periods in Parkinson's disease. *Parkinsonism Relat Disord* 2019; 64: 175–180.

LeWitt PA, RA Hauser, R Pahwa, SH Isaacson, HH Fernandez, M Lew, M Saint-Hilaire, E Pourcher, L Lopez-Manzanares, C Waters,

L

M Rudzínska, A Sedkov, R Batycky, C Oh. Safety and efficacy of CVT-301 (levodopa inhalation powder) on motor function during off periods in patients with Parkinson's disease: a randomised, double-blind, placebo-controlled phase 3 trial. *Lancet Neurol* 2019; 18(2): 145–154.

References

Hampson NB, KD Kieburtz, PA LeWitt, M Leinonen, MI Freed. Prospective evaluation of pulmonary function in Parkinson's disease patients with motor fluctuations. *Int J Neurosci* 2017; 127(3): 276–284.

Levodopa. In: Brayfield A (Ed.), *Martindale: The Complete Drug Reference*. London: The Royal Pharmaceutical Society of Great Britain. Accessed on 11 March 2023 via www.medicinescomplete.com.

Levodopa. In: DRUGDEX® System (electronic version). Truven Health Analytics, Greenwood Village, Colorado, USA. Accessed on 11 March 2023 via www.micromedexsolutions.com.

LeWitt PA, R Pahwa, A Sedkov, A Corbin, R Batycky, H Murck. Pulmonary safety and tolerability of inhaled levodopa (CVT-301) Administered to Patients with Parkinson's disease. *J Aerosol Med Pulm Drug Deliv* 2018; 31(3): 155–161.

Lipp MM, R Batycky, J Moore, M Leinonen, MI Freed. Preclinical and clinical assessment of inhaled levodopa for OFF episodes in Parkinson's disease. *Sci Transl Med* 2016; 8(360): 360ra136.

LEVODOPA, INHALED

LUBIPROSTONE

Therapeutics
Chemical Name and Structure
Lubiprostone ((–)-7-[(2R,4aR,5R,7aR)-2-(1,1-difluoropentyl)-2-hydroxy-6-oxooctahydrocylcopenta[b]pyran-5-yl]heptanoic acid) has a molecular weight of 390.5 and a molecular formula of $C_{20}H_{32}F_2O_5$.

Brand Names
• **Amitiza** (*Canada, Japan, Singapore, Switzerland, USA*).
• **Lubigut, Lubilax, Lubowel** (*Bangladesh, India*).

Generics Available
• No.

Licensed Indications for Parkinson's Disease
• None.

Licensed Indications for Other Conditions
• Chronic idiopathic constipation (FDA).
• Constipation-predominant irritable bowel syndrome (adult women) (FDA).
• Opioid-induced constipation in patients with chronic non-cancer-related pain, including patients with chronic pain related to prior cancer or its treatment who do not require frequent (e.g. weekly) opioid dosage escalation (diphenylheptane opioids are excluded) (FDA).

Non-Licensed Use for Parkinson's Disease
• Constipation.

Non-Licensed Use for Other Conditions
• None.

Ineffective
• Not reported.

Mechanism of Action
• Lubiprostone is a locally acting chloride channel 2 activator, which increases the secretion of chloride-rich fluid, resulting in the softening of stools and the enhancement of intestinal motility.
• Lubiprostone acts at the apical surface of intestinal epithelial cells.

Efficacy Profile
• Lubiprostone has been characterized as 'likely efficacious' and 'possibly useful' in the treatment of constipation in Parkinson's disease (MDS EBM Committee).

- A multi-centre RCT examining the effect of lubiprostone on constipation among Parkinson's disease patients has demonstrated a significant improvement in all measured parameters (global impression, constipation scales) without compromising motor performance.
- Available data from well-organized studies, including phase III trials for chronic constipation in non-Parkinson's disease patients, support the short-term efficacy of lubiprostone for no longer than 4 weeks of therapy. Only anecdotal reports are currently available considering a good clinical response to lubiprostone for months or years.
- Lubiprostone has also been found efficacious on constipation-related symptoms of abdominal bloating, pain, and staining.

Pharmacokinetics
Absorption and Distribution
- Oral bioavailability: low systemic availability with negligible (not calculable) plasma concentration after oral administration.
- Food co-ingestion: a high-fat meal decreases lubiprostone plasma concentration. The clinical relevance of the food effect on lubiprostone pharmacokinetics is not clear.
- Tmax (M3 metabolite): 1 h (not reliably calculated).
- Time to steady state: not reported.
- Protein binding: 94% (in vitro studies).
- Volume of distribution: not reported.

Metabolism
- Probably metabolized in the stomach and jejunum by carbonyl reductase.
- Hepatic CYP450 system is not implicated in lubiprostone metabolism.
- M3 is the only measurable, active metabolite of lubiprostone.

Elimination
- Lubiprostone plasma half-life is not calculable, while the half-life of M3 is 0.9–1.4 h.
- Studies using radiolabelled lubiprostone demonstrate that it is nearly completely eliminated in 48 h.

Drug Interaction Profile
Pharmacokinetic Drug Interactions
- Pharmacokinetic interactions with lubiprostone are highly unlikely due to low plasma concentration.

Pharmacodynamic Drug Interactions
- Not reported.

L

Adverse Effects

How Drug Causes Adverse Effects
- Adverse effects of lubiprostone usually result from the local action of the drug on the GI system and are usually dose-dependent.

Common Adverse Effects
- Very common (≥1/10):
  ○ Nausea, diarrhoea, headache.
- Common (≥1/100 to <1/10):
  ○ Neuropsychiatric: dizziness.
  ○ Cardiovascular: chest pain/discomfort.
  ○ Respiratory: dyspnoea.
  ○ GI: abdominal pain/discomfort or distension, flatulence, vomiting, loose stools, dyspepsia, dry mouth.
  ○ Other: oedema, fatigue.

Life-Threatening or Dangerous Adverse Effects
- Ischaemic colitis.
- Hypersensitivity reactions.
- Hypotension, syncope, tachycardia.

Rare and Not Life-Threatening Adverse Effects
- Muscle cramps/spasms.

Weight Change
- Not reported.

What to Do About Adverse Effects
- Before introducing lubiprostone, discuss common or life-threatening adverse effects with patients and/or caregivers, including symptoms that should be reported to the physician.
- Clinical trials and current administration recommendations include taking with food to reduce risk of adverse events likely through reducing maximum plasma concentration.
- Patients should be informed that lubiprostone may cause nausea or diarrhoea during therapy. If it occurs, lubiprostone dose should be reduced, as these symptoms may predispose to hypotension and syncope (especially at a dose of 24 micrograms BID).
- Patients on lubiprostone therapy may experience difficulty in breathing or chest tightness within 30–60 min of taking the first dose. Despite the fact that these symptoms are usually transient and resolve within a few hours, patients are instructed to immediately seek medical help. Recurrence of these symptoms on subsequent lubiprostone administration has also been reported.

ADVERSE EFFECTS

L

LUBIPROSTONE

Dosing and Use

Usual Dosage Range
• 24–48 micrograms.

Available Formulations
• Capsules: 8 micrograms, 24 micrograms.

How to Dose
• An initial dose of 24 micrograms OD is suggested for one week, followed by an increase to 24 micrograms BID, which is the usual maintenance dose. If not well-tolerated, the dose can be decreased once again to 24 micrograms OD.
• The duration of lubiprostone therapy is typically 2–4 weeks.
• If no improvement in constipation occurs after 2 weeks of therapy, consider stopping treatment.

Dosing Tips
• Lubiprostone should be administered with food and water to decrease the risk of nausea (preferably after breakfast and after supper).

How to Withdraw Drug
• No tapering is needed.
• Lubiprostone withdrawal was not found to cause a rebound effect.

Overdose
• Only limited cases of lubiprostone overdose have been described (most of them in healthy volunteers) without any reported major complications.

Tests and Therapeutic Drug Monitoring
• No special monitoring is required.

Other Warnings/Precautions
• If there is any suspicion of a potential mechanical GI obstruction, a thorough evaluation should be performed to exclude this possibility before initiating lubiprostone therapy.
• Caution is advised with lubiprostone administration in patients with hypotension due to the possibility of diarrhoea during therapy, which may lead to hypovolaemia and syncope, especially in patients with pre-existing low blood pressure.

Do Not Use (contraindications)
• Known sensitivity to lubiprostone or to any of its excipients.
• (History of) mechanical GI obstruction.
• Severe diarrhoea.

Special Populations

Renal Impairment
- No dose adjustments are needed.

Hepatic Impairment
- Mild impairment: no dosage adjustments required.
- Moderate impairment (Child–Pugh B): a maximum initial dose of 16 micrograms BID is suggested. If tolerated and an adequate response has not been obtained, consider escalation to a full standard dose with appropriate patient monitoring.
- Severe impairment (Child–Pugh C): a maximum initial dose of 8 micrograms BID is suggested. If tolerated and an adequate response has not been obtained, consider escalation to a full standard dose with appropriate patient monitoring.

Elderly
- No differences reported.

Pregnancy
- Pregnancy category C (FDA).
- No data are currently available on the effect of lubiprostone on fetus development.
- Lubiprostone therapy is not recommended during pregnancy, as adverse effects cannot be excluded.

Breastfeeding
- It is not known whether lubiprostone is excreted in human milk.
- Lubiprostone therapy is not recommended during breastfeeding, as adverse effects on nursing infants or milk production cannot be excluded.

Costs
- Not available in the UK.

The Overall Place of Lubiprostone in the Treatment of Parkinson's Disease

Lubiprostone, an intestinal chloride secretagogue, is used for the short-term treatment of chronic constipation in the general population (usual duration of 4 weeks). Considering its use for the treatment of constipation in the context of Parkinson's disease, there is only one RCT available demonstrating a positive effect on Parkinson's disease patients' symptoms without any major safety issues reported. These results are further supported by data from high-quality studies, which did include elderly in their samples, but not Parkinson's disease patients specifically. Lubiprostone is suggested to be used as a last-line option in patients

L

THE TREATMENT OF PARKINSON'S DISEASE

L

with resistant and troublesome constipation, who do not respond to lifestyle changes (e.g. increase of fibre and fluid intake), probiotics or laxatives, such as macrogol. It is generally considered well-tolerated.

Potential Advantages
• No rebound effects have been described after cessation of therapy.

Potential Disadvantages
• Lubiprostone is a relatively expensive treatment option, which is not available in many countries around the world.

Clinical Box
A 67-year-old woman with an 8-year history of Parkinson's disease presented at the Movement Disorders Outpatients Clinic. The patient was recently hospitalized and initiated on clozapine therapy and was scheduled for a follow-up appointment after her discharge. Both her and her partner reported a good response of her psychotic symptoms to clozapine; however, she mentioned a deterioration of her constipation with very few bowel movements during the week. She was already on probiotics and polyethylene glycol 17 g OD and was aware of the necessary lifestyle changes (higher fluid and fibre intake, routine physical exercise), which she had been following; however, her efforts were futile. She was then prescribed lubiprostone 24 micrograms BID. After 2 weeks of therapy, the patient reported she was able to have regular bowel movements.

Suggested Reading
Ondo WG, C Kenney, K Sullivan, A Davidson, C Hunter, I Jahan, A McCombs, A Miller, TA Zesiewicz. Placebo-controlled trial of lubiprostone for constipation associated with Parkinson disease. *Neurology* 2012; 78(21): 1650–1654.

References
Li F, T Fu, WD Tong, BH Liu, CX Li, Y Gao, JS Wu, XF Wang, AP Zhang. Lubiprostone is effective in the treatment of chronic idiopathic constipation and irritable bowel syndrome: a systematic review and meta-analysis of randomized controlled trials. *Mayo Clin Proc* 2016; 91(4): 456–468.
Lubiprostone. In: Brayfield A (Ed.), *Martindale: The Complete Drug Reference*. London: The Royal Pharmaceutical Society of Great Britain. Accessed on 18 December 2022 via www.medicinescomplete.com.
Lubiprostone. In: DRUGDEX® System (electronic version). Truven Health Analytics, Greenwood Village, Colorado, USA. Accessed on 18 December 2022 via www.micromedexsolutions.com.

MACROGOL

M

Therapeutics

Chemical Name and Structure
Polyethylene glycol or macrogol 4,000 (2-(1-benzothiophene-2-car-bonylamino)ethyl-diethylazanium;chloride) is an osmotic laxative with a molecular weight of 312.9 and a molecular formula of $C_{15}H_{21}ClN_2OS$ (although these parameters may be slightly different between different macrogol preparations).

Brand Names
★Some of these preparations might contain macrogol in combination with electrolytes.

- **Accualaxan** (*Equador*); **Aetoxisclerol** (*France*); **Atolaxant** (*Spain*); **AuroGo** (*Poland*).
- **Barex Unipeg** (*Argentina*).
- **Casenjunior** (*Italy*); **Cadenlax** (*Italy*); **Casenlax** (*Netherlands, Portugal, Spain, Turkey*); **Chang Song** (*China*); **Clearlax** (*Canada*); **Comfilax** (*Canada*); **Contumax** (*Chile, Mexico*).
- Diagnol (*Ukraine*); Dulcolax Balance (*UK, USA*).
- **Emolax** (*Canada*); **Ezlax** (*India*).
- **Femlax** (*Spain*); **Forlax** (*Austria, Belgium, China, Czech Republic, Estonia, France, Hong Kong, Hungary, Lithuania, Malaysia, Netherlands, Poland, Portugal, Russian Federation, Singapore, South Africa, Sweden, Thailand, Tunisia, Ukraine*); **Fortese** (*Russian Federation*).
- **GaviLAX** (*USA*).
- **Hydralax** (*Canada*).
- **Idrolax** (*Ireland*).
- **Klean-Prep** (*France, Hong Kong, Ireland, Netherlands, New Zealand, Poland, South Africa, Tunisia, UK*); **Kronys** (*Italy*).
- **Lax 3350** (*Chile*); **Laxaclear** (*Ireland*); **Laxbene** (*Germany*); **Laxido** (*Ireland, South Africa*); **Laxipeg** (*Switzerland*); **Laxofalk** (*Germany*); **Laxogol** (*Austria*); **Laxopeg** (*India*); **Laxuave** (*Argentina*); **Lax-a-Day** (*Canada*); **Legkolax** (*Ukraine*); **Lumencol** (*Argentina*).
- **Macrolief** (*Ireland*); **MiraLax** (*Greece, USA*), **Molaxole** (*Australia, Austria, Cyprus, Estonia, Ireland, Lithuania, Netherlands, New Zealand, Spain*); **Movicol** (*Australia, Austria, Finland, France, Ireland, New Zealand, South Africa, Spain, Tunisia, UK*); **Movicolon** (*Netherlands*); **Muvinlax** (*Brazil*).
- **Normalax** (*Israel*).
- **Olopeg** (*Austria, Estonia, Finland, Lithuania, Poland*); **Onlipeg** (*Italy*); **Osmogol** (*Russian Federation*); **OsmoLax** (*Australia*).
- **Paxabel** (*Italy*); **Pegalax** (*Canada*); **Peglax** (*Ireland, Israel, UK*); **PegLax** (*UK*); **Pegorion** (*Finland, Poland*); **Pegulos** (*Finland*); **Pergidal** (*Italy*); **Plenvu** (*Finland, Ireland, New Zealand, Poland*); **Policol** (*Turkey*); **Polyoxidin** (*Russian Federation*).
- **Realaxan** (*Russian Federation*); **Regulax** (*Israel*); **Relexa** (*Canada*); **Restoralax** (*Canada*); **Run Ke Long** (*China*).

- **Solostin** (*Mexico*); **Sulizol** (*Mexico*); **Surelax** (*Philippines*).
- **Tanesa** (*Argentina*); **Tanilas** (*Greece*); **TransiSoft** (*UK*).
- **Wecol** (*Ireland*).
- **You Sai Le** (*China*).

Generics Available
- Yes.

Licensed Indications for Parkinson's Disease
- None.

Licensed Indications for Other Conditions
- Bowel preparation before surgery or colonoscopy (FDA).
- Chronic constipation (FDA, EMA, EMC).
- Faecal impaction (EMC).

Non-Licensed Use for Parkinson's Disease
- Constipation.

Non-Licensed Use for Other Conditions
- Not reported.

Ineffective
- Not reported.

Mechanism of Action
- Macrogol is an osmotic laxative; it causes water retention in stools, which results in more frequent bowel movements and softer stools to facilitate an easier passage.
- Some of the available macrogol products also contain electrolytes to ensure that there is no overall gain or loss of water, potassium, or sodium.
- Effects of macrogol therapy are expected to occur 24–96 h after consumption.

Efficacy Profile
- Macrogol has been characterized as 'likely efficacious' and 'possibly useful' in the treatment of constipation in Parkinson's disease (MDS EBM Committee).
- The role of macrogol on constipation in Parkinson's disease has been explored in a double-blind RCT, which demonstrated a positive effect of macrogol plus electrolytes on the frequency of bowel movements and stool consistency.
- The above findings were also supported by a small open-label study assessing the effect of macrogol on chronic constipation in Parkinson's disease and MSA patients.
- The efficacy profiles of macrogol 4,000 and macrogol 3,350 are generally considered similar.

MACROGOL

Pharmacokinetics
Absorption and Distribution
- Oral bioavailability: not absorbed.
- Food co-ingestion: no food interactions have been described.
- Tmax: not applicable.
- Time to steady state: not applicable.
- Pharmacokinetics: most of the drug stays unchanged in the GI tract, so pharmacokinetic analysis is not relevant.
- Protein binding: not applicable.
- Volume of distribution: not applicable.

Metabolism
- Not applicable.

Elimination
- About 93% of an administered dose is excreted unchanged in faeces and 0.2% in the urine (which is the small percentage of the drug that enters the systemic circulation).

Drug Interaction Profile
Pharmacokinetic Drug Interactions
- Effects by macrogol:
  - The absorption of other medicinal products (e.g. anti-epileptics) may be transiently impaired due to a macrogol-associated increase in GI transit rate.

Pharmacodynamic Drug Interactions
- Co-medication with starch-based thickeners reduces the viscosity of the starch-thickened liquid.
- Co-medication with ACE inhibitors, NSAIDs, diuretics, angiotensin receptor blockers, and other agents affecting renal function may pre-dispose to renal impairment.

Adverse Effects
How Drug Causes Adverse Effects
- Adverse effects of macrogol usually result from the local action of the drug on the GI system or impairment of fluid/electrolyte balance, for example hyperkalaemia.

Common Adverse Effects
- Unknown frequency:
- Neuropsychiatric: headache.
  - GI: abdominal pain, diarrhoea, vomiting/nausea, dyspepsia, abdominal distension, flatulence, aphthous ulcerations.

- Skin: erythema.
- Other: peripheral oedema, electrolyte disturbances, particularly hyper-/hypokalaemia (higher risk with prolonged use).

Life-Threatening or Dangerous Adverse Effects
- Ischaemic colitis.
- Allergic reactions, including anaphylaxis, angioedema, dyspnoea, rash, urticaria, pruritus.

Rare and Not Life-Threatening Adverse Effects
- Not reported.

Weight Change
- Rare reports of anorexia and weight decrease.

What to Do About Adverse Effects
- Before introducing macrogol, discuss common or life-threatening adverse effects with patients and/or caregivers, including symptoms that should be reported to the physician.
- If fluid/electrolyte impairment occurs (e.g. oedema, shortness of breath, fatigue, dehydration, cardiac failure) macrogol should be discontinued and appropriate therapy should be implemented.

Dosing and Use
Usual Dosage Range
- Depending on the product details.

Available Formulations
★These are indicative formulations; many more might be available with different concentrations of macrogol and electrolytes.
- Oral packet: 17 g/packet.
- Oral powder (sodium sulphate/sodium bicarbonate/sodium chloride/potassium chloride): 119 g, 238 g, 255 g, 510 g, 527 g, 850 g.
- Powder for solution (sodium bicarbonate/sodium chloride/potassium chloride): 5.72 g/11.2 g/1.48 g (240 g), 5.72 g/11.2 g/1.48 g (420 g).
- Sachets: 13.125 g (sodium chloride 350.7 mg, sodium hydrogen carbonate 178.5 mg, potassium chloride 46.6 mg).
- Sachets: 200 g.

How to Dose
- 17 g packet or one heaped spoon of oral powder in 120–240 ml (4–8 oz) of beverage per day.
- 1–3 sachets daily in divided doses according to individual response.
- It is necessary for macrogol products to be diluted with water; products should not be consumed directly.

- Macrogol therapy should not be prolonged beyond 1–2 weeks.
  - Extended use may be necessary in patients with chronic or resistant constipation secondary to Parkinson's disease.
  - In case of extended use, a lower dose is suggested.

Dosing Tips
- Refrigerate before administration to improve palatability.
- Patients should fast for a minimum of 3–4 h before consuming macrogol.
- Patients should be instructed to drink macrogol preparations rapidly.
- It is important that patients are properly hydrated during macrogol therapy.
- Macrogol should not be mixed directly into milk/juice/flavoured drink, as it needs to be diluted in water first. However, the resultant liquid after water addition can be mixed with something (e.g. yogurt) that encourages the patient to consume it.
- Macrogol 4,000 is considered to taste better than macrogol 3,350+electrolytes; thus, it may increase compliance.

How to Withdraw Drug
- Macrogol can be abruptly discontinued.

Overdose
- Macrogol overdose can manifest with vomiting or diarrhoea, leading to extensive fluid loss and electrolyte imbalance, which should be treated accordingly.
- In case of severe distension or abdominal pain, consider applying nasogastric aspiration.

Tests and Therapeutic Drug Monitoring
- Before initiation of macrogol therapy:
  - An ECG should be performed in patients at high risk for cardiac arrhythmias.
  - Blood tests to monitor renal function including electrolytes should be performed in patients with renal impairment.
- During macrogol therapy:
  - Consider ongoing monitoring of renal function and electrolytes in patients with renal impairment.

Other Warnings/Precautions
- There have been reports of generalized tonic–clonic seizures and/ or loss of consciousness due to subjacent macrogol-related fluid and electrolyte abnormalities. Caution is advised with macrogol administration in patients with a history of epilepsy or at increased risk for seizures; macrogol may lower seizure threshold.
- Caution is advised when macrogol is administered in unconscious or semiconscious patients, those with impaired gag reflex/swallowing

problems, or patients who are prone to regurgitation/aspiration, especially if macrogol is given through a nasogastric tube.
- Macrogol use predisposes to electrolyte abnormalities, which may result in arrhythmias, seizures, and renal impairment, especially in vulnerable patients.
- Caution is advised in case of macrogol administration in patients at risk of cardiac arrhythmia, including unstable angina, congestive heart failure, recent MI, uncontrolled arrhythmias, or cardiomyopathy.
- Macrogol products are considered high in sodium; thus, caution is advised in case of patients who follow a low-salt diet; consider macrogol preparations that do not contain electrolytes.
- Patients should not take any other orally administered medications 1 h before or after macrogol administration, as macrogol may interfere with their absorption.

Do Not Use (Contraindications)
- Known sensitivity to macrogol or any of its excipients.
- History of mechanical GI obstruction.
- Gastric retention.
- Bowel perforation.
- Severe inflammatory disease of the intestinal tract (e.g. ulcerative colitis, Crohn's disease, toxic megacolon).
- Co-administration of stimulant laxatives, as it may predispose to ischaemic colitis.
- Co-administration with starch-based thickeners, as it might predispose to aspiration.

Special Populations
Renal Impairment
- Caution is advised in case of macrogol administration in patients with renal impairment; patients should be advised to remain sufficiently hydrated.
- No dosage modifications are suggested.

Hepatic Impairment
- No dosage adjustment is necessary.

Elderly
- Caution is advised in elderly patients vulnerable to electrolyte abnormalities.

Pregnancy
- Some macrogol products can be used during pregnancy as systemic exposure to macrogol is considered negligible.
  - The decision should be taken on a case-by-case basis.

Breastfeeding
- It is not known whether macrogol is excreted in human milk.
- Macrogol therapy is not recommended during breastfeeding, as adverse effects on nursing infants or milk production cannot be excluded.

Costs
- NHS indicative price 18 December 2022:

This is just macrogol; many more formulations are available with different concentrations of macrogol and electrolytes.
  - TransiSoft oral powder 8.5 g sachets (HFA Healthcare Ltd) – 28 sachets: £99.85.

The Overall Place of Macrogol in the Treatment of Parkinson's Disease

Constipation is a common non-motor symptom among Parkinson's disease patients, even from the prodromal phase. If it cannot be managed with non-pharmacological measures, initiation of osmotic agents, such as macrogol, is considered a reasonable and conservative treatment option in the general population, as it has been associated with marked improvement of relevant symptoms. Macrogol is also considered an efficient and safe laxative in the management of chronic constipation in Parkinson's disease, and it is commonly regarded as a first-line treatment, particularly for those suffering from slow transit constipation. More specifically, a high-quality study of 8 weeks' duration has demonstrated the beneficial effect of macrogol on constipation in Parkinson's disease patients, resulting in an increased number of bowel movements and better stool consistency, whereas no participants on macrogol had to use rectal laxatives as a rescue therapy. It was also shown that macrogol therapy was well tolerated by the vast majority of the study population with minor adverse events occurring (nausea, diarrhoea) and without any impact on the course of Parkinson's disease.

Potential Advantages
- The amount of macrogol detected in the systemic circulation is negligible thus, it has few adverse effects and drug–drug interactions.
- No other laxatives, such as lactulose, milk of magnesia or glycerin, have been formally assessed in Parkinson's disease.

Potential Disadvantages
- The taste or volume of macrogol preparations may discourage patients from adhering to macrogol therapy.

M

MACROGOL

Clinical Box

A 56-year-old man with a 5-year history of Parkinson's disease presented at his GP due to an aggravation of already existent constipation. The patient reported 1–2 bowel movements per week, which significantly affected his daily routine. The rest of his medical history was unremarkable. The patient was initially given instructions on lifestyle changes, including an increase of fluids and fibre intake, plus regular physical exercise, although without success. Therefore, he was given the option of following a 2-week course of macrogol, which markedly improved his symptoms. The same course was re-introduced after 3 months when the patient reported a similar aggravation of his constipation.

Suggested Reading

Zangaglia R, E Martignoni, M Glorioso, M Ossola, G Riboldazzi, D Calandrella, G Brunetti, C Pacchetti. Macrogol for the treatment of constipation in Parkinson's disease. A randomized placebo-controlled study. *Mov Disord* 2007; 22(9): 1239–1344.

References

Eichhorn TE, WH Oertel. Macrogol 3350/electrolyte improves constipation in Parkinson's disease and multiple system atrophy. *Mov Disord* 2001; 16(6): 1176–1177.

Joint Formulary Committee. British National Formulary (online). London: BMJ Group and Pharmaceutical Press. Accessed on 18 December 2022 via www.medicinescomplete.com.

Macrogol. In: Brayfield A (Ed.), *Martindale: The Complete Drug Reference*. London: The Royal Pharmaceutical Society of Great Britain. Accessed on 18 December 2022 via www.medicinescomplete.com.

Macrogol. In: DRUGDEX® System (electronic version). Truven Health Analytics, Greenwood Village, Colorado, USA. Accessed on 18 December 2022 via www.micromedexsolutions.com.

MELATONIN

M

Therapeutics

Chemical Name and Structure

Melatonin (*N*-acetyl-5-methoxytryptamine or *N*-[2-(5-methoxy-1H-indol-3-yl)ethyl]acetamide) is a tryptophan-derived hormone and an antioxidant, produced primarily in the pineal gland. Exogenous melatonin is an amphiphilic, white–cream to yellowish crystalline powder, unchanged in the entire pH range. It has a molecular weight of 232.28 and an empirical formula of $C_{13}H_{16}N_2O_2$, while its chemical structure resembles serotonin.

Brand Names

- **Adaflex** (*UK*); **Aritonin** (*Sweden*); **Armonia** (*Italy*); **Armonil Noche** (*Argentina*).
- **Benedorm** (*Mexico*); **Bio-Melatonin** (*Hungary*); **Buenas Noches** (*Argentina*).
- **Ceyesto** (*UK*); **Circadin** (*Argentina, Australia, Austria, Belgium, Cyprus, Czech Republic, Denmark, Ecuador, Estonia, Finland, France, Germany, Greece, Hungary, Ireland, Israel, Lithuania, Netherlands, New Zealand, Norway, Poland, Portugal, Russian Federation, Singapore, South Africa, Spain, Sweden, Switzerland, Thailand, UK*); **Cronocaps** (*Mexico*).
- **Easymagnevie** (*France*).
- **Mecastrin** (*Denmark, Finland, Sweden*); **Melabiorytm** (*Poland*); **Melarena, Melaritm** (*Russian Federation*); **Melatal** (*Denmark*); **Melatin** (*Singapore*); **Melatol** (*Argentina, Ecuador*); **Melatonite** (*Spain*); **Melatrix** (*Argentina*); **Melaxen** (*Russian Federation, Ukraine*); **Mellozzan** (*Sweden*); **Melnoc** (*South Africa*); **Meloset** (*India*); **Melotin** (*New Zealand*); **Melsoma** (*Singapore*).
- **Normolem** (*Mexico*).
- **Pillow Mint** (*Canada*); **Pineal Notte Fast** (*Italy*).
- **Remedin, Revenox** (*Mexico*).
- **Sental** (*Poland*); **Siesta** (*Canada*); **SleepEasy, Sleepwell** (*Philippines*); **Sleep Right** (*Canada*); **Slenyto** (*Austria, Denmark, Estonia, Finland, France, Ireland, Lithuania, Netherlands, New Zealand, Norway, Poland, Spain, UK*); **Sonella** (*Ukraine*); **Sonnovan** (*Russian Federation*); **Sub-Z** (*Mexico*); **Syncrodin** (*UK*).
- **Transzone** (*USA*).
- **Vigisom** (*New Zealand, Venezuela*).

Generics Available

- Yes.

Licensed Indications for Parkinson's Disease

- None.

Licensed Indications for Other Conditions
- As a monotherapy for short-term treatment of primary insomnia for individuals over 55 years old (EMA, only for PR tablets).
- Short-term treatment of jet-lag disorder in adults (EMC).

Non-Licensed Use for Parkinson's Disease
- Sleep disorders and wakefulness, including insomnia in Parkinson's disease.
- RBD.

Non-Licensed Use for Other Conditions
- Insomnia (American Academy of Family Physicians, AAFP) and other sleep disorders.
- Primary insomnia.
- Age-related insomnia.
- Jet lag disorder.
- Shift work sleep disorder.
- Post-traumatic brain injury.
- Alzheimer's disease.
- Benzodiazepine or nicotine withdrawal.
- Cancer (adjunctive therapy) and chemo-induced thrombocytopenia.
- Headache (prevention).
- Winter depression.
- Tardive dyskinesia.

Ineffective
- Depressive symptoms.

Mechanism of Action
- Melatonin synthesis and secretion are enhanced by darkness and inhibited by light (luminous information transferred to the pineal gland via the retina and the suprachiasmatic nucleus of the hypothalamus). Nearly 80% of melatonin is synthesized at night.
- Melatonin is believed to exert its action via the membrane receptors conventionally called MT1-, MT2-, and MT3-R.
- Modulation of GABAergic inhibition and inhibition of calmodulin, which might then affect skeletal muscle ACh receptors, are believed to be involved in the role of melatonin in RBD.
- Other biological mechanisms of action include but are not limited to:
  - Bone deposition via MT2 found on osteoblasts.
  - Anti-oxidative and anti-inflammatory effects, regulation of cellular and humoral immunity.
  - Regulation of lipid and glucose metabolism.
  - Antihypertensive, anxiolytic, and analgesic effects.
  - Activation of mitochondrial cell survival pathways and regulation of apoptosis in neurodegenerative disorders, including Parkinson's disease.

M

Efficacy Profile
- Melatonin has been characterized as 'possibly useful' in the management of sleep disorders and wakefulness in Parkinson's disease, including insomnia, at doses of 3–5 mg (MDS EBM Committee).
- A range of 3–12 mg, with an average effective dose of 6 mg, in symptomatic RBD with co-morbid sleep apnoea or sleep problems, has also been suggested and has been associated with reduced injury potential.
- Preliminary findings in Parkinson's disease-related nocturia.
- Recent studies in animal models and cell cultures have shown a neuroprotective effect of melatonin in neurodegenerative diseases, stroke, brain and spinal cord trauma injury, including subarachnoid haemorrhage.

Pharmacokinetics
Absorption and Distribution (Oral Formulations)
- Oral bioavailability: ~15%.
- Food co-ingestion: limited data; food intake may increase melatonin absorption almost twofold.
- Tmax: ~50 min.
- Pharmacokinetics: linear over the dose range of 2–8 mg (IR).
- Protein binding: 50–60%.
- Volume of distribution: 1602 l (4 mg) (bioavailability corrected value).

Metabolism
- About 90% is metabolized in the liver, primarily by CYP1A2, CYP1A1, and possibly CYP2C19.
- Mainly hydroxylated to 6-hydroxymelatonin (~90%), which is converted to sulphate (70–90%) or glucuronide conjugates (10–30%) prior to urinary excretion (inactive metabolites). Melatonin is metabolized to a lesser extent to *N*-acetylserotonin (~10%).

Elimination
- Plasma elimination half-life is about 45 min.
- Limited data suggest that Cmax and AUC of IR melatonin may be higher in women compared to men, although plasma half-life is not significantly different.
- Renal excretion: approximately 90% of an administered dose is excreted as 6-hydroxymelatonin conjugates and about 1% as unchanged active substance in the urine.
- A small amount is excreted in the faeces.

Drug Interaction Profile
Pharmacokinetic Drug Interactions★
- Effects by melatonin:
  - The excretion of *pravastatin, piperacillin* can be decreased.
  - The metabolism of *dicoumarol* can be decreased.
- Effects on melatonin:
  - CYP1A2 inhibitors, including oestrogen therapy (e.g. contraceptives, hormone replacement therapy) and quinolones, increase melatonin levels.
  - CYP1A2 inducers, including *carbamazepine* and *rifampicin*, reduce melatonin levels.
  - Cigarette smoking may decrease melatonin levels due to induction of CYP1A2.
  - *Fluvoxamine, 5-* or *8-methoxypsoralen, cimetidine* increase melatonin levels by inhibiting its metabolism via CYP enzymes.
  - *Valsartan, irbesartan, triamterene, ticlopidine, clopidogrel, acetylsalicyclic acid, simvastatin, sildenafil, acetaminophen, celecoxib, piroxicam, diclofenac, naproxen, meloxicam, cimetidine, cisplatin, cyclophosphamide, acyclovir, ranitidine, selegiline* can decrease the metabolism of melatonin.
  - *Omeprazole* can increase the metabolism of melatonin.

Pharmacodynamic Drug Interactions
- Co-medication with CNS depressants, including benzodiazepines (e.g. *midazolam, temazepam*), opiates (e.g. *tramadol*), *baclofen* and other hypnotics (e.g. *zaleplon, zolpidem, zopiclone*) may increase their sedative effects.
- Co-medication with anti-parkinsonian medication, including *pramipexole* and *dopamine*, may increase their sedative effects.
- Co-medication with *warfarin, fondaparinux, heparin*, or *dabigatran* may affect the anticoagulation activity.
- Co-medication with antidepressants (e.g. *citalopram, sertraline, venlafaxine, amitriptyline, mirtazapine*), neuroleptics (e.g. *olanzapine, alprazolam*), triptans (e.g. *electriptan, zolmitriptan, sumatriptan*), *dihydroergotamine, linezolid*, and *acetazolamide* can increase the risk or severity of adverse effects.
- Co-medication with anti-seizure medicines (e.g. *phenytoin, valproic acid, lamotrigine*) might alter their efficacy.

Adverse Effects
How Drug Causes Adverse Effects
- Melatonin is generally considered safe, even in extreme doses, although mild complications have been described with higher doses, ER formulations, and when used long-term.
- Adverse effects are mediated by the activity of melatonin on MT1-R (expressed in the retina, ovary, testis, mammary gland, coronary circulation, aorta, gallbladder, liver, kidney, skin, and the immune system)

and MT2-R (expressed in the CNS, lung, heart, coronary circulation, aorta, myometrium, duodenum, immune cells, and adipocytes).
- The most common adverse events are usually a result of the sedative properties of melatonin.

Common Adverse Effects
- Common (≥1/100 to <1/10):
  - Nervous system disorders: headache, somnolence.
- Uncommon (≥1/1,000 to <1/100):
  - Neuropsychiatric: dizziness, irritability, restlessness, abnormal dreams, anxiety.
  - Cardiovascular: hypertension.
  - GI: nausea, abdominal pain, dyspepsia, dry mouth, oral ulcers.
  - Skin: pruritus, rash, dry skin.
  - Renal/urinary: glycosuria, proteinuria.
  - Other: chest pain, malaise, increased weight, hypothermia.

Life-Threatening or Dangerous Adverse Effects
- None.

Rare and Not Life-Threatening Adverse Effects
- Leukopenia, thrombocytopenia, hypertriglyceridemia, polyuria, haematuria, abnormal blood electrolytes.
- Aggressive behaviour, disorientation, increased libido, syncope/fainting, memory impairment, RLS.
- Reduced visual acuity or blurred vision, increased lacrimation.
- Palpitations, hot flushes.
- Gastritis, salivary hypersecretion.

Weight Change
- Increased body weight has been reported as an uncommon sequelae of melatonin use (0.1–1%).

What to Do About Adverse Effects
- Discuss common adverse events with patients or caregivers before starting medication, including symptoms that should be reported to the physician.
- Most adverse effects usually resolve spontaneously within a few days, without any dose adjustments of melatonin.
- In case of persistent or troublesome adverse events, consider lowering the dose or discontinuing melatonin therapy; most adverse effects are expected to resolve immediately after melatonin withdrawal.
- Serious adverse events are rare and mostly constitute aggravations of pre-existing conditions, for example worsening migraine or mood swings in patients with behavioural disorders.

M

ADVERSE EFFECTS

MELATONIN

Dosing and Use

Usual Dosage Range
- 0.1–12 mg daily.

Available Formulations
- IP tablets: 1 mg, 2 mg, 3 mg, 4 mg, 5 mg.
- IR capsules: 1 mg, 3 mg, 5 mg, 10 mg, 20 mg.
- ER tablets: 2 mg, 5 mg, 10 mg.
- Soluble tablet: 3 mg, 5 mg, 10 mg, 12 mg, 500 micrograms.
- Sublingual tablet: 5 mg.
- Oral solution: 1 mg/ml.
- Intravenous, nasal spray, anal suppository, skin patches, cream.

How to Dose
- Effective melatonin dosing in the context of Parkinson's disease is not well defined.
- An initial dose of 2–6 mg, depending on the severity of symptoms, is generally necessary to achieve a clinical effect, although an initial dose range of 1–10 mg is considered safe.
- Consider increasing the dose in case of inadequate response.

Dosing Tips
- Tablets should be taken 1–2 h before bedtime.
- Patients should not consume food for 2 h before and 2 h after melatonin intake.
- Tablets should be swallowed whole with fluid.
- In case of persistent RBD symptoms, co-medication with a low dose of clonazepam could also be considered.

How to Withdraw Drug
- Melatonin can be abruptly withdrawn without any tapering.

Overdose
- Exogenous melatonin is remarkably non-toxic, with up to 3,200 mg/kg described as the lethal dose in rats.
- Daily consumption of 300 mg by healthy adults did not cause any significant complications.
- In case of overdose, the most commonly reported symptoms include drowsiness, headache, dizziness, and nausea.
- Gastric lavage and administration of activated charcoal may be considered.
- General supportive measures are advised.
- Elimination of the active substrate is expected within 12 h.

Tests and Therapeutic Drug Monitoring
- None.

M

Other Warnings / Precautions
- Patients should not drive or use hazardous machinery for 4–5 h after taking melatonin.
- Melatonin should be used with caution if its sedative effects impose a risk to the patient's safety.
- Use with caution in patients with epileptic disorders, as it might precipitate seizures.
- High doses of melatonin may inhibit ovulation.
- Preliminary data suggest that long-term melatonin administration is associated with decreased semen quality in healthy men, probably via aromatase inhibition at the testicular level.
- Melatonin should be taken at least 3 h after food ingestion in patients with impaired glucose tolerance or diabetes, as it might impair blood glucose control.

Do Not Use (Contraindications)
- Known hypersensitivity to the active substance or to any of its excipients.
- It should not be administered to patients with rare hereditary problems of galactose intolerance, total lactase deficiency, or glucose–galactose malabsorption.
- In autoimmune disorders (e.g. rheumatoid arthritis, post-organ transplant), as melatonin might stimulate the immune system through promoting the production of IL-1, -2, -6, and -12, IFNγ, and inflammatory cells.
- Co-medication with the SSRI fluvoxamine, alcohol, and other CNS depressants.

Special Populations
Renal Impairment
- Caution is advised when used in patients with renal impairment.
- Not recommended in severe renal impairment, although no melatonin accumulation was detected in patients on haemodialysis.

Hepatic Impairment
- Not recommended in moderate to severe hepatic impairment.

Elderly
- Night-time endogenous melatonin plasma levels are lower in the elderly.
- No dosage adjustments are suggested.

Pregnancy
- Melatonin readily crosses the placenta, with the levels found in umbilical blood of full-term newborns being only slightly lower than their mothers' following ingestion of a 3-mg dose.

SPECIAL POPULATIONS

M

- No direct or indirect harmful effects during pregnancy have been identified in animal studies.
- Melatonin use should be avoided during pregnancy.

Breastfeeding
- Exogenous melatonin is probably secreted into human milk. It has been detected in milk in animal studies.
- Melatonin use should be avoided during breastfeeding.

Costs

NHS indicative prices accessed 4 December 2022:
- Adaflex 1 mg tablets (AGB-Pharma) – 30 tablets: £13.30.
- Adaflex 2 mg tablets (AGB-Pharma) – 30 tablets: £15.30.
- Adaflex 3 mg tablets (AGB-Pharma) – 30 tablets: £17.60.
- Adaflex 4 mg tablets (AGB Pharma) – 30 tablets: £20.23.
- Adaflex 5 mg tablets (AGB Pharma) – 30 tablets: £23.27.
- Ceyesto 3 mg tablets (Alturix Ltd) – 30 tablets: £10.99.
- Slenyto 1 mg modified-release tablets (Flynn Pharma Ltd) – 30 tablets: £41.20.
- Slenyto 5 mg modified-release tablets (Flynn Pharma Ltd) – 30 tablets: £103.00.
- Syncrodin 3 mg tablets (Pharma Nord (UK) Ltd) – 30 tablets: £14.95.
- Circadin 2 mg modified-release tablets (Flynn Pharma Ltd) – 30 tablets: £15.39.
- Melatonin 3 mg tablets – 30 tablets: £14.95–£19.81.
- Melatonin 2 mg modified-release tablets – £12.25–£15.39.
- Melatonin 1 mg/ml oral solution – 60 ml: £60.00; 100 ml: £86.67–£137.79; 150 ml: £130.00–£152.53.

The Overall Place of Melatonin in the Treatment of Parkinson's Disease

Melatonin is a neurohormone, which is believed to be involved in numerous biological functions, including the circadian rhythm, sleep quality, the stress response, aging, and immunity. Its best-known purpose is the promotion of sleep. There are no licensed indications for melatonin use in Parkinson's disease; however, various reports suggest its efficacy in Parkinson's disease-related sleep disorders, including insomnia and RBD. Compared to other sedative agents, its use is favoured in the elderly and those with dementia or obstructive sleep apnoea, although very commonly a trial with melatonin will be the initial therapeutic approach before prescribing clonazepam. Melatonin formulations are available over the counter, while the FDA has not given official approval for any indication. The actual melatonin content of different products on the market has been found to vary significantly from the stated content, which might

M

explain why reported efficacy varies widely. Melatonin is considered relatively safe with a low risk of side effects, even in high doses.

Potential Advantages
- Compared to clonazepam, which is also a first-line therapeutic option in Parkinson's disease-related RBD, melatonin is considered more efficacious in preventing RBD-related injuries and has a better safety profile. It reduces REM sleep without atonia (RSWA), a prerequisite for a polysomnographic RBD diagnosis, and does not exacerbate co-morbid obstructive sleep apnoea or cognitive impairment.
- Good tolerability profile for elderly patients.

Potential Disadvantages
- No official indications for melatonin use in Parkinson's disease.
- Great heterogeneity in studies investigating the effect of melatonin in Parkinson's disease-related problems, including sleep disorders.
- Limited data on long-term efficacy of melatonin.

Clinical Box
A 70-year-old man with a 2-year history of Parkinson's disease presented with symptoms of polysomnography-diagnosed RBD and vivid dreams. A diagnosis of obstructive sleep apnoea was excluded. His current medication included levodopa/carbidopa 100 mg/25 mg QID. His medical history included hypercholesterolaemia and hypertension. A low dose of clonazepam 0.5 mg OD at bedtime was initially prescribed. At the 1-month follow-up visit, the patient reported a reduction of nights with dream acting out and vocalizations; however, he mentioned memory dysfunction and trouble thinking and requested clonazepam discontinuation. Initiation of melatonin 6 mg OD was suggested as an alternative option. Within the first week of melatonin therapy, the patient reported an improvement of his symptoms, including frightening dreams, without any significant side effects. The beneficial effect was maintained at the 4-month follow-up assessment.

Suggested Reading
Ma H, J Yan, W Sun, M Jiang, Y Zhang. Melatonin treatment for sleep disorders in Parkinson's disease: a meta-analysis and systematic review. *Front Aging Neurosci* 2022; 14: 784314.

Medeiros CA, PFC de Bruin, LA Lopes, MC Magalhães, M de Lourdes Seabra, VMS de Bruin. Effect of exogenous melatonin on sleep and motor dysfunction in Parkinson's disease. A randomized, double blind, placebo-controlled study. *J Neurol* 2007; 254(4): 459–464.

St Louis EK, AR Boeve, BF Boeve. REM sleep behavior disorder in Parkinson's disease and other synucleinopathies. *Mov Disord* 2017; 32(5): 645–658.

SUGGESTED READING

References

AHFS Drug information, 2012. Bethesda: American Society of Health-System Pharmacists. Accessed on 4 December 2022 via www.medicinescomplete.com.

Batla A, S Simeoni, T Uchiyama, L deMin, J Baldwin, C Melbourne, S Islam, KP Bhatia, M Pakzad, S Eriksson, JN Panicker. Exploratory pilot study of exogenous sustained-release melatonin on nocturia in Parkinson's disease. *Eur J Neurol* 2021; 28(6): 1884–1892.

Besag FMC, MJ Vasey, KSJ Lao, ICK Wong. Adverse events associated with melatonin for the treatment of primary or secondary sleep disorders: a systematic review. *CNS Drugs* 2019; 33(12): 1167–1186.

Biggio G, F Biggio, G Talani, MC Mostellino, A Aguglia, E Aguglia, L Palagini. Melatonin: from neurobiology to treatment. *Brain Sci* 2021; 11(9): 1121.

Carrillo-Vico A, PJ Lardone, N Alvarez-Sánchez, A Rodríguez-Rodríguez, JM Guerrero. Melatonin: buffering the immune system. *Int J Mol Sci* 2013; 14(4): 8638–8683.

Erland LAE, PK Saxena. Melatonin natural health products and supplements: presence of serotonin and significant variability of melatonin content. *J Clin Sleep Med* 2017; 13(2): 275–281.

Filali S, C Bergamelli, ML Tall, D Salmon, D Laleye, C Dhelens, E Diouf, C Pivot, F Pirot. Formulation, stability testing, and analytical characterization of melatonin-based preparation for clinical trial. *J Pharm Anal* 2017; 7(4): 237–243.

Hansen MV, AK Danielsen, I Hageman, J Rosenberg, I Gögenur. The therapeutic or prophylactic effect of exogenous melatonin against depression and depressive symptoms: a systematic review and meta-analysis. *Eur Neuropsychopharmacol* 2014; 24(11): 1719–1728.

Harpsøe NG, LP Anderson, I Gögenur, J Rosenberg. Clinical pharmacokinetics of melatonin: a systematic review. *Eur J Clin Pharmacol* 2015; 71(8): 901–909.

Jiménez-Delgado A, GG Ortiz, DL Delgado-Lara, HA González-Usigli, LJ González-Ortiz, M Cid-Hernández, JA Cruz-Serrano, FP Pacheo-Moisés. Effect of melatonin administration on mitochondrial activity and oxidative stress markers in patients with Parkinson's disease. *Oxid Med Cell Longev* 2021; 2021: 5577541.

Joint Formulary Committee. British National Formulary (online). London: BMJ Group and Pharmaceutical Press. Accessed on 4 December 2022 via www.medicinescomplete.com.

Li C, D Ma, M Li, T Wei, X Zhao, Y Heng, D Ma, EO Anto, Y Zhang, M Niu, W Zhang. The therapeutic effect of exogenous melatonin on depressive symptoms: a systematic review and meta-analysis. *Front Psychiatry* 2022; 13: 737972.

Luboshitzky R, Z Shen-Orr, R Nave, S Lavi, P Lavie. Melatonin administration alters semen quality in healthy men. *J Androl* 2002; 23(4): 572–578.

McGrane IR, JG Leung, EK St Louis, BF Boeve. Melatonin therapy for REM sleep behavior disorder: a critical review of evidence. *Sleep Med* 2015; 16(1): 19–26.

Melatonin. In: Brayfield A (Ed.), *Martindale: The Complete Drug Reference*. London: The Royal Pharmaceutical Society of Great Britain. Accessed on 4 December 2022 via www.medicinescomplete.com.

Melatonin. In: DRUGDEX® System (electronic version). Truven Health Analytics, Greenwood Village, Colorado, USA. Accessed on 4 December 2022 via www.micromedexsolutions.com.

Summary of product characteristics – Adaflex 1 mg tablets. AGB-Pharma AB. Electronic Medicines Compendium: Adaflex 1 mg tablets – summary of product characteristics (SmPC) – (emc). Accessed on 4 December 2022 via www.medicines.org.uk.

Xu C, Z He, J Li. Melatonin as a potential neuroprotectant: mechanisms in subarachnoid hemorrhage-induced early brain injury. *Front Aging Neurosci* 2022; 14: 899678.

M

M MEMANTINE

Therapeutics

Chemical Name and Structure

Memantine (1-amino-3,5-dimethyladamantane hydrochloride) is a
white to off-white fine powder or a clear and colourless to light yellowish solution, with a molecular weight of 215.76 and an empirical
formula of $C_{12}H_{21}$ N•HCl.

Brand Names

- **Abixa** (*Indonesia, Philippines, Ukraine*); **Acepter** (*Ecuador*); **Adaxor**
(*Finland*); **Admenta** (*Ecuador, India, Singapore, Ukraine*); **Akatinol**
(*Argentina, Ecuador, Mexico, Russian Federation*); **Albix** (*Hong Kong*);
Alceba (*Turkey*); **Almenta** (*Turkey*); **Almerzac** (*Greece*); **Alois**
(*Brazil*); **Alzant** (*Turkey*); **Alzedem** (*Cyprus*); **Alzeim** (*Russian
Federation*); **Alzer** (*Turkey*); **Alzia** (*Turkey*); **Amint** (*Philippines*);
Appelom (*Tunisia*); **Auranex** (*Russian Federation*); **Avanten**
(*Singapore*); **Axura** (*Austria, Germany, Netherlands, Poland, Portugal,
Spain, Switzerland*).
- **Biomentin** (*Poland*).
- **Carrier** (*Argentina, Ecuador*); **Ceramin** (*Turkey*); **Cissor** (*Turkey*);
Cogito (*Turkey*); **Cognimet** (South Africa); **Cognitine** (*Philippines*);
Cognomem (*Estonia, Greece, Lithuania, Poland*); **Cognum** (*Ecuador*);
Conexine (*Argentina*).
- **Demax** (*Turkey*); **Demenco** (*Italy*); **Denigma** (*Philippines, Ukraine*).
- **Ebantina** (*Chile*); **Ebimem** (*Greece*); **Ebitex** (*Turkey*); **Ebitine** (*South
Africa*); **Ebix** (*Brazil*); **Ebixa** (*Argentina, Australia, Austria, Belgium,
Canada, Chile, China, Cyprus, Czech Republic, Denmark, Estonia,
Finland, France, Germany, Greece, Hong Kong, Hungary, Ireland, Israel,
Italy, Malaysia, Mexico, Netherlands, New Zealand, Norway, Poland,
Portugal, Singapore, South Africa, Spain, Switzerland, Thailand, Tunisia,
Turkey, UK*); **Emaxin** (*Turkey*); **Esmirtal** (*Ecuador*); **Eutebrol** (*Chile,
Ecuador, Mexico*); **Exem** (*Argentina*); **Exemantis** (*Italy*); **Ezagun**
(*Mexico*); **Ezemantis** (*Italy*).
- **Fentina** (*Argentina*); **Fixrem** (*Turkey*).
- **Gnotrin** (*Cyprus*).
- **Heimer** (*Brazil*).
- **Kamppi** (*Brazil*); **Korint** (*Turkey*).
- **Lonrela** (*Spain*); **Lucidex** (*Argentina, Ecuador*).
- **Maizher** (*Brazil*); **Mantinex** (*Spain*); **Mantomed** (*Cyprus,
Czech Republic, Estonia, Greece, Lithuania, Netherlands*); **Marbodin**
(*Denmark, Finland, Netherlands, Poland*); **Marixino** (*Austria, Cyprus,
Czech Republic, Estonia, Greece, Hong Kong, Ireland, Lithuania,
Malaysia, Netherlands, Poland, Singapore, Spain, UK*); **Maruxa**
(*Russian Federation, UK*); **Marvedol** (*Russian Federation*); **Maryzola**
(*Lithuania*); **Maxiram** (*Turkey*); **Mealz** (*Brazil*); **Mebral** (*Chile*);
Melanda (Turkey); **Mema** (*Ukraine*); **Memabix** (*Czech Republic,*

M

Poland); **Memadem** (*Philippines*); **Memamed** (*Ukraine*); **Memando** (*Germany*); **Memanurin** (*Russian Federation*); **Memantal** (*Russian Federation*); **Memantinol** (*Russian Federation*); **Memanvitae** (*Chile, Ecuador*); **Memanxa** (*Australia*); **Memanzaks** (*Turkey*); **Memary** (*Japan*); **Memasolv** (*Greece*); **Mematex** (*South Africa*); **Memax** (*Chile*); **Membral** (*Ukraine*); **Memicar** (*Russian Federation*); **Memigmin** (*Czech Republic, Lithuania, Poland*); **Memikare** (*Chile*); **Memini** (*Cyprus, Greece*); **Meminist** (*South Africa*); **Memixa** (*Czech Republic, Tunisia*); **Memolan** (*Austria, Czech Republic, Germany*); **Memolek** (*Poland*); **Memor** (*South Africa*); **Memorall** (*Brazil*); **Memorel** (*Russian Federation*); **Memorix** (*Turkey*); **Memotec** (*Turkey*); **Memox** (*Israel, Ukraine*); **Memry** (*Philippines*); **Memxa** (*Hong Kong, Malaysia, Thailand*); **Mentadem** (*India*); **Mentax** (*Turkey*); **Mentifar** (*Cyprus, Greece*); **Mentium** (*Chile*); **Mentixa** (*Denmark, Finland*); **Merital** (*Argentina, Chile, Ecuador*); **Mentra** (*India, Philippines*); **Merandex** (*Poland*); **Mevitan** (*Philippines*); **Mexia** (*Turkey*); **Mimetix** (*Chile*); **Mirvedol** (*Hungary, Poland, Ukraine*); **Mobius** (*Greece*); **Modualz** (*Ecuador*); **Moriale ODT** (*Brazil*); **Morysa** (*Czech Republic, Hungary, Poland*).
- **Nabila** (*Spain*); **Namecip** (*Venezuela*); **Namenda** (*USA*); **Nemdatine** (*Austria, Cyprus, Czech Republic, Estonia, Greece, Hungary, Ireland, Lithuania, Netherlands, Norway, Poland, Portugal, Singapore, Spain*); **Nemedan** (*Poland*); **Neumantine** (*Thailand*); **Neurontin** (*Ukraine*); **Neuroplus** (*Argentina, Ecuador*); **Neuropron FT** (*Chile*); **Noojerone** (*Russian Federation*).
- **Perduquan** (*Mexico*); **Polmatine** (*Czech Republic, Estonia, Poland*); **Precel** (*Argentina*); **Prilben** (*Argentina*); **Protalon** (*Spain*).
- **Recorine** (*Argentina*); **Remem** (*Thailand*).
- **Solemantis** (*Italy*); **Sytine** (*Mexico*).
- **Timantil** (*Ecuador, Venezuela*); **Tingrex** (*Russian Federation, Ukraine*); **Tonibral** (*Argentina*); **Tormoro** (*Poland*).
- **Uxamax** (*Spain*).
- **Valios** (*UK*); **Vexil** (*Venezuela*); **Vilimen** (*Greece*); **Vivimex** (*Chile*); **Viximem** (*Turkey*).
- **Xapimant** (*Estonia, Lithuania, Netherlands, Philippines, Poland*); **Xeimer** (*Turkey*).
- **Zemertinex** (*Estonia, Poland*); **Zenmem** (*Poland*); **Zider** (*Brazil*); **Zimerz** (*Philippines*); **Zolmemin** (*Greece*).

Generics Available
- Yes.

Licensed Indications for Parkinson's Disease
- None.

Licensed Indications for Other Conditions
- Moderate to severe Alzheimer's type dementia (FDA, EMA, EMC).

THERAPEUTICS

Non-Licensed Use for Parkinson's Disease
• Parkinson's disease-related dementia (immediate release formulations).

Non-Licensed Use for Other Conditions
• Mild to moderate Alzheimer's disease.
• Mild to moderate vascular dementia.
• LBD.
• Chronic pain.
• Psychiatric disorders.
• MCI.

Ineffective
• Parkinson's disease-related MCI.
• Age-associated cognitive impairment.
• HIV-associated cognitive impairment.
• Cognitive impairment in HD and FTD.

Mechanism of Action
• Memantine is a low to moderate affinity, partial and non-competitive antagonist of the NMDA glutamate receptor subtype.
  • NMDA receptors are voltage-gated cation channels.
  • Memantine blocks NMDA receptors when excessive stimulation is occurring but without suppressing normal physiological transmission.
• Memantine is also thought to have an antagonist effect at the serotonergic type 3 (5-HT3) and nicotinic ACh receptors.

Efficacy Profile
• Memantine may confer some cognitive improvement in PDD and LBD, including behavioural symptoms (e.g. aggression).
  • Memantine may produce an overall improvement in clinical global impression in patients with either LBD or PDD, including cognitive tests of attention and episodic recognition memory.

Pharmacokinetics
Absorption and Distribution
• Oral bioavailability: about 100%.
• Food co-ingestion: no effect of food on immediate release formulations.
• Tmax: 3–8 h (immediate release).
• Time to steady state: about 2 weeks.
• Pharmacokinetics: linear for a dose range of 10–40 mg.
• Protein binding: 45%.
• Volume of distribution: 9–11 l/kg.

Metabolism
- Main metabolites are *N*-3,5-dimethyl-gludantan, the isomeric mixture of 4- and 6-hydroxy-memantine, and 1-nitroso-3,5-dimethyladamantane (inactive metabolites).
- Memantine undergoes partial hepatic metabolism. It is not metabolized by the CYP450 system.

Elimination
- Elimination half-life is 60–80 h.
- Renal excretion: about 50% of an administered dose is excreted unchanged in the urine, involving active tubular secretion, which is moderated by pH-dependent tubular reabsorption.
  - Alkaline urine pH reduces excretion; therefore, factors raising urine pH (e.g. drastic diet changes from carnivore to vegetarian diet, ingestion of alkaline buffers, renal tubular acidosis, and severe infection by *Proteus* bacteria) might have an effect on memantine excretion and plasma levels.

Drug Interaction Profile
Pharmacokinetic Drug Interactions
- Effects by memantine:
  - Memantine may reduce plasma levels of *hydrochlorothiazide.*
- Effects on memantine:
  - Agents that use the same renal cationic transport system as memantine (e.g. *cimetidine, procainamide, quinidine, quinine, nicotine*) may lead to increased plasma concentrations of memantine.

Pharmacodynamic Drug Interactions
- Co-medication with other NMDA antagonists (e.g. *amantadine, dextromethorphan, ketamine*) might cause additive adverse effects, mainly from the CNS, such as psychosis.
- Co-medication with levodopa, dopaminergic agonists, and anticholinergics might lead to an enhanced effect of the above medications.
- Co-medication with neuroleptics or barbiturates might reduce these medications' effect.
- Co-medication with antispasmodic agents (e.g. *dantrolene, baclofen*) might modify their effects and dose adjustments might be needed.

Adverse Effects
How Drug Causes Adverse Effects
- In contrast to other NMDA-receptor antagonists (e.g. *ketamine*), memantine has a much safer profile, although it is not clear why.
- Although there have been some case reports of memantine causing more severe adverse effects, such as hallucinations or delirium, it is

M

ADVERSE EFFECTS

difficult to distinguish the roles of concomitantly administered medications and the underlying neurological disease.

Common Adverse Effects
- Common (≥1/100 to <1/10):
  ○ Nervous/psychiatric: somnolence, dizziness, balance impairment, headache.
  ○ Cardiovascular: hypertension.
  ○ Respiratory: dyspnoea.
  ○ Gastrointestinal: constipation.
  ○ Other: drug hypersensitivity, elevated liver function test.
- Uncommon (≥1/1,000 to <1/100):
  ○ Nervous: confusion, hallucinations, fatigue.
  ○ Other: fungal infections.

Life-Threatening or Dangerous Adverse Effects
- Uncommon (≥1/1,000 to <1/100):
  ○ Cardiac failure, venous thrombosis/thromboembolism, TIA.
  ○ Intracranial haemorrhage.
  ○ NMS.
- Very rare (<1/10,000):
  ○ Seizures.
- Unknown frequency:
  ○ Acute renal failure.
  ○ Hepatitis, liver failure, pancreatitis.
  ○ Stevens–Johnson syndrome.
  ○ Suicidal ideation.
  ○ Agranulocytosis, leukopenia, pancytopenia, thrombocytopenia, thrombotic thrombocytopenic purpura.

Rare and Not Life-Threatening Adverse Effects
  ○ Psychotic reactions.

Weight Change
  ○ None.

What to Do About Adverse Effects
  ○ Before introducing memantine, discuss common or life-threatening adverse effects with patients and/or caregivers, including symptoms that should be reported to the treating physician.
  ○ Memantine should only be prescribed if a caregiver is available to regularly monitor the drug intake for the patient and the occurrence of adverse effects.
  ○ Adverse effects are usually mild to moderate in severity and memantine discontinuation due to adverse reactions is considered unusual. However, in case of troublesome side effects, consider withdrawing memantine.

M

Dosing and Use
Usual Dosage Range
- 10–20 mg (IR).

Available Formulations
- Tablets: 5 mg, 10 mg, 15 mg, 20 mg.
- Soluble tablets: 10 mg, 20 mg.
- ODT: 5 mg, 10 mg, 15 mg, 20 mg.
- Capsules, ER: 7 mg, 14 mg, 21 mg, 28 mg.
- Oral solution: 2 mg/ml, 10 mg/ml.

How to Dose
- Tablets or oral solution: initial dose of 5 mg OD; increase by increments of 5 mg/day every week until the target dose of 10 mg BID.
- Maintenance therapy can be continued for as long as a therapeutic benefit exists and the drug is well tolerated.

Dosing Tips
- Tablets can be taken with or without food and should not be chewed, crushed, or divided.
- The oral solution is withdrawn from the bottle with a syringe and can be swallowed directly or dosed onto a spoon or into a glass of water. It should not be mixed with any other liquid.
- If a dose is missed, the next dose should be taken as scheduled. If dosing is interrupted for a few days, patients should inform their treating physician, as they might need to resume a gradual titration scheme starting from lower doses, according to the patient's tolerance.
- Memantine use can be combined with acetylcholinesterase inhibitors.
  - Due to the serotonergic blocking activity, memantine might result in fewer GI adverse effects than acetylcholinesterase inhibitors.

How to Withdraw Drug
- A dose reduction from a total dose of 10 mg BID to 10 mg OD and a complete discontinuation of treatment after 4 weeks is suggested.
- The recommended tapering schedule may be tailored according to circumstances. In case of severe adverse events, memantine can be discontinued without tapering.

Overdose
- If symptomatic, overdose might present with symptoms of confusion, drowsiness, somnolence, vertigo, agitation, aggression, hallucinations, gait impairment, vomiting, and diarrhoea.
- There have been limited reports of memantine overdose cases who have recovered and survived even after oral intake of large quantities of memantine (up to 2,000 mg).
- General supportive measures are suggested.
- No specific antidote is available.

DOSING AND USE

- Procedures to remove the active substance (e.g. gastric lavage, carbo medicinalis, acidification of urine, forced diuresis) can be applied as appropriate.

Tests and Therapeutic Drug Monitoring
- The tolerance and dosing of memantine should be preferably reassessed within 3 months after treatment initiation and on a regular basis afterwards.

Other Warnings / Precautions
- Caution is advised in patients with a medical history of epilepsy or convulsions or predisposing factors for epilepsy.
- Close monitoring of patients with conditions predisposing to alkaline urine pH is advised.
- Close monitoring of patients treated with oral anticoagulants is advised, as there have been reports of increased INR in co-medication with memantine.
- The ability of patients on memantine to drive or operate machinery should be regularly monitored, not only because it can cause dizziness and somnolence, but also due to the patients' background of dementia.

Do Not Use (Contraindications)
- Known hypersensitivity to memantine or any of the formulation excipients.
  - The oral solution contains sorbitol; therefore, it should not be consumed by patients with rare hereditary problems of fructose intolerance.
- Recent myocardial infarction, uncompensated congestive heart failure (NYHA III or IV), uncontrolled hypertension.
- Co-medication with other NMDA antagonists should be avoided.

Special Populations
Renal Impairment
- No dose adjustments are necessary in mild or moderate renal impairment.
- In severe renal impairment (CrCl 2–29 ml/min) a maximum dose of 5 mg BID is recommended.

Hepatic Impairment
- No dose adjustments are necessary in mild or moderate hepatic impairment.
- Memantine use is not recommended in patients with severe hepatic impairment (Child–Pugh C).

Elderly
- No dose adjustments are required.

MEMANTINE

Pregnancy
- ∘ Some complications from memantine use during pregnancy have been reported in animal studies, although there are no available data in humans.
- ∘ Memantine should not be used during pregnancy.

Breastfeeding
- ∘ It is unclear whether memantine is excreted in human milk, although this would be a reasonable possibility due to the lipophilicity of the drug.
- ∘ Women on memantine should not breastfeed.

Costs
NHS indicative price accessed 19 July 2022:
- • Tablets:
  - • Ebixa (Lundbeck Ltd) – 28 × 10 mg tablets: £34.50; 28 × 20 mg tablets: £69.01.
  - • Marixino (Consilient Health Ltd) – 28 × 10 mg tablets: £29.32; 28 × 20 mg tablets: £58.65.
  - • Generic formulations – 28 × 10 mg tablets: £1.20–£34.50; 28 × 20 mg tablets: £1.45–£69.01.
- • Soluble tablets:
  - • Memantine soluble tablets sugar free (Zentiva Pharma UK Ltd) – 28 × 10 mg tablets: £18.74; 28 × 20 mg tablets: £37.49.
- • Orodispersible tablets:
  - • Valios orodispersible tablets sugar free (Dr Reddy's Laboratories (UK) Ltd) – 28 × 10 mg tablets: £24.99; 28 × 20 mg tablets: £49.98.
- • Oral solution:
  - • Ebixa 5 mg/0.5 ml pump actuation oral solution (Lundbeck Ltd) – 50 ml £61.61; 100 ml £123.23.
- • Generic formulations: 10 mg/ml oral solution × 50 ml £7.38–£61.61; 10 mg/ml oral solution × 100 ml £15.47–£123.23.

The Overall Place of Memantine in the Treatment of Parkinson's Disease

Memantine is an NMDA receptor antagonist, which has been typically used in moderate to severe Alzheimer's disease and is thought to exert its beneficial effect on dementia by normalizing glutamatergic neurotransmission. Although the clinical role of memantine in Parkinson's disease-related dementia has been characterized as 'investigational' by the MDS EBM Committee, there are some indications that it might be beneficial in improving cognitive function in patients with either PDD or LBD. Other reported potential benefits of memantine in PDD include behavioural symptoms and levodopa-induced dyskinesias, although the data supporting the above are scarce and based on case reports. There is insufficient evidence to consider the use of memantine in Parkinson's disease-related dementia and gait disorders. Memantine is generally well-tolerated, with mostly mild or moderate adverse effects, and can be combined with acetylcholinesterase inhibitors, which have been typically used in PDD.

Potential Advantages
- It can be administered as an oral solution formulation in patients who have swallowing difficulties or who might otherwise be less cooperative with drug administration.
- It has a good safety profile with minimal reports of individuals discontinuing memantine due to side effects.

Potential Disadvantages
- The therapeutic benefit of memantine in PDD or other parameters of Parkinson's disease are disputable.

Clinical Box

An 86-year-old lady with advanced Parkinson's disease and moderate to severe Parkinson's disease-related dementia presented at the Neurology Department Outpatient Clinic with her daughter for her scheduled follow-up appointment. The patient was receiving LCIG infusion therapy, a transdermal rivastigmine patch of 9.5 mg/24 h and clonazepam 0.5 mg OD. The rest of her medical history included coronary artery disease with mild heart failure (NYHA II) and a past ischaemic stroke due to large-artery atherosclerosis, leaving the patient with a mild functional deficit (mRS = 2). Considering her motor symptoms, the patient's daughter mentioned that her mother was relatively stable during the past 3 months, although she did mention a few OFF periods occurring during the day, which were successfully addressed with extra levodopa doses. Her cognitive state seemed to be stable or slightly worse. She had also developed some behavioural issues, with the patient often being nervous, agitated, or even aggressive, which was troublesome for her caregiver. Due to the behavioural problems and the cognitive impairment, a gradually increasing dose of memantine was prescribed (target dose of 10 mg BID) according to standard tapering instructions. Because of her cardiovascular medical history and the dementia background, other medications that might have been suitable to address behavioural issues (e.g. low-dose antipsychotic therapy) were avoided.

M

Suggested Reading

Moreau C, A Delval, V Tiffreau, L Defebvre, K Dujardin, A Duhamel, G Petyt, C Hossein-Foucher, D Blum, B Sablonnière, S Schraen, D Allorge, A Destée, R Bordat, D Devos. Memantine for axial signs in Parkinson's disease: a randomised, double-blind, placebo-controlled pilot study. *J Neurol Neurosurg Psychiatry* 2013; 84(5): 552–555.

Ondo WG, L Shinawi, A Davidson, D Lai. Memantine for non-motor features of Parkinson's disease: a double-blind placebo controlled exploratory pilot trial. *Parkinsonism Relat Disord* 2011; 17(3): 156–159.

Wang HF, JT Yu, SW Tang, T Jiang, CC Tan, XF Meng, C Wang, MS Tan, L Tan. Efficacy and safety of cholinesterase inhibitors and memantine in cognitive impairment in Parkinson's disease, Parkinson's disease dementia, and dementia with Lewy bodies: systematic review with meta-analysis and trial sequential analysis. *J Neurol Neurosurg Psychiatry* 2015; 86(2): 135–143.

References

Aarsland D, C Ballard, Z Walker, F Bostrom, G Alves, K Kossakowski, I Leroi, F Pozo-Rodriguez, L Minthon, E Londos. Memantine in patients with Parkinson's disease dementia or dementia with Lewy bodies: a double-blind, placebo-controlled, multicentre trial. *Lancet Neurol* 2009; 8(7): 613–618.

AHFS Drug information, 2012. Bethesda: American Society of Health-System Pharmacists. Accessed on 19 July 2022 via www.medicinescomplete.com.

Emre M, M Tsolaki, U Bonuccelli, A Destée, E Tolosa, A Kutzelnigg, A Ceballos-Baumann, S Zdravkovic, A Bladström, R Jones ; 11018 Study Investigators. Memantine for patients with Parkinson's disease dementia or dementia with Lewy bodies: a randomised, double-blind, placebo-controlled trial. *Lancet Neurol* 2010; 9(10): 969–977.

Gomolin IH, C Smith, TM Jeitner. Once-daily memantine: pharmacokinetic and clinical considerations. *J Am Geriatr Soc* 2010; 58(9): 1812–1813. https://cdpc.sydney.edu.au/wp-content/uploads/2019/06/deprescribing-guideline.pdf.

Joint Formulary Committee. British National Formulary (online). London: BMJ Group and Pharmaceutical Press. Accessed on 19 July 2022 via www.medicinescomplete.com.

Kavirajan H. Memantine: a comprehensive review of safety and efficacy. *Expert Opin Drug Saf* 2009; 8(1): 89–109.

Kawashima S, N Matsukawa. Memantine for the patients with mild cognitive impairment in Parkinson's disease: a pharmacological fMRI study. *BMC Neurol* 2022; 22(1): 175.

Kuns B, A Rosani, V Varghese. Memantine. [Updated 2022 May 2]. In: StatPearls [Internet]. Treasure Island (FL): StatPearls Publishing; 2022. Available from: www.ncbi.nlm.nih.gov/books/NBK500025/

Leroi I, R Overshott, EJ Byrne, E Daniel, A Burns. Randomized controlled trial of memantine in dementia associated with Parkinson's disease. *Mov Disord* 2009; 24(8): 1217–1221.

Mirabegron. In: Brayfield A (Ed.), *Martindale: The Complete Drug Reference*. London: The Royal Pharmaceutical Society of Great Britain. Accessed on 19 July 2022 via www.medicinescomplete.com.

Mirabegron. In: DRUGDEX® System (electronic version). Truven Health Analytics, Greenwood Village, Colorado, USA. Accessed on 10 March 2023 via www.micromedexsolutions.com.

Rogawski MA, GL Wenk. The neuropharmacological basis for the use of memantine in the treatment of Alzheimer's disease. *CNS Drug Rev* 2003; 9(3): 275–308.

Summary of Product Characteristics – Ebixa 10 mg film-coated tablets. Lundbeck Limited. Electronic Medicines Compendium: Ebixa 10 mg film-coated tablets – summary of product characteristics (SmPC) – (emc). Accessed on 19 July 2022 via www.medicines.org.uk.

Varanese S, J Howard, A Di Rocco. NMDA antagonist memantine improves levodopa-induced dyskinesias and "on-off" phenomena in Parkinson's disease. *Mov Disord* 2010; 25(4):508–510.

Vidal EI, FB Fukushima, AP Valle, PJF Villas Boas. Unexpected improvement in levodopa-induced dyskinesia and on-off phenomena after introduction of memantine for treatment of Parkinson's disease dementia. *J Am Geriatr Soc* 2013; 61(1): 170–172.

Wesnes KA, D Aarsland, C Ballard, E Londos. Memantine improves attention and episodic memory in Parkinson's disease dementia and dementia with Lewy bodies. *Int J Geriatr Psychiatry* 2015; 30(1): 46–54.

MEMANTINE

MIDODRINE

M

Therapeutics

Chemical Name and Structure

Midodrine hydrochloride (2-amino-*N*-(β-hydroxy-2,5-dimethoxy-phenethyl)acetamide hydrochloride or (*RS*)-*N*-(β-hydroxy-2,5-dimeth-oxyphenethyl)glycinamide hydrochloride), molecular weight 290.74 and a molecular formula of $C_{12}H_{18}N_2O_4$,HCl.

Brand Names
- **Abalnate** (*Japan*); **An De Lin** (*China*).
- **Bramox** (*UK*).
- **Dortrenin** (*Japan*).
- **Gutron** (*Argentina, Austria, Chile, China, Czech Republic, Estonia, France, Germany, Greece, Hong Kong, Hungary, Italy, Netherlands, New Zealand, Poland, Portugal, Singapore, Spain, Thailand*).
- **Hypotron** (*Denmark, Finland, Norway, Sweden, Switzerland*).
- **Metligine** (*Japan*); **Midon** (*Ireland*); **Midorine** (*Thailand*); **Mi Wei** (*China*).
- **Orvaten** (*USA*).
- **ProAmatine** (*USA*).

Generics Available
- Yes.

Licensed Indications for Parkinson's Disease
- None.

Licensed Indications for Other Conditions
- Symptomatic orthostatic hypotension due to autonomic dysfunction (FDA, EMA, EMC).

Non-Licensed Use for Parkinson's Disease
- Severe orthostatic hypotension.

Non-Licensed Use for Other Conditions
- Stress incontinence.
- An adjunct therapy in the management of urinary incontinence.
- Retrograde ejaculation.

Ineffective
- Severely fluctuating blood pressure.

Mechanism of Action
- Midodrine is an alpha-1 selective adrenergic agonist, which increases peripheral vascular resistance.

THERAPEUTICS

- The increase in arteriolar and venous tone results in higher values of sitting, standing, and supine systolic and diastolic blood pressure in patients with orthostatic hypotension.
- Midodrine acts on both the arterial and venous system, but has no direct cardiac effect.
- Midodrine does not cross the blood–brain barrier.
- No accumulation of midodrine is observed after repeated dosing.

Efficacy Profile
- Midodrine has been characterized as 'possibly useful' for the treatment of orthostatic hypotension in Parkinson's disease, although there is currently 'insufficient evidence' to support its use (MDS EBM Committee).
- No studies focusing on the effect of midodrine on orthostatic hypotension in Parkinson's disease are currently available. There is indirect evidence on midodrine efficacy from studies including Parkinson's disease patients in their sample.
- Limited data are available on the long-term effects of midodrine.
- The initial effect of midodrine appears about 45–90 min after administration with maximum effected reported at an average of 1 h.

Pharmacokinetics
Absorption and Distribution
- Oral bioavailability: 93%.
- Food co-ingestion increases midodrine concentration and shortens Tmax.
- Tmax: 15–30 min (midodrine); 1–2 h (desglymidodrine).
- Protein binding: <30%.
- Volume of distribution: <1.66 l/kg.

Metabolism
- Midodrine undergoes extensive enzymatic hydrolysis in the systemic circulation producing the active metabolite desglymidodrine.
  - Desglymidodrine is a relatively long-acting alpha-1 selective adrenergic agonist. It is 15 times more potent than midodrine and is primarily responsible for the drug effects.
  - Desglymidodrine is also a substrate of CYP2D6.

Elimination
- Half-life is 25–30 min and 3–4 h for midodrine and desglymidodrine, respectively.
- More than 90% of midodrine, desglymidodrine, and their metabolites are excreted in urine in conjugated or non-conjugated form within 24 h.
- Midodrine is also detected in small amounts in the faeces (1–2%).

M

Drug Interaction Profile

Pharmacokinetic Drug Interactions
- Effects by midodrine:
  - Midodrine is a CYP2D6 inhibitor and may increase serum levels of relevant substrates, such as tricyclic antidepressants, beta blockers, SSRIs, antiarrhythmics class 1A/1B/1C, and MAOIs type B.
- Effects on midodrine:
  - *Amiodarone, digoxin, metformin, triamterene, sulfamethoxazole, verapamil,* and *memantine* may increase the levels or effects of midodrine via basic (cationic) drug competition for renal tubular clearance.
  - CYP2D6 inhibitors (e.g. *quinidine, paroxetine, fluoxetine, bupropion*) may increase plasma levels of desglymidodrine, the active metabolite of midodrine.

Pharmacodynamic Drug Interactions
- Tricyclic antidepressants (e.g. *amitriptyline*) may alter the effect of midodrine by blocking norepinephrine reuptake.
- Co-medication with phenothiazines, particularly *thioridazine*, may predispose to cardiac arrhythmia or sudden death, especially in vulnerable individuals.
- Co-medication with ergots (e.g. *dihydroergotamine*), sympathomimetic agents (e.g. *phenylephrine, pseudoephedrine, droxidopa*), MAOIs (e.g. *linezolid, phenelzine, selegiline, rasagiline*), corticosteroids, *bromocriptine, trazodone, safinamide, caffeine,* and other vasoconstrictive agents (including over-the-counter remedies available without prescription) may potentiate the pressor effects of droxidopa.
  - Co-medication with *droxidopa* or *fludrocortisone* may increase the risk for supine hypertension.
- Midodrine may antagonize the effects of some antihypertensive agents (e.g. *hydralazine*).
- Co-medication with corticosteroids (including *fludrocortisone*) may cause increased intraocular pressure/glaucoma.

Adverse Effects

How Drug Causes Adverse Effects
- Midodrine causes adverse effects through its adrenergic activity.
- Symptoms of urinary urgency can occur by stimulation of the trigone and sphincter of the urinary bladder.
- Pilomotor effects and pupillary dilation can occur by stimulation of the pilomotor muscles and the radial muscle of the iris, respectively.

Common Adverse Effects
- Very common (≥1/10):
  - Paraesthesia, piloerection, pruritus, chills, flushing, rash, supine hypertension, urinary retention/urgency.

ADVERSE EFFECTS

- Common (≥1/100 to <1/10):
  - Neuropsychiatric: headache.
  - GI: nausea, dyspepsia, stomatitis.
  - Other: pain (including abdominal pain).
- Uncommon (≥1/1,000 to <1/100):
  - Neuropsychiatric: dry mouth, anxiety, dizziness, confusion, insomnia, somnolence, weakness, irritability, excitability.
  - Cardiovascular: reflex bradycardia.
  - Skin: dry skin, erythema multiforme.

Life-Threatening or Dangerous Adverse Effects
- Rare (≥1/10,000 to <1/1,000):
  - Tachycardia, palpitations.
  - Hepatic impairment, raised liver enzymes.

Rare and Not Life-Threatening Adverse Effects
- Diarrhoea.

Weight Change
  - An increase in body weight has been reported, probably due to extracellular fluid volume expansion.

What to Do About Adverse Effects
  - Before introducing midodrine therapy, discuss common or life-threatening adverse effects with patients and/or caregivers, including symptoms that should be reported to the physician.
  - Patients should be instructed to elevate the head of their bed at least 30–45° at night when sleeping in order to lower the risk of supine hypertension. If supine hypertension occurs despite this manoeuvre, consider dose reduction or cessation of midodrine.
  - Patients should be instructed to report any symptoms suggestive of supine hypertension, such as chest pain, palpitations, shortness of breath, headache, or blurred vision.
  - If signs or symptoms of bradycardia appear, midodrine therapy should be stopped.
  - If concomitant administration with drugs that increase blood pressure cannot be avoided, close monitoring of blood pressure is recommended.

Dosing and Use
Usual Dosage Range
  - 5–30 mg.

Available Formulations
  - Tablets: 2.5 mg, 5 mg, 10 mg.

M

How to Dose
- An initial dose of 2.5 mg BID or TID is suggested; weekly increases by increments of 2.5 mg TID can be applied depending on the patient's response and the measurements of supine and standing blood pressure up to a total dose of 30 mg divided in three doses.
  - The usual maintenance dose is 10 mg TID.
  - Depending on patient's needs, midodrine can also be administered every 12 h (initial scheme of 2.5 mg BID and dose increases by increments of 2.5 mg BID every week).
- A total dose of 40 mg per day should not be exceeded.
- Careful assessments of the patient's clinical response to therapy along with tolerability issues should take place before any increases in midodrine dosage or in prolonged midodrine therapy.

Dosing Tips
- The first dose should be received upon rising in the morning, the second at midday, and the third late in the afternoon (before 6 p.m.) at least 4 h before bedtime to lower the risk for supine hypertension.
  - Midodrine should be given at the same time schedule every day.
  - An interval of at least 3–4 h between doses is needed.
- Midodrine should be taken during a meal and with sufficient fluid.
- Midodrine tablets should be taken during daytime when patients perform their daily activities in upright position.

How to Withdraw Drug
- Due to short half-life, midodrine can be tapered off relatively quickly.

Overdose
- Midodrine overdose may manifest with hypertension, piloerection, feeling cold, bradycardia, and urinary retention.
- Induced vomiting and the administration of an alpha-sympatholytic agent (e.g. *nitroglycerine, phentolamine*) are recommended (vasodilation).
- If bradycardia and/or bradycardic conduction disturbances occur, consider administration of atropine.
- Supportive measures and close monitoring are recommended. No antidote is available.

Tests and Therapeutic Drug Monitoring
- Before initiation of midodrine therapy:
  - Supine, sitting, and 3-min standing blood pressure should be measured.
  - Heart rate should be monitored.
  - Renal and hepatic function should be assessed.
- During midodrine therapy:

DOSING AND USE

M

MIDODRINE

• Supine, sitting, and 3-min standing blood pressure should be regularly monitored (at least twice a week), especially in dosage increases. Night measurements should also be included.
  • Patients should be instructed to measure blood pressure 1 h after midodrine administration.
• Regular assessment of heart rate is advised.
• Hepatic and renal function should be assessed at regular intervals.

Other Warnings / Precautions
○ Midodrine has a black box warning for causing supine hypertension, which, if left untreated, can predispose to cardiovascular events, particularly strokes.
○ Caution is advised when midodrine is used in patients with diabetes mellitus or vision problems.
○ Caution is advised when midodrine is used in patients with atherosclerotic disease, including those with symptoms of intestinal angina or claudication of the legs.
○ In patients with severe disturbances of the autonomic nervous system midodrine may cause a further decrease of blood pressure and therapy should be discontinued.
○ Midodrine may slow heart rate due to vagal reflex; co-administration with cardiac glycosides (including digitalis preparations), β-blockers or other agents with negative chronotropic action is not recommended.
○ Close monitoring is needed if co-administered with antihypertensive agents due to opposing effects on blood pressure control.
○ Close monitoring is needed if co-administered with *bromocriptine* due to increased risk of hypertension or ventricular tachycardia.
○ Close monitoring is needed if co-administered with *safinamide* due to potential additive effects on blood pressure and heart rate.
○ Close monitoring is needed if co-administered with antipsychotics, benzodiazepines, opiates, *mirtazapine*, *topiramate*, or other sedatives due to opposing effects on sedation.
○ Patients with orthostatic hypotension who experience symptoms of dizziness or light-headedness while on midodrine therapy should avoid driving or operating dangerous machinery.

Do Not Use (Contraindications)
○ Known sensitivity to midodrine or to any of the excipients.
○ Severe organic heart disease, including bradycardia, congestive heart failure, cardiac conduction disturbances, aortic aneurysm, heart attack.
○ Severe obliterative blood vessel disease, cerebrovascular occlusion, vessel spasms.
○ Already known supine hypertension.
○ Urinary retention or acute kidney disease.
○ Pheochromocytoma.

M

- Thyrotoxicosis/hyperthyroidism.
- Serious prostate disorder (high risk for urinary retention).
- Proliferative diabetic retinopathy.
- Narrow-angle glaucoma.
- Co-administration with tricyclic antidepressants, selective and non-selective MAOIs, ergots, and *trazodone* is contraindicated due to risk of acute hypertensive episode.

Special Populations
Renal Impairment
- Midodrine is contraindicated in severe renal impairment and acute renal impairment.
- Caution is advised when administered in patients with renal impairment.

Hepatic Impairment
- No specific dose modifications are suggested.
- Caution is advised, midodrine use has not been studied in patients with hepatic impairment.

Elderly
- No specific dose modifications are suggested for the elderly.
- Caution is recommended during dose titration for potential adverse events.

Pregnancy
- Pregnancy category C: use with caution if benefits outweigh risks (FDA).
- Midodrine should not be used during pregnancy or in women of childbearing potential who do not use contraception (UK SPC, EMA).

Breastfeeding
- It is unknown whether midodrine is excreted in human milk.
- Midodrine therapy is not recommended during breastfeeding, as a toxic effect on milk production or on nursing infants cannot be excluded.

Costs
NHS indicative pricing on 29 December 2022:
- Bramox tablets (Brancaster Pharma Ltd) – 100 × 2.5 mg tablets: £33.91; 100 × 5 mg tablets: £49.05; 100 × 10 mg tablets: £83.32.
- Midodrine 2.5 mg tablets – 100 × 2.5 mg tablets: £48.85–£53.35.
- Midodrine 5 mg tablets – 100 × 5 mg tablets: £70.27–£81.25.

The Overall Place of Midodrine in the Treatment of Parkinson's Disease

Midodrine is an orally available, short-acting selective α1-adrenergic agonist used for the treatment of symptomatic orthostatic hypotension due to autonomic dysfunction. Midodrine is a prodrug whose function is mediated through its primary metabolite, desglymidodrine. Both increase blood pressure via inducing vasoconstriction and decreasing venous pooling. Due to the high risk of severe adverse reactions, midodrine therapy should only be introduced in severe cases of orthostatic hypotension, when corrective factors have been excluded and no therapeutic alternatives are available. However, if a patient can stand for predictable short periods of time, it is reasonable to introduce midodrine to enhance orthostatic tolerance.

Despite the fact that there are no high-quality studies focusing on the efficacy of midodrine in Parkinson's disease patients specifically, midodrine could be considered as a treatment option in clinical practice, as Parkinson's disease patients were included in the study populations of two level-I studies. Careful monitoring for the development of supine hypertension or other cardiovascular adverse reactions is recommended.

Potential Advantages
- Midodrine can be a useful tool for acute needs in blood pressure control.
- Unlike most vasopressors, midodrine has virtually no stimulant effect on β-adrenergic receptors.

Potential Disadvantages
- Due to the safety profile of midodrine, its use should be restricted to patients with significantly impaired and refractory orthostatic hypotension despite standard clinical care.
- Regular monitoring is required.

Clinical Box

A 65-year-old woman with a 5-year history of Parkinson's disease was referred to the Movement Disorders Outpatient Clinic due to severe orthostatic hypotension which significantly impaired her daily life. She was receiving levodopa/carbidopa 100 mg/25 mg TID. She also had a history of depression and diabetes mellitus type II for which she was taking escitalopram 20 mg OD and metformin 850 mg BID, respectively. Non-pharmacologic measures and fludrocortisone therapy had no effect on her symptoms. Droxidopa was not available in the patient's country, so midodrine therapy at a dose of 2.5 mg BID was suggested. Regular follow-up assessments and instructions for blood pressure measurements were given to the patient. Despite the fact that fludrocortisone did not improve her symptoms, she did not experience any adverse reactions, so it was continued. The patient reported alleviation of symptoms at a midodrine dose of 7.5 mg BID.

M

Suggested Reading

Jankovic J, JL Gilden, BC Hiner, H Kaufmann, DC Brown, CH Coghlan, M Rubin, FM Fouad-Tarazi. Neurogenic orthostatic hypotension: a double-blind, placebo-controlled study with midodrine. *Am J Med* 1993; 95(1): 38–48.

Low PA, JL Gilden, R Freeman, KN Sheng, MA McElligott. Efficacy of midodrine vs placebo in neurogenic orthostatic hypotension. A randomized, double-blind multicenter study. Midodrine Study Group. *JAMA* 1997; 277(13): 1046–1051.

References

AHFS Drug information, 2012. Bethesda: American Society of Health-System Pharmacists. Accessed on 29 December 2022 via www.medicinescomplete.com.

Joint Formulary Committee. British National Formulary (online). London: BMJ Group and Pharmaceutical Press. Accessed on 29 December 2022 via www.medicinescomplete.com.

Midodrine. In: Brayfield A (Ed.), *Martindale: The Complete Drug Reference*. London: The Royal Pharmaceutical Society of Great Britain. Accessed on 29 December 2022 via www.medicinescomplete.com.

Midodrine. In DRUGDEX® System (electronic version). Truven Health Analytics, Greenwood Village, Colorado, USA. Accessed on 29 December 2022 via www.micromedexsolutions.com.

Smith W, H Wan, D Much, AG Robinson, P Martin. Clinical benefit of midodrine hydrochloride in symptomatic orthostatic hypotension: a phase 4, double-blind, placebo-controlled, randomized, tilt-table study. *Clin Auton Res* 2016; 26(4): 269–277.

Summary of product characteristics – Bramox 2.5 mg tablets. Brancaster Pharma Limited. Electronic Medicines Compendium: Bramox 2.5 mg tablets – summary of product characteristics (SmPC) – (emc). Accessed on 29 December 2022 via www.medicines.org.uk.

MIRABEGRON

Therapeutics

Chemical Name and Structure

Mirabegron (2-(2-amino-1,3-thiazol-4-yl)-*N*-[4-(2-{[(2*R*)-2-hydroxy-2-phenylethyl]amino}ethyl)phenyl]acetamide) has a molecular weight of 396.5 and a molecular formula of $C_{21}H_{24}N_4O_2S$.

Brand Names

- **Betanis** (*Japan*); **Betmiga** (*Australia, Austria, Belgium, China, Cyprus, Czech Republic, Denmark, Estonia, Finland, France, Germany, Greece, Hong Kong, Hungary, Indonesia, Ireland, Israel, Lithuania, Malaysia, Netherlands, Norway, Philippines, Poland, Portugal, Russian Federation, Singapore, South Africa, Spain, Sweden, Switzerland, Thailand,* UK, Ukraine).
- **Myrbetric** (*Argentina, Brazil*); **Myrbetriq** (*Canada, USA*).

Generics Available

- No.

Licensed Indications for Parkinson's Disease

- None.

Licensed Indications for Other Conditions

- Overactive bladder (urinary incontinence, urgency, increased micturition), either as a monotherapy or in combination with the muscarinic antagonist solifenacin succinate (FDA, EMA, EMC).

Non-Licensed Use for Parkinson's Disease

- Overactive bladder.

Non-Licensed Use for Other Conditions

- Ureteral stent-related symptoms.

Ineffective

- Not reported.

Mechanism of Action

- Mirabegron is a selective and potent beta-3 adrenergic receptor agonist, which causes relaxation of the detrusor smooth muscle of the urinary bladder and, thus, increases bladder capacity.

Efficacy Profile

- Two recent double-blind RCTs assessed the effect of mirabegron 50 mg and 25–50 mg on overactive bladder symptoms in a small number of Parkinson's disease patients for a short time, demonstrating a positive effect of mirabegron with minor adverse effects.

THE MOVEMENT DISORDERS PRESCRIBER'S GUIDE TO PARKINSON'S DISEASE

- Another recent double RCT (PaDoMi study) has assessed the effect of mirabegron on overactive bladder symptoms in patients with parkinsonism for 12 weeks, also demonstrating a favourable effect of mirabegron with acceptable adverse events.
- These findings were further supported by a retrospective analysis examining the effect of mirabegron 50 mg on overactive bladder symptoms in Parkinson's disease patients for 6 weeks.

Pharmacokinetics
Absorption and Distribution
- Oral bioavailability: 29% (25 mg tablets) and 35% (50 mg tablets).
- Food co-ingestion: high-/low-fat meals will reduce mirabegron serum concentration.
- Tmax: 3.5 h.
- Time to steady state: 7 days.
- Pharmacokinetics: linear after IV dosing (7.5–50 mg), but increased more than proportionally after oral dosing (25–150 mg).
- Protein binding: about 71%.
- Volume of distribution: 1670 l.

Metabolism
- Mirabegron undergoes hepatic metabolism and is transported and metabolised via numerous routes. Specifically, it is a substrate for CYP2D6, CYP3A4, butyrylcholinesterase, uridine diphospho-glucuronosyl-transferases (UGT), the efflux transporter P-gp, and the influx organic cation transporters OCT1, OCT2, and OCT3.
- Mirabegron is a moderate CYP2D6 and a weak CYP3A inhibitor.
  - CYP2D6 activity is expected to recover within 15 days after mirabegron discontinuation.
- Mirabegron is a weak P-gp inhibitor.

Elimination
- Half-life of mirabegron is approximately 50 h.
- About 55% of an administered dose is excreted in the urine and 34% is detected in faeces.

Drug Interaction Profile
Pharmacokinetic Drug Interactions
- Effects by mirabegron:
  - Mirabegron may increase the levels or effects of CYP2D6 substrates, such as *amitriptyline, aripiprazole, captopril, carvedilol, chloroquine, chlorpromazine, citalopram, clozapine, desipramine, duloxetine, flecainide, fluoxetine, haloperidol, imipramine, metoprolol, mirtazapine, nebivolol, nortriptyline, paroxetine, procainamide, promethazine, propranolol, risperidone, sertraline, timolol, tramadol, venlafaxine*, and others.

M

- Mirabegron may increase the levels or effects of *digoxin, dabigatran* and other sensitive P-gp substrates.
- Mirabegron may decrease the levels or effects of *tamoxifen*, as the latter is a prodrug metabolized to active metabolites by CYP2D6.
- Effects on mirabegron:
  - Strong CYP3A or P-gp inhibitors (e.g. *ketoconazole, itraconazole*) may increase mirabegron levels.
  - CYP3A or P-gp inducers (e.g. *rifampicin*) may decrease mirabegron levels.

Pharmacodynamic Drug Interactions
- Co-medication with antimuscarinic drugs increases the risk of urinary retention.

Adverse Effects
How Drug Causes Adverse Effects
- Beta-3 adrenergic receptors located on skeletal muscle and myocardial tissue may be responsible for the cardiovascular effects of mirabegron.
- Higher than recommended doses of mirabegron may stimulate beta-one adrenergic receptors.

Common Adverse Effects
- Very common (≥1/10):
  - Increased blood pressure (especially in patients with pre-existing hypertension).
- Common (≥1/100 to <1/10):
  - Neuropsychiatric: headache, dizziness.
  - Eye/ear: blurred vision.
  - Cardiovascular: tachycardia.
  - GI: dry mouth, constipation, diarrhoea, nausea.
  - Respiratory: nasopharyngitis, sinusitis.
  - Renal/urinary: urinary tract infections, cystitis.
  - Other: back pain, arthralgia, fatigue, reports of neoplasms.
- Uncommon (≥1/1,000 to <1/100):
  - Eye/ear: glaucoma.
  - Cardiovascular: palpitations, atrial fibrillation.
  - GI: gastritis, dyspepsia, abdominal distension.
  - Respiratory: rhinitis.
  - Renal/urinary: nephrolithiasis, bladder pain, cystitis.
  - Reproductive: vulvovaginal pruritus, vaginal infection.
  - Skin: urticaria, leucocytoclastic vasculitis, rash, pruritus, purpura.
  - Other: elevated hepatic enzymes, joint swelling.

Life-Threatening or Dangerous Adverse Effects
- Angioedema of the face, lips, tongue, and larynx.
- Urinary retention.
- Hypertensive crisis.

Rare and Not Life-Threatening Adverse Effects
- Eyelid or lip oedema.
- Insomnia.

Weight Change
- Not reported.

What to Do About Adverse Effects
- Before introducing mirabegron, discuss common or life-threatening adverse effects with patients and/or caregivers, including symptoms that should be reported to the physician.
- In case of angioedema, which may occur after the initial dose or after multiple doses, mirabegron therapy should be discontinued and appropriate treatment should be applied to ensure a patent airway.
- In case of troublesome or persistent adverse effects, consider therapy discontinuation.
  - Changes in heart rate and blood pressure are reversible upon discontinuation of mirabegron therapy.

Dosing and Use
Usual Dosage Range
- 25–50 mg.

Available Formulations
- ER tablets: 25 mg, 50 mg.
- Mirabegron granules are also available, but they are not substitutable on a mg for mg basis with the tablets. Granules do not have an approved indication for overactive bladder management.

How to Dose
- An initial dose of 25 mg OD is suggested; consider increasing to 50 mg OD depending on the patient's clinical response and drug tolerability after 4–8 weeks.

Dosing Tips
- Mirabegron tablets may be taken with or without food.
- Mirabegron therapy should be taken at the same time every day.
- In case of a missed dose:
  - <12 h since missed dose: take as soon as remembered.
  - >12 h since missed dose: skip dose and take next dose at usual time.

How to Withdraw Drug
- Mirabegron discontinuation can be abrupt.

Overdose
- Mirabegron overdose may present with palpitations and increased heart rate.

M

MIRABEGRON

- Supportive measures, close monitoring of blood pressure/pulse rate, and ECG monitoring is suggested.

Tests and Therapeutic Drug Monitoring
- Before initiation of mirabegron therapy:
  - Blood pressure should be measured.
- During mirabegron therapy:
  - Blood pressure should be measured at regular intervals, especially in hypertensive patients.

Other Warnings/Precautions
- Caution is advised in patients with hypertension.
- Caution is advised in patients with congenital or acquired QT prolongation, although the effect of mirabegron on these patients is not clear.
- Caution is advised in patients with bladder outlet obstruction or those already taking antimuscarinic agents, as they might be prone to urinary retention.
- Because mirabegron is a moderate CYP2D6 inhibitor, close monitoring is advised if co-administering with those CYP2D6 substrates that have a narrow therapeutic index, such as *thioridazine*, tricyclic antidepressants, and type 1C antiarrhythmics; dose adjustments might also be considered.
- If co-administering with *digoxin*, the lowest initial dose of digoxin is suggested; monitoring of serum digoxin levels and dose titration based on desired clinical effect is necessary.

Do Not Use (Contraindications)
- Hypersensitivity to mirabegron or any of its excipients.
- Severe uncontrolled hypertension.

Special Populations
Renal Impairment
- Mild to moderate impairment (eGFR ≥ 30 ml/min/1.73 m^2): no dosage modifications are needed.
- Moderate to severe impairment (eGFR 15–29 ml/min/1.73 m^2): a maximum dose of 25 mg per day is recommended.
- Severe impairment (eGFR < 15 ml/min/1.73 m^2) or dialysis: not recommended.

Hepatic Impairment
- Mild impairment (Child–Pugh A): no dosage modification needed.
- Moderate (Child–Pugh B): a maximum dose of 25 mg per day is recommended.
- Severe (Child–Pugh C): not recommended.

Elderly
- No differences reported.

Pregnancy
- No data are available on the use of mirabegron during pregnancy.
- Mirabegron use is not recommended during pregnancy, as potential risks for the fetus cannot be excluded.

Breastfeeding
- It is not known whether mirabegron is excreted in human milk.
- No data are available on the effect of mirabegron on nursing infants or milk production.
- Mirabegron use is not recommended during breastfeeding, as potential risks for the nursing infant cannot be excluded.

Costs
NHS indicative price accessed on 29 December 2022
- Betmiga modified-release tablets (Astellas Pharma Ltd) – 30 × 25 mg tablets: £29.00; 30 × 50 mg tablets: £29.00.

The Overall Place of Mirabegron in the Treatment of Parkinson's Disease
Mirabegron is a selective and potent beta-3 adrenergic agonist, which is approved for the management of overactive bladder. Although antimuscarinic agents are considered first-line drugs for the treatment of overactive bladder, mirabegron may be an appropriate alternative for those in whom antimuscarinic agents were not beneficial or tolerated due to troublesome anticholinergic adverse effects. Human bladder smooth muscle relaxation is thought to be mediated principally by the beta-3 adrenergic receptors; therefore, mirabegron results in an increase of the bladder capacity. Unlike antimuscarinic agents, which affect neural control of the voiding phase of micturition, mirabegron acts on the neural control of the storage phase of micturition. It can be combined with antimuscarinic agents due to its different mechanism of action. The efficacy of mirabegron on Parkinson's disease-related urinary urgency/incontinence was recently demonstrated in two double-blind RCTs and in a retrospective study (maximum of 12 weeks of therapy) with minor adverse effects.

Potential Advantages
- In contrast to antimuscarinic agents, mirabegron is free of adverse anticholinergic effects, which are particularly problematic among elderly patients and those with cognitive impairment.

- A recent, large Canadian population-based case–control study found that patients taking some anticholinergic medications for overactive bladder symptoms had a higher risk of dementia compared to those on mirabegron.
- In contrast to antimuscarinic agents, mirabegron does not have any effect on bladder contraction during the voiding phase, thus, it is not expected to increase post-voiding residual urine volume.

Potential Disadvantages
- According to a recent study of real-life data, mirabegron use has been associated with a higher risk for hypertension compared to other medications used to treat overactive bladder symptoms.
- Experience from routine clinical practice has shown that mirabegron may be used in the long term; however, no relevant studies are currently available to support long duration of mirabegron therapy in Parkinson's disease patients.

Clinical Box

A 75-year-old woman with a 14-year history of Parkinson's disease presented at the Movement Disorders Outpatient Clinic for her regular follow-up assessment. The patient had undergone DBS surgery about 5 years ago; she was also receiving levodopa/carbidopa 50 mg/12.5 mg QID, amantadine 100 mg BID, rotigotine transdermal patch 4 mg/24 h and fluoxetine 20 mg OD, and had a medical history of diabetes mellitus type II and hypertension for which she received metformin 850 mg BID and olmesartan/hydrochlorothiazide 20 mg/12.5 mg. The patient reported symptoms of an overactive bladder with increased micturition and urged urination, including episodes of unintentional loss of urine during the day. After a thorough assessment, her symptoms were thought to be related to Parkinson's disease. Due to her age, mirabegron therapy seemed preferable to an antimuscarinic agent and she was, therefore, prescribed mirabegron 25 mg OD. Her blood pressure was well controlled; however, she was given instructions concerning regular assessments of her blood pressure and heart rate while on mirabegron therapy. She reported an improvement of her symptoms after 5 weeks of therapy without any undesirable effects.

Suggested Reading

Cho SY, SJ Jeong, S Lee, J Kim, SH Lee, MS Choo, SJ Oh. Mirabegron for treatment of overactive bladder symptoms in patients with Parkinson's disease: s double-blind, randomized placebo–controlled trial (Parkinson's Disease Overactive bladder Mirabegron, PaDoMi Study). *Neurourol Urodyn* 2021; 40(1): 286–294.

Madan A, T Brown, S Ray, P Agarwal, I Roy-Faderman, D Burdick. A novel trial of mirabegron and behavioral modification including

M

pelvic floor exercise for overactive bladder in Parkinson's disease (MAESTRO). *Cureus* 2022; 14(11): e31818.

Moussa M, MA Chakra, B Dabboucy, Y Fares, A Dellis, A Papatsoris. The safety and effectiveness of mirabegron in Parkinson's disease patients with overactive bladder: a randomized controlled trial. *Scand J Urol* 2022; 56(1): 66–72.

Peyronnet B, G Vurture, JA Palma, DR Malacarne, A Feigin, RD Sussman, MC Biagioni, R Palmerola, R Gilbert, N Rosenblum, S Frucht, H Kaufmann, VW Nitti, BM Brucker. Mirabegron in patients with Parkinson disease and overactive bladder symptoms: a retrospective cohort. *Parkinsonism Relat Disord* 2018; 57: 22–26.

References

AHFS Drug Information, 2012. Bethesda: American Society of Health-System Pharmacists. Accessed on 29 December 2022 via www.medicinescomplete.com.

Eltink C, J Lee, M Schaddelee, W Zhang, V Kerbusch, J Meijer, S van Marle, N Grunenberg, D Kowalski, T Drogendijk, S Moy, H Iitsuka, M van Gelderen, H Matsushima, T Sawamoto. Single dose pharmacokinetics and absolute bioavailability of mirabegron, a β_3-adrenoceptor agonist for treatment of overactive bladder. *Int J Clin Pharmacol Ther* 2012; 50(11): 838–850.

Joint Formulary Committee. British National Formulary (online). London: BMJ Group and Pharmaceutical Press. Accessed on 29 December 2022 via www.medicinescomplete.com.

Matta R, T Gomes, D Juurlink, K Jarvi, S Herschorn, RK Nam. Receipt of overactive bladder drugs and incident dementia: a population-based case–control study. *Eur Urol Focus* 2022; 8(5): 1433–1440.

Mirabegron. In: Brayfield A (Ed.), *Martindale: The Complete Drug Reference*. London: The Royal Pharmaceutical Society of Great Britain. Accessed on 29 December 2022 via www.medicinescomplete.com.

Mirabegron. In: DRUGDEX® System (electronic version). Truven Health Analytics, Greenwood Village, Colorado, USA. Accessed on 29 December 2022 via www.micromedexsolutions.com.

Nunzio CDE, A Nacchia, C Gravina, B Turchi, G Gallo, A Trucchi, FDI Giacomo, G Disabato, A Franco, L Rovesti, R Lombardo, A Cicione, A Tubaro. Adverse events related to antimuscarinics and beta-3-agonist: "real-life" data from the Eudra-Vigilance database. *Minerva Urol Nephrol* 2022; 74(6): 761–779.

Summary of product characteristics – Betmiga 25 mg prolonged-release tablets. Astellas Pharma Ltd. Electronic Medicines Compendium: Betmiga 25 mg prolonged-release tablets – summary of product characteristics (SmPC) – (emc). Accessed on 29 December 2022 via www.medicines.org.uk.

REFERENCES

MIRTAZAPINE

Therapeutics

Chemical Name and Structure

Mirtazapine (2-methyl-1,2,3,4,10,14b-hexahydropyrazino[2,1-*a*]pyrido[2,3-*c*][2]benzazepine) is an atypical antidepressant with a molecular weight of 265.35 and an empirical formula of $C_{17}H_{19}N_3$.

Brand Names

- **Adco-Mirteron** (*South Africa*); **Afloyan** (*Spain*); **Amirel** (*Chile*); **Aurozapine**, **Avanza**, **Axit** (*Australia*); **Azapin** (*Greece*).
- **Beron** (*South Africa*); **Bilanz** (*Argentina*); **Blumirtax** (*Italy*).
- **Calixta** (*Russian Federation*); **Ciblex** (*Chile*); **Combar** (*Denmark*); **Comenter** (*Argentina, Mexico, Venezuela*).
- **Depreram** (*Greece*); **Divaril** (*Chile*).
- **Esprital** (*Czech Republic, Estonia, Lithuania, Russian Federation, Ukraine*); **Eufotina** (*Argentina*).
- **Matiz**, **Maz** (*India*); **Menelat** (*Brazil, Philippines*); **Merdaten** (*Germany, Greece*); **Mi Er Ning** (*China*); **Milivin** (*Australia*); **Minelza** (*Turkey*); **Miradep** (*South Africa*); **Mirap** (*Ireland*); **Miramind** (*India*); **Mirastad** (*Hong Kong*); **Miraz** (*India*); **Mirazep** (*India, Philippines, Ukraine*); **Mirnite** (*Hong Kong, India*); **Miro** (*Israel*); **Mirpine** (*India*); **Mirrador** (*Greece*); **Mirstar, Mirt** (*India*); **Mirtabene** (*Austria*); **Mirtacin**, **Mirtadep** (*India*); **Mirtadepi** (*Hungary*); **Mirtagav** (*Finland*); **Mirtagen** (*Poland*); **Mirtalan** (*Russian Federation*); **Mirtalich** (*Germany*); **Mirtamor** (*Greece*); **Mirtanor** (*Denmark*); **Mirtanza** (*Australia*); **Mirtapan** (*Hong Kong*); **Mirtapax** (*Ecuador*); **Mirtapil** (*Greece*); **Mirtaron** (*Turkey*); **Mirtastad** (*Estonia, Hungary, Lithuania*); **Mirtastadin** (*Ukraine*); **Mirtaz** (*India*); **Mirtazafer** (*Greece*); **Mirtazap** (*Switzerland*); **Mirtazelon** (*Germany*); **Mirtazon** (*Australia*); **Mirtazonal** (*Russian Federation*); **Mirtel** (*Austria, Ukraine*); **Mirtin** (*Denmark, Sweden*); **Mirtor** (*Poland*); **Mirzalux** (*Ecuador, Mexico*); **Mirzap** (*Indonesia*); **Mirzasna** (*Netherlands*); **Mirzaten** (*Czech Republic, Estonia, Hungary, Lithuania, Poland, Russian Federation*); **Mirzest** (*India*); **Mitabor** (*Netherlands*); **Mitocent** (*India*); **Mizapin** (*Hungary*); **Molrem** (*Turkey*); **Motofen** (*Greece*); **Mytra** (*South Africa*).
- **Nassa** (*India*); **Norset** (*France*); **Noxibel** (*Argentina, Ecuador, Russian Federation*); **Nutaz** (*India*).
- **Onvi** (*Lithuania*).
- **Paidisheng** (*China*); **Promyrtil** (*Chile*); **Psidep** (*Portugal*).
- **Ramure** (*South Africa*); **Razapina** (*Brazil*); **Redepra** (*Turkey*); **Reflex** (*Japan*); **Remergil** (*Estonia, Germany*); **Remergon** (*Belgium*); **Remeron** (*Argentina, Australia, Brazil, Canada, China, Cyprus, Ecuador, Estonia, Germany, Greece, Hong Kong, Hungary, Indonesia, Italy, Japan, Lithuania, Malaysia, Mexico, Netherlands, Norway, Philippines, Portugal, Russian Federation, Singapore, South Africa, Switzerland, Thailand, Turkey, Ukraine, USA, Venezuela*); **Remirta** (*Hong Kong, Poland*); **Rexer** (*Spain*).
- **Saxib** (*Greece*); **Segmir** (*Mexico*).

M

- **Tazeron** (*South Africa*); **Tetrazic** (*Argentina*); **Trovia** (*Venezuela*).
- **Velorin** (*Turkey*).
- **Yarocen** (*Hungary*).
- **Zamir** (*Hong Kong*); **Zapex** (*Mexico*); **Zapsy** (*Brazil*); **Zaritim** (*Denmark*); **Zestat** (*Turkey*); **Zismirt, Zispin** (*Ireland*); **Zymron** (*Thailand*).

Generics Available
- Yes.

Licensed Indications for Parkinson's Disease
- None.

Licensed Indications for Other Conditions
- Major depressive disorder (FDA, EMA, EMC).

Non-Licensed Use for Parkinson's Disease
- Parkinson's disease-related depression.

Non-Licensed Use for Other Conditions
- Post-traumatic stress disorder.
- Other anxiety disorders, including panic disorder, undifferentiated somatoform disorder, obsessive-compulsive disorder, generalized anxiety disorder, and social anxiety disorder.
- Hot flushes.
- Insomnia.

Ineffective
- Not reported.

Mechanism of Action
- Mirtazapine has a tetracyclic structure, which differs from that of SSRIs, TCAs, and MAOIs.
  - Through central presynaptic alpha2-adrenergic antagonist activity, mirtazapine stimulates norepinephrine and serotonin release. Serotonergic neurotransmission enhancement is specifically mediated by 5-HT1 receptors, as mirtazapine is a potent antagonist of 5-HT2 and 5-HT3 receptors.
  - Mirtazapine is a potent antagonist of histamine receptors and a moderate antagonist of alpha1-adrenergic and muscarinic receptors.

Efficacy Profile
- Mirtazapine is an effective and well-tolerated treatment option for Parkinson's disease-related depression.
  - The antidepressant effect typically appears after 1–2 weeks of therapy, but it may take as long as 4 weeks.
  - Mirtazapine is considered as effective as other antidepressants and it is a rational option for elderly patients with depression.

THERAPEUTICS

283

- In contrast to SSRIs, mirtazapine improves sleep efficiency, increases total sleep time and shortens sleep latency in patients with depression and insomnia, without suppressing REM sleep.
- A potential benefit of mirtazapine on parkinsonian tremor has been reported, which is believed to be mediated via serotonergic mechanisms.

Pharmacokinetics
Absorption and Distribution
- Oral bioavailability: 50%.
- Food co-ingestion does not impair mirtazapine absorption.
- Tmax: 2 h.
- Time to steady state: 4–6 days.
- Pharmacokinetics: linear over a dose range of 15–80 mg.
- Protein binding: 85%.
- Volume of distribution: 4.5 l/kg.

Metabolism
- Metabolized in the liver by CYP1A2, CYP2D6, and CYP3A4.
- All metabolites are inactive.

Elimination
- Half-life ranges between 20 h and 40 h.
  - Approximately 75% and 15% of an administered dose is excreted in urine and faeces, respectively.

Drug Interaction Profile
Pharmacokinetic Drug Interactions
- Effects by mirtazapine:
  - Mirtazapine is a very weak inhibitor of CYP1A2, CYP2D6, and CYP3A4 and is unlikely to affect the concentrations of drugs metabolized by these isoenzymes.
- Effects on mirtazapine:
  - CYP3A4 inhibitors (e.g. *ketoconazole, citalopram, escitalopram*) may significantly increase plasma levels of mirtazapine.
  - CYP3A4 inducers (e.g. *carbamazepine, phenytoin*) may significantly decrease plasma levels of mirtazapine.
- Smoking can significantly lower serum concentrations of mirtazapine.

Pharmacodynamic Drug Interactions
- Co-medication with drugs causing electrolyte imbalance or increasing QT interval, such as Class IA and III antiarrhythmics, antipsychotics (e.g. *haloperidol, phenothiazine* derivatives, *pimozide*), tricyclic antidepressants, certain antimicrobial agents (e.g. *moxifloxacin, erythromycin*), certain antihistamines (e.g. *astemizole, mizolastine*), and others

MIRTAZAPINE

M

may lead to potentially fatal Torsade de Pointes arrhythmias and is considered a risk factor for sudden cardiac death.

- Co-medication with CNS depressants (e.g. benzodiazepines, most antipsychotics, antihistamines H1 antagonists, opioids) or alcohol might lead to synergistic sedative effects, including somnolence and dizziness.
- In doses of mirtazapine higher than 30 mg per day, co-medication with warfarin might increase INR.
- Co-medication with MAOIs is contraindicated, while caution is advised in co-medication with other serotonergic drugs (e.g. *triptans, SSRIs, tramadol, lithium, venlafaxine*) due to an increased risk of serotonin syndrome.
- Mirtazapine decreases effects of *clonidine* by pharmacodynamic antagonism.

Adverse Effects
How Drug Causes Adverse Effects
- Symptoms of a serotonin syndrome, including hyperthermia, rigidity, myoclonus, autonomic instability, and mental status change, are a result of mirtazapine's serotonergic activity, especially when used concomitantly with other serotonergic active substances.
- Somnolence is believed to be mediated by potent histamine H1 receptor antagonist action.
- Anti-cholinergic adverse reactions are minimal.
- Hyponatraemia may occur rarely, probably due to SIADH.

Common Adverse Effects
- Very common ($\geq 1/10$):
  ○ Somnolence, headache, xerostomia, increased appetite/ weight, constipation.
- Common ($\geq 1/100$ to $<1/10$):
  ○ Nervous/psychiatric: dizziness, lethargy, dream disorder, thinking disturbance, confusion, anxiety, insomnia, tremor.
  ○ Cardiovascular: orthostatic hypotension.
  ○ GI: nausea/vomiting, diarrhoea.
  ○ Respiratory: dyspnoea.
  ○ Musculoskeletal: myalgia, arthralgia, back pain.
  ○ Other: asthenia, weakness, increased triglycerides, increased transaminases, peripheral oedema, fatigue.
- Uncommon ($\geq 1/1,000$ to $<1/100$):
  ○ Nervous/psychiatric: mania, hallucinations, psychomotor restlessness (including akathisia, hyperkinesia), paraesthesia, syncope.

Life-Threatening or Dangerous Adverse Effects
- Uncommon ($\geq 1/1,000$ to $<1/100$):
- Grand mal seizure (uncommon).

ADVERSE EFFECTS

- Rare (≥1/10,000 to <1/1,000):
  - Suicidal thoughts, suicide.
  - Agranulocytosis, neutropenia.
  - Torsade de Pointes.
  - Serotonin syndrome.
  - Hyponatraemia.
  - QT prolongation.
  - Pancreatitis.

Rare and Not Life-Threatening Adverse Effects
- Myoclonus.

Weight Change
- Weight gain and increased appetite are common, especially in paediatric patients.

What to Do About Adverse Effects
- Before introducing mirtazapine, discuss common or life-threatening adverse effects with patients and/or caregivers, including symptoms that should be reported to the physician.
- Patients and their caregivers should be informed about the possibility of mirtazapine causing suicidal ideation/behaviour. If such signs/symptoms emerge, patients should urgently seek medical advice and be treated accordingly. Mirtazapine should be discontinued.
  - Due to suicidality risk, consider providing patients with a limited number of mirtazapine tablets.
- Patients should be advised to report immediately any signs or symptoms compatible with agranulocytosis (e.g. fever, sore throat, stomatitis, weakness, lethargy, infection with low WBC count) during mirtazapine therapy (usually after 4–6 weeks of treatment). If agranulocytosis is suspected, consider discontinuing mirtazapine and closely monitor the patient.
- In case of akathisia/psychomotor restlessness, which usually appears during the first weeks of therapy, do not increase the mirtazapine dose. Mirtazapine discontinuation might be considered if the symptoms persist or become troublesome to the patient.
- In case of jaundice, mirtazapine should be discontinued.

Dosing and Use
Usual Dosage Range
- 15–45 mg.

Available Formulations
- Tablets: 7.5 mg, 15 mg, 30 mg, 45 mg.
- Disintegrating tablets: 15 mg, 30 mg, 45 mg.

M

How to Dose
- Initial dose of 15 mg or 30 mg OD, preferably in the evening, immediately before bedtime.
- May increase by 15 mg every 1–2 weeks; maximum dose of 45 mg.

Dosing Tips
- Mirtazapine may be administered with or without food.
- The daily dose can be divided into two doses taken in the morning and at bedtime (larger dose at bedtime).
- After achieving an optimal clinical effect and if the patient is free of symptoms, mirtazapine should be continued for 4–6 months and then a gradual withdrawal can be considered.
- If no clinical response is seen within 2–4 weeks of therapy with the maximum dose, mirtazapine should be gradually discontinued.
- Smokers might need higher doses of mirtazapine than non-smokers.

How to Withdraw Drug
- A gradual tapering is necessary.
- Mirtazapine withdrawal, especially if abrupt, may cause dizziness, abnormal dreams, sensory disturbances (including paraesthesia and electric shock sensations), agitation, anxiety, fatigue, confusion, headache, tremor, nausea, vomiting, and sweating.

Overdose
- Symptoms of overdose are usually mild, although disorientation, prolonged sedation, tachycardia, and mild hyper-/hypotension have been reported.
- In severe cases (at doses higher than the therapeutic range or with mixed overdose), mirtazapine overdose can lead to QT prolongation, torsade de pointes, ventricular tachycardia and sudden cardiac death.
- General supportive measures are suggested.
- There is no known antidote for mirtazapine overdosage.
- Treatment with activated charcoal is suggested. Gastric lavage may be considered if necessary.

Tests and Therapeutic Drug Monitoring
- Before initiation of mirtazapine therapy:
  - A baseline ECG should be performed to check for QT prolongation.
  - A metabolic panel should be performed, including electrolytes, renal and hepatic function.
- During mirtazapine therapy:
  - Patients should be regularly evaluated for worsening of depression, suicidality, behaviour changes, or other common adverse effects, especially for the first few months after introducing therapy or during dose modifications.
  - INR monitoring is advised if co-administering with *warfarin*.

DOSING AND USE

Other Warnings / Precautions

- Patients with depression might experience an initial worsening of their symptoms, emergence of suicidal ideation/behaviour or unusual behaviour changes. This risk might persist until significant remission occurs.
- There is a black box warning for young adults (less than 24 years old) who take mirtazapine for depression and other psychiatric disorders concerning suicidal thinking and behaviour.
  - A slight increase in suicidal thinking has also been seen in the elderly (>65 years old) receiving mirtazapine.
  - Patients with a history of suicide-related events are at higher risk and careful monitoring during treatment is required, especially early in therapy and following changes in dose.
- Close monitoring is recommended in patients with a history of bipolar disorder, as mirtazapine may trigger a manic episode.
  - Mirtazapine should be withdrawn in any patient entering a manic phase.
- An aggravation of psychotic symptoms, including paranoid thoughts, may occur in patients with schizophrenia or other psychoses.
- Careful monitoring is advised in patients at high risk of prolonged cardiac repolarization (e.g. co-medication with drugs increasing QT interval, patients with cardiovascular disease, family history of QT prolongation, congenital long QT syndrome, congestive heart failure, heart hypertrophy, hypokalaemia or hypomagnesemia), especially the elderly.
- Caution is advised in patients with a history of epilepsy or organic brain syndrome due to the possibility of triggering status epilepticus.
- Careful monitoring is advised in patients with hypotension.
- Despite the weak anticholinergic effects of mirtazapine, caution is advised in patients with micturition disturbances, including prostatic hyperplasia, acute narrow-angle glaucoma, and elevated intraocular pressure.
- An angle-closure attack may be triggered in patients with anatomically narrow angles without iridectomy due to mirtazapine causing pupillary dilation.
- Mirtazapine may alter glycaemic control in patients with diabetes mellitus. Alterations in insulin and/or hypoglycaemic formulations may be considered.
- Caution is advised in the elderly or in patients treated with medication known to cause hyponatraemia (e.g. diuretics or antiseizure medicines), as mirtazapine may aggravate this effect.
- The initial dose of mirtazapine might cause psychomotor impairment, affecting the ability to drive or operate dangerous machinery; however, this effect is not sustained as therapy continues.
- In the case of co-administration with strong CYP3A4 inhibitors, a dose reduction of mirtazapine may be necessary.
- Caution is advised in co-medication with CNS depressants, including alcohol.
  - Alcoholic beverages should be avoided.

MIRTAZAPINE

Do Not Use (Contraindications)
- Known sensitivity to mirtazapine or to any of the excipients, including lactose.
  - Patients with rare hereditary problems of galactose intolerance, total lactase deficiency, or glucose–galactose malabsorption.
- Co-medication with *clonidine* should be avoided.
- Mirtazapine should not be co-administered with MAOIs or within 2 weeks after their discontinuation due to increased risk of potentially fatal serotonin syndrome.
- Co-administration with linezolid or methylene blue IV.
  - If *linezolid* administration is necessary, mirtazapine should be discontinued immediately, and the patient should be monitored for CNS toxicity. Mirtazapine therapy can be resumed 24 h after last linezolid dose or after 2 weeks of monitoring, whichever applies first.

Special Populations

Renal Impairment
- The clearance of mirtazapine may be decreased in patients with moderate to severe renal impairment, caution is advised in prescribing. In patients with moderate (creatinine clearance < 40 ml/min) and severe (creatinine clearance ≤ 10 ml/min) impairment, clearance of mirtazapine was about 30% and 50% decreased, respectively. No significant differences are reported in mild renal impairment.

Hepatic Impairment
- The clearance of mirtazapine may be decreased in patients with hepatic impairment. Close monitoring is advised.

Elderly
- Changes in dose should be applied cautiously and under close supervision.

Pregnancy
- Mirtazapine should only be used during pregnancy if clearly indicated.
  - Consider the risk of untreated depression in the case of discontinuation or change of treatment during pregnancy.
- Prolonged exposure to mirtazapine therapy during pregnancy has not reliably identified a drug-associated risk of major birth defects, miscarriage, or adverse maternal/fetal outcomes.

Breastfeeding
- Low levels of mirtazapine have been identified in human milk; no adverse effects on breastfed infant have been reported.
- Health benefits of breastfeeding should be considered along with mother's need for mirtazapine therapy and any potential effects on breastfed infant either from the drug or from the mother's underlying condition.

Costs

Costs: NHS indicative price 4 December 2022:
- Mirtazapine 15 mg tablets – 28 tablets: £1.07–£3.95.
- Mirtazapine 30 mg tablets – 28 tablets: £1.06–£4.50.
- Mirtazapine 45 mg tablets – 28 tablets: £1.32–£4.95.
- Mirtazapine 15 mg orodispersible tablets – 30 tablets: £1.29–£3.95.
- Mirtazapine 30 mg orodispersible tablets – 30 tablets: £1.34–£4.50.
- Mirtazapine 45 mg orodispersible tablets – 30 tablets: £2.01–£4.95.
- Mirtazapine 15 mg/ml oral solution – 66 ml: £117.00.

The Overall Place of Mirtazapine in the Treatment of Parkinson's Disease

Mirtazapine is an atypical antidepressant, primarily used for the treatment of major depression. Data derived mostly from case reports suggest that mirtazapine might be efficacious in co-morbid depression in Parkinson's disease, especially in patients with sleep disturbance. Mirtazapine does worsen extrapyramidal features, as it has a low affinity for dopamine receptors. Mirtazapine may have a beneficial effect on parkinsonian tremor. Mirtazapine is the most frequently used antidepressant in Parkinson's disease after SSRIs, reflecting the treatment of depression in the psychogeriatric population. Although an SSRI might be the initial choice in Parkinson's disease, mirtazapine is a reasonable alternative if sedation or an increased appetite is required or in the case of treatment failure. A small number of published case reports have also suggested a positive effect of mirtazapine on Parkinson's disease-related hallucinations. Finally, mirtazapine has been found moderately effective in diminishing LID, either as a monotherapy or in combination with amantadine, and may be of use in patients who do not respond or are intolerant to amantadine.

Potential Advantages
- Mirtazapine lacks the undesirable anticholinergic effects of the TCAs, which might be particularly marked in older patients.
- It may exhibit a more rapid onset of action compared to SSRIs.
- The availability of an ODT formulation makes mirtazapine suitable for patients with swallowing difficulties, GI disorders, or those who concurrently receiving multiple other oral medications.

Potential Disadvantages
- Only limited data are currently available considering the use of mirtazapine in Parkinson's disease.

M

Clinical Box
A 63-year-old woman with a diagnosis of Parkinson's disease presented with depressive symptoms, weight loss, and sleep disturbances in the form of insomnia, significantly interfering with her daily functioning. Her current medication included levodopa–carbidopa 100 mg/25 mg QID and rasagiline 1 mg OD. Her past and current medical history was unremarkable. In order to simultaneously address the above symptoms, mirtazapine 15 mg OD at night was prescribed.

Suggested Reading
Agüera-Ortiz L, R García-Ramos, FJ Grandas Pérez, J López-Álvarez, JM Montes Rodríguez, FJ Olazarán Rodríguez, J Olivera Pueyo, C Pelegrín Valero, J Porta-Etessam. Focus on depression in Parkinson's disease: a Delphi consensus of experts in psychiatry, neurology, and geriatrics. *Parkinsons Dis* 2021; 2021: 6621991.

Gordon PH, SL Pullman, ED Louis, SJ Frucht, S Fahn. Mirtazapine in Parkinsonian tremor. *Parkinsonism Relat Disord* 2002; 9(2): 125–126.

Meco G, E Fabrizio, S Di Rezze, A Alessandri, L Pratesi. Mirtazapine in L-dopa-induced dyskinesias. *Clin Neuropharmacol* 2003; 26(4): 179–181.

Sid-Otmane L, P Huot, M Panisset. Effect of antidepressants on psychotic symptoms in Parkinson disease: a review of case reports and case series. *Clin Neuropharmacol* 2020; 43(3): 61–65.

References
AHFS Drug information, 2012. Bethesda: American Society of Health-System Pharmacists. Accessed on 4 December 2022 via www.medicinescomplete.com.

Croom KF, CM Perry, GL Plosker. Mirtazapine: a review of its use in major depression and other psychiatric disorders. *CNS Drugs* 2009; 23(5): 427–452.

Haasum Y, J Fastbom, K Johnell. Use of antidepressants in Parkinson's disease: a Swedish register-based study of over 1.5 million older people. *Parkinsonism Relat Disord* 2016; 27: 85–88.

Joint Formulary Committee. British National Formulary (online). London: BMJ Group and Pharmaceutical Press. Accessed on 4 December 2022 via www.medicinescomplete.com.

Mirtazapine. In: Brayfield A (Ed.), *Martindale: The Complete Drug Reference*. London: The Royal Pharmaceutical Society of Great Britain. Accessed on 4 December 2022 via www.medicinescomplete.com.

Mirtazapine. In: DRUGDEX® System (electronic version). Truven Health Analytics, Greenwood Village, Colorado, USA. Accessed on 4 December 2022 via www.micromedexsolutions.com.

REFERENCES

Summary of product characteristics – Mirtazapine 15 mg tablets. Aurobindo Pharma – Milpharm Ltd. Electronic Medicines Compendium: Mirtazapine 15 mg tablets – summary of product characteristics (SmPC) – (emc). Accessed on 4 December 2022 via www.medicines.org.uk.

Timmer CJ, JM Sitsen, LP Delbressine. Clinical pharmacokinetics of mirtazapine. *Clin Pharmacokinet* 2000; 38(6): 461–474.

MIRTAZAPINE

MODAFINIL

M

Therapeutics

Chemical Name and Structure
Modafinil (2-[(diphenylmethyl)sulfinyl]acetamide) is a white to off-white crystalline powder with a molecular weight of 273.4 and a molecular formula of $C_{15}H_{15}NO_2S$.

Brand Names
- **Actimodan** (*Poland*); **Alertec** (*Canada*); **Alertex** (*Chile, Equador*); **Aspendos** (*Cyprus, Greece, Netherlands*).
- **Carim** (*Equador*).
- **Intensit** (*Argentina*).
- **Mentix** (*Chile*); **Modafin** (*Australia*); **Modalert** (*India, South Africa*); **Modasomil** (*Austria, Switzerland*); **Modavigil** (*Australia, New Zealand*); **Modfil** (*India*); **Modiodal** (*Cyprus, Denmark, Estonia, France, Greece, Japan, Mexico, Netherlands, Norway, Portugal, Spain, Tunisia, Turkey*); **Modiogen** (*Turkey*); **Modiva** (*South Africa*); **Modivigil** (*Turkey*); **Modiwake** (*Turkey*); **Movigil** (*Chile*); **Myldamo** (*Denmark, Sweden*).
- **Prolert** (*South Africa*); **Prosentio** (*Ireland*); **Provigil** (*Belgium, Denmark, Estonia, Ireland, Israel, Italy, South Africa, UK, USA*).
- **Resotyl** (*Chile*).
- **Sleepex** (*Turkey*); **Stavigile** (*Brazil*).
- **Vigicer** (*Argentina*); **Vigil** (*Czech Republic, Germany*); **Vigimax** (*Chile*); **Visper** (*Argentina*).
- **Zalux** (*Chile*).

Generics Available
- Yes.

Licensed Indications for Parkinson's Disease
- None.

Licensed Indications for Other Conditions
- Excessive sleepiness, associated with:
  - Narcolepsy, with or without cataplexy (FDA, EMA, EMC).
  - Obstructive sleep apnoea, as an adjunct to CPAP (FDA).
  - Shift work sleep disorder (FDA).

  *Excessive sleepiness is defined as difficulty maintaining wakefulness and an increased likelihood of falling asleep in inappropriate situations.

Non-Licensed Use for Parkinson's Disease
- Excessive daytime somnolence and sudden onset of sleep.
- Fatigue.

THERAPEUTICS

MODAFINIL

Non-Licensed Use for Other Conditions
- Acute unipolar and bipolar depressive episodes.
- Depression-related fatigue.
- Cocaine dependence (mixed results).
- Cancer-related fatigue (mixed results).
- MS-related fatigue.
- Attention-deficit hyperactive disorder.

Ineffective
- Not reported.

Mechanism of Action
- Modafinil, a benzhydryl sulfinylacetamide derivative, is a central stimulant, which is structurally and pharmacologically distinct from other currently available CNS stimulants (e.g. amphetamines, caffeine).
- Its mechanism of action in producing stimulatory effects is not known; it does not appear to act as a sympathomimetic agent.
- Modafinil may increase dopamine levels in the brain by binding to the dopamine transporter and inhibiting dopamine reuptake, including in the nucleus accumbens; drugs with such activity are generally associated with abuse potential.
- Animal studies have shown that modafinil inhibits the release of GABA and increases the release of glutamate from the cerebral cortex, hippocampus, nucleus accumbens, medial preoptic area, and posterior hypothalamus. The relevance to its mode of action in man is unknown.

Efficacy Profile
- Modafinil has been characterized as 'possibly useful' in the treatment of excessive daytime somnolence and sudden sleep onset in the context of Parkinson's disease.
- There is insufficient evidence to support modafinil use in Parkinson's disease–related fatigue.
- Two small, crossover, double-blind RCTs have found a positive effect of modafinil on daytime sleepiness, while one larger double-blind RCT found no significant improvement of modafinil on daytime sleepiness among Parkinson's disease patients, as assessed by the Epworth Sleepiness Scale.
- According to a meta-analysis of the above trials, modafinil was found to significantly decrease sleepiness. A small open-label study further supported these findings.
- One small, double-blind, placebo-controlled pilot study has found that modafinil use did not significantly improve Parkinson's disease-related fatigue.

Pharmacokinetics
Absorption and Distribution
- Oral bioavailability: not determined due to its aqueous insolubility preventing intravenous use for comparison.
- Food co-ingestion: no effect on overall modafinil bioavailability, but absorption may be delayed by about 1 h if taken with food.
- Tmax: 2–4 h.
- Time to steady state: 2–4 days.
- Pharmacokinetics: linear over the range of 200–600 mg.
- Protein binding: about 60% (mainly to albumin).
- Volume of distribution: 0.9 l/kg.

Metabolism
- Modafinil undergoes hepatic metabolism, mostly by CP3A4 and CYP3A5. Its two primary metabolites are modafinil acid and modafinil sulfone, both of which lack pharmacological activity.
- Modafinil may induce its own metabolism via CYP3A4/5; this effect is modest and unlikely to have clinically significance.

Elimination
- Half-life is 15 h.
- Renal excretion: 80% of an administered dose is excreted in the urine (<10% of the parent drug is excreted unchanged).

Drug Interaction Profile
Pharmacokinetic Drug Interactions
- Effects by modafinil:
  - Modafinil is a moderate CYP3A4/5 inducer and may decrease levels and effects of CYP3A4/5 substrates (e.g. contraceptives, *cyclosporine*, *midazolam*, *triazolam*).
  - Modafinil is a weak CYP2C19 inhibitor and may increase levels and effects of CYP2C19 substrates (e.g. *phenytoin*, *diazepam*, *clozapine*, *propranolol*, *omeprazole*, *amitriptyline*, *citalopram*, *escitalopram*, *clobazam*, *olanzapine*).
  - Modafinil may decrease levels and effects of *clopidogrel* by affecting CYP2C19 metabolism.
  - Modafinil appears to produce a concentration-related inhibition of CYP2C9 activity.
  - Modafinil may decrease levels and effects of *duloxetine* and *lidocaine* by affecting CYP1A2 metabolism.
- Effects on modafinil:
  - *Clarithromycin*, *phenobarbital*, *ritonavir*, *istradefylline*, *itraconazole*, and others may increase levels and effects of modafinil by inhibiting CYP3A4 metabolism.
  - *Carbamazepine*, *fosphenytoin*, *phenytoin*, *primidone*, *rifabutin* may decrease levels and effects of modafinil by inducing CYP3A4 metabolism.

Pharmacodynamic Drug Interactions
- Co-medication with drugs having sedative properties, such as neuroleptics (e.g. *alprazolam, aripiprazole, chlorpromazine, haloperidol, quetiapine, risperidone*), benzodiazepines (e.g. *lorazepam, midazolam*), opiates (e.g. *oxycodone, tramadol*), *mirtazapine, topiramate,* or *melatonin* will have opposing effects on sedation.
- Co-medication with MAOIs (e.g. *rasagiline, linezolid, selegiline*) may lead to pharmacodynamic synergism and high risk of an acute hypertensive episode and/or cardiovascular reactions.
- Modafinil may reduce effectiveness of steroidal contraceptives, even 1 month after discontinuation of drug therapy.

Adverse Effects
How Drug Causes Adverse Effects
- Modafinil-induced side effects are usually dose-related.

Common Adverse Effects
- Very common (≥1/10):
  - Headache, rhinitis, decreased appetite, nausea, abdominal pain.
- Common (≥1/100 to <1/10):
  - Neuropsychiatric: nervousness, dizziness, somnolence, paraesthesia, insomnia, anxiety, depression, abnormal thinking, confusion, irritability.
  - Eye/ear: blurred vision.
  - Cardiovascular: syncope, tachycardia, palpitations, vasodilation, chest pain.
  - GI: dry mouth, diarrhoea, dyspepsia, constipation.
  - Other: asthenia, abnormal liver function tests, dose-related increases in alkaline phosphatase and gamma glutamyl transferase.
- Uncommon (≥1/1,000 to <1/100):
  - Neuropsychiatric: sleep disorder, emotional lability, decreased libido, hostility, depersonalization, personality disorder, abnormal dreams, agitation, aggression, suicidal ideation, psychomotor hyperactivity, dyskinesia, hypertonia, hyperkinesia, amnesia, migraine, tremor, vertigo, hypoesthesia, incoordination, speech disorder, taste perversion.
  - Eye/ear: abnormal vision, dry eye.
  - Respiratory: pharyngitis, sinusitis, dyspnoea, increased cough, asthma, epistaxis.
  - Cardiovascular: arrhythmia, bradycardia, hypertension, hypotension, abnormal ECG.
  - GI: flatulence, reflux, vomiting, dysphagia, glossitis, mouth ulcers.
  - Renal/urinary: abnormal urine, urine frequency.
  - Endocrine: hyperglycaemia, diabetes mellitus, menstrual disorder.
  - Skin: sweating, rash, acne, pruritus.

M

- Musculoskeletal: back/neck pain, myalgia, myasthenia, leg cramps, arthralgia, twitch.
- Other: eosinophilia, leukopenia, minor allergic reactions, hypercholesterolaemia, increased appetite, peripheral oedema, thirst.

Life-Threatening or Dangerous Adverse Effects
- Uncommon (≥1/1,000 to <1/100):
  - Suicide-related behaviours, including suicide attempts and suicidal ideation.
- Rare (≥1/10,000 to <1/1,000):
  - Serious or life-threatening hypersensitivity reactions, including anaphylaxis, angioedema, Stevens–Johnson syndrome, toxic epidermal necrolysis, and drug rash with eosinophilia and systemic symptoms (DRESS).
- Very rare (<1/10,000):
  - Multi-organ hypersensitivity reaction (very rare).

Rare and Not Life-Threatening Adverse Effects
- Hallucinations, mania, psychosis.

Weight Change
- Weight increases and decreases have been reported (uncommon) with modafinil use.

What to Do About Adverse Effects
- Before introducing modafinil, discuss common or life-threatening adverse effects with patients and/or caregivers, including symptoms that should be reported to the physician.
- Due to the potential of modafinil to cause severe skin or other hypersensitivity reactions, modafinil therapy should be discontinued at the first sign of serious rash or development of symptoms suggestive of angioedema or anaphylaxis.
- In cases where depression, anxiety, psychosis, mania, bipolar disorders, aggressive/hostile behaviour, or suicide-related symptoms are evident, modafinil should be discontinued.
- Modafinil should be discontinued in patients who develop arrhythmia or moderate to severe hypertension and not reintroduced until the condition has been adequately treated.
- Modafinil use may alter judgement, thinking, or motor skills. Patients with abnormal levels of somnolence who take modafinil should be advised to avoid driving or operating hazardous machinery, until they are reasonably certain that modafinil does not adversely affect their ability to engage in such activities.
  - Co-administration with CNS depressants or alcohol should be avoided.

ADVERSE EFFECTS

Dosing and Use

Usual Dosage Range
- 100–400 mg daily.

Available Formulations
- Tablets: 100 mg, 200 mg.

How to Dose
- An initial dose of 200 mg is suggested. The total dose may be taken as a single dose in the morning or as two doses, one in the morning and one at noon, according to physician's assessment and the patient's response.
  - In patients with shift work sleep disorder, modafinil should be taken 1 h prior to the start of their work shift.
- Dose can be increased up to 400 mg in one or two divided doses, according to the patient's response.

Dosing Tips
- Modafinil can be administered without regard to meals.
- Patients should be advised that modafinil is not a replacement for sleep and good sleep hygiene is a priority.

How to Withdraw Drug
- Modafinil needs to be discontinued gradually to lower the risk for potential withdrawal symptoms, which may include shaking, sweating, chills, nausea, vomiting, and confusion.

Overdose
- Death has been reported with modafinil overdose alone or in combination with other drugs.
- Modafinil overdose may present with insomnia, restlessness, disorientation, confusion, agitation, anxiety, excitation, hallucinations, digestive changes (e.g. nausea, diarrhoea), and cardiovascular changes (e.g. tachycardia, bradycardia, hypertension, chest pain).
- Induced emesis or gastric lavage should be considered.
- Patient should be closely monitored for abnormal psychomotor or cardiovascular findings until symptoms have fully resolved.

Tests and Therapeutic Drug Monitoring
- Before initiation of modafinil therapy:
  - An ECG should be performed.
  - Blood pressure and heart rate should be evaluated at baseline.
- During modafinil therapy:
  - Blood pressure and heart rate should be regularly monitored.
  - Periodic assessment of sleepiness is suggested.
  - Periodic assessment for suicide-related behaviours, psychiatric disorders, or signs of misuse/abuse, especially after modafinil dose adjustments and in patients with a prior history of psychiatric disorder.

M

- If modafinil is used concomitantly with CPAP, periodic assessment of CPAP compliance is necessary.

Other Warnings / Precautions
- A potential of modafinil causing dependence cannot be excluded.
- Caution is advised in patients with a prior history or active depression, anxiety, psychosis, mania, or alcohol/drug/illicit substance abuse, as it may exacerbate these conditions.
- Caution is advised in patients with Tourette syndrome, as modafinil may unmask tics.
- Close monitoring is advised in co-administration with CYP3A4/5, CYP1A2, or CYP2C19 substrates. Consider dose adjustments or an alternative therapeutic option, if possible.
- Close monitoring is advised in co-administration with a CYP3A4 inhibitor/inducer. Consider an alternative therapeutic option, if possible.
- Close monitoring is advised in co-administration with *phenytoin* for signs of phenytoin toxicity. Repeated measurements of phenytoin plasma levels are needed upon initiation or discontinuation of modafinil treatment.
- A number of tricyclic antidepressants and SSRIs are largely metabolized by CYP2D6 or CYP2C19 in patients deficient in CYP2D6, which is 10% of a Caucasian population. Lower doses of antidepressants may be needed in this latter group of patients, as modafinil may inhibit CYP2C19.
- Close monitoring is advised in co-administration with drugs with similar effects on sedation, such as *dobutamine* or *metaproterenol*.
- Frequent monitoring of INR/PT/APTT is advised in co-administration with *warfarin*, as modafinil may decrease warfarin clearance by suppressing CYP2C9.
- Close monitoring is advised in co-administration with MAOIs due to high risk of acute hypertensive episode. Consider an alternative therapeutic option, if possible.
  - Co-administration with linezolid and transdermal selegiline is contraindicated.
- Women of childbearing potential should be established on a contraceptive programme before taking modafinil. Because the effectiveness of steroidal contraceptives may be reduced with concomitant modafinil use, alternative or concomitant methods of contraception are recommended, and for 2 months after modafinil discontinuation.

Do Not Use (Contraindications)
- Known sensitivity to modafinil or any of its excipients, including lactose.
  - Patients with rare hereditary problems of galactose intolerance, total lactase deficiency, or glucose–galactose malabsorption.
- Patients with cardiac arrhythmias, angina, cardiac ischemia, recent history of MI, left ventricular hypertrophy, or mitral valve prolapse.
- Uncontrolled moderate to severe hypertension.

DOSING AND USE

MODAFINIL

Special Populations

Renal Impairment
- There is insufficient information considering modafinil efficacy and safety among patients with renal impairment.

Hepatic Impairment
- Severe hepatic impairment: a maximum dose of 100 mg OD is recommended.

Elderly
- Due to the potential for lower clearance and increased systemic exposure, a maximum dose of 100 mg OD is recommended.

Pregnancy
- Intrauterine growth restriction, congenital malformations, and spontaneous abortion have been reported with modafinil use.
- Animal studies have shown that modafinil at clinically relevant plasma concentrations may lead to developmental toxicity.
- Although findings from well-controlled studies are not currently available, modafinil use is not recommended during pregnancy.
- Women of childbearing potential taking modafinil must use effective contraception.

Breastfeeding
- It is not known whether modafinil is excreted in human milk or whether it has any effect on milk production or the nursing infant.
- Modafinil use is not recommended during breastfeeding.

Costs
NHS indicative pricing as of 30 December 2022:
- Provigil 100 mg tablets (Teva UK Ltd) – 30 × 100 mg tablets: £52.60.
- Modafinil 100 mg tablets – 30 × 100 mg tablets: £2.81–£4.30.
- Modafinil 200 mg tablets – 30 × 200 mg tablets: £6.88–£9.12.

The Overall Place of Modafinil in the Treatment of Parkinson's Disease

Modafinil is a psychostimulant drug, whose efficacy in excessive daytime somnolence in Parkinson's disease remains controversial. It appears to promote wakefulness by enhancing dopaminergic transmission, although its exact mechanism of action is unclear. According to available studies, Parkinson's disease patients treated with modafinil may experience an improvement in sleep perception without an actual improvement in objective sleep parameters, meaning that modafinil may not be a definitive solution. Although there is no conclusive evidence, modafinil treatment may be considered for excessive daytime sleepiness when other treatable causes, such as drug-related sleep problems, sleep apnoea, insomnia, or depression, have been excluded or properly addressed. Modafinil has generally been found to be well-tolerated among Parkinson's disease patients with minimal adverse effects reported.

Potential Advantages
- Modafinil may be a reasonable option for Parkinson's disease patients with concomitant obstructive sleep apnoea.
- There are limited options in the management of excessive daytime sleepiness in Parkinson's disease.

Potential Disadvantages
- Modafinil efficacy on Parkinson's disease-related somnolence remains unclear.
- Long-term use of modafinil (>9 weeks) has not been evaluated.
- A number of drug–drug interactions need to be considered before introducing modafinil therapy.

Clinical Box

A 50-year-old man with a 5-year history of Parkinson's disease presented at the Movement Disorders Outpatient Clinic for his regular follow-up appointment. The patient complained of excessive daytime sleepiness during the past month, leading him to fall asleep in inappropriate situations, such as in the middle of social encounters or while driving. The patient was on a stable drug regimen for his Parkinson's disease over the past 6 months, including levodopa/carbidopa 200 mg/50 mg QID and rotigotine 8 mg/24 h, and he reported no sleep problems during the night, such as insomnia or RBD. He gradually discontinued the rotigotine use, while a diagnosis of depression and sleep apnoea were excluded. After rotigotine cessation, his somnolence was slightly improved, although still troublesome; a low dose of modafinil 200 mg OD in the morning was prescribed.

Suggested Reading

Adler CH, JN Caviness, JG Hentz, M Lind, J Tiede. Randomized trial of modafinil for treating subjective daytime sleepiness in patients with Parkinson's disease. *Mov Disord* 2003; 18(3): 287–293.

Högl B, M Saletu, E Brandauer, S Glatzl, B Frauscher, K Seppi, H Ulmer, G Wenning, W Poewe. Modafinil for the treatment of daytime sleepiness in Parkinson's disease: a double-blind, randomized, crossover, placebo-controlled polygraphic trial. *Sleep*, 2002; 25(8): 905–909.

Lou JS, DM Dimitrova, BS Park, SC Johnson, R Eaton, G Arnold, JG Nutt. Using modafinil to treat fatigue in Parkinson disease: a double-blind, placebo-controlled pilot study. *Clin Neuropharmacol* 2009; 32(6): 305–310.

M

SUGGESTED READING

Ondo WG, R Fayle, F Atassi, J Jankovic. Modafinil for daytime somnolence in Parkinson's disease: double blind, placebo controlled parallel trial. *J Neurol, Neurosurg, Psychiatry* 2005; 76(12): 1636.

Rodrigues TM, A Castro Caldas, JJ Ferreira. Pharmacological interventions for daytime sleepiness and sleep disorders in Parkinson's disease: Systematic review and meta-analysis. *Parkinsonism Relat Disord* 2016; 27: 25–34.

References

AHFS Drug information, 2012. Bethesda: American Society of Health-System Pharmacists. Accessed on 30 December 20 via www.medicinescomplete.com.

Joint Formulary Committee. British National Formulary (online). London: BMJ Group and Pharmaceutical Press. Accessed on 30 December 20 via www.medicinescomplete.com.

Modafinil. In: Brayfield A (Ed.), *Martindale: The Complete Drug Reference*. London: The Royal Pharmaceutical Society of Great Britain. Accessed on 30 December 2022 via www.medicinescomplete.com.

Modafinil. In DRUGDEX® System (electronic version). Truven Health Analytics, Greenwood Village, Colorado, USA. Accessed on 30 December 2022 via www.micromedexsolutions.com.

Nieves AV, AE Lang. Treatment of excessive daytime sleepiness in patients with Parkinson's disease with modafinil. *Clin Neuropharmacol* 2002; 25(2): 111–114.

Robertson P, Jr, ET Hellriegel. Clinical pharmacokinetic profile of modafinil. *Clin Pharmacokinet* 2003; 42(2): 123–137.

Summary of Product Characteristics – Modafinil 100 mg tablets. Aurobindo Pharma – Milpharm Ltd. Electronic Medicines Compendium: Modafinil 100 mg tablets – summary of product characteristics (SmPC) – (emc). Accessed on 30 December 2022 via www.medicines.org.uk.

MODAFINIL

NALTREXONE

N

*Information provided below applies to naltrexone use in the context of Parkinson's disease and not for opioid/alcohol dependence or IM administration.

Therapeutics

Chemical Name and Structure

Naltrexone ((5*R*)-9*a*-Cyclopropylmethyl-3,14–dihydroxy-4,5–epoxymorphinan-6-one; 17-(cyclopropylmethyl)-4,5α-epoxy-3,14–dihydroxymorphinan-6-one) has a molecular weight of 341.4 and a molecular formula of $C_{20}H_{23}NO_4$.

Brand Names
- **Abernil** (*Cyprus*); **Adepend** (*Denmark, Estonia, Hungary, Lithuania, Poland, UK*); **Altrex** (*South Africa*); **Antaxone** (*Italy, Russian Federation, Ukraine*).
- **Basinal** (*Portugal*).
- **Dependex** (*Austria*); **Destoxican** (*Portugal*).
- **Ethylex** (*Austria, Ireland, Turkey*).
- **Nalcotrex** (*Argentina*); **Nalerona** (*Chile*); **Nalorex** (*Greece, Hong Kong, Italy, UK*); **Naltima** (*India, South Africa*); **Naltraccord** (*New Zealand*); **Naltrex** (*Poland*); **Naltrexin** (*Austria, Switzerland, Venezuela*); **Narcoral** (*China, India*); **Narpan** (*Malaysia, Singapore*); **Nodict** (*Estonia, India*); **Nuo Xin Sheng** (*China*); **Nutrexon** (*Indonesia*).
- **Opizone** (*UK*).
- **Phaltrexia** (*Indonesia*); **Prodetoxon** (*Russian Federation*).
- **Revia** (*Australia, Brazil, Canada, Thailand*); **Revez** (*Argentina*).
- **Tranalex** (*Spain*); **Trexan** (*Singapore, USA*).
- **Uninaltrex** (*Brazil*).
- **Vivitrol** (*Russian Federation, Ukraine, USA*).

Generics Available
- Yes.

Licensed Indications for Parkinson's Disease
- None.

Licensed Indications for Other Conditions
- Opioid dependence (FDA, EMA, EMC).
- Alcohol dependence (FDA).

Non-Licensed Use for Parkinson's Disease
- Impulse control and related disorders in Parkinson's disease.

Non-Licensed Use for Other Conditions
- Autoimmune hepatitis (orphan).

THERAPEUTICS

- Post-herpetic neuralgia (orphan).
- Obesity (co-administration with bupropion).
- Bulimia nervosa.
- Self-injurious behaviour.
- Schizophrenia (mixed results).
- Hallucinogen persisting perception disorder (flashbacks) in patients with a prior history of LSD abuse.
- Kleptomania.
- Nicotine dependence (mixed results).
- Fibromyalgia.
- Gilles de la Tourette's syndrome.
- Chorea in Huntington's disease.
- Crohn's disease.
- Prophylaxis for morphine adverse reactions.
- Erectile dysfunction.
- Polycystic ovary syndrome (mixed results).
- Premenstrual syndrome.
- Secondary physiologic amenorrhea (mixed results).

Ineffective
- Motor performance in Parkinson's disease.

Mechanism of Action
- Naltrexone is a competitive, non-selective opioid receptor antagonist. Its presumed efficacy on ICDs is believed to be mediated by the potential modulation of the mesolimbic circuitry.
- It has minimal or no opioid agonist activity.
- Naltrexone may inhibit the effects of endogenous endorphins.
- Naltrexone treatment does not lead to physical or mental dependence. No tolerance for the opioid antagonizing effect is seen.

Efficacy Profile
- Naltrexone use in Parkinson's disease-related impulse control disorders has been characterized as 'investigational'.
- An 8-week, double-blind RCT in Parkinson's disease patients with one ICD has shown that a flexible dose of naltrexone (50–100 mg/day) had a beneficial effect on ICDs when assessed by a patient-completed Parkinson's disease-specific ICD rating scale, but not using a clinician-based global assessment scale, which was the primary outcome of the study.
- A small case series of Parkinson's disease patients with dopamine agonist-induced pathological gambling reported a beneficial effect of naltrexone on these symptoms.
- A controlled study has demonstrated a beneficial response of pathological gambling to naltrexone doses up to 250 mg per day in the general population, while various case reports have suggested a benefit for other ICDs with daily doses up to 150 mg.

- Onset of naltrexone action begins at 15–30 min and lasts for 24 h.
- In a case series of non-Parkinson's disease male gamblers treated with different drugs, 40% of those treated with naltrexone relapsed after 6 months of follow-up.

Pharmacokinetics

Absorption and Distribution
- (Oral) bioavailability: 5–40%.
- Food co-ingestion does not interfere with naltrexone pharmacokinetics.
- Tmax: 1 h.
- According to daily measurements, steady state is achieved rapidly after the first dose of naltrexone.
- Pharmacokinetics: linear for doses of 50–200 mg.
- Protein binding: 21–28%.
- Volume of distribution: 1,350 l.

Metabolism
- Naltrexone undergoes hepatic metabolism by dihydrodiol dehydrogenase, a cytosolic enzyme family, producing numerous metabolites with 6-β-naltrexol being the primary metabolite.
- Extra-hepatic sites of naltrexone metabolism may also exist.

Elimination
- Half-life is 4 h for the parent drug and 13 h for 6-β-naltrexol.
- The half-life of naltrexone appears to be biphasic; in the first 24 h following administration of a single dose, half-life ranges between 3.9 h and 10.3 h. About 24 h following an oral dose of naltrexone, another, extremely slow decline in plasma concentration occurs, with the estimated half-life of this terminal phase being 96 h, suggesting sequestration of naltrexone in tissues and slow release into the circulation.
- Renal excretion: naltrexone is mainly excreted in the urine with less than 2% of the parent drug excreted unchanged.

Drug Interaction Profile

Pharmacokinetic Drug Interactions
- Neither naltrexone nor 6-β-naltrexol are metabolized by or affect CYP450 enzymes; therefore, no relevant drug–drug interactions are observed.

Pharmacodynamic Drug Interactions
- Augmentation of naltrexone-induced lethargy and somnolence have been reported following initial doses of naltrexone in several patients stabilized on *phenothiazine* therapy.

DRUG INTERACTION PROFILE

N

NALTREXONE

Adverse Effects

How Drug Causes Adverse Effects

- Adverse effects of naltrexone usually result from its opiate antagonist action.
- At oral doses of 30–50 mg per day, naltrexone generally produces minimal analgesia, slight drowsiness, and no respiratory depression.
- Some naltrexone-related adverse effects, like hepatotoxicity, are dose-dependent.

Common Adverse Effects

*Some of the following adverse effects have occurred in patients who took naltrexone for opioid dependence and may be a result of opioid withdrawal, rather than naltrexone use; therefore, a causal relationship for many adverse events is not clearly established.

- Very common (≥1/10):
  - Headache, restlessness, insomnia, nervousness, anxiety, dizziness, anxiety, nausea, upper respiratory tract infection, pharyngitis, decreased appetite, nausea, vomiting, diarrhoea, abdominal pain, arthralgia, myalgia, increased CPK, asthenia.
- Common (≥1/100 to <1/10):
  - Neuropsychiatric: depression, somnolence, irritability, affective disorders, dizziness.
  - Eye/ear: increased lacrimation.
  - Cardiovascular: tachycardia, palpitations, ECG changes, chest pain.
  - GI: dry mouth, constipation.
  - Skin: rash.
  - Other: muscle cramps, back pain, delayed ejaculation, erectile dysfunction, thirst, chills, hyperhidrosis, increased energy.
- Uncommon (≥1/1,000 to <1/100):
  - Neuropsychiatric: hallucinations, confusion, depression, paranoia, disorientation, nightmares, agitation, libido disorder, abnormal dreams, tremor.
  - Eye/ear: blurred vision, eye irritation/pain, photophobia, eye swelling, ear discomfort/pain, tinnitus, vertigo.
  - Cardiovascular: increased systolic and diastolic blood pressure, flushing.
  - Respiratory: dyspnoea, nasal congestion, oropharyngeal pain, dysphonia, cough, yawning, sinus disorder, increased sputum.
  - GI: hepatocellular injury/hepatitis, increased bilirubin, liver function abnormalities flatulence, haemorrhoids, ulcer.
  - Renal/urinary: dysuria.
  - Skin: seborrhoea, pruritus, acne, alopecia.
  - Other: oedema, phlebitis, lymphadenopathy, groin pain, oral herpes, tinea pedis, increased appetite, pyrexia, peripheral coldness, feeling hot.

Life-Threatening or Dangerous Adverse Effects
- Rare (≥1/10,000 to <1/1,000):
  - Hypersensitivity reactions, including anaphylaxis.
  - Idiopathic thrombocytopenic purpura.
- Very rare (<1/10,000):
  - Rhabdomyolysis.
- Unknown frequency:
  - Suicidality.
  - Eosinophilic pneumonia.

Weight Change
- Weight increase or decrease have been reported as uncommon adverse events of naltrexone use.

What to Do About Adverse Effects
- Before introducing naltrexone, discuss common or life-threatening adverse effects with patients and/or caregivers, including symptoms that should be reported to the physician.
- At usual oral doses, adverse effects of naltrexone are generally mild to moderate in severity and usually subside within a few days.
- Patients and their caregivers should be informed about the possibility of naltrexone causing suicidal ideation/behaviour.
- Naltrexone should be discontinued if signs/symptoms of acute hepatitis develop. Naltrexone use may cause an increase of liver transaminases, which usually subsides to baseline within several weeks of naltrexone discontinuation.

Dosing and Use
Usual Dosage Range
- 50–100 mg.

Available Formulations
- Tablets: 50 mg.
- Microspheres for IM injection: 380 mg.

How to Dose
- An initial dose of 50 mg OD is suggested. If the patient does not respond after 4 weeks of therapy, the dose can be further increased to 100 mg OD.

Dosing Tips
- Naltrexone tablets should be taken with a drink.
- Adverse effects from the GI system may be minimized if naltrexone is taken with food or antacids or after meals.

N

How to Withdraw Drug
- There is limited information of withdrawal of naltrexone in Parkinson's disease, and while it is likely there is no need for gradual discontinuation of naltrexone, it is advisable to withdraw slowly if possible.

Overdose
- There is limited experience with naltrexone overdose.
- No evidence of toxicity was found in volunteers receiving daily doses of up to 800 mg for 7 days.
- Close monitoring and supportive measures are recommended. Usual measures to decrease GI absorption, such as induced emesis or gastric lavage, should be employed.

Tests and Therapeutic Drug Monitoring
- Before initiation of naltrexone therapy:
  - Assessment of liver and renal function.
  - A naloxone challenge test is recommended if opioid use is suspected; a withdrawal syndrome precipitated by naloxone hydrochloride will be of shorter duration compared to naltrexone. This test should not be performed in patients who test positive for opioids in the urine.
- During naltrexone therapy:
  - Regular assessments of liver and renal function.

Other Warnings/Precautions
- Abnormal liver function values have been reported with naltrexone use in obese patients with no history of drug abuse.
- Patients should be advised against the concomitant use of opioids (e.g. opioids in cough medication, antidiarrhoeal drugs, analgesics), including over-the-counter drugs. High-dose opioid intake concomitantly to naltrexone treatment can lead to life-threatening opioid poisoning from respiratory and circulatory impairment.
  - During naltrexone treatment, painful conditions should be treated with non-opioid analgesics. If opioid analgesics are used, larger doses than usual will be probably needed, thus increasing the risk for opioid-related adverse events.
  - Naltrexone should be stopped 48–72 h before elective surgery involving opioid analgesia.
- Naltrexone may cross-react with some immunoassay methods for the detection of opioids in the urine.
- Co-administration with central anti-hypertensives (e.g. α-*methyldopa*) should be avoided.
- Close monitoring is advised with co-administration of benzodiazepines, hypnotics, sedative antidepressants (e.g. *amitriptyline*, *doxepin*), sedative antihistamines, neuroleptics (e.g. *clozapine*, *droperidol*), *lithium*, or *amantadine*, as it might lead to a higher risk of adverse events.

N

- Naltrexone and *disulfiram* are potentially hepatotoxic drugs; thus, co-administration should better be avoided.
- Naltrexone may negatively affect the ability to drive a car or operate hazardous machinery due to impairment of mental and/or physical abilities required.

Do Not Use (Contraindications)
- Known sensitivity to naltrexone or to any of its excipients, including lactose.
  - Patients with rare hereditary problems of galactose intolerance, total lactase deficiency, or glucose–galactose malabsorption.
- Acute hepatitis, liver failure.
- Patients who are currently dependent on opioids, have a positive screen for opioids, or have failed the naloxone provocation test.
- Concurrent use with an opioid-containing medication or methadone.

Special Populations
Renal Impairment
- Close monitoring is recommended in renal impairment.
- Naltrexone use is contraindicated in patients with severe renal impairment.

Hepatic Impairment
- Close monitoring is recommended in hepatic impairment.
- Naltrexone use is contraindicated in patients with acute hepatitis or liver failure.

Elderly
- Safe naltrexone use in the elderly has not been established.
- Abnormal liver function values have been reported with naltrexone use in geriatric patients with no history of drug abuse.

Pregnancy
- Available data are insufficient to identify a drug-associated risk of major birth defects, miscarriage, or adverse maternal or fetal outcomes.

Breastfeeding
- Naltrexone and its metabolites are detected in human milk.
- There are no available data on the effect of naltrexone on the nursing infant or on milk production.

COSTS

Costs
NHS indicative costs accessed on 30 December 22:
- Adepend 50 mg tablets (AOP Orphan Ltd) – 28 × 50 mg tablets: £47.43.
- Naltrexone 50 mg tablets: 28 × 50 mg tablets: £23.00–£92.36.

The Overall Place of Naltrexone in the Treatment of Parkinson's Disease

ICDs are a common complication of dopaminergic therapy in Parkinson's disease, particularly in association with dopamine agonist use either alone or in combination with levodopa. The initial step in ICD management is a reduction or even cessation of the prescribed dopamine agonist or a switch to another dopamine agonist less prone to causing the development of ICDs, such as the rotigotine patch. However, ICDs may be associated with the total levodopa equivalent dose, irrespective of the drug category, and it can be challenging to maintain a balance between motor control and behavioural issues. In this context, available pharmacologic options are limited with SSRIs and antipsychotic agents having mixed results. Naltrexone is an opioid antagonist, which can be considered in cases of ICDs resistant to the adjustment of dopaminergic therapy. Efficacy results are mixed, with a high-quality study showing a lack of effect of naltrexone on ICDs, as assessed by the treating physicians, although the subjective impression of the patients was positive. Naltrexone is generally considered to be well tolerated. However, experience of naltrexone use is limited.

Potential Advantages
• Naltrexone may prove beneficial in the treatment of ICDs, as other therapeutic options are currently limited and have controversial results.

Potential Disadvantages
• Naltrexone efficacy on Parkinson's disease-related ICDs is unclear with mixed reports published.

Clinical Box

A 52-year-old patient with a 5-year history of Parkinson's disease and no prior psychiatric history presented with pathological gambling behaviours and increased sexual urges after 6 months of pramipexole use. Pramipexole was tapered off and replaced by a levodopa/carbidopa scheme; however, his ICD persisted, along with worsening of his motor performance. The patient was initially prescribed sertraline 100 mg OD and started cognitive-behavioural therapy without significant improvement after 6 months, while the total levodopa equivalent dose had to be increased due to poor motor performance. Naltrexone 50 mg OD was subsequently added with full resolution of his symptoms after 1 month. In the meantime, the patient was scheduled for DBS surgery.

Suggested Reading

Bosco D, M Plastino, C Colica, F Bosco, S Arianna, A Vecchio, F Galati, D Cristiano, A Consoli, D Consoli. Opioid antagonist naltrexone for the treatment of pathological gambling in Parkinson disease. *Clin Neuropharmacol* 2012; 35(3): 118–120.

Papay K, SX Xie, M Stern, H Hurtig, A Siderowf, JE Duda, J Minger, D Weintraub. Naltrexone for impulse control disorders in Parkinson disease: a placebo-controlled study. *Neurology* 2014; 83(9): 826–833.

References

AHFS Drug information, 2012. Bethesda: American Society of Health-System Pharmacists. Accessed on 30 December 2022 via www.medicinescomplete.com.

Dannon PN, K Lowengrub, E Musin, Y Gonopolsky, M Kotler. 12-Month follow-up study of drug treatment in pathological gamblers: a primary outcome study. *J Clin Psychopharmacol* 2007; 27(6): 620–624.

Grant JE, SW Kim. A case of kleptomania and compulsive sexual behavior treated with naltrexone. *Ann Clin Psychiatry* 2001; 13(4): 229–231.

Joint Formulary Committee. British National Formulary (online). London: BMJ Group and Pharmaceutical Press. Accessed on 30 December 2022 via www.medicinescomplete.com.

Kim SW, JE Grant, DE Adson, YC Shin. Double-blind naltrexone and placebo comparison study in the treatment of pathological gambling. *Biol Psychiatry* 2001; 49(11): 914–921.

Naltrexone. In: Brayfield A (Ed.), *Martindale: The Complete Drug Reference*. London: The Royal Pharmaceutical Society of Great Britain. Accessed on 30 December 2022 via www.medicinescomplete.com.

Naltrexone. In: DRUGDEX® System (electronic version). Truven Health Analytics, Greenwood Village, Colorado, USA. Accessed on 30 December 2022 via www.micromedexsolutions.com.

Neumeister A, A Winkler, C Wöber-Bingöl. Addition of naltrexone to fluoxetine in the treatment of binge eating disorder. *Am J Psychiatry* 1999; 156(5): 797.

Rascol O, N Fabre, O Blin, J Poulik, U Sabatini, JM Senard, M Ané, JL Montastruc, A Rascol. Naltrexone, an opiate antagonist, fails to modify motor symptoms in patients with Parkinson's disease. *Mov Disord* 1994; 9(4): 437–440.

Summary of Product Characteristics – Adepend 50 mg film coated tablets. AOP Orphan Ltd. Electronic Medicines Compendium: Adepend 50 mg film coated tablets – summary of product characteristics (SmPC) – (emc). Accessed on 30 December 2022 via www.medicines.org.uk.

Verebey K, J Volavka, SJ Mulé, RB Resnick. Naltrexone: disposition, metabolism, and effects after acute and chronic dosing. *Clin Pharmacol Ther* 1976; 20(3): 315–328.

NORTRIPTYLINE

Therapeutics

Chemical Name and Structure

Nortriptyline hydrochloride (3-(10,11-dihydro-5H-dibenzo[*a*,*d*]cyclo-hepten-5-ylidene)propyl(methyl)amine hydrochloride) is a dibenzocy-clohexadiene tricyclic antidepressant with a molecular weight of 299.8 and an empirical formula of $C_{19}H_{21}N$,HCl.

Brand Names

- **Allegron** (*Australia, UK*); **Aventyl** (*Canada*).
- **Norfenazin** (*Spain*); **Noritren** (*Denmark, Finland, Italy, Japan, Norway*); **Norline** (*Thailand*); **Norpress** (*New Zealand*); **Norterol** (*Portugal*); **Nortrilen** (*Belgium, Czech Republic, Germany, Hong Kong, Netherlands, Switzerland*); **Nortritabs** (*Australia*); **Nortylin** (*Israel*); **Nortyline** (*Thailand*); **N-Trip** (*Thailand*).
- **Ortrip** (*Thailand*).
- **Pamelor** (*Brazil, USA*); **Paxtibi** (*Spain*).
- **Sensaval** (*Sweden*); **Sensival** (*India*).

Generics Available

- Yes.

Licensed Indications for Parkinson's Disease

- None.

Licensed Indications for Other Conditions

- Depression (FDA, EMA, EMC).

Non-Licensed Use for Parkinson's Disease

- Depressive symptoms in Parkinson's disease.

Non-Licensed Use for Other Conditions

- Postpartum depression, premenstrual dysphoric disorder.
- Depressive symptoms in brain injury, bereavement, heart disease.
- Depressive symptoms as a complication of electroshock therapy.
- Smoking cessation.
- Attention Deficit Hyperactivity Disorder.
- Chronic urticaria, nocturnal pruritus, angioedema.
- Post-herpetic neuralgia.
- Neuropathic pain (including diabetic neuropathy, chemotherapy-induced pain).
- Cancer pain.
- Pain in sickle cell anaemia.
- Irritable bowel syndrome.
- Bulimia nervosa.
- Neurogenic bladder, nocturnal enuresis.
- Tinnitus.

Ineffective
• Not reported.

Mechanism of Action
• Nortriptyline is the primary active metabolite of amitriptyline and their mechanism of action is very similar.
• It inhibits serotonin and norepinephrine reuptake in the presynaptic neuronal membrane, thus increasing the concentration of these neurotransmitters in the synapse.
  • It is a more potent inhibitor of norepinephrine than of serotonin uptake.
• It blocks the effects of histamine and acetylcholine, which is responsible for the most common adverse effects.
• It increases and decreases the pressor effects of norepinephrine and phenethylamine, respectively.

Efficacy Profile
• The MDS EBM Committee has characterized nortriptyline as 'likely efficacious' and 'possibly useful' in the management of depressive symptoms in Parkinson's disease patients (MDS EBM Committee).
• Two placebo-controlled studies, one of them randomized, have shown a beneficial effect of nortriptyline on depressive symptoms in Parkinson's disease patients.
• The effect of nortriptyline on depression becomes apparent about 1–3 weeks after therapy initiation.
• There is preliminary evidence that nortriptyline might be effective in the management of anxiety in Parkinson's disease.

Pharmacokinetics
Absorption and Distribution
• Oral bioavailability: about 60%.
• Food co-ingestion: no effect on nortriptyline bioavailability.
• Tmax: 7–8.5 h.
• Time to steady state: about 1 week.
• Pharmacokinetics: a great variance is observed between individuals, which cannot be described by simple correlation.
• Protein binding: 86–95%.
• Volume of distribution: 15–27 l/kg.

Metabolism
• Nortriptyline undergoes extensive hepatic metabolism, mostly by CYP2D6, producing the active hydroxymetabolite 10-hydroxynortriptyline (thought to have similar therapeutic but fewer anticholinergic and cardiotoxic effects).

N

PHARMACOKINETICS

- Nortriptyline is metabolized to a small extent by CYP1A2 and CYP3A4.
- Nortriptyline metabolism is subject to genetic polymorphism (CYP450 isoenzymes).

Elimination
- Half-life of nortriptyline is 15–39 h.
- A small amount of the administered dose is excreted unchanged in the urine and faeces.

Drug Interaction Profile
Pharmacokinetic Drug Interactions
- Effects by nortriptyline:
  - Nortriptyline may inhibit *tramadol* metabolism and increase its concentration.
- Effects on nortriptyline:
  - CYP2D6 inhibitors (e.g. neuroleptics, SSRIs/SNRIs, beta-blockers, antiarrhythmics) may lower plasma concentration of nortriptyline.
  - Oral contraceptives, *rifampicin, phenytoin, barbiturates*, and *carbamazepine* may lower plasma concentration of nortriptyline.
  - Inhibitors of other CYP350 isoenzymes, including *cimetidine, methylphenidate, ethanol, valproic acid*, and calcium-channel blockers (e.g. *diltiazem, verapamil*), may increase plasma concentration of nortriptyline.
  - Strong CYP1A2 (e.g. *fluvoxamine*) and CYP3A4 inhibitors (e.g. *ketoconazole, itraconazole, ritonavir*) may increase plasma concentration of nortriptyline.

Pharmacodynamic Drug Interactions
- Co-medication with other serotonergic agents, including SSRIs/SNRIs, tricyclic antidepressants, opioids, *lithium, buspirone*, amphetamines, and triptans, can lead to potentially life-threatening serotonin syndrome.
- Co-medication with drugs causing electrolyte imbalance or increasing QT interval, such as Class IA and III antiarrhythmics, antipsychotics (e.g. *haloperidol, phenothiazine derivatives*), tricyclic antidepressants, certain antimicrobial agents (e.g. *moxifloxacin, erythromycin*), certain antihistamines (e.g. *astemizole, mizolastine*), pimozide, and others may lead to potentially fatal Torsade de Pointes arrhythmias and is considered a risk factor for sudden cardiac death.
- Co-administration with diuretics might increase the risk of hyponatremia or hypokalaemia (e.g. *furosemide*).
- Co-medication with CNS depressants (e.g. benzodiazepines, most antipsychotics, antihistamines H1 antagonists, opioids) or alcohol might lead to synergistic sedative effects, including somnolence and dizziness.

Adverse Effects

How Drug Causes Adverse Effects
- Although the activity of nortriptyline is mediated by a number of neuronal actions, its anticholinergic effects are responsible for the most common adverse effects.
- About 3–10% of the general population are considered poor CYP2D6 metabolizers, which might lead to elevated plasma concentrations of nortriptyline at usual doses and an increased risk of side effects.

Common Adverse Effects
- Very common (≥1/10):
  - Aggression, tremor, dizziness, headache, accommodation disorder, palpitations, tachycardia, congested nose, dry mouth, constipation, nausea, increased perspiration.
- Common (≥1/100 to <1/10):
  - Nervous/psychiatric: confusion, agitation, decreased libido, attention disturbance, dysgeusia, paraesthesia, ataxia.
  - Eye/ear: mydriasis.
  - Cardiovascular: orthostatic hypotension, atrioventricular or bundle branch block, ECG abnormalities (prolonged QT or QRS complex).
  - Renal/urinary: micturition disorders.
  - Reproductive: erectile dysfunction.
  - Other: fatigue, feeling thirsty, hyponatraemia.
- Uncommon (≥1/1,000 to <1/100):
  - Nervous/psychiatric: (hypo)mania, anxiety, insomnia, nightmares, convulsions.
  - Eye/ear: tinnitus, increased intraocular pressure.
  - Cardiovascular: hypertension, worsening of cardiac failure, collapse.
  - Gastrointestinal: diarrhoea, vomiting, tongue oedema, hepatic impairment.
  - Skin: rash, urticaria, face oedema.
  - Renal/urinary: urinary retention.
  - Reproductive: galactorrhoea.

Life-Threatening or Dangerous Adverse Effects
- Rare (≥1/10,000 to <1/1,000):
  - Bone marrow suppression, agranulocytosis, leukopenia, eosinophilia, thrombocytopenia.
  - Delirium (in the elderly).
  - Arrhythmia.
  - Ileus paralytic.
  - Pyrexia.
- Very rare (<1/10,000):
  - Acute glaucoma.
  - Cardiomyopathy, torsade de pointes.
  - Alveolitis.

N

ADVERSE EFFECTS

- Unknown frequency:
  - SIADH.
  - Suicidal ideation/behaviour.
  - Hypersensitivity myocarditis.
  - Hepatitis.

Rare and Not Life-Threatening Adverse Effects
- Decreased appetite.
- Akathisia, dyskinesia.
- Extrapyramidal disorder.
- Salivary gland enlargement.
- Jaundice.
- Alopecia, photosensitivity reaction.
- Gynaecomastia.

Weight Change
- Weight increase is very common with nortriptyline therapy.
- Weight loss has been reported rarely with nortriptyline therapy.

What to Do About Adverse Effects
- Before introducing nortriptyline, discuss common or life-threatening adverse effects with patients and/or caregivers, including symptoms that should be reported to the physician.
- Patients and their caregivers should be informed about the possibility of nortriptyline causing suicidal ideation/behaviour, especially in the early phase of recovery. If such signs/symptoms emerge, patients should urgently seek medical advice and be treated accordingly. Nortriptyline should be discontinued.
  - Due to suicidality risk, consider giving the patient a limited supply of nortriptyline.
- Patients and caregivers should be informed and be particularly vigilant for anticholinergic side effects of nortriptyline, including dry mouth, constipation, blurred vision, confusion, and seizures.
- In case a patient using nortriptyline reports bone pain, swelling, bruising or point tenderness, the possibility of a subjacent bone fracture should be excluded.
- Tricyclic antidepressants might aggravate RBD in Parkinson's disease patients; consider removing nortriptyline before initiating treatment for RBD.
- Regular dental assessments are advised, as dry mouth is a common side effect of nortriptyline use.

Dosing and Use

Usual Dose Range
- 10–150 mg daily.

Available Formulations
- Capsules: 10 mg, 25 mg, 50 mg, 75 mg.
- Tablets: 10 mg, 25 mg, 50 mg.
- Oral solution: 10 mg/5 ml, 25 mg/5 ml.

How to Dose
- Initial dose of 10 mg TID or QID, which is gradually increased as required, typically to 25 mg TID or QID; dosage can be increased at minimum intervals of 2–4 weeks; a maximum dose of 150 mg per day should not be exceeded.
- Maintenance dose should be the lowest effective dose for the shortest possible duration.
- The total dose can also be administered as a single dose, usually at night before bedtime.
- Nortriptyline can be discontinued if not tolerated or if considered ineffective after 12 weeks of therapy.
- Nortriptyline dose scheme should be carefully individualized; when introducing therapy, the lowest possible dose is generally suggested.

Dosing Tips
- Lower dosage is suggested in outpatients due to a lack of close monitoring.
- Plasma levels of nortriptyline are difficult to measure and treating physicians should consult their local laboratory staff.
- If nortriptyline therapy is effective, it should be applied for a minimum of 6 months to ensure that the patient is free of symptoms and lower the risk of relapse.
- Due to the potential for adverse effects, regular assessments and review of nortriptyline dose is advised.

How to Withdraw Drug
- Dose tapering over a period of several weeks is necessary to lower the risk of withdrawal symptoms, especially in case of high dose or long-term treatment (more than 8 weeks).
- A minimum of 4 weeks of tapering is suggested, depending on the initial dose and the duration of therapy (higher dose and longer periods of treatment need longer tapering, which might be as long as 6 months).
- Withdrawal symptoms usually manifest as one of the following distinct syndromes:
  - GI disturbances and generalized symptoms, such as malaise, chills, headache, increased sweating, agitation, and anxiety.
  - Sleep impairment with insomnia, followed by vivid dreams.

N

DOSING AND USE

- Parkinsonism or akathisia.
- Hypomania or mania.
- Cardiac arrhythmias might also be a consequence of abrupt discontinuation of nortriptyline.
- In case of severe or prolonged symptoms during dose reduction or withdrawal, consider resuming the previously prescribed dose and follow a longer tapering period.
- Treating physicians need to be aware of the possibility of withdrawal symptoms to avoid misinterpretation of such symptoms as indications of relapse.

Overdose
- Nortriptyline overdose might present with blurred vision, confusion, restlessness, agitation, dizziness, hypo-/hyperthermia, fever, vomiting, hyperactive reflexes, dilated pupils, hypotension, tachycardia, cardiac arrhythmias, dry mouth, decreased bowel sounds, inability to void, myoclonic jerks, seizures, respiratory depression, myoglobinuric renal failure, nystagmus, ataxia, dysarthria, choreoathetosis, coma.
  - QRS complex exceeding 100 ms is predictive of more severe toxicity.
- Supportive measures, close monitoring and maintenance of a clear airway with adequate ventilation are recommended.
- Activated charcoal can be more helpful than emesis or gastric lavage. Diuresis and dialysis are not effective.
- Ventricular arrhythmias may respond to alkalinization by hyperventilation or administration of sodium bicarbonate. Refractory arrhythmias may respond to propranolol, bretylium, or lignocaine. Quinidine and procainamide should be avoided.
- Seizures may respond to diazepam and phenytoin.
- Phenytoin might antagonize atrial tachycardia, gut motility, myoclonic jerks, and somnolence, although its effects are short-lived.

Tests and Therapeutic Drug Monitoring
- Before initiation of nortriptyline therapy:
  - A baseline ECG should be performed to check for QT prolongation.
  - A metabolic panel should be performed, including electrolytes and hepatic function.
- During nortriptyline therapy:
  - Plasma concentrations of nortriptyline should be monitored when a daily dosage of 100 mg is exceeded. Plasma levels should be maintained between 50 and 150 nanograms/ml.
  - Patients should be regularly evaluated for worsening of depression, suicidality, behaviour changes, or other common adverse effects, especially after introducing therapy or during dose modifications.

Other Warnings / Precautions
- There is a black box warning for young adults (less than 24 years old) who take nortriptyline for depression and other psychiatric disorders concerning suicidal thinking and behaviour.
  - A slight increase in suicidal thinking has also been seen in the elderly (>65 years old) receiving nortriptyline.
  - Patients with a history of suicide-related events are at higher risk and careful monitoring during treatment is required, especially early in therapy and following changes in dose.
- Close monitoring is advised in patients with benign prostate hyperplasia, urinary or GI retention, respiratory impairment, hepatic or renal impairment.
- Caution is advised in patients with a history of epilepsy or brain tumour because nortriptyline might lower the seizure threshold, especially in simultaneous use of neuroleptics.
- Caution is advised in patients with hyperthyroidism or those taking thyroid medication, as nortriptyline might precipitate cardiac arrhythmias.
- Caution is advised in patients with mania, bipolar disorder, or schizophrenia, as it may induce or aggravate psychosis.
- Close monitoring is recommended in patients with a history of bipolar disorder, as nortriptyline may trigger a manic episode.
  - Nortriptyline should be withdrawn in any patient entering a manic phase.
- Nortriptyline might aggravate anxiety and agitation when introduced in overactive or agitated patients.
- Caution is advised in patients with diabetes mellitus, because nortriptyline might affect glycaemic control; insulin or other antidiabetic regimes might need to be modified accordingly.
- Close monitoring is advised in patients with frequent hypotensive episodes, including those with cardiovascular disease, hypovolaemia, or simultaneous use of medication predisposing to hypotension or bradycardia.
- Hyponatraemia and/or SIADH have been reported with nortriptyline therapy, especially in dehydrated or volume-depleted patients.
- An angle-closure attack may be triggered in patients with high intraocular pressure or those at risk of angle-closure glaucoma (e.g. anatomically narrow angles without a patent iridectomy).
- Nortriptyline might cause CNS depression, affecting the ability to drive or operate dangerous machinery.
  - Co-administration with CNS depressants or alcohol should be avoided.
- Nortriptyline should be discontinued, before the patient undergoes electroconvulsive therapy, because it might worsen potential complications of this intervention.

N

DOSING AND USE

- Nortriptyline should be discontinued before the patient undergoes elective surgery due to potential drug-to-drug interactions with anaesthesia or predisposition to cardiac arrhythmias.
- In case of co-administration with CYP2D6 inhibitors, dose adjustments of nortriptyline might be necessary.
- Clinical monitoring is recommended in case of co-administration with valproic acid.
- Caution is advised in case of co-administration with diuretics that induce hypokalaemia.

Do Not Use (Contraindications)
- Known sensitivity to nortriptyline or to any of its excipients.
  - Nortriptyline formulations contain sodium bisulphite, which might precipitate allergic reactions, especially in asthmatic individuals.
  - Hypersensitivity to other dibenzazepine derivatives due to potential cross-sensitivity reactions.
- During recovery after a recent MI or in coronary artery insufficiency.
- In confirmed or suspected Brugada syndrome, as fatal cases have been reported.
- Patients with any degree of heart block or cardiac rhythm disorders.
- Co-administration with drugs that predispose to QT prolongation.
- Co-administration with MAOIs (including *selegiline* and *rasagiline*) or within 2 weeks after their discontinuation due to increased risk of potentially fatal serotonin syndrome. MAOIs should not be administered for 1 week after nortriptyline discontinuation. The same applies for co-administration of *safinamide*.
- Co-administration with *linezolid* or methylene blue IV:
  - If *linezolid* administration is necessary, nortriptyline should be discontinued immediately, and the patient should be monitored for CNS toxicity. Nortriptyline therapy can be resumed 24 h after last linezolid dose or after 2 weeks of monitoring, whichever applies first.
- Co-administration with sympathomimetic agents (e.g. *adrenaline, ephedrine, isoprenaline, noradrenaline, phenylephrine, phenylpropanolamine*), often included in anaesthetics and nasal decongestants, and adrenergic neuron blockers/centrally active antihypertensives (e.g. *clonidine, reserpine*).
- Co-medication with anticholinergic agents might enhance their effects and should be avoided.
- Co-medication with strong CYP1A2 and CYP3A4 inhibitors should be avoided.
- Co-medication with *tramadol* might lead to opioid toxicity and should be avoided.

Special Populations

Renal Impairment
• Patients with severe renal impairment may require reduced doses.

Hepatic Impairment
• Dosage modification and careful monitoring may be necessary in case of hepatic impairment; measurement of nortriptyline plasma levels is suggested.

Elderly
• Elderly patients may exhibit a delayed (up to 6 weeks) response to nortriptyline therapy.
• Nortriptyline half-life may be more than 90 h in the elderly.
• Nortriptyline use in the elderly is better avoided due to anticholinergic and sedative effects, particularly in those with a history of falls or fractures, cognitive impairment, and those at high risk of delirium or syncope.
• If it is used, a maximum dose of 50 mg should not be exceeded. If a higher dose is considered necessary, regular monitoring with ECG and plasma levels of nortriptyline are needed.

Pregnancy
• The safety of nortriptyline during pregnancy has not been established. Use in life-threatening emergencies when no safer drug is available.
• Neonates exposed to nortriptyline late in the third trimester might develop withdrawal symptoms, such as irritability, hypertonia, tremor, irregular breathing, weak suckling, and anticholinergic symptoms.

Breastfeeding
• Nortriptyline is excreted in human milk in low concentrations.
• Breastfeeding is not recommended during nortriptyline therapy unless the potential benefits of nortriptyline therapy clearly outweigh potential risks; close monitoring of the infant is advised, especially for the first 4 weeks after birth.

Costs
NHS indicative price accessed 20 November 2022:
• Nortriptyline 10 mg tablets – 100 × 10 mg tablets: £0.95–£33.41; 30 × 10 mg tablets: £1.00–£11.79; 28 × 10 mg tablets: £2.14; 84 × 10 mg tablets: £6.42.
• Nortriptyline 25 mg tablets – 100 × 25 mg tablets: £0.95–£35.22; 30 × 25 mg tablets: £1.00–£12.43; 28 × 25 mg tablets: £2.46; 84 × 25 mg tablets: £7.38.
• Nortriptyline 50 mg tablets – 30 × 50 mg tablets: £21.13–£84.50.
• Nortriptyline 10 mg/5 ml oral solution – 250 ml: £80.00–£246.00.
• Nortriptyline 25 mg/5 ml oral solution – 250 ml: £324.00.

The Overall Place of Nortriptyline in the Treatment of Parkinson's Disease

Nortriptyline, a dual serotonin and noradrenaline reuptake inhibitor with mild anticholinergic activity, is a tricyclic antidepressant that can be effectively used for the treatment of moderate to severe depression in Parkinson's disease. Nortriptyline has been associated with fewer side effects than amitriptyline. However, similarly to other tricyclic antidepressants, its initiation requires vigilance for adverse effects and careful evaluation of patients for comorbidities and simultaneous medications for drug–drug interactions, which are common and significantly increase the risk for serious complications. Due to tolerability issues, nortriptyline is not commonly used as a first-line therapy in Parkinson's disease-related depression.

Potential Advantages
• Nortriptyline is one of the less-sedating tricyclic antidepressants with mild antimuscarinic effects, which are responsible for its more common adverse effects.

Potential Disadvantages
• Administration of tricyclic antidepressants to Parkinson's disease patients might precipitate or worsen psychosis, sedation, somnolence, cognitive impairment, or delirium, especially in those with impaired cognition.
• A long list of drug–drug interactions accompanies nortriptyline administration.
• Nortriptyline formulations are not available in numerous countries.

Clinical Box

A 52-year-old man with a diagnosis of Parkinson's disease was referred to the Movement Disorders Outpatient Clinic due to a constantly low mood, feelings of hopelessness, and episodes of crying. The patient had been diagnosed with moderate depression and had been treated with citalopram at first and then venlafaxine, which he had to discontinue due to side effects. The patient was currently taking pramipexole 2.1 mg OD and levodopa/benserazide 100 mg/25 mg QID. The rest of his medical history was unremarkable. Based on his motor performance, the patient was considered relatively stable. No contraindications for nortriptyline therapy were found, so a low dose of nortriptyline 25 mg OD at night was suggested, which was gradually increased to 75 mg within 2 months. The patient reported a significant improvement of his depressive symptoms, but also a decrease in drooling, which had been troubling him for the past few months.

N

Suggested Reading

Andersen J, E Aabro, N Gulmann, A Hjelmsted, HE Pedersen. Anti-depressive treatment in Parkinson's disease. A controlled trial of the effect of nortriptyline in patients with Parkinson's disease treated with L-DOPA. *Acta Neurol Scand* 1980; 62(4): 210–219.

Menza M, RD Dobkin, H Marin, MH Mark, M Gara, S Buyske, K Bienfait, A Dicke. A controlled trial of antidepressants in patients with Parkinson disease and depression. *Neurology* 2009; 72(10): 886–892.

References

AHFS Drug information, 2012. Bethesda: American Society of Health-System Pharmacists. Accessed on 20 November 2022 via www.medicinescomplete.com.

Joint Formulary Committee. British National Formulary (online). London: BMJ Group and Pharmaceutical Press. Accessed on 20 November 2022 via www.medicinescomplete.com.

Nortriptyline. In: Brayfield A (Ed.), *Martindale: The Complete Drug Reference*. London: The Royal Pharmaceutical Society of Great Britain. Accessed on 20 November 2022 via www.medicinescomplete.com.

Nortriptyline. In: DRUGDEX® System (electronic version). Truven Health Analytics, Greenwood Village, Colorado, USA. Accessed on 20 November 2022 via www.micromedexsolutions.com.

Prange S, H Klinger, C Laurencin, T Danaila, S Thobois. Depression in patients with Parkinson's disease: current understanding of its neurobiology and implications for treatment. *Drugs Aging* 2022; 39(6): 417–439.

Summary of product characteristics – Nortriptyline 10 mg film-coated tablets. Advanz Pharma. Electronic Medicines Compendium: Nortriptyline 10 mg film-coated tablets – summary of product characteristics (SmPC) – (emc). Accessed on 20 November 2022 via www.medicines.org.uk.

Troeung L, SJ Egan, N Gasson. A meta-analysis of randomised placebo-controlled treatment trials for depression and anxiety in Parkinson's disease. *PLoS One* 2013; 8(11): e79510.

REFERENCES

OPICAPONE

Therapeutics

Chemical Name and Structure

Opicapone (2,5-dichloro-3-[5-(3,4-dihydroxy-5-nitrophenyl)-1,2,4-oxadiazol-3-yl]-4,6-dimethylpyridine *N*-oxide) is a yellow powder/crystalline solid with poor aqueous solubility. It has a molecular weight of 413.2 and an empirical formula of $C_{15}H_{10}Cl_2N_4O_6$.

Brand Names
• **Ongentys** (*Austria, Finland, Germany, Ireland, Netherlands, Poland, Portugal, Switzerland, UK, USA*).

Generics Available
• No.

Licensed Indications for Parkinson's Disease
• An adjunctive therapy to levodopa/DDI preparations in Parkinson's disease patients, who experience end-of-dose motor fluctuations or OFF episodes and cannot be stabilized with levodopa/DDI combination alone (FDA, EMA, EMC).

Licensed Indications for Other Conditions
• None.

Non-Licensed Use for Parkinson's Disease
• None.

Non-Licensed Use for Other Conditions
• None.

Ineffective
• Patients not receiving levodopa therapy.

Mechanism of Action
• A potent, third-generation, peripheral, selective, and reversible COMT inhibitor (as assessed by inhibition of COMT activity in erythrocytes), which mediates the peripheral degradation of levodopa. Opicapone binds tightly to S-COMT and only slowly dissociates, which explains the long duration of effect despite a short plasma half-life. When levodopa decarboxylation has already been prevented by DDI, opicapone administration leads to increased levodopa plasma levels and levodopa delivery to the brain, increased levodopa elimination half-life, and an improved clinical response to levodopa treatment compared to levodopa/DDI alone.
• Opicapone serves to improve the bioavailability and duration of action of levodopa.
• Opicapone has a long duration of action, lasting for more than 24 h (50 mg).

Efficacy Profile
- Opicapone use has been associated with an average reduction of about 60 min daily in end-of-dose fluctuations and OFF time compared to placebo (BIPARK I & II studies).
- Opicapone was found non-inferior to adjunctive entacapone in improving OFF time (BIPARK I study).
- Switching of entacapone to opicapone was associated with a further OFF time reduction (about 39 min).
- Both doses of opicapone (25 mg and 50 mg) were associated with significant OFF and ON time improvements in a sample of Japanese Parkinson's disease patients, while the 50-mg dose was also associated with a significant enhancement of motor performance during the ON phase (COMFORT-PD study).
- According to the OPTIPARK study, there is preliminary evidence of a positive effect of opicapone on sleep/fatigue and mood/cognition (OPTIPARK study).
- Opicapone shows potential efficacy on total non-motor symptoms burden, including sleep/fatigue, mood/apathy and GI symptoms (OPTIPARK & OPEN-PD studies).
- A clinically meaningful effect was found with up to 1 year of opicapone treatment (OPTIPARK & BIPARK II studies).
- Opicapone use was found to be well tolerated and consistently effective in decreasing OFF time in Japanese Parkinson's disease patients with motor fluctuations over a follow-up period of 52 weeks (open-label extension of COMFORT-PD study).

Pharmacokinetics
Absorption and Distribution
- Oral bioavailability: about 20%.
- Food co-ingestion: delays absorption and reduces peak plasma concentrations.
- Tmax: average of 2 h (range 1–4 h).
- Time to steady state: no statistical evaluation could be performed as trough concentrations of opicapone have been found to be below the lower limit of quantification. However, there are indications that, in a multiple dose regimen, maximum exposure is achieved after the first administration of opicapone.
- Pharmacokinetics: rapidly absorbed, linear in dose range of 25–50 mg daily.
- Protein binding: >99%, regardless of drug concentration.
- Volume of distribution: 29 l (at a dose of 50 mg daily).

Metabolism
- Metabolized primarily by sulphation in the liver, yielding the inactive metabolite opicapone sulphate (BIA 9–1103), followed by methylation (BIA 9–1104). Minor contributions by glucuronidation, reduction (BIA 0–1079, active metabolite), and glutathione conjugation (generally not detectable metabolites in plasma samples).

PHARMACOKINETICS

- Largely excreted by faeces (59–76%).
  - About 22% excreted as unchanged parent drug.
- About 20% excreted in exhaled air and about 5% in the urine (<1% as unchanged).
  - Glucuronide metabolite is the primary detectable metabolite in the urine.

Elimination
- Half-life value in healthy adults is 1–2 h.
- Despite the short half-life, the observed half-life of opicapone-induced COMT inhibition in human red blood cells was 61.6±37.6 h (because of tight binding to COMT and slow dissociation), so allowing once daily administration.
- No clinically significant pharmacokinetics differences related to age.
- Following termination of treatment, COMT inhibition slowly returns to baseline levels with >35% inhibition still observed 5 days after the last dose.

Drug Interaction Profile
Pharmacokinetic Drug Interactions
- Effects by opicapone:
  - Minor inhibition of CYP1A2 and CYP2B6 at the highest concentrations of opicapone in in-vitro studies. Indications of CYP3A4, CYP2C8, and CYP2C9 inhibition, although no clinical interactions with *warfarin*, a CYP2C9 substrate, or *repaglinide*, a CYP2C8 substrate, were confirmed.
- Effects on opicapone:
  - Isolated reports that *quinidine* may reduce opicapone exposure.

Pharmacodynamic Drug Interactions
- Peak and overall levodopa exposure increased by about 43% and 62–94%, respectively, in Parkinson's disease patients after a single daily dose of opicapone at bedtime with levodopa/carbidopa administered every 3–4 h compared to administration of levodopa/carbidopa alone.
- Co-medication with non-selective MAOIs (e.g. *isocarboxazid, phenlzine, tranylcypromine, moclobemide*) may increase catecholamine concentrations and predispose to increased heart rate, arrhythmias, and excessive blood pressure.
- Co-medication with selective MAO-B inhibitors (e.g. *selegiline, rasagiline*) was not found to bear important clinical effects in opicapone pharmacokinetics; therefore, they can be used concomitantly.
- Potential pharmacokinetic interactions with drugs metabolized by COMT (e.g. inotropes, vasopressors, SSRIs/SNRIs).
  - Co-medication with sympathomimetic (adrenergic) agents (e.g. *dobutamine, epinephrine, norepinephrine, dopamine, dopexamine, isoproterenol, rimiterol, isoprenaline*) may increase heart rate and induce arrhythmias and excessive blood pressure changes.

OPICAPONE

Adverse Effects

How Drug Causes Adverse Effects
• Mainly (but not solely) through increasing dopaminergic activity.

Common Adverse Effects
• Very common (≥1/10):
  ○ Dyskinesias.
• Common (≥1/100 to <1/10):
  ○ Neuropsychiatric: abnormal dreams, hallucinations, insomnia, dizziness, headache, somnolence.
  ○ Cardiovascular: orthostatic hypotension.
  ○ GI: constipation, dry mouth, vomiting.
  ○ Musculoskeletal: muscle spasms.
  ○ Other: increased CPK.
• Uncommon (≥1/1,000 to <1/100):
  ○ Neuropsychiatric: anxiety, depression, nightmares, sleep disorders, ICDs, dysgeusia.
  ○ Eye/ear: dry eye, ear congestion.
  ○ Cardiovascular: palpitations, hypertension, syncope.
  ○ Respiratory: dyspnoea.
  ○ GI: abdominal distension/pain, dyspepsia.
  ○ Musculoskeletal: muscle twitching/stiffness, myalgia.
  ○ Renal/urinary: chromaturia, nocturia.
  ○ Other: decreased appetite, hypertriglyceridaemia.

Life-Threatening or Dangerous Adverse Effects
• Episodes of sudden sleep onset.

Rare and Not Life-Threatening Adverse Effects
• None.

Weight Change
• Opicapone use has been reported to decrease body weight (4%).

What to Do About Adverse Effects
• Discuss common adverse events with patients or caregivers before starting medication, including symptoms that should be reported to the physician.
• Patients on opicapone and their caregivers should be specifically asked about the development of somnolence or new-onset or increased ICDs (e.g. gambling, sexual urges, uncontrolled spending), as patients may not recognize these behaviours as abnormal.
• In case of new-onset or exacerbation of pre-existing dyskinesia, consider lowering each levodopa dose (or selected doses of levodopa if dyskinesia appears at specific times during the day) or extend the dosing intervals, without discontinuing opicapone.
  • According to an open-label, randomized, modified cross-over study comparing opicapone combinations with four- or five-intake

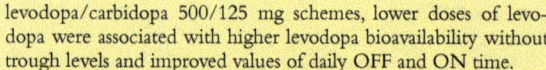

levodopa/carbidopa 500/125 mg schemes, lower doses of levo-dopa were associated with higher levodopa bioavailability without trough levels and improved values of daily OFF and ON time.
- Prior to opicapone initiation, consider other factors that may increase somnolence risk. In case of daytime sleepiness or episodes of patient falling asleep during activities requiring active participation (e.g. con-versations, eating, driving), consider adjusting other dopaminergic agents (e.g. dopamine agonists) or sedative drugs regimens, or discon-tinuing opicapone.
  - If continuing opicapone therapy, patients should be advised to avoid driving or other activities, which require their full attention.
- In case of hypotension or syncope, consider adjusting dosage of other agents that can lower blood pressure or discontinuing opicapone.
- Consider withdrawing therapy if adverse effects are troublesome (e.g. hallucinations, ICD, dyskinesias).

Dosing and Use

Usual Dosage Range
- 50 mg daily at bedtime.

Available Formulations
- Capsules: 25 mg, 50 mg.

How to Dose
- An initial dose of 50 mg OD is suggested; no gradual increase is needed.

Dosing Tips
- Opicapone should be taken at bedtime.
- Patients should not eat food for 1 h before and 1 h after opicapone intake.
- If a dose is missed, the next dose should be taken next day at the scheduled time.
- Opicapone is administered as an adjunct therapy to levodopa/DDI preparations and is expected to enhance levodopa effects. It is, thus, often necessary to adjust levodopa dosing schemes within the first days or weeks of introducing opicapone (extend levodopa dosing intervals and/or reduce the amount of levodopa per dose).

How to Withdraw Drug
- Opicapone can be discontinued without tapering or gradual withdrawal.
- Patient's monitoring is required, as abrupt withdrawal can cause hyperpyrexia and confusion.
- Consider adjustment of other agents commonly used in Parkinson's disease as needed, including increasing levodopa dose or frequency.

OPICAPONE

Overdose
- Close monitoring, along with symptomatic and supportive treatment, should be applied as appropriate.
- In case of opicapone overdose, consider removing it by gastric lavage and/or inactivation by administering activated charcoal.
- No specific antidotes are known.

Tests and Therapeutic Drug Monitoring
- Opicapone has not been linked to serum liver enzymes elevation or cases of clinically apparent liver injury, so regular monitoring of serum enzymes is not recommended.
- Consider general medical evaluation, including assessment of liver function, in patients experiencing progressive anorexia, asthenia, and weight decrease within a relatively short period.

Other Warnings/Precautions
- Opicapone should be avoided in patients with a major psychotic disorder due to increased risk of exacerbating psychosis because of an increase in central dopaminergic tone.
- Caution is advised in patients with suspected or diagnosed DDS due to risk of exacerbation.
  - Caution is advised in co-administration with sympathomimetic (adrenergic) agents due to potential cardiovascular complications; close monitoring of heart rate/rhythm and blood pressure is recommended.
- There is no experience with concomitant use of opicapone and the MAO-B inhibitor *safinamide*; therefore, caution is advised.
- Careful monitoring is advised when opicapone is co-administered with drugs metabolized by COMT.
- Caution is advised when opicapone is co-administered with TCAs and SNRIs due to limited experience with this combination; monitor for potential side effects.
- Opicapone may cause daytime sleepiness or episodes of falling asleep during daily activities with no preceding warning signs, affecting the patients' ability to drive and safely operate machinery.

Do Not Use (Contraindications)
- Hypersensitivity to the active substance or to any of its excipients, including lactose.
  - Patients with rare hereditary problems of galactose intolerance, total lactase deficiency, or glucose–galactose malabsorption.
- Diagnosis of pheochromocytoma, paraganglioma, or other catecholamine-secreting neoplasms.
- Severe hepatic impairment or end-stage renal disease (CrCl < 15 ml/min).
- History of NMS and/or non-traumatic rhabdomyolysis.
- Co-administration with non-selective MAO inhibitors.

DOSING AND USE

Special Populations

Renal Impairment
- Minor to moderate renal impairment (CrCl > 30 ml/min): no dosage modifications needed.
- Severe renal impairment (CrCl < 30 ml/min): caution is advised; monitor for adverse events and discontinue therapy if tolerability issues arise.
- End-stage renal disease (CrCl < 15 ml/min): contraindicated.

Hepatic Impairment
- Mild hepatic impairment (Child–Pugh A): no dose adjustments are necessary.
- Moderate hepatic impairment (Child–Pugh B): a dose of 25 mg OD is suggested.
- Severe hepatic impairment (Child–Pugh C): contraindicated.

Elderly
- No dose adjustments are required, although increased sensitivity to adverse reactions has been reported (BIPARK extension studies). Limited experience in those older than 85 years old.

Pregnancy
- Opicapone use is not recommended during pregnancy.
- Women of childbearing potential are advised to use contraception during opicapone therapy.
- Embryo–fetal abnormalities have been observed in animal studies.

Breastfeeding
- Women are advised not to breastfeed during opicapone treatment.
- It is not known whether opicapone is excreted in human milk or whether it has any effect on the nursing infant or milk production.
- In lactating rats, opicapone and its metabolites were detected in breast milk.

Costs
NHS indicative price accessed 22 April 2022:
- 30 × 50 mg caps: £93.90.

The Overall Place of Opicapone in the Treatment of Parkinson's Disease
Opicapone, a third-generation COMT inhibitor, can overcome the limitations of other marketed COMT inhibitors (*tolcapone, entacapone*), including safety issues, suboptimal pharmacokinetics, and a short duration of effect. Numerous high-quality studies have shown an improved levodopa plasma profile and a significant benefit on motor fluctuations

and OFF time reduction when opicapone was used as an adjunctive therapy to levodopa/DDI preparations in Parkinson's disease patients, even in the long term (up to 1 year). Opicapone is generally well tolerated, with the most commonly reported adverse events being dyskinesia, constipation, and insomnia, usually occurring early after therapy initiation (first 4 weeks).

Potential Advantages
- Once daily administration, improving adherence.
- Independent adjustment of levodopa dose, regardless of opicapone dose.
- Opicapone has not been associated with severe diarrhoea.
- Opicapone has not been associated with hepatotoxicity, so no liver toxicity monitoring is required.

Potential Disadvantages
- A relatively novel agent; thus, there is limited clinical experience with opicapone use.
- Not available globally.
- May cause or exacerbate dyskinesia, postural hypotension, and somnolence.

Clinical Box

A 50-year-old woman with an 8-year history of Parkinson's disease reported end-of-dose deterioration and increased OFF time. The patient was also experiencing mild dyskinesia, especially during the afternoon, which was not bothersome. Her current medications included levodopa/benserazide 200 mg/50 mg QID and rotigotine 8 mg/24 h. Her medical history included irritable bowel syndrome with frequent episodes of diarrhoea. Opicapone 50 mg OD at bedtime was prescribed. OFF time improved, but the patient's dyskinesia exacerbated, becoming troublesome to the patient. A reduction of levodopa/benserazide to 1 × 200 mg/50 mg tablet at 8 a.m. and 1 × 100 mg/25 mg and 1 × 50 mg/12.5 mg TDS (at 12 p.m., 4 p.m., and 8 p.m.) led to improvement of dyskinesia without an increase in daily OFF time.

Suggested Reading

Fabbri M, JJ Ferreira, A Lees, F Stocchi, W Poewe, E Tolosa, O Rascol. Opicapone for the treatment of Parkinson's disease: a review of a new licensed medicine. *Mov Disord* 2018; 33(10): 1528–1539.

Ferreira JJ, A Lees, JF Rocha, W Poewe, O Rascol, P Soares-da-Silva; Bi-Park 1 Investigators. Opicapone as an adjunct to levodopa in patients with Parkinson's disease and end-of-dose motor fluctuations: a randomised, double-blind, controlled trial. *Lancet Neurol* 2016; 15(2): 154–165.

SUGGESTED READING

Jenner, P., JF Rocha, JJ Ferreira, O Rascol, P Soares-da-Silva. Redefining the strategy for the use of COMT inhibitors in Parkinson's disease: the role of opicapone. *Expert Rev Neurother* 2021; 21(9): 1019–1033.

Leta, V., DJ van Wamelen, A Sauerbier, S Jones, M Parry, A Rizos, KR Chaudhuri. Opicapone and levodopa–carbidopa intestinal gel infusion: the way forward towards cost savings for healthcare systems? *J Parkinsons Dis* 2020; 10(4): 1535–1539.

Reichmann H, A Lees, JF Rocha, D Magalhães, P Soares-da-Silva; OPTIPARK Investigators. Effectiveness and safety of opicapone in Parkinson's disease patients with motor fluctuations: the OPTI-PARK open-label study. Transl Neurodegener. 2020 Mar 4; 9(1):9. doi: 10.1186/s40035-020-00187-1.

References

AHFS Drug information, 2012. Bethesda: American Society of Health–System Pharmacists. Accessed on 22 April 2022 via www.medicinescomplete.com.

Ferreira, JJ. , W Poewe, O Rascol, F Stocchi, A Antonini, J Moreira, B Guimarães, JF Rocha, P Soares-da-Silva. Effect of opicapone on levodopa pharmacokinetics in patients with fluctuating Parkinson's disease. *Mov Disord* 2022; 37(11): 2272–2283.

Joint Formulary Committee. British National Formulary (online). London: BMJ Group and Pharmaceutical Press. Accessed on 22 April 2022 via www.medicinescomplete.com.

Lees AJ, J Ferreira, O Rascol, W Poewe, JF Rocha, M McCrory, P Soares-da-Silva. Opicapone as adjunct to levodopa therapy in patients with Parkinson disease and motor fluctuations: a randomized clinical trial. *JAMA Neurol* 2017; 74(2): 197–206.

Opicapone. In: Brayfield A (Ed.), *Martindale: The Complete Drug Reference*. London: The Royal Pharmaceutical Society of Great Britain. Accessed on 22 April 2022 via www.medicinescomplete.com.

Opicapone. In: DRUGDEX® System (electronic version). Truven Health Analytics, Greenwood Village, Colorado, USA. Accessed on 22 April 2022 via www.micromedexsolutions.com.

Scott LJ. Opicapone: a review in Parkinson's disease. *CNS Drugs* 2021; 35(1): 121–131.

Summary of product characteristics – Ongentys 25 mg hard capsules. Bial Pharma UK Ltd. Electronic Medicines Compendium: Ongentys 25 mg hard capsules – summary of product characteristics (SmPC) – (emc). Accessed on 22 April 2022 via www.medicines.org.uk.

Takeda A, R Takahashi, Y Tsuboi, M Nomoto, T Maeda, A Nishimura, K Yoshida, N Hattori. Long-term safety and efficacy of opicapone in Japanese Parkinson's patients with motor fluctuations. *J Neural Transm (Vienna)* 2021; 128(3): 337–344.

Takeda A, R Takahashi, Y Tsuboi, M Nomoto, T Maeda, A Nishimura, K Yoshida, N Hattori. Randomized, controlled study of opicapone in Japanese Parkinson's patients with motor fluctuations. *Mov Disord* 2021; 36(2): 415–423.

OPICAPONE

OXYBUTYNIN

Therapeutics

Chemical Name and Structure

Oxybutynin (4-diethylaminobut-2-ynyl 2-cyclohexyl-2-phenylglycolate; 4-(diethylamino)-2-butynyl α-phenylcyclohexaneglycolic acid ester) has a molecular weight of 357.5 and a molecular formula of $C_{22}H_{31}NO_3$.

Brand Names
- **Anrushan** (*China*); **Ao Ning** (*China*).
- **Cobapolas** (*Japan*); **Cystrin** (*Ireland*).
- **Delak** (*Argentina*); **Detrusan** (*Austria*); **Ditropan** (*Argentina, Australia, Austria, Canada, Czech Republic, France, Greece, Hungary, Ireland, Italy, Poland, Portugal, South Africa, Spain, Sweden, UK, USA*); **Diutropan** (*Thailand*); **Dresplan** (*Cyprus, Spain*); **Dridase** (*Germany, Netherlands*); **Driptan** (*Ukraine*); **Driptane** (*Estonia, France, Lithuania, Philippines, Poland, Russian Federation, Tunisia*).
- **Frenurin** (*Brazil*).
- **Gelnique** (*USA*).
- **Halarase** (*Japan*).
- **Incontinol** (*Brazil*); **Innobase** (*Japan*).
- **Jie Sai** (*China*).
- **Kentera** (*Austria, Belgium, Denmark, Estonia, Finland, Germany, Greece, Ireland, Lithuania, Netherlands, Norway, Poland, Spain, Switzerland, Turkey, UK*).
- **Lenditro** (*South Africa*); **Lyrinel** (*Greece, Israel, Mexico, South Africa, Thailand, UK*); **Lyrinel XL** (*Ireland*).
- **Nefryl** (*Mexico*); **Neoxy** (*Japan*); **Nourin** (*Brazil*); **Novitropan** (*Israel, Russian Federation*).
- **Obutin** (*Singapore*); **Orivate** (*Japan*); **Oxybtan** (*Tunisia*); **Oxybugamma** (*Germany*); **Oxytrol** (*Australia, Canada, New Zealand, USA*); **Oxyrest** (*South Africa*); **Oxyspas** (*South Africa*).
- **Palnaxol** (*Japan*); **Pollakisu** (*Japan*); **Porabutin** (*Japan*); **Poratile** (*Japan*).
- **Retemic** (*Brazil*); **Retevan** (*Venezuela*).
- **Shuang Miao** (*China*); **Sibutin** (*Ukraine*).
- **Tavor** (*Mexico*).
- **Uralex** (*Poland*); **Urazol** (*Chile*); **Urequin** (*Argentina*); **Uricont** (*Chile*); **Urihexal** (*South Africa*); **Uropan** (*Turkey*); **Uroxal** (*Czech Republic, Hungary*).
- **Vesolox** (*Netherlands*); **Vesoxx** (*Austria, Germany, Poland, Switzerland*).
- **Yi Jing** (*China*).

Generics Available
- Yes.

Licensed Indications for Parkinson's Disease
• None.

Licensed Indications for Other Conditions
• Overactive bladder symptoms in the context of uninhibited neurogenic or reflex neurogenic bladder (FDA).
• Symptomatic treatment of urge incontinence and/or increased urinary frequency and urgency in patients with unstable bladder (EMA).
• Overactive bladder symptoms in the context of idiopathic overactive bladder or neurogenic bladder dysfunction (detrusor over activity) (EMC).
• Detrusor overactivity-related nocturia in conjunction with non-pharmaceutical therapy when other treatments have failed to relieve symptoms (EMC).

Non-Licensed Use for Parkinson's Disease
• Overactive bladder.

Non-Licensed Use for Other Conditions
• Bladder pain/spasms provoked by indwelling ureteral stents or Foley catheters.
• Primary hyperhidrosis.

Ineffective
• As a monotherapy in nocturnal enuresis.

Mechanism of Action
• Oxybutynin is a synthetic tertiary amine that is a competitive antagonist of ACh at post-ganglionic muscarinic receptors with a higher affinity for M1 and M3 receptors.
• Oxybutynin exhibits both a direct spasmolytic and an antimuscarinic action on smooth muscle of the bladder, resulting in relaxation of the detrusor muscle of the bladder.
  • Oxybutynin appears to have little/no effect on smooth muscle of blood vessels.
  • No antinicotinic effect has been described.
• Oxybutynin use leads to increased bladder capacity, less uninhibited contraction, reduced frequency and urgency, and delayed desire to void.
• Oxybutynin crosses the blood–brain barrier to a significant degree.
• N-desethyloxybutynin, the active metabolite of oxybutynin, has similar pharmacologic profile to oxybutynin.

Efficacy Profile
• Up to now, there are no published studies investigating the effect of oxybutynin on Parkinson's disease-related urinary symptoms. High-quality studies concerning oxybutynin efficacy on overactive bladder

symptoms in the general population, including elderly patients, have been used by regulatory authorities to grant the relevant approvals for its use. Based on these indications, oxybutynin can also be used by Parkinson's disease patients, as Parkinson's disease is not listed as a contraindication.

- The onset of oxybutynin action is expected to be about 30–60 min after administration and lasts 6–10 h with peak efficacy at around 3–6 h.
- The efficacy of oxybutynin in treating overactive bladder symptoms persists for at least 12 weeks.

Pharmacokinetics

Absorption and Distribution

- Oral bioavailability: about 6% in IR formulations (1.5–2 times higher for ER formulations).
- Concurrent consumption of food does not affect the plasma pharmacokinetics of oxybutynin ER, but it has been reported that it may increase bioavailability of oxybutynin IR by 25% due to delayed absorption.
- Tmax: <1 h in IR formulations, ~12 h in ER formulations and 36–48 h in transdermal application.
- Time to steady state: within 3 days (ER formulation) and after the second patch in transdermal application.
- Protein binding: >99% (mainly to α-1 acid glycoprotein).
- Volume of distribution: 193 l (100–200 l) (IV administration).

Metabolism

- Oxybutynin is extensively metabolized in the liver and intestinal wall, mostly by CYP3A4.
- It is converted to the active metabolite *N*-desethyloxybutynin (mainly in the gut) and to the inactive metabolite phenylcyclohexylglycolic acid.
- On transdermal administration, the levels of *N*-desethyloxybutynin are lower than those found after oral dosing.
- Lower metabolism of oxybutynin was found in healthy Japanese individuals compared to Caucasians.

Elimination

- Plasma half-life is 2–3 h for IR formulations (including oral solution) and 12–13 h for ER formulations.
- Following removal of the oxybutynin transdermal patch, oxybutynin and its active metabolite are removed from plasma after 7–8 h.
- Renal excretion: 100% of an administered dose is excreted in urine.
  - <0.1% of the administered dose is excreted unchanged in urine.

PHARMACOKINETICS

Drug Interaction Profile

Pharmacokinetic Drug Interactions

- Effects by oxybutynin:
  - Oxybutynin increases levels and effects of CYP3A4 substrates (e.g. *carbamazepine*).
  - Oxybutynin decreases levels of *aripiprazole, clozapine, haloperidol, olanzapine, quetiapine, risperidone* by inhibition of GI absorption.
  - Oxybutynin decreases levels of *acetaminophen* by unspecified interaction mechanism.
- Effects on oxybutynin:
  - CYP3A4 inhibitors (e.g. *acetazolamide, clarithromycin, diltiazem, itraconazole, ketoconazole, verapamil*) increase levels and effects of oxybutynin.
  - CYP3A4 inducers (e.g. *carbamazepine, cortisone, dexamethasone, fosphenytoin, phenytoin, prednisone, rifampin, topiramate*), including grapefruit, decrease levels and effects of oxybutynin.

Pharmacodynamic Drug Interactions

- Co-medication with *abobotulinumtoxinA, onabotulinumtoxinA, amantadine*, tricyclic antidepressants, and other agents with anticholinergic properties (e.g. *trazodone*) may enhance potential systemic anticholinergic effects (synergistic action).
- Co-medication with cholinergic agents (e.g. anticholinesterase inhibitors, *pilocarpine, pyridostigmine*) leads to opposing results; effect of interaction is not clear.
- Oxybutynin may reduce the effect of medicinal products, which stimulate GI motility (e.g. *metoclopramide, cisapride*).

Adverse Effects

How Drug Causes Adverse Effects

- Oxybutynin undesirable effects are mostly mediated by its anticholinergic activity.

Common Adverse Effects

- Very common (≥1/10):
  - Dry mouth, constipation, somnolence, nausea, dizziness, headache, fatigue, facial flushing, dry skin/decreased sweating.
- Common (≥1/100 to <1/10):
  - Neuropsychiatric: confusion.
  - Eye/ear: blurred vision, dry eyes.
  - Respiratory: rhinitis.
  - GI: diarrhoea, dyspepsia, vomiting.
  - Renal/urinary: urinary retention.
  - Other: asthenia, pain.
- Uncommon (≥1/1,000 to <1/100):
  - Neuropsychiatric: drowsiness.
  - Eye/ear: light hypersensitivity.

- ○ Cardiovascular: chest discomfort.
- ○ GI: dysphagia, frequent bowel movements, abdominal discomfort.
- ○ Other: anorexia, thirst, fluid retention, dysphonia.

Life-Threatening or Dangerous Adverse Effects
- Rare (≥1/10,000 to <1/1,000):
  - ○ GI obstruction (ER formulations).
- Unknown frequency:
  - ○ Angioedema.
  - ○ Delirium.
  - ○ Hypertension, tachycardia, cardiac arrhythmias.
  - ○ QT prolongation.
  - ○ Seizures.
  - ○ Heat stroke.

Rare and Not Life-Threatening Adverse Effects
- Concentration/memory impairment.
- Excitation.
- Phototoxicity.
- Erectile dysfunction.
- Anxiety, hallucinations, nightmares, paranoia.
- Symptoms of depression and/or dependence in patients with a history of substance abuse.
- Mydriasis, cycloplegia.
- Urinary tract infections.
- Nasal congestion.
- Gastro-oesophageal reflux disease.
- Skin rash, decreased perspiration.

Weight Change
- Not reported.

What to Do About Adverse Effects
- Before introducing oxybutynin, discuss common or life-threatening adverse effects with patients, including symptoms that should be reported to the physician.
  - Patients should be particularly aware of potential CNS adverse reactions related to the drugs antimuscarinic activity, especially after oxybutynin initiation or after dose increase. If such side effects occur, consider dose reduction or complete cessation of therapy.
  - Patients should also be aware that oxybutynin might increase the risk of heat prostration during hot weather due to decreased sweating.
  - Due to high risk of narrow-angle glaucoma, patients should be advised to immediately seek medical help in case of sudden loss of visual acuity or ocular pain.
- If diarrhoea occurs, the possibility of (partial) intestinal obstruction should be excluded, especially in vulnerable patients.

ADVERSE EFFECTS

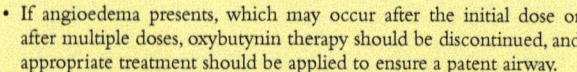

- If angioedema presents, which may occur after the initial dose or after multiple doses, oxybutynin therapy should be discontinued, and appropriate treatment should be applied to ensure a patent airway.
- Regular dental check-ups are advisable during oxybutynin therapy due to high risk of the drug causing dry mouth, which predisposes to dental caries, parodontosis, or oral candidiasis.

OXYBUTYNIN

Dosing and Use

Usual Dosage Range
- IR: 10–20 mg daily.
- ER: 5–30 mg daily.

Available Formulations
- Tablets: 2.5 mg, 5 mg.
- Tablets, extended-release: 5 mg, 10 mg, 15 mg.
- Oral solution: 5 mg/5 ml.
- Transdermal patch: 3.9 mg/24 h.
- Topical gel: 10% weight per weight ethanol-based.

How to Dose
- IR (or oral solution): initial dose of 2.5–5 mg BID or TID; usual maintenance dose is 10–15 mg divided into 2–3 doses; total dose of 20 mg divided in 2–4 doses should not be exceeded.
- ER: initial dose of 5–10 mg OD; may be increased by 5 mg/day at weekly intervals: not to exceed 30 mg/day.
  - Doses of more than 10 mg/day are not often used in practice.
- A personalized scheme with the lowest effective dose should be followed.
- Patient should be reassessed if symptoms do not improve after 2 weeks of therapy.

Dosing Tips
- The 5 mg tablets can be divided into equal halves.
- If IR oxybutynin is not well tolerated, a transdermal or ER formulation can be considered.
  - ER preparations of oxybutynin may be preferred to IR preparations due to lower risk of dry xerostomia.
- Considering the oxybutynin transdermal system:
  - The patch should be applied to intact skin and replaced every 3–4 days.
  - Absorption of oxybutynin is similar following application of the transdermal system to the abdomen, buttock, or hip.
  - Reapplication to the same site should be avoided for 7 days.
- ER tablets are designed to remain intact and slowly release oxybutynin from a non-absorbable shell during passage through the GI tract. Patients should be advised not to be concerned if they notice a tablet-like substance in their stools.

How to Withdraw Drug
- A gradual discontinuation by 25–50% of the daily dose every 1–4 weeks is suggested.
- Consider faster tapering if discontinuing due to adverse events.

Overdose
- Oxybutynin overdose can potentially present with severe anticholinergic effects, including CNS disturbances (from restlessness to excitement and psychotic behaviour), circulatory changes (flushing, hypotension), respiratory failure, paralysis, and coma; clinical manifestations may be prolonged due to delayed absorption in the setting of anticholinergic ileus.
- Immediate gastric lavage and physostigmine administration by slow IV injection are suggested; activated charcoal, as well as a purgative may also be administered.
  - IV physostigmine: 0.5–2 mg; repeat after 5 min if considered necessary up to a maximum total dose of 2 mg.
- In pronounced restless/excitation, consider administering IV diazepam 10 mg.
- In case of tachycardia, consider administering IV propranolol.
- Supportive measures, close monitoring of core temperature, vital signs, mental status, and maintenance of a clear airway with adequate ventilation are recommended.
  - Protect airway early in patients with severe intoxication, as these patients may develop paralysis of respiratory muscles.
- In overdose of ER formulations, patients should be monitored for 24 h.
- Following overdose with the oxybutynin patch, the patch(es) should be removed, and patients should be monitored until any symptoms have resolved.

Tests and Therapeutic Drug Monitoring
- Before initiation of oxybutynin therapy:
  - The diagnosis of neurogenic bladder should be confirmed by cystometry and other appropriate diagnostic procedures before oxybutynin therapy is applied.
- During oxybutynin therapy:
  - The patient's response to therapy should be periodically evaluated by cystometry.

Other Warnings/Precautions
- Caution is advised in male patients with lower urinary tract symptoms or benign prostatic hyperplasia, as oxybutynin use may cause reduced urinary flow and urinary retention.
  - Prostatic hypertrophy is a contraindication of oxybutynin use.
- Close monitoring is advised in mild-to-moderate ulcerative colitis and partial obstructive uropathy, as oxybutynin may aggravate these conditions.

DOSING AND USE

OXYBUTYNIN

- Close monitoring is advised in decreased GI motility, hiatus hernia/gastro-oesophageal reflux, or for those concurrently treated with medicinal products that may trigger or aggravate oesophagitis/high risk for gastric retention.
- Caution is advised in autonomic neuropathy (including relevant cases of Parkinson's disease), as oxybutynin may exacerbate symptoms of decreased GI motility.
- Close monitoring is recommended in hypertension, coronary heart disease, cardiac arrhythmias, heart failure, or hyperthyroidism, as oxybutynin use might aggravate tachycardia.
- Oxybutynin use should be avoided in elderly patients with delirium or at high risk of delirium, or in patients with dementia or cognitive impairment.
- Close monitoring is advised when co-administered with medicinal compounds, which are CYP3A4 substrates or induce/inhibit CYP3A4 metabolism.
- Caution is advised when co-administered with other drugs with anticholinergic properties. A 1-week interval is suggested after discontinuation of oxybutynin therapy before introducing another anticholinergic agent.
- Caution is advised when co-administered with cholinergic agents due to opposing effects and doubtful therapeutic results.
- When concomitant treatment with medicinal products administered sublingually (e.g. sublingual nitrates) is employed, patients should be informed that absorption may be impaired due to a high risk of oxybutynin causing dry mouth. Patients should be advised to moisten their mouth with a little water before taking a sublingual tablet.
- Concurrent use with alcohol or other sedative drugs may enhance drowsiness and should be avoided.
- Oxybutynin may cause blurred vision and somnolence; therefore, driving or operating dangerous machinery is not advised, at least until patients know how therapy affects them.

Do Not Use (Contraindications)
- Known sensitivity to oxybutynin or to any of its excipients, including lactose.
  - Patients with rare hereditary problems of galactose intolerance, total lactase deficiency, or glucose–galactose malabsorption.
- Functional or organic gastric or urinary obstruction or retention, including paralytic ileus and pyloric stenosis.
- Severe GI condition, including history of ileostomy, colostomy, toxic megacolon, or severe ulcerative colitis.
- Frequent urination at night caused by heart or kidney disease.
- Narrow-angle glaucoma or shallow anterior chamber.
- Myasthenia gravis.
- Tachycardia secondary to cardiac insufficiency or thyrotoxicosis.
- Cholinergic subtype of Parkinson's disease where use of anticholinergics can be hazardous owing to worsening cognitive function.

Special Populations
Renal Impairment
- No data are available.
- Caution is advised if oxybutynin is administered in patients with renal impairment.

Hepatic Impairment
- No data are available.
- Caution is advised if oxybutynin is administered in patients with hepatic impairment.

Elderly
- Elimination half-life increases 3–5 times in geriatric patients.
- An initial dose of 2.5 mg BID is suggested, especially in frail patients, which might also be adequate as a maintenance dose. A maximum dose of 5 mg BID can be used.
- There is some evidence that transdermal formulations may be better tolerated in the elderly, although direct comparative studies are not currently available.

Pregnancy
- No data are available on the use of oxybutynin during pregnancy in humans.
- Results from animal studies have not demonstrated any direct negative effects of oxybutynin on fetal development, miscarriage, rate or parturition.
- Oxybutynin should not be used during pregnancy, unless clearly necessary, as potential risks for the fetus cannot be excluded.

Breastfeeding
- Oxybutynin is excreted in human milk in small amounts.
- No data are available on the effect of oxybutynin on nursing infants or milk production.
- Oxybutynin use is not recommended during breastfeeding.

Costs
NHS indicative costs accessed on 31 December 2022:
- Ditropan tablets (Neon Healthcare Ltd) – 84 × 2.5 mg tablets: £1.60; 84 × 5 mg tablets: £2.90.
- Kentera 3.9 mg/24 h patches (Accord Healthcare Ltd) – 8 patches: £27.20.
- Oxybutynin 2.5 mg tablets – 56 × 2.5 mg tablets: £1.42–£6.58; 84 × 2.5 mg tablets: £1.60–£7.00.
- Oxybutynin 3 mg tablets – 56 × 3 mg tablets: £14.00–£24.80.
- Oxybutynin 5 mg tablets – 56 × 5 mg tablets: £1.41–£5.53, 84 × 5 mg tablets: £2.00–£6.50.

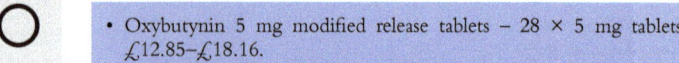

- Oxybutynin 5 mg modified release tablets – 28 × 5 mg tablets: £12.85–£18.16.
- Oxybutynin 10 mg modified release tablets – 28 × 10 mg tablets: £25.70–£36.33.
- Oxybutynin 2.5 mg/5 ml oral solution – 150 ml solution: £150.39–£214.84.
- Oxybutynin 5 mg/5 ml oral solution – 150 ml solution: £173.94–£247.00.

OXYBUTYNIN

The Overall Place of Oxybutynin in the Treatment of Parkinson's Disease

Oxybutynin is the longest-established antimuscarinic drug that is approved and indicated for the treatment of overactive bladder symptoms, including urinary frequency and urgency, and for patients with detrusor instability related to neurogenic bladder. Anticholinergic agents are marketed as a first-line treatment option for overactive bladder symptoms; despite being characterized as 'peripheral' anticholinergics, their use has been associated with cognitive deterioration and other central anticholinergic effects, especially in geriatric patients. Oral oxybutynin is not commonly prescribed in older adults (particularly if they are cognitively impaired), as it has been associated with the worst effect on cognitive deterioration among antimuscarinic agents. Moreover, oxybutynin dosage higher than 10 mg/day is of questionable value in clinical practice due to safety concerns. New formulations of oxybutynin have been introduced to the market in order to enhance the adverse effect profile. ER preparations of oxybutynin may be preferred over IR preparations, as they are associated with a lower risk of dry mouth without any apparent loss of efficacy. On the other hand, the transdermal system of oxybutynin may be a useful therapeutic option, especially among Parkinson's disease patients with dysphagia and drooling, as it does not carry the same risk of worsening cognition compared to other marketed antimuscarinic agents and has a comparable tolerability profile with fewer side effects from the GI system. Local skin reactions may appear though.

Potential Advantages
- Oxybutynin offers the option of transdermal application.
- The total cost of oxybutynin therapy is favourable compared to other antimuscarinic agents.
- Oxybutynin may be useful in patients with overactive bladder and concurrent Parkinson's disease-related drooling.

Potential Disadvantages
- Among antimuscarinic drugs, high doses of oxybutynin (>10 mg) have been associated with significantly more side effects.
- Oxybutynin is less well tolerated than *solifenacin* in older patients.

- According to a recent, large retrospective cohort study, oxybutynin, among antimuscarinic agents, was significantly more likely to cause cognitive decline.
- Oxybutynin may aggravate symptoms of Parkinson's disease.

Clinical Box

A 65-year-old man with advanced Parkinson's disease presented at the Neurology Department Outpatient Clinic for his regular follow-up assessment. The patient had been recently treated with mirabegron for overactive bladder symptoms; however, he had to discontinue therapy due to hypertension. Because he was cognitively intact and was also complaining of dysphagia, the patient was prescribed transdermal oxybutynin 3.9 mg with good response of his symptoms.

Suggested Reading

Herschorn S, L Stothers, K Carlson, B Egerdie, JB Gajewski, P Pommerville, J Schulz, S Radomski, H Drutz, J Barkin, F Paradiso-Hardy. Tolerability of 5 mg solifenacin once daily versus 5 mg oxybutynin immediate release 3 times daily: results of the VECTOR trial. *J Urol* 2010; 183(5): 1892–1898.

Wagg A, M Dale, R Tretter, B Stow, G Compion. Randomised, multicentre, placebo-controlled, double-blind crossover study investigating the effect of solifenacin and oxybutynin in elderly people with mild cognitive impairment: the SENIOR study. *Eur Urol* 2013; 64(1): 74–81.

References

AHFS Drug information, 2012. Bethesda: American Society of Health-System Pharmacists. Accessed on 31 December 2022 via www.medicinescomplete.com.

Buser N, S Ivic, TM Kessler, AG Kessels, LM Bachmann. Efficacy and adverse events of antimuscarinics for treating overactive bladder: network meta-analyses. *Eur Urol*, 2012; 62(6): 1040–1060.

Joint Formulary Committee. British National Formulary (online). London: BMJ Group and Pharmaceutical Press. Accessed on 31 December 2022 via www.medicinescomplete.com.

Kessler TM, LM Bachmann, C Minder, D Löhrer, M Umbehr, HJ Schünemann, AG Kessels. Adverse event assessment of antimuscarinics for treating overactive bladder: a network meta-analytic approach. *PLoS One* 2011; 6(2): e16718.

Oxybutynin. In: Brayfield A (Ed.), *Martindale: The Complete Drug Reference*. London: The Royal Pharmaceutical Society of Great Britain. Accessed on 31 December 2022 via www.medicinescomplete.com.

REFERENCES

Oxybutynin. In: DRUGDEX® System (electronic version). Truven Health Analytics, Greenwood Village, Colorado, USA. Accessed on 31 December 2022 via www.micromedexsolutions.com.

Summary of product characteristics – Ditropan 2.5 mg tablets. Neon Healthcare Ltd. Electronic Medicines Compendium: Ditropan 2.5 mg tablets – summary of product characteristics (SmPC) – (emc). Accessed on 31 December 2022 via www.medicines.org.uk.

Vouri SM, CD Kebodeaux, PM Stranges, BF Teshome. Adverse events and treatment discontinuations of antimuscarinics for the treatment of overactive bladder in older adults: a systematic review and meta-analysis. *Arch Gerontol Geriatr* 2017; 69: 77–96.

Wagg A, W Gibson, J Ostaszkiewicz, T Johnson 3rd, A Markland, MH Palmer, G Kuchel, G Szonyi, R Kirschner-Hermanns. Urinary incontinence in frail elderly persons: report from the 5th International Consultation on Incontinence. *Neurourol Urodyn* 2015; 34(5): 398–406.

Welk B, JA McClure. The impact of anticholinergic use for overactive bladder on cognitive changes in adults with normal cognition, mild cognitive impairment, or dementia. *Eur Urol Open Sci* 2022; 46: 22–29.

Yoo DS, JY Han, KS Lee, MS Choo. Prescription pattern of oxybutynin ER in patients with overactive bladder in real life practice: a multicentre, open-label, prospective observational study. *Int J Clin Pract* 2012; 66(2): 132–138.

OXYBUTYNIN

PIMAVANSERIN

P

Therapeutics

Chemical Name and Structure

Pimavanserin (1-[(4-fluorophenyl)methyl]-1-(1-methylpiperidin-4-yl)-3-[[4-(2-methylpropoxy)pneyl]methyl]urea) has a molecular weight of 427.6 and an empirical formula of $C_{25}H_{34}FN_3O_2$ (free base).

Brand Names
- **Nuplazid** (*USA*).

Generics Available
- No.

Licensed Indications for Parkinson's Disease
- Hallucinations and delusions associated with Parkinson's disease psychosis (FDA).

Licensed Indications for Other Conditions
- None.

Non-Licensed Use for Parkinson's Disease
- None.

Non-Licensed Use for Other Conditions
- Dementia-related psychosis (including Alzheimer's disease, LBD, FTD, or vascular dementia).
- Primitive findings on refractory psychosis in the context of schizophrenia and schizoaffective disorder.

Ineffective
- Agitation in dementia.

Mechanism of Action
- Pimavanserin's beneficial effect on psychosis is believed to be mediated by a selective serotonin inverse agonist activity, preferentially targeting 5-HT2A serotonergic receptors, and maybe to a lesser extent the 5-HT2C serotonergic and sigma-1 receptors.
  - In contrast to an antagonist, which would not change any intrinsic characteristics of the receptor, pimavanserin causes a response opposite to an agonist.
- Pimavanserin exhibits no effect on dopaminergic, muscarinic, adrenergic, and histaminergic receptors.
- An open-label, 8-week study has shown that pimavanserin was associated with early and sustained improvement of depressive symptoms in Parkinson's disease patients.

THERAPEUTICS

P

Efficacy Profile
- According to the MDS EBM Committee, pimavanserin is 'efficacious' and 'clinically useful' for treating psychosis in Parkinson's disease over a 6-week period.
- Results from two double-blind RCTs showed a beneficial effect of pimavanserin on Parkinson's disease-related psychosis without significant side effects or deterioration of motor performance.
- Results from a pivotal randomized study showed pimavanserin had a beneficial effect both on cognitively intact and cognitively impaired Parkinson's disease patients, while this effect seemed to be amplified when pimavanserin was co-administered with cognition-enhancing drugs, such as cholinesterase inhibitors. However, the use of the latter was associated with more serious side effects and therapy discontinuations.
- An open-label study showed the efficacy of pimavanserin was maintained for a period of 10 weeks.
- Pimavanserin may ameliorate nocturnal sleeping without causing diurnal sedation.
- According to a retrospective cohort study directly comparing quetiapine to pimavanserin, pimavanserin may be more clinically useful for the treatment of Parkinson's disease-related psychosis due to lower rates of early discontinuation.
- Pimavanserin use has been associated with a decrease in the perceived burden of Parkinson's disease patients' caregivers.

Pharmacokinetics

Absorption and Distribution
- Oral bioavailability: about 99%.
- Food co-ingestion: a prolongation of Tmax was observed (~4 h), although this was not found to be clinically relevant.
  - In the presence of high-fat meals maximum plasma concentration and AUC decrease by 9% and increase by 8%, respectively; not clinically meaningful.
- Tmax: 6 h (4–24 h).
- Time to steady state: about 12–14 days with continuous once daily treatment.
- Pharmacokinetics: linear in single oral doses ranging from 17 mg to 225 mg.
- Protein binding: about 91–97%.
- Volume of distribution: 2,021 l.

Metabolism
- Pimavanserin is mainly metabolized by CYP3A4 and CYP3A5.
- CYP3A4 metabolism produces the major active *N*-desmethylated metabolite (AC-279).

- Pimavanserin is metabolized to a lesser extent by CYP2J2 and CYP2D6.
- Neither pimavanserin nor AC-279 act as clinically significant CYP inhibitors or inducers.

Elimination
- Half-life is 57 h for the parent drug and about 200 h for the active metabolite.
- Approximately 0.5% of an administered dose is excreted unchanged in the urine and about 1.5% is found unchanged in faeces.

Drug Interaction Profile
Pharmacokinetic Drug Interactions
- Effects on pimavanserin:
  - Co-administration with CYP3A4 inhibitors (e.g. *chloramphenicol, clarithromycin, isoniazid, ketoconazole*), including grapefruit consumption, might increase the levels of pimavanserin.
  - Co-administration with CYP3A4 inducers (e.g. *carbamazepine, phenytoin, rifampin*), might decrease the levels of pimavanserin.

Pharmacodynamic Drug Interactions
- Co-medication with drugs causing electrolyte imbalance or increasing QT interval, such as Class IA and III antiarrhythmics, antipsychotics (e.g. *haloperidol, phenothiazine* derivatives, *pimozide*), tricyclic antidepressants, certain antimicrobial agents (e.g. *moxifloxacin, erythromycin*), certain antihistamines (e.g. *astemizole, mizolastine*), and others may lead to potentially fatal Torsade de Pointes arrhythmias and is considered a risk factor for sudden cardiac death.

Adverse Effects
How Drug Causes Adverse Effects
- Not reported.

Common Adverse Effects
- Common (≥1/100 to <1/10):
  - Neuropsychiatric: dizziness, somnolence, confusion, hallucinations, gait disturbance, headache, fatigue.
  - GI: nausea, constipation, diarrhoea.
  - Other: peripheral oedema, falls, urinary tract infections.

Life-Threatening or Dangerous Adverse Effects
- Angioedema.

Rare and Not Life-Threatening Adverse Effects
- Not reported.

P

Weight Change
• Not reported.

What to Do About Adverse Effects
• Before introducing pimavanserin, discuss common or life-threatening adverse effects with patients and/or caregivers, including symptoms that should be reported to the physician, such as new-onset palpitations, syncope, or near-syncope, which might refer to QTc prolongation.
• If adverse events are troublesome or persist, consider withdrawing pimavanserin.

Dosing and Use

Usual Dosage Range
• 17–34 mg daily.

Available Formulations
Only available as immediate-release formulations.
• Capsule 34 mg.
• Tablet 17 mg.

How to Dose
• The recommended dose is 34 mg, taken as either one 34 mg capsule or two 17 mg tablets OD, without titration.

Dosing Tips
• It may be consumed with or without food.
• In case of inability to swallow pimavanserin capsules, contents may be sprinkled over 15 ml of applesauce, yogurt, pudding, or liquid nutritional supplement, or the capsule may be consumed immediately without chewing as a mixture with food.
• Treating physicians should be aware that occasionally pimavanserin might cause a paradoxical worsening of psychosis, early after treatment initiation.
• In case of switching to pimavanserin from a low dose of quetiapine (<100 mg), full-dose pimavanserin (34 mg) should be added to quetiapine for a period of 4 weeks. Quetiapine can be subsequently reduced by half every week until the dose of 12.5 mg OD is reached, and then withdrawn.
• In case of switching to pimavanserin from a low dose of clozapine (<100 mg), full dose pimavanserin (34 mg) should be added to clozapine for a period of 6 weeks. Clozapine can be subsequently reduced by 6.25 mg per week until complete withdrawal. Tapering should not last less than 4 weeks.
  • If the antipsychotic effect diminishes during quetiapine or clozapine tapering, consider returning to the previous quetiapine or clozapine dose level and reintroduce tapering after 1 week.

How to Withdraw Drug
• Due to its long half-life, pimavanserin can be abruptly discontinued.

Overdose
• No available information to date considering Parkinson's disease patients. Dose-limiting nausea and vomiting have been observed in healthy subjects.
• There is no specific antidote available.

Tests and Therapeutic Drug Monitoring
• Before initiation of pimavanserin therapy:
  • A baseline ECG should be performed.

Other Warnings/Precautions
• Caution is advised when administering pimavanserin in patients at high risk of prolonged cardiac repolarization (e.g. co-medication with drugs increasing QTc interval, symptomatic bradycardia and other cardiac arrhythmias, family history of QT prolongation, congenital long QT syndrome, bradycardia, congestive heart failure, recent history of MI, heart hypertrophy, hypokalaemia, or hypomagnesaemia), especially in the elderly.
• When co-administered with strong CYP3A4 inhibitors, a dose reduction of pimavanserin at 17 mg OD is suggested.
• When co-administered with strong CYP3A4 inducers, an increase in pimavanserin dosage may be needed.

Do Not Use (Contraindications)
• Known sensitivity to the active substance or any of its excipients.
• In elderly patients with dementia-related psychosis, as it has been associated with an increased all-cause risk of death (black box warning).
• Grapefruit consumption.

Special Populations
Renal Impairment
• Mild to moderate (CrCl > 30 ml/min): no dose adjustment is necessary.
• Severe (CrCl < 30 ml/min) or end-stage renal impairment: contraindicated.

Hepatic Impairment
• No available data.
• Not recommended with any degree of hepatic impairment.

Elderly
• No dose adjustment is needed.

P

Pregnancy
- No reports of pimavanserin-associated risk of major congenital malformations or miscarriage in humans.
- No adverse events have been reported in animal studies.
- If pimavanserin administration is needed during pregnancy, close observation is necessary.

Breastfeeding
- It is not known whether pimavanserin is distributed into human milk.
- Potential benefits and risks from the drug or the mother's subjacent condition should be weighed before deciding if pimavanserin should be discontinued or the mother should not breastfeed.

Costs
- Not available in the UK for comparative costs.

The Overall Place of Pimavanserin in the Treatment of Parkinson's Disease

Pimavanserin is the only FDA-approved atypical antipsychotic for hallucinations and delusions in the context of Parkinson's disease-related psychosis, an entity that is difficult to manage due to lack of effective and safe therapeutic options. Being a serotonin 5-HT2A inverse agonist without any effect on other neurotransmitter receptors, pimavanserin has a unique pharmacological profile and constitutes a major breakthrough in the pharmacotherapy of Parkinson's disease-related non-motor symptoms. In contrast to other antipsychotic medication, it does not aggravate motor performance due to the lack of any activity on dopaminergic receptors. Although there are currently no other approved indications for pimavanserin, numerous ongoing studies explore its therapeutic potential in other conditions, including Alzheimer's disease. Pimavanserin is generally considered safe with a relatively benign tolerability profile. According to a recently published, large retrospective cohort study, pimavanserin use among community-dwelling Parkinson's disease patients with psychosis was associated with 35% lower mortality compared to other atypical antipsychotics during the first 6 months of therapy.

Potential Advantages
- Special monitoring is not necessary.
- Once per day administration, which might improve patients' adherence.
- No exacerbation of Parkinson's disease motor symptoms.
- No dose reduction of concomitant antiparkinsonian dopaminergic medication.

- Pimavanserin use carries a lower risk for orthostatic hypotension, sedation, and metabolic syndrome compared to quetiapine and clozapine.
- There have been no reports of pimavanserin-related NMS, tardive dyskinesias, or serotonin syndrome.

Potential Disadvantages
- It currently lacks approval in Europe and is not commercially available in numerous countries around the globe.
- Lack of controlled safety data beyond 6 weeks of therapy and long-term experience in routine clinical practice, although the analysis of post-marketing reports has not revealed any unexpected side effects.
- Increased cost.
- Compared to clozapine or quetiapine, it may take longer (a minimum of 2 weeks, typically 4–6 weeks) to demonstrate any clinical benefit. The time to onset of therapeutic action is crucial when considering switching from drugs with shorter half-lives to pimavanserin.

Clinical Box
A 72-year-old woman with a 10-year history of Parkinson's disease was urgently assessed by her treating neurologist due to troublesome visual hallucinations and paranoid ideation, occurring a few days after replacing levodopa/carbidopa with levodopa/carbidopa/entacapone tablets due to end-of-dose OFF phenomena. The patient was instructed to discontinue entacapone and reintroduce the previous scheme of levodopa/carbidopa; however, the psychotic features persisted. The rest of her medical history included hypertension, hypercholesterolaemia, and diabetes mellitus type 2. Other causes of hallucinations were excluded (e.g. subjacent infection) and pimavanserin 17 mg BID was prescribed. Targeted symptoms resolved in 3 weeks without the patient reporting any side effects.

Suggested Reading
Black, K.J., et al., *Guidance for switching from off-label antipsychotics to pimavanserin for Parkinson's disease psychosis: an expert consensus.* CNS Spectr, 2018. **23**(6): p. 402–413.

Bozymski, K.M., D.K. Lowe, K.M. Pasternak, T.L. Gatesman, and E.L. Crouse. *Pimavanserin: A Novel Antipsychotic for Parkinson's Disease Psychosis.* Ann Pharmacother, 2017. **51**(6): p. 479–487.

Cummings, J., S. Isaacson, R. Mills, H. Williams, K. Chi-Burris, A. Corbett, R. Dhall, and C. Ballard, *Pimavanserin for patients with Parkinson's disease psychosis: a randomised, placebo-controlled phase 3 trial.* Lancet, 2014. **383**(9916): p. 533–40.

P

P

Mosholder, A.D., et al., *Mortality Among Parkinson's Disease Patients Treated With Pimavanserin or Atypical Antipsychotics: An Observational Study in Medicare Beneficiaries.* Am J Psychiatry, 2022. **179**(8): p. 553–561.

Sahli, Z.T. and F.I. Tarazi, *Pimavanserin: novel pharmacotherapy for Parkinson's disease psychosis.* Expert Opin Drug Discov, 2018. **13**(1): p. 103–110.

References

Ballard C, C Banister, Z Khan, J Cummings, G Demos, B Coate, JM Youakim, R Owen, S Stankovic. Evaluation of the safety, tolerability, and efficacy of pimavanserin versus placebo in patients with Alzheimer's disease psychosis: a phase 2, randomised, placebo-controlled, double-blind study. *Lancet Neurol* 2018; 17(3): 213–222.

Bozymski KM, DK Lowe, KM Pasternak, TL Gatesman, EL Crouse. Pimavanserin: a novel antipsychotic for Parkinson's disease psychosis. *Ann Pharmacother* 2017; 51(6): 479–487.

Cummings J, C Ballard, P Tariot, R Owen, E Foff, J Youakim, J Norton, S Stankovic. Pimavanserin: potential treatment for dementia-related psychosis. *J Prev Alzheimers Dis* 2018; 5(4): 253–258.

DeKarske D, G Alva, JL Aldred, B Coate, M Cantillon, L Jacobi, R Nunez, JC Norton, V Abler. An open-label, 8-week study of safety and efficacy of pimavanserin treatment in adults with Parkinson's disease and depression. *J Parkinsons Dis* 2020; 10(4): 1751–1761.

Espay AJ, MT Guskey, JC Norton, B Coate, JA Vizcarra, C Ballard, SA Factor, JH Friedman, AE Lang, NJ Larsen, C Andersson, D Fredericks, D Weintraub. Pimavanserin for Parkinson's disease psychosis: effects stratified by baseline cognition and use of cognitive-enhancing medications. *Mov Disord* 2018; 33(11): 1769–1776.

Hawkins T, BD Berman. Pimavanserin: a novel therapeutic option for Parkinson disease psychosis. *Neurol Clin Pract* 2017; 7(2): 157–162.

Horn S, H Richardson, SX Xie, D Weintraub, N Dahodwala. Pimavanserin versus quetiapine for the treatment of psychosis in Parkinson's disease and dementia with Lewy bodies. *Parkinsonism Relat Disord* 2019; 69: 119–124.

Isaacson SH, B Coate, J Norton, S Stankovic. Blinded SAPS-pd assessment after 10 weeks of pimavanserin treatment for Parkinson's disease psychosis. *J Parkinsons Dis* 2020; 10(4): 1389–1396.

Meltzer HY, R Mills, S Revell, H Williams, A Johnson, D Bahr, JH Friedman. Pimavanserin, a serotonin(2A) receptor inverse agonist, for the treatment of Parkinson's disease psychosis. *Neuropsychopharmacology* 2010; 35(4): 881–892.

Nasrallah HA, R Fedora, R Morton. Successful treatment of clozapine-nonresponsive refractory hallucinations and delusions with pimavanserin, a serotonin 5HT-2A receptor inverse agonist. *Schizophr Res* 2019; 208: 217–220.

PIMAVANSERIN

P

Pimavanserin. In: Brayfield A (Ed.), *Martindale: The Complete Drug Reference*. London: The Royal Pharmaceutical Society of Great Britain. Accessed on 4 December 2022 via www.medicinescomplete.com.

Schneider LS. The safety of pimavanserin for Parkinson's disease and efforts to reduce antipsychotics for people with dementia. *Am J Psychiatry* 2022; 179(8): 519–521.

Tariot PN, JL Cummings, ME Soto-Martin, C Ballard, D Erten-Lyons, DL Sultzer, DP Devanand, D Weintraub, B McEvoy, JM Youakim, S Stankovic, EP Foff. Trial of pimavanserin in dementia-related psychosis. *N Engl J Med* 2021; 385(4): 309–319.

Webster P. Pimavanserin evaluated by the FDA. *Lancet* 2018; 391(10132): 1762.

P

PIRIBEDIL

Therapeutics

Chemical Name and Structure

Piribedil (2-(4-piperonylpiperazin-1-yl)pyrimidine) is a non-ergot dopamine agonist with a molecular weight of 298.34 and an empirical formula of $C_{16}H_{18}N_4O_2$.

Brand Names

* **Clarium** (*Germany*).
* **Pronokognil** (*Russian Federation*); **Pronoran** (*Greece, Lithuania, Poland, Russian Federation, Ukraine*).
* **Trastal** (*China*); **Trivastal** (*Argentina, Brazil, France, Greece, India, Malaysia, Philippines, Portugal, Singapore, Tunisia, Turkey, Venezuela*); **Trivastan** (*Italy*); **Tivastal** (*Egypt, Tunisia*).

Generics Available

* Not reported.

Licensed Indications for Parkinson's Disease

* As a monotherapy in Parkinson's disease (especially in cases with pre-dominant tremor) (EMA).
* As an adjunct therapy to levodopa preparations, amantadine and anticholinergic agents (especially in cases with predominant tremor) (EMA).

Licensed Indications for Other Conditions

* As an adjunctive symptomatic therapy in elderly individuals with chronic cognitive and neurosensorial deficits.
* As an adjunctive therapy in cases of intermittent claudication in chronic obliterating arteriopathies of the lower limbs (stage 2).
* Suggested use in ischaemic symptoms in ophthalmology.

Non-Licensed Use for Parkinson's Disease

* Parkinson's disease-related apathy.

Non-Licensed Use for Other Conditions

* As an adjunctive symptomatic therapy in elderly individuals with chronic cognitive and neurosensorial deficits, including MCI.
* As an adjunctive therapy in cases of intermittent claudication in chronic obliterating arteriopathies of the lower limbs (stage 2).
* Suggested use in ischaemic symptoms in ophthalmology.

Ineffective

* Alzheimer's disease and other dementias.

P

Mechanism of Action
- Piribedil is a selective, non-ergot, partial agonist of D2 and D3 dopaminergic receptors (similar to ropinirole and pramipexole).
  - Piribedil affinity for D2 and D3 dopaminergic receptors is lower compared to ropinirole and pramipexole.
  - The characterization of piribedil as 'partial' is controversial and is believed to be associated with decreased anti-parkinsonian potency compared to full agonists.
- Both piribedil and its main metabolite, the catechol S584, are thought to act at D1 dopaminergic receptors as well (D3 > D2 > D1).
- Piribedil also has antagonistic effects at α2-adrenergic receptors, low affinity for 5-HT serotonergic receptors, and negligible affinity for histaminergic and cholinergic receptors, which are thought to mediate its efficacy in non-motor Parkinson's disease symptoms.
  - Cholinergic mechanisms are thought to mediate the benefit of piribedil on apathy, cognitive performance, and on excessive daytime sleepiness in Parkinson's disease.
  - α2-Adrenergic antagonism is thought to mediate any antidepressant effects of piribedil and promote neurogenesis at the hippocampus.
- The action of piribedil on peripheral circulation is mediated by dopaminergic receptors in the femoral vascular bed; administration of piribedil leads to an increase in femoral blood flow.

Efficacy Profile
- According to the MDS EBM Committee:
  - piribedil has been characterized as 'efficacious' and 'clinically useful':
    - For symptomatic monotherapy in Parkinson's disease.
    - As an adjunct therapy to levodopa in early or stable Parkinson's disease patients.
  - Piribedil has been characterized as 'likely efficacious' and 'possibly useful' in the treatment of Parkinson's disease-related apathy, including apathy occurring in the context of STN-DBS and post-operative discontinuations of anti-Parkinson's disease medications.
  - There are insufficient data to support the use of piribedil in the management of:
    - Motor fluctuations in Parkinson's disease.
    - Sleep disorders and wakefulness in Parkinson's disease.
- In a randomized study, it was shown that switching from pramipexole or ropinirole to piribedil reduced daytime sleepiness to a clinically relevant degree, while maintaining the same therapeutic motor effect.
- Piribedil has been found to be beneficial on parkinsonian tremor.
- According to pilot studies, sublingual and IV formulations of piribedil were found efficacious in the management of fluctuations in Parkinson's disease. However, no trials are available on oral ER formulations.
- Early uncontrolled studies have shown a positive effect of piribedil on Parkinson's disease-related depressive symptoms, although these results are exploratory.

THERAPEUTICS

- There are some indications that piribedil might exert a beneficial effect on memory and cognition; however, further investigation is necessary.
- Human kinetic studies have shown that the therapeutic coverage of piribedil ER exceeds 24 h.
- The anti-parkinsonian effects are usually observed 2–4 weeks after piribedil initiation.

Pharmacokinetics
Limited information on piribedil pharmacokinetics is available in the literature.

Absorption and Distribution
- Oral bioavailability: less than 10%.
- Food co-ingestion: not reported.
- Tmax: 1 h after oral administration.
- Time to steady state: not reported.
- Pharmacokinetics: IV infusion of escalating doses of piribedil (2–16 mg) has shown linear pharmacokinetics.
- Protein binding: 70–80%.
- Volume of distribution: not reported.

Metabolism
- Piribedil undergoes extensive metabolism in the liver (primarily demethylation, *p*-hydroxylation, and *N*-oxidation), producing several metabolites, one of which is pharmacologically active (1-(3,4-dihydroxybenzyl) 4-(2-pyrimidinyl)-piperazine).

Elimination
- Plasma elimination is biphasic and is composed of a first phase characterized by a half-life of 1.7 h and a second, slower phase characterized by a half-life of 6.9 h. Elimination half-life is about 21 h.
- Excretion: 68% of an administered dose is excreted by the renal route in the form of metabolites and 25% is excreted in bile.
  - No unchanged parent compound is found in the urine.

Drug Interaction Profile
Pharmacokinetic Drug Interactions
- Not reported.

Pharmacodynamic Drug Interactions
- Co-medication with antipsychotics (with the exclusion of *clozapine*) will result in antagonistic effects.
- Co-medication with CNS depressants (e.g. sedatives) or alcohol might exacerbate their sedative effects.

P

Adverse Effects

How Drug Causes Adverse Effects
- Mainly (but not solely) through increasing dopaminergic activity.
- There are indications from animal studies that some adverse events, including hypotension and somnolence, could be mediated by piribedil-induced α2-antagonism.

Common Adverse Effects
- Common (≥1/100 to <1/10):
  - Neuropsychiatric: confusion, hallucinations, agitation, dizziness, somnolence.
  - GI: nausea, vomiting, flatulence.
- Uncommon (≥1/1,000 to <1/100) or unknown frequency:
  - Neuropsychiatric: syncope, dyskinesias, ICDs (e.g. pathological gambling, hypersexuality, increased libido, compulsive spending or shopping, excessive food consumption/food disorders).
  - Cardiovascular: (orthostatic) hypotension, unstable blood pressure, peripheral oedema.
  - Other: allergic reactions (due to the presence of cochineal red).

Life-Threatening or Dangerous Adverse Effects
- Aggression, delusions, delirium.
- Sudden sleep attacks without prodromal signs.
- Neuroleptic malignant syndrome.

Rare and Not Life-Threatening Adverse Effects
- Peripheral oedema.

What to Do About Adverse Effects
- Before introducing piribedil, discuss common or life-threatening adverse effects with patients and/or caregivers, including symptoms that should be reported to the physician.
  - Before therapy initiation, patients should be asked for somnolence or other factors that increase somnolence risk (e.g. CNS depressants, sleep disorders).
- On a regular basis, monitor for sleepiness (which might occur without preceding warning signs, even later in therapy, e.g. after 1 year), drowsiness, hypotension (especially during dosing escalation), ICDs, hallucinations, or psychotic-like behaviours with focused and direct questions to patients and caregivers, as patients might not acknowledge such symptoms as abnormal to report them.
- Minor GI disturbances, such as nausea, vomiting, or flatulence, might disappear by adjusting piribedil dosage, especially by following a stepwise up-titration (50 mg every 2 weeks).
- If patients on piribedil experience somnolence and/or episodes of sudden-onset sleep during activities that require active participation, they should refrain from driving or operating machines and inform their treating physician. Therapy discontinuation is generally advised.

- Patients and their caregivers should be made aware about the possibility of developing ICDs, usually in higher doses. This complication is generally reversible following dose reduction of piribedil or discontinuation of therapy.
- In the case of confusion, agitation, delusion, hallucinations, or delirium, discontinuation of treatment is advised.
- Dyskinesias might occur in advanced-stage Parkinson's disease patients, when piribedil is co-administered with levodopa, especially when first introducing piribedil, although it is generally considered to have a low dyskinetic potential. If dyskinesias occur, the dose of piribedil should be reduced.
- In case of any troublesome side effects, consider lowering piribedil dose or withdrawing therapy.

Dosing and Use

Usual Dosage Range
- ER formulations: 150–250 mg/day, divided at 3–5 equal doses.

Available Formulations
- ER tablets: 50 mg.

How to Dose
- As a monotherapy:
  - Initial dose of 50 mg OD; increase by 50 mg every 3–7 days until a maximum of 150–250 mg per day divided in 3–5 equal doses, respectively.
- As an add-on to levodopa:
  - Initial dose of 50 mg OD; increase by 50 mg every 3–7 days until a maximum of 150 mg/day divided in 3 equal doses (approximately 50 mg of piribedil per 250 mg of levodopa).
- The minimum effective dose is suggested to avoid the risk of ICDs.

Dosing Tips
- Piribedil tablets should be swallowed whole (not chewed) with half a glass of water, at the end of meals.

How to Withdraw Drug
- A gradual withdrawal of piribedil is suggested to limit the possibility of side effects.

Overdose
- Given the emetic effect of piribedil at high doses, overdose of orally administered tablets seems unlikely.
- Overdose might present as blood pressure instability (either hypertension or hypotension) and GI symptoms (nausea, vomiting).

P

- Overdose symptoms are expected to respond to piribedil discontinuation.
- There is no known antidote for dopamine agonists' overdose. General supportive measures are suggested.

Tests and Therapeutic Drug Monitoring
- Monitoring of blood pressure is advised, particularly at the beginning of piribedil therapy and/or when it is used as an add-on to levodopa preparations or in patients with cardiovascular disease.

Other Warnings / Precautions
- Patients should be advised that piribedil may cause somnolence and they should not drive a car or operate complex machinery until they have gained sufficient experience with the drug to determine whether it affects their mental and/or motor performance.

Do Not Use (Contraindications)
- Hypersensitivity to the active substance or to any of its excipients, including sucrose.
  - Patients with fructose intolerance, glucose or galactose malabsorption, or sucrase–isomaltase deficiency.
- During the acute phase of MI or cardiovascular shock.
- Co-medication with CNS depressants or alcohol should be avoided due to additive sedative effects.
- Co-medication with antipsychotics (with the exception of *clozapine*) or antiemetics with extrapyramidal effects (e.g. *metoclopramide*) is not advisable.

SPECIAL POPULATIONS

Special Populations

Renal Impairment
- Not reported.
- Caution is recommended when using piribedil in this group of patients.

Hepatic Impairment
- Not reported.
- Caution is recommended when using piribedil in this group of patients.

Elderly
- No dose adjustments are reported.

Pregnancy
- Piribedil use is not recommended.
- Data on animal models show that piribedil passes the placental barrier and is distributed in fetal organs.

Breastfeeding
- Piribedil use is not recommended.

P

PIRIBEDIL

Costs
• Not available in the UK for comparison.

The Overall Place of Piribedil in the Treatment of Parkinson's Disease

Piribedil was the first marketed dopamine agonist for the treatment of Parkinson's disease in the early 1970s. It exhibits partial agonist properties at D2 and D3 dopaminergic receptors coupled to antagonist actions at α2-adrenoreceptors. Piribedil use is not authorized in the UK or the USA, and it is mostly used in Argentina and other Latin American countries. Its efficacy on motor symptoms of Parkinson's disease, both as a monotherapy and as an adjunctive therapy to levodopa, amantadine, or anticholinergic medications, has been confirmed in high-quality studies, and open-label studies, further supported by ad-hoc clinical observations, have shown a distinctive benefit on parkinsonian tremor compared to levodopa. Its effect on fluctuations remains controversial. Piribedil is one of the few medications that have been considered efficacious for the management of Parkinson's disease-related apathy. There are also preliminary indications that piribedil might exert a beneficial effect on Parkinson's disease-related depressive symptoms, cognitive function, and daytime somnolence; however, these aspects need to be investigated further. In general, piribedil use has been associated with significant side effects, including ICDs, hallucinations, orthostatic hypotension, somnolence, and nausea/vomiting, especially with higher doses. As it is not available in many countries, piribedil is not a first-line option for Parkinson's disease management, even in countries where it has been available for many years. Given the age of the population treated, the risks including falls (whether related to hypotension or not), episodes of sudden-onset sleep, and delirium must be taken into account before therapy initiation.

Potential Advantages
• The alleged partial dopaminergic agonism of piribedil is thought to be sufficient to achieve clinical efficacy, while avoiding dopaminergic hyperstimulation, which might induce dyskinesias and cognitive deterioration in Parkinson's disease patients.
• Piribedil is effective at all Parkinson's disease stages, both as a monotherapy and as an adjunctive therapy to levodopa, while it can be particularly beneficial on parkinsonian tremor, a symptom that occasionally responds poorly to first-line antiparkinsonian drugs.
• Piribedil is one of the very few drugs to be effective on Parkinson's disease-related apathy based on the results of good-quality studies.
• Piribedil may be less prone to cause somnolence compared to other dopamine agonists, but this is not proven.
• Piribedil can be titrated to its common therapeutic efficacy range in less time than other dopamine agonists.

P

Potential Disadvantages
- Piribedil is not available in all countries.
- Piribedil has an unfavourable adverse events profile.
- In contrast to other ER formulations, piribedil is prescribed three times daily.
- Similarly to other dopamine agonists, development of ICDs, hallucinations or psychotic-like behaviour, sudden sleep attacks, and orthostatic hypotension is a possibility among patients treated with piribedil and might lead to severe sequelae in patients' life (e.g. financial difficulties, injuries).

Clinical Box

A 50-year-old man was referred to the Movement Disorders Outpatient Clinic due to unilateral tremor of the left arm. He also reported having lost interest in his surroundings and lacking any motivation to engage in activities, a behaviour which was quite prominent during the last few months and was not typical of his personality. The rest of his medical history included hypercholesterolaemia and hypothyroidism. Clinical examination revealed mild bilateral bradykinesia and rigidity, more pronounced on the left side. Apathy was also detected, without any signs of depressive symptoms, and, upon targeted questioning, the patient reported anosmia and constipation over the past few years. He mentioned no history of ICDs, somnolence or psychotic behaviour. A clinical diagnosis of Parkinson's disease was made, while the results of a scheduled brain MRI scan were unremarkable. Piribedil ER tablets 50 mg OD were prescribed and the patient was given instructions for gradual weekly increases (50 mg per week) until the dose of 50 mg TID was reached.

Suggested Reading

Perez-Lloret S, O Rascol. Piribedil for the Treatment of Motor and Non-motor Symptoms of Parkinson Disease. *CNS Drugs* 2016; 30(8): 703–717.

Thobois S, E Lhommée, H Klinger, C Ardouin, E Schmitt, A Bichon, A Kirstner, A Castrioto, J Xie, V Fraix, P Pelissier, S Chabardes, P Mertens, JL Quesada, JL Bosson, P Pollak, E Broussolle, P Krack. Parkinsonian apathy responds to dopaminergic stimulation of D2/D3 receptors with piribedil. *Brain* 2013: 136(Pt 5): 1568–1577.

References

Czernecki V, M Schüpbach, S Yaici, R Lévy, E Bardinet, J Yelnik, B Dubois, Y Agid. Apathy following subthalamic stimulation in Parkinson disease: a dopamine responsive symptom. *Mov Disord* 2008: 23(7): 964–969.

REFERENCES

P

Deleu D, MG Northway, Y Hanssens. Clinical pharmacokinetic and pharmacodynamic properties of drugs used in the treatment of Parkinson's disease. *Clin Pharmacokinet* 2002; 41(4): 261–309.

Eggert K, C Öhlwein, J Kassubek, M Wolz, A Kupsch, A Ceballos-Baumann, R Ehret, U Polzer, F Klostermann, J Schwartz, G Fuchs, W Jost, A Albert, A Haag, A Hermsen, K Lohmüller, K Kuhn, M Wangemann, W Hoertel. Influence of the nonergot dopamine agonist piribedil on vigilance in patients with Parkinson disease and excessive daytime sleepiness (PiViCog-PD): an 11-week randomized comparison trial against pramipexole and ropinirole. *Clin Neuropharmacol* 2014; 37(4): 116–122.

Jenner P. Parkinson's disease: pathological mechanisms and actions of piribedil. *J Neurol* 1992; 239(Suppl 1): S2–S8.

Lebrun-Frenay C, M Borg. Choosing the right dopamine agonist for patients with Parkinson's disease. *Curr Med Res Opin* 2002; 18(4): 209–214.

Mentenopoulos G, Z Katsou, S Bostantjopoulou, J Logothetis. Piribedil therapy in Parkinson's disease. Use of the drug in the retard form. *Clin Neuropharmacol* 1989; 12(1): 23–28.

Millan MJ. From the cell to the clinic: a comparative review of the partial D_2/D_3receptor agonist and $\alpha2$-adrenoceptor antagonist, piribedil, in the treatment of Parkinson's disease. *Pharmacol Ther* 2010; 128(2): 229–273.

Nagaraja D, S Jayashree. Randomized study of the dopamine receptor agonist piribedil in the treatment of mild cognitive impairment. *Am J Psychiatry* 2001; 158(9): 1517–1519.

Nyholm D. Pharmacokinetic optimisation in the treatment of Parkinson's disease: an update. *Clin Pharmacokinet* 2006; 45(2): 109–136.

Piribedil. In: Brayfield A (Ed.), *Martindale: The Complete Drug Reference*. London: The Royal Pharmaceutical Society of Great Britain. Accessed on 4 December 2022 via www.medicinescomplete.com.

Rondot P, M Ziegler. Activity and acceptability of piribedil in Parkinson's disease: a multicentre study. *J Neurol* 1992; 239(Suppl 1): S28–S34.

Rota S, I Boura, L Batzu, N Titova, P Jenner, C Falup-Pecurariu, KR Chaudhuri. 'Dopamine agonist phobia' in Parkinson's disease: when does it matter? Implications for non-motor symptoms and personalized medicine. *Expert Rev Neurother* 2020; 20(9): 953–365.

PIRIBEDIL

PRAMIPEXOLE★

★Pramipexole doses reported in the literature and the following chapter refer to pramipexole salt, unless stated otherwise.

Therapeutics

Chemical Name and Structure

Pramipexole ((S)-2-amino-4,5,6,7-tetrahydro-6(propylamino)benzo-thiazole dihydrochloride monohydrate) is a white to off-white powder, freely soluble in water. It is a dopamine agonist with a molecular weight of 302.3 and an empirical formula of $C_{10}H_{17}N_3S,2HCl,H_2O$.

Brand Names

- **Apoxole** (*South Africa*); **Astepen, Axalanz** (*Greece*).
- **Biopsol** (*Chile*); **BI-Sifrol** (*Japan*).
- **Calmolan** (*Austria, Czech Republic, Hungary, Lithuania*).
- **Derinik** (*Sweden*).
- **Erimexol** (*Hungary*); **Ezaprev** (*Estonia, Italy, Lithuania*).
- **Frodix** (*Greece*).
- **Glepark** (*Czech Republic, Denmark, Germany, Greece, Netherlands*).
- **Hitoff** (*Poland*).
- **Intaxel** (*Chile*).
- **Mariprax** (*Greece, Italy*); **Maxtenk** (*Argentina*); **Medopexol** (*Cyprus, Czech Republic, Greece, Lithuania*); **Mepimer** (*Mexico*); **Minergi** (*Brazil*); **Miparkan** (*Italy*); **Mipexole** (*Russian Federation*); **Miraleton** (*Greece*); **Miramel** (*Ireland*); **Miraparkin** (*Greece*); **Miraper** (*Italy*); **Mirapex** (*Canada, Ecuador, Hong Kong, Japan, Russian Federation, Ukraine, USA, Venezuela*); **Mirapexin** (*Austria, Belgium, Cyprus, Estonia, Germany, Greece, Hungary, Ireland, Italy, Netherlands, Poland, Portugal, Spain, Sweden, UK*); **Mirapezol** (*Greece*), **Miraxol** (*Ukraine*), **Miviren** (*Italy*), **Movial** (*Greece*), **Muvend** (*Chile*).
- **Nervius** (*Greece*); **Neurosomat** (*Argentina*); **Newmirex** (*Greece*); **Nixol** (*Argentina*); **Noxopran** (*Argentina*); **Nulipar** (*Argentina, Ecuador*).
- **Oprymea** (*Austria, Cyprus, Czech Republic, Denmark, Estonia, Finland, France, Germany, Greece, Hungary, Ireland, Lithuania, Netherlands, Norway, Poland, Portugal, Russian Federation, Spain, Sweden, UK*); **Oxpola** (*South Africa*).
- **Pacto, Parim** (*Turkey*); **Parmital** (*Chile, Venezuela*); **Parkipex, Parkizol** (*Turkey*); **Parkpex** (*Ecuador, Mexico*); **Parkyn** (*Turkey*); **Parxamil** (*Greece*); **Pazoram** (*South Africa*); **Pexa** (*Turkey*); **Pexasp** (*South Africa*); **Pexiplan** (*South Africa*); **Pexol** (*Ecuador*); **Pexola** (*South Africa, Turkey*); **Pexoleg** (*Venezuela*); **Pexomir, Pexson** (*South Africa*); **Pipexus** (*UK*); **Pisa** (*Brazil*); **Portiv** (*Argentina*); **Pradose** (*Turkey*); **Pramex** (*South Africa*); **Pramexol** (*Hong Kong, Thailand*); **Pramifer** (*Greece*); **Pramigen** (*Italy*); **Pramip** (*Argentina*); **Pramiperal** (*Italy*); **Pramipex** (*Ukraine*); **Pramipezan** (*Brazil*); **Pramithon** (*Estonia*);

P

Pramivex (*Indonesia*); Pramixil (*Poland*); Pramixol (*Greece*); Pranow (*Turkey*); Praxis (*Chile*); Primizol (*Greece*); Proxegol (*South Africa*).
- Quera (*Brazil*).
- Ramipex (*New Zealand, Philippines, Turkey, Ukraine*); Ramixole (*Italy*); Rapexole (*Cyprus, Greece*); Redipex (*Venezuela*).
- Sifrol (*Argentina, Australia, Austria, Belgium, Brazil, Chile, China, Denmark, Estonia, Finland, France, Germany, Indonesia, Ireland, Israel, Lithuania, Malaysia, Mexico, Netherlands, Norway, Philippines, Poland, Singapore, Sweden, Switzerland, Thailand, Tunisia*); Simipex, Simpral (*Australia*); Stabil (*Brazil*).
- Treatson (*Indonesia*).
- X-Tremble (*Greece*).
- Zymipex (*South Africa*).

Generics Available
- Yes.

Licensed Indications for Parkinson's Disease
- As monotherapy or adjunctive therapy to levodopa preparations in the treatment of Parkinson's disease from early and right up to late stages when the effect of levodopa is considered inadequate and fluctuations occur (FDA, EMA, EMC).

Licensed Indications for Other Conditions
- Symptomatic therapy of moderate to severe idiopathic RLS (dosage up to 0.54 mg, only IR formulations) (FDA, EMA, EMC).

Non-Licensed Use for Parkinson's Disease
- Depression and depressive symptoms in Parkinson's disease.

Non-Licensed Use for Other Conditions
- A potentially beneficial role in idiopathic RBD.

Ineffective
- To prevent/delay Parkinson's disease progression.

Mechanism of Action
- Pramipexole dihydrochloride is a non-ergot dopamine receptor agonist that selectively binds with full intrinsic activity to D_2-like receptors (D_2, D_3, D_4 subtypes). It has a higher affinity for D_3 compared to D_2 or D_4 receptor subtypes. Pramipexole does not interact with D_1-like receptors (D_1, D_5 subtypes).
- The selectivity of pramipexole for D_3 receptors may explain its anti-depressant effect, as these receptors are predominant in the limbic system, which is involved in emotional and reward functions.
- It binds with moderate affinity to α_2-adrenergic receptors (agonist) and has little or no affinity for α_1- or β-adrenergic, acetylcholine, or serotonin receptors.

- Its effect on motor symptoms in Parkinson's disease are believed to be mainly due to post-synaptic dopamine receptor stimulation in the striatum.
- Its exact mechanism of action in RLS remains unknown, although it is thought to be dopaminergic.

Efficacy Profile
- According to the MDS EBM Committee, pramipexole was characterized as:
  - 'Efficacious' as monotherapy in early Parkinson's disease, as adjunct therapy in early or stable Parkinson's disease patients, and for motor fluctuations (both IR and ER preparations).
  - 'Efficacious' in preventing/delaying motor fluctuations or dyskinesia (IR preparations).
  - 'Efficacious' in the treatment of depression and depressive symptoms in Parkinson's disease.
- According to the MDS EBM Committee there is 'insufficient evidence' considering pramipexole efficacy on existing dyskinesia.
- Pramipexole might exhibit a potentially beneficial role in idiopathic RBD.
  - In the context of personalized medicine, and because there are currently no firm recommendations considering the treatment of Parkinson's disease-related RBD, a trial with a low dose of pramipexole IR could be suggested.
- There are some preliminary indications that pramipexole alone or in combination with levodopa might be efficacious on Parkinson's disease-related apathy, although no strong evidence to date.

Pharmacokinetics
Absorption and Distribution
- Oral bioavailability: approximately 90%.
- Food co-ingestion: food increases Tmax by 1 h for IR preparations and by 2 h for ER formulations, and Cmax by 20%.
- Tmax: about 2 h in fasting patients and about 3 h with food consumption (IR formulations); about 6 h (ER formulations).
- Time to steady state: within 2 days of dosing.
- Pharmacokinetics: linear with therapeutic doses.
- Protein binding: less than 20%.
- Volume of distribution: 400–500 l.

Metabolism
- Less than 10% of the administered dose is metabolized.
  - No discernible metabolites in plasma or urine.
- No interactions with CYP enzymes are described at therapeutic doses.

Elimination
- Elimination half-life values in adults range from 8 h (in younger patients) to 12 h (in the elderly).
- Renal excretion: more than 90% of an administered dose is excreted unchanged in the urine.
  - Less than 2% is found in the faeces.

Drug Interaction Profile
Pharmacokinetic Drug Interactions
- Effects by pramipexole:
  - Pramipexole may increase the level or effect of *verapamil* and *triamterene* by basic (cationic) drug competition for renal tubular clearance.
- Effects on pramipexole:
  - Drugs that inhibit the cationic secretory transport system of the renal tubules or are eliminated by this pathway, such as *cimetidine, memantine, amantadine, mexiletine, zidovudine, cisplatin, quinine, procainamide, digoxin* may result in reduced clearance of pramipexole,; thus, a reduced dose of pramipexole should be considered on such occasions.
  - Antacids may decrease oral clearance of pramipexole, although histamine H_2-receptor blockers, anticholinergics, prokinetics, and PPIs are thought to have little effect on pramipexole clearance.

Pharmacodynamic Drug Interactions
- Co-medication with CNS depressants (e.g. opiates, benzodiazepines, antidepressants, triptans, anti-seizure medicines, *baclofen*) or alcohol might exacerbate their sedative effects.

Adverse Effects
How Drug Causes Adverse Effects
- Mainly (but not solely) through increasing dopaminergic activity.
- Drug interactions through cationic competition for renal tubular clearance.

Common Adverse Effects
- Very common (≥1/10):
  - Somnolence (especially at doses > 1.5 mg/day), dizziness, dyskinesia, nausea.
- Common (≥1/100 to <1/10):
  - Neuropsychiatric: headache, insomnia, hallucinations, abnormal dreams, confusion, ICDs (e.g. pathological gambling, compulsive shopping, binge eating, hypersexuality, dopamine dysregulation syndrome).

P

- ○ Eye: visual impairment (e.g. diplopia, blurred vision, reduced visual acuity).
- ○ Cardiovascular: hypotension.
- ○ GI: constipation, vomiting.
- ○ Other: fatigue, malaise, peripheral oedema, weight loss/decreased appetite.
- Uncommon (≥1/1,000 to <1/100):
  - ○ Neuropsychiatric: episodes of sudden sleep onset, amnesia, hyperkinesia, syncope, libido disorder, delusion, paranoia, delirium.
  - ○ Cardiovascular: cardiac failure.
  - ○ Respiratory: pneumonia, dyspnoea, hiccups.
  - ○ Endocrine: inappropriate antidiuretic hormone secretion.
  - ○ General: hypersensitivity, pruritus, rash, weight increase.

Life-Threatening or Dangerous Adverse Effects
- DAWS has been reported with pramipexole cessation, especially if it is discontinued abruptly. Patients may develop neuropsychiatric or autonomic symptoms, which do not respond to levodopa. In severe cases, DAWS can be life-threatening.
- NMS (fever, muscular rigidity, altered consciousness, autonomic instability) during rapid dosage reduction or abrupt pramipexole withdrawal.
- Rhabdomyolysis.
- Fibrotic complications (e.g. peritoneal, pleural, or pulmonary fibrosis), although a causal association has not been confirmed.

Rare and Not Life-Threatening Adverse Effects
- Mania.
- Postural deformities, including antecollis, camptocormia, pleurothotonus (Pisa syndrome), even later in therapy (after several months).

Weight Change
- Weight changes, especially weight loss, might occur.

What to Do About Adverse Effects
- Before introducing pramipexole, discuss common or life-threatening adverse effects with patients and/or caregivers, including symptoms that should be reported to the physician.
  - Before therapy initiation, patients should be asked about somnolence or other factors that increase somnolence risk, such as co-administration with sedating medications (see above on pharmacodynamic interactions), obstructive sleep apnoea, or sleep deprivation.
- The majority of adverse effects usually occur early in pramipexole therapy and tend to disappear as therapy continues.
- On a regular basis, monitor for sleepiness (which might occur without preceding warning signs, even later in therapy, e.g. after 1 year), drowsiness, hypotension (especially during dosing escalation), ICDs,

ADVERSE EFFECTS

P

hallucinations, or psychotic-like behaviours. Treating physicians should address these manifestations with focused and direct questions to patients and caregivers, as patients might not acknowledge such symptoms as abnormal to report them.

- If patients taking pramipexole experience somnolence and/or episodes of sudden-onset sleep during activities that require active participation, they should refrain from driving or operating machinery and inform their treating physician. Therapy discontinuation is generally advised.
- Patients on pramipexole should avoid rising rapidly after sitting or lying down, especially if they have been in a seated or recumbent position for prolonged time periods or if they have just begun pramipexole therapy.
- Patients and their caregivers should be made aware about the possibility of developing ICDs or mania/delirium. In this case, a reduction of pramipexole dose or discontinuation of therapy should be considered.
- If dyskinesias occur in advanced Parkinson's disease patients taking levodopa and pramipexole during the initial titration of pramipexole, at first consider reducing the levodopa dose.
- If dystonia or postural deformities occur, all dopaminergic medications should be reviewed and a pramipexole dose reduction or even discontinuation should be considered.
- In case of severe or persistent DAWS, temporary re-administration of pramipexole at the lowest effective dose may be considered.
- In case of peripheral oedema as a side effect to pramipexole, consider lowering the dose or discontinuing therapy. Use of diuretics is not recommended due to the risk of aggravating orthostatic hypotension.
- Periodic assessment for augmentation is advised in RLS cases.

Dosing and Use
Usual Dosage Range
- IR: 0.088–1.1 TID (mg of base) equal to 0.125–1.5 mg TID (mg of salt).
- ER: 0.26–3.15 mg OD equal to 0.375–4.5 mg OD (mg of salt).

Available Formulations
- Immediate-release tablets (mg of salt): 0.125 mg, 0.25 mg, 0.5 mg, 0.75 mg, 1 mg, 1.5 mg.
- Immediate-release tablets (mg of base): 0.088 mg, 0.18 mg, 0.35 mg, 0.7 mg.
- Extended-release tablets (mg of salt): 0.375 mg, 0.75 mg, 1.5 mg, 2.25 mg, 3 mg, 3.75 mg, 4.5 mg.
- Extended-release tablets (mg of base): 0.26 mg, 0.52 mg, 1.05 mg, 2.1 mg, 3.15 mg.

How to Dose
- Based on response and tolerability, the lowest possible dose should be used.
- Patients may be switched overnight from IR to ER tablets at the same total daily dosage. Following conversion, dosage can be adjusted, if necessary, based on response and tolerability.

Gradual dose increase of pramipexole IR tablets				
Week	Dose (mg of base)	Total daily dose (mg of base)	Dose (mg of salt)	Total daily dose (mg of salt)
1	3 × 0.088	0.264	3 × 0.125	0.375
2	3 × 0.18	0.54	3 × 0.25	0.75
3	3 × 0.35	1.1	3 × 0.5	1.50
4	3 × (0.35 + 0.18)	1.57	3 × 0.75	2.25
5	3 × 0.7	2.1	3 × 1.0	3.0
6	3 × (0.7 + 0.18)	2.64	3 × (1.0 + 0.25)	3.75
7	3 × (0.7 + 0.35)	3.3	3 × 1.5	4.5

Gradual dose increase of pramipexole ER tablets		
Week	Daily dose (mg of base)	Daily dose (mg of salt)
1	0.26	0.375
2	0.52	0.75
3	1.05	1.50
4	1.05+0.52	2.25
5	2.1	3.00
6	2.1+0.52	3.75
7	3.15	4.50

Dosing Tips
- The ER tablets should be swallowed whole (do not chew, crush, or divide).
- Pramipexole may be taken with or without food.
  - Taking pramipexole with food may reduce nausea.

P

- May switch overnight from IR to ER tablets at the same daily dose, although dose adjustments might be necessary for some patients.
- IR and ER tablets should not be taken concurrently.
- If an IR tablet is missed, patients should be advised to continue with their regular dosing schedule without any adjustments.
- If an ER tablet is missed, patients should be advised to take the dose as soon as possible, but no later than 12 h after the regularly scheduled time; after 12 h have passed, the missed dose should be skipped and the next dose should be taken the following day at the regularly scheduled time.
- Some patients taking the ER tablets may notice a residue resembling swollen pieces of the original tablet in their stool. Patients should be informed about this possibility and should be instructed to notify their treating physician if this occurs, as this event might be associated with a worsening of their parkinsonian symptoms.
- If pramipexole therapy is interrupted for a substantial time period, re-titration may be required.
- It has been suggested that if Parkinson's disease-related depressive symptoms do not correspond to a dosage of up to 3 mg of pramipexole, it should be replaced by other pharmacological alternatives, including antidepressants.

How to Withdraw Drug
- A total daily dose reduction of 0.375 mg every second day is suggested.
  - In case of serious adverse events (e.g. delirium) and a pramipexole dose of more than 3 mg/day, an initial daily reduction of 0.75 mg is suggested until the level of 3 mg/day is reached and then the standard reduction process of 0.375 every second day can be followed.
  - If the pramipexole dose is higher than 4.5 mg/day, then the initial reduction could be 1.5 mg/day until the level of 4.5 mg/day and then the same steps as above apply.
  - This suggested withdrawal scheme can be further slowed down depending on the patient's response.
- DAWS can occur independently of the rate of dose reduction. Regular monitoring of patients during the withdrawal period is essential.
- A potential deterioration in motor performance following pramipexole reduction usually has to be compensated with levodopa preparations.

Overdose
- Experience on pramipexole overdose is limited.
- Pramipexole overdose might lead to manifestations of central dopaminergic stimulation, including nausea, vomiting, hypotension, hallucinations, agitation, confusion, involuntary movements and seizures, or even coma.
- There is no known antidote for dopamine agonist overdose. General supportive measures are suggested, along with gastric lavage,

intravenous fluid, activated charcoal administration and electrocardio-gram monitoring.

Tests and Therapeutic Drug Monitoring
- Ophthalmologic monitoring is recommended at regular intervals or if vision abnormalities occur.
- Periodic skin examinations by qualified clinicians should be performed to monitor for melanoma.
- Careful monitoring of blood pressure is advised in patients with severe cardiovascular disease due to reported hypotension, especially at the initiation of treatment.

Other Warnings / Precautions
- Pramipexole should not be used in patients with a history of psychotic disorders unless the potential benefits outweigh the risks.
- Patients should be advised that pramipexole may cause somnolence and they should not drive a car or operate complex machinery until they have gained sufficient experience with the drug to determine whether it affects their mental and/or motor performance.

Do Not Use (Contraindications)
- Hypersensitivity to the active substance or to any of its excipients.
- Co-medication with CNS depressants or alcohol should be avoided due to additive sedative effects.
- Co-medication with antipsychotic drugs or antiemetics with extrapyramidal effects (e.g. *metoclopramide*) should be avoided.

Special Populations
Renal Impairment
- Increases are applied at least at 7 days intervals.
- FDA (IR):
  - CrCl 30–50 ml/min: 0.125 mg BID initially; not to exceed a maximum daily dose of 0.75 mg TID.
  - CrCl 15–29 ml/min: 0.125 mg OD; not to exceed 1.5 mg OD.
  - CrCl <15 ml/min or patients on haemodialysis: not recommended.
- FDA (ER):
  - CrCl 30–50 ml/min: 0.375 mg every second day; increase to 0.375 mg every day; further increase if needed, not to exceed 2.25 mg OD.
  - CrCl <30 ml/min or patients on haemodialysis: not recommended.
- EMA, EMC (IR):
  - CrCl 20–50 ml/min: 0.088 mg of base (0.125 mg of salt) BID; increase if needed, not to exceed 1.57 mg of base (2.25 mg of salt) BID.
  - CrCl <20 ml/min: 0.088 mg of base (0.125 mg of salt) OD; increase if needed, not to exceed 1.1 mg of base (1.5 mg of salt) OD.
  - CrCl <15 ml/min or patients on haemodialysis: not recommended.

P

SPECIAL POPULATIONS

- EMA, EMC (ER):
  - CrCl 30–50 ml/min: 0.26 mg of base (0.375 mg of salt) OD; increase if needed by 0.26 mg/week; not to exceed 1.57 mg of base (2.25 mg of salt) OD.
  - CrCl >30 ml/min or patients on haemodialysis: not recommended.
- If renal function declines during maintenance therapy, pramipexole dosage should be adjusted accordingly.

Hepatic Impairment
- No dosage adjustments are recommended, although the effect of pramipexole on hepatic function has not been fully investigated.

Elderly
- Pramipexole plasma levels were found to be higher in patients older than 65 years compared to younger individuals, possibly due to renal function reduction. It is suggested that pramipexole should be withdrawn or reduced in dose more slowly in older patients.
- Geriatric patients might be more prone to developing hallucinations or psychotic-like behaviour on pramipexole therapy.

Pregnancy
- The teratogenic potential of pramipexole in animal studies has not been fully investigated and there are insufficient data on pregnant women.
- Pramipexole should not be used during pregnancy unless clearly necessary.

Breastfeeding
- It is not known whether pramipexole is distributed into human milk.
- According to studies in rats, pramipexole was distributed into breast milk.
- Pramipexole is expected to inhibit lactation due to inhibition of prolactin secretion.
- Pramipexole should not be used during breastfeeding; if its use is necessary, breastfeeding should be discontinued.

Costs
NHS indicative price accessed 9 June 2022:
- Branded:
  ○ Mirapexin tablets (Boehringer Ingelheim Ltd) – 30 × 0.088 mg tablets: £11.24; 30 × 0.18 mg tablets: £22.49; 100 × 0.18 mg tablets: £74.95; 30 × 0.35 mg tablets: £44.97; 100 × 0.35 mg tablets: £149.90; 30 × 0.7 mg tablets: £89.94; 100 × 0.7 mg tablets: £299.82.
  ○ Oprymea tablets (Consilient Health Ltd) – 30 × 0.088 mg tablets: £3.23; 30 × 0.18 mg tablets: £6.09; 100 × 0.18 mg tablets: £15.46;

30 × 0.35 mg tablets: £32.47; 100 × 0.35 mg tablets: £108.23; 30 × 0.7 mg tablets: £18.26; 100 × 0.7 mg tablets: £117.63.
- ∘ Mirapexin modified-release tablets (Boehringer Ingelheim Ltd); 30 × 0.26 mg tablets: £32.49; 30 × 0.52 mg tablets: £64.98; 30 × 1.05 mg tablets: £129.96; 30 × 1.05 mg tablets:£129.96; 30 × 1.57 mg tablets: £202.36; 30 × 2.1 mg tablets :£259.91; 30 × 2.62 mg tablets: £337.27; 30 × 3.15 mg tablets: £389.87.
- ∘ Oprymea modified-release tablets (Consilient Health Ltd) – 30 × 0.26 mg tablets:£25.56; 30 × 0.52 mg tablets:£51.14; 30 × 1.05 mg tablets:£102.28; 30 × 1.57 mg tablets: £159.26; 30 × 2.1 mg tablets: £204.56; 30 × 2.62 mg tablets:£337.27; 30 × 3.15 mg tablets:£389.87.
- ∘ Pipexus modified-release tablets (Ethypharm UK Ltd) – 30 × 0.26 mg tablets:£16.25; 30 × 0.52 mg tablets:£32.49; 30 × 105 mg tablets: £64.98; 30 × 1.57 mg tablets: £101.18; 30 × 2.1 mg tablets: £246.57; 30 × 2.62 mg tablets:£168.64; 30 × 3.15 mg tablets: £194.94.
- • Generic:
  - ∘ Pramipexole tablets – 30 × 88 microgram tablets: £2.10–£9.55; 30 × 180 microgram tablets:£1.49–£19.12; 100 × 180 microgram tablets:£5.17–£7.32; 30 × 350 microgram tablets:£13.89–£38.22; 100 × 350 microgram tablets: £49.30; 30 × 700 microgram tablets: £1.87–£68.76; 100 × 700 microgram tablets: £6.23–£10.62.
  - ∘ Pramipexole modified-release tablets – 30 × 260 microgram tablets: £13.00–£30.87; 30 × 520 microgram tablets: £25.99–£61.73; 30 × 1.05 mg tablets: £51.98–£123.46; 30 × 1.57 mg tablets: £80.94–£192.24; 30 × 2.1 mg tablets: £103.97–£246.91; 30 × 2.62 mg tablets: £134.95–£320.41; 30 × 3.15 mg tablets: £155.95–£370.38.

The Overall Place of Pramipexole in the Treatment of Parkinson's Disease

Pramipexole use has been approved for all stages of Parkinson's disease as monotherapy, or as an adjunct therapy to levodopa preparations in both early and advanced Parkinson's disease. It is also considered efficacious for the treatment of Parkinson's disease-related depression or depressive symptoms. Pramipexole may also have a potentially beneficial role in the treatment of RBD and apathy, although no high-quality data are currently available to support this effect. Finally, pramipexole has a role in the management of RLS. Pramipexole is generally well-tolerated, even in non-demented older patients, although with lower daily doses. Patients, their caregivers, and treating physicians should be aware of particular adverse events, including ICDs, somnolence and sleep attacks, hallucinations and psychotic-like behaviour, and orthostatic hypotension.

P

THE TREATMENT OF PARKINSON'S DISEASE

Potential Advantages

- Because SSRIs might worsen tremor and parkinsonism, pramipexole might be a beneficial alternative in Parkinson's disease-related depression, as long as patients are monitored for ICDs and somnolence.
- Although rotigotine has been recommended for the treatment of night-time disabilities in Parkinson's disease, especially in early morning OFF phenomena, pramipexole might constitute a better option in patients with concomitant depressive symptoms.
- The once daily administration of ER formulations of pramipexole might contribute to patients' better adherence, especially in Parkinson's disease patients with complicated drug schemes, and provide continuous drug delivery.
- Pramipexole is mostly metaboliszd in the kidneys, so it is not expected to affect or be affected by CYP450 isoenzymes inducers or inhibitors in the liver.
- Selective D_3 stimulation may be associated with a lower frequency of LID.

Potential Disadvantages

- Similarly to other dopamine agonists, the development of ICDs, hallucinations or psychotic-like behaviour, sudden sleep attacks, and orthostatic hypotension is a possibility in patients treated with pramipexole and might lead to severe life-changing outcomes (e.g. financial difficulties, injuries). Somnolence is particularly an issue among older patients taking pramipexole.
- Selective D_3 stimulation may be associated with a higher risk of ICDs.
- Pramipexole is extensively cleared by the kidneys and, therefore, therapeutic or toxic levels might be reached at lower doses in case of renal impairment.

Clinical Box

A 45-year-old woman presented at the Neurology Department Outpatient Clinic with bilateral bradykinesia and tremor of the upper limbs, more pronounced on the left side, and hypomimia. She reported prodromal symptoms of constipation, anosmia, and RBD over the past few years, with the latter getting worse during the last few months. She also mentioned mild depressive symptoms and insomnia. She had been initially prescribed a low dose of antidepressant by her GP, which she did not start. The rest of her medical history was unremarkable. She reported no history of ICDs, somnolence, or psychotic behaviour. A clinical diagnosis of Parkinson's disease was made and a brain MRI scan and a DaTSCAN were scheduled. The results were supportive to the diagnosis of Parkinson's disease. Pramipexole ER tablets 0.26 mg OD were prescribed and the patient was given instructions for gradual weekly increases of dose according to response and tolerance, and follow-up assessments via the phone were scheduled. Bearing in mind the

P

anticipated antidepressant effect of pramipexole, the initially prescribed antidepressant was not deemed necessary. She was also instructed to regularly measure her blood pressure, as she reported some occasional episodes of hypotension. At a dose of 1.05 mg OD, the patient reported significant improvement of her symptoms, including tremor and non-motor symptoms, without any adverse events. The patient was scheduled to be reassessed after 6 months.

Suggested Reading

Barone P, W Poewe, S Albrecht, C Debieuvre, D Massey, O Rascol, E Tolosa, D Weintraub. Pramipexole for the treatment of depressive symptoms in patients with Parkinson's disease: a randomised, double-blind, placebo-controlled trial. *Lancet Neurol* 2010: 9(6): 573–580.

Rizos A, A Sauerbier, C Falup-Pecurariu, A Antonini, P Martinez-Martin, B Kessel, T Henriksen, M Silverdale, G Durner, KR Chaudhuri ; EUROPAR and the IPMDS Non-Motor PD Study Group. Tolerability of non-ergot oral and transdermal dopamine agonists in younger and older Parkinson's disease patients: an European multicentre survey. *J Neural Transm (Vienna)* 2020; 127(6): 875–879.

Rota S, I Boura, L Batzu, N Titova, P Jenner, C Falup-Pecurariu, KR Chaudhuri. 'Dopamine agonist phobia' in Parkinson's disease: when does it matter? Implications for non-motor symptoms and personalized medicine. *Expert Rev Neurother* 2020; 20(9): 953–365.

Silindir M, AY Ozer. The benefits of pramipexole selection in the treatment of Parkinson's disease. *Neurol Sci* 2014; 35(10): 1505–1511.

Wang Y, DQ Jiang, CS Lu, MX Li, LL Jiang. Efficacy and safety of combination therapy with pramipexole and levodopa vs levodopa monotherapy in patients with Parkinson disease: a systematic review and meta-analysis. *Medicine (Baltimore)* 2021; 100(44): e27511.

References

Agüera-Ortiz L, R García-Ramos, FJG Pérez, J Lopez-Álvarez, JMM Rodríguez, FJA Rodríguez, JO Pueyo, CP Valero, J Porta-Etessam. Focus on depression in Parkinson's Disease: a Delphi consensus of experts in psychiatry, neurology, and geriatrics. *Parkinson's Dis* 2021; 2021: 6621991.

AHFS Drug information, 2012. Bethesda: American Society of Health-System Pharmacists. Accessed on 9 June 2022 via www.medicinescomplete.com.

Cardon-Dunbar A, T Robertson, MS Roberts, GK Isbister. Pramipexole overdose associated with visual hallucinations, agitation and myoclonus. *J Med Toxicol* 2017; 13(4): 343–346.

Contin M, G Lopane, S Mohamed, G Callandra-Buonaura, S Capellini, P De Massis, S Nassetti, A Perrone, R Riva, L Sambati, C Scaglione,

P

PRAMIPEXOLE

P Cortelli. Clinical pharmacokinetics of pramipexole, ropinirole and rotigotine in patients with Parkinson's disease. *Parkinsonism Relat Disord* 2019; 61: 111–117.

Joint Formulary Committee. British National Formulary (online). London: BMJ Group and Pharmaceutical Press. Accessed on 19 February 2023 via www.medicinescomplete.com.

Koschel J, KR Chaudhuri, L Tönges, M Thiel, V Raeder, WH Jost. Implications of dopaminergic medication withdrawal in Parkinson's disease. *J Neural Transm (Vienna)* 2022; 129(9): 1169–1178.

Latt MD, S Lewis, O Zekry, VSC Fung. Factors to consider in the selection of dopamine agonists for older persons with Parkinson's disease. *Drugs Aging* 2019; 36(3): 189–202.

Lazcano-Ocampo C, YM Wan, DJ van Wamelen, L Batzu, I Boura, N Titova, V Leta, M Qamar, P Martinez-Martin, KR Chaudhuri. Identifying and responding to fatigue and apathy in Parkinson's disease: a review of current practice. *Expert Rev Neurother* 2020; 20(5): 477–495.

Oguro H, K Kadota, M Ishihara, K Okada, S Yamaguchi. Efficacy of pramipexole for treatment of apathy in Parkinson's disease. *Int J Clin Med* 2014; 5: 885–889.

Pramipexole. In: Brayfield A (Ed.), *Martindale: The Complete Drug Reference*. London: The Royal Pharmaceutical Society of Great Britain. Accessed on 9 June 2022 via www.medicinescomplete.com.

Pramipexole. In: DRUGDEX® System (electronic version). Truven Health Analytics, Greenwood Village, Colorado, USA. Accessed on 9 June 2022 via www.micromedexsolutions.com.

Seier M, A Hiller. Parkinson's disease and pregnancy: an updated review. *Parkinsonism Relat Disord* 2017; 40: 11–17.

Summary of product characteristics – Mirapexin 0.18 mg tablets. Boehringer Ingelheim Ltd. Electronic Medicines Compendium: MIRAPEXIN 0.18 mg tablets – summary of product characteristics (SmPC) – (emc). Accessed on 9 June 2022 via www.medicines.org.uk.

Wilson SM, MG Wurst, MF Whatley, RN Daniels. Classics in chemical neuroscience: pramipexole. *ACS Chem Neurosci* 2020; 11(17): 2506–2512.

QUETIAPINE

Q

Therapeutics

Chemical Name and Structure

Quetiapine fumarate (2-[2-(4-benzo[b][1,4]benzothiazepin-6-ylpiperazin-1-yl)ethoxy]ethanol;(*E*)-but-2-enedioic acid) is an atypical antipsychotic with a molecular weight of 883.1 and an empirical formula of $(C_{21}H_{25}N_3O_2S)_2, C_4H_4O_4$.

Brand Names

- **Aebol** (*Brazil*); **Afidat** (*Argentina*); **Alaquet** (*UK*); **Alcreno** (*Poland*); **Alvoquel** (*Hong Kong, Singapore*); **Alzen** (*Portugal*); **Anaquetan** (*Greece*); **ApoTiapina** (*Poland*); **Aretaeus** (*Mexico*); **Arezil** (*Greece*); **Aroquet** (*South Africa*); **As-Kalmeks** (*Turkey*); **Asicot** (*Chile*); **Atip** (*Brazil*); **Atipina** (*Argentina*); **Atrolak** (*Poland, UK*).
- **Biatrix** (*Argentina*); **Bipresso** (*Japan*); **Biquelle** (*UK*); **Biquetan** (*Denmark, Finland*); **Bonogren** (*Poland*); **Brancico** (*UK*).
- **Cedrina** (*Turkey*); **Cizyapine** (*Turkey*).
- **Delucon** (*Australia*); **Dendritex** (*Argentina*); **Derin** (*Czech Republic*); **Dominium** (*Argentina*); **Dopaquel** (*South Africa*).
- **Ebesque** (*UK*); **Etiaben** (*Greece*); **Etiagen** (*Poland*); **Etiapin** (*Greece*); **Etiasel** (*Argentina*); **Etipin** (*Turkey*).
- **Gedonin** (*Russian Federation*); **Geldoren** (*Poland*); **Geroquel** (*Ireland*); **Gofyl** (*Chile*); **Gyrex** (*Turkey*).
- **Hedonin** (*Czech Republic, Estonia, Lithuania*).
- **Inquetia** (*Argentina*).
- **Kaptan** (*Australia*); **Keday** (*Turkey*); **Kefrenex** (*Poland*); **Kemoter** (*Argentina*); **Kenantis** (*Argentina*); **Kesaquil** (*Hong Kong*); **Ketap** (*Turkey*); **Ketian** (*Ecuador*); **Ketiap** (*Poland*); **Ketidose** (*Turkey*); **Ketilept** (*Czech Republic, Hungary, Lithuania, Philippines, Poland, Portugal, Turkey, Ukraine*); **Ketinel** (*Turkey*); **Ketipina** (*Ecuador*); **Ketipine** (*Cyprus, Greece*); **Ketipinor** (*Denmark, Estonia, Finland, Lithuania, Malaysia, Poland, Singapore, Sweden*); **Ketrel** (*Poland*); **Ketya** (*Turkey*); **Kitapen** (*Brazil*); **Kizofrin** (*South Africa*); **Kronalt** (*Ecuador*); **Kvelux** (*Poland*); **Kventiax** (*Czech Republic, Estonia, Hungary, Lithuania, Poland, Portugal*); **Kwetaplex** (*Poland*); **Kwetax** (*Poland*).
- **Laquel** (*Russian Federation*).
- **Matepil** (*Greece*); **Matisse** (*Ecuador*); **Megazon** (*Greece*); **Mintreleq** (*UK*).
- **Nantarid** (*Lithuania, Russian Federation*); **Neotiapim** (*Brazil*); **Neutapin** (*Thailand*); **Norsic** (*Chile*); **Notiabolfen** (*Ireland*).
- **Orocuelia** (*Greece*).
- **Pinexet** (*Poland*); **Poetra** (*Poland*); **Psicotric** (*Spain*); **Psyquet** (*South Africa*).
- **Qi Wei** (*China*); **Q-mind** (*Mexico*); **Qpine** (*Philippines*); **Qtipine** (*Philippines*); **Quentaxin** (*Greece*); **Quantia** (*Hong Kong, Thailand*); **Quantiax** (*Ireland, Italy*); **Quapianol** (*Greece*); **Qudix** (*Spain*);

QUETIAPINE

Quekline (*Philippines, Venezuela*); Quel (*India*); Quental (*Greece*); Quentapil (*Poland*); Quentiax (*Greece, Ireland, Italy, Spain*); Queopine (*Brazil*); Quepimax (*Chile*); Quepin (*Greece*); Quepina (*Ecuador*); Quepine (*Australia*); Quepsia LP (*Brazil*); Querok (*Brazil*); Queropax (*Brazil*); Quesara (*South Africa*); Quesero (*Hong Kong*); Questax (*Czech Republic, Poland*); Quet (*Brazil, Ecuador*); Quetact (*Venezuela*); Quetadin (*Philippines*); Quetamed (*Italy*); Quetap (*Tunisia*); Quetapel (*New Zealand*); Quetapo (*Czech Republic*); Queteper (*Italy*); Quetex (*Chile, Ireland*); Quetia (*Australia, Venezuela*); Quetiaccord (*Australia*); Quetiafair (*Netherlands*); Quetialan (*Austria*); Quetiap (*Russian Federation*); Quetiapro (*Philippines*); Quetiaros (*Argentina*); Quetiateg (*Ecuador*); Quetiazic (*Argentina, Chile, Ecuador*); Quetibux (*Brazil*); Quetidin (*Chile, Ecuador, Venezuela*); Quetin (*Australia*); Quetiapin (*Brazil, Ukraine*); Quetirel (*Ecuador, Venezuela*); Quetiron (*Ukraine*); Quetiser (*Poland*); Quetitex (*Russian Federation*); Quetium (*Ecuador, Chile*); Quetixol (*Ukraine*); Quetkare (*Chile*); Quetoser (*South Africa*); Quetrina (*Poland*); Quetros (*Brazil*); Quetvell (*Indonesia*); Quin (*Venezuela*); Qurax (*Chile*); Qutero (*Malaysia*); Quitipin (*Ecuador*); Qutipine (*Russian Federation*); Q-win (*Philippines*).
- Realiquel (*South Africa*); Rocoz (*Spain*); Rostrum (*Argentina*).
- Secuelia (*Greece*); Seotiapim (*UK*); Sequa (*Turkey*); Sequase (*Australia, Switzerland*); Serapine (*Australia*); Serendra (*Philippines*); Serex (*Turkey*); Serez (*South Africa*); Seroc (*Ecuador*); Serogen (*Hong Kong*); Seromind (*South Africa*); Seronia (*Australia*); Seronova (*Venezuela*); Seropia (*Ireland*); Seropin (*Greece*); Seroquel (*Argentina, Australia, Austria, Belgium, Brazil, Canada, Chile, China, Cyprus, Denmark, Ecuador, Estonia, Finland, Germany, Greece, Hong Kong, Hungary, Indonesia, Ireland, Israel, Italy, Japan, Lithuania, Malaysia, Mexico, Netherlands, New Zealand, Norway, Philippines, Poland, Portugal, Russian Federation, Singapore, South Africa, Spain, Sweden, Switzerland, Thailand, Tunisia, Turkey, UK, Ukraine, USA, Venezuela*); Seroquin (*India*); Serotia (*Philippines*); Serotiapin (*Greece*); Servitel (*Russian Federation*); Setinin (*Hong Kong, Poland*); Shu Si (*China*); Siquel (*Ecuador*); Sizocam, Sizonorm (*South Africa*); Socalm (*India*); Sondate (*UK*); Squro (*Thailand*); Stadaquel (*Denmark, Hungary, Poland*); Symquel (*Poland*); Syquet (*Australia*).
- Tevaquel (*Ireland*); Tevatiapine (*Australia*); Tiapinan (*Venezuela*); Tiaquel (*Greece*); Tim ASF (*Mexico*); Tiquepin (*Ecuador*); Tomel (*Cyprus*); Tracox (*Brazil*); Truvalin (*South Africa*).
- Vesparax (*Argentina*); Victoel (*Russian Federation*); Victus (*Philippines*); Vipocerex (*Ecuador*); Vorta (*Poland*).
- Xeroquel (*France*); Xetamed (*Italy*).
- Zaluron (*UK*); Zambiquet (*South Africa*); Zoqit (*South Africa*).

Generics Available
- Yes.

Licensed Indications for Parkinson's Disease
• None.

Licensed Indications for Other Conditions
• Schizophrenia (FDA, EMC).
• Bipolar I disorder:
  • Moderate to severe manic episodes (FDA, EMA, EMC).
  • Major depressive episodes (FDA, EMA, EMC).
  • Prevention of recurrence of manic/depressive episodes in patients who previously responded to quetiapine therapy (FDA, EMA, EMC).
• Major depressive disorder (only ER formulations, as an adjunctive therapy to antidepressants) (FDA, EMA, EMC).

Non-Licensed Use for Parkinson's Disease
• Parkinson's disease-related psychosis.
• DLB-related psychosis.

Non-Licensed Use for Other Conditions
• Alcohol dependence.
• Insomnia.
• Generalized anxiety disorder.
• PTSD.
• As an add-on to SSRIs in OCD.
• Borderline personality disorder.
• To decrease aggression in psychiatric illness.

Ineffective
• Dementia-related psychosis.

Mechanism of Action
• Quetiapine is reported to have affinity for serotonin (5-HT2), 5-HT1A, histamine (H1), and adrenergic (A1 and A2) receptors as well as dopamine D1 and D2 receptors.
• The active metabolite norquetiapine has similar activity to quetiapine with greater activity at 5HT2A receptors and antagonizes muscarinic M1 and norepinephrine receptors.
• It is believed that the efficacy of quetiapine in schizophrenia and the mood stabilization effects are mediated by its combined antagonist activity of D2 and 5HT2 receptors.
• The partial agonist activity at 5HT1A and norepinephrine antagonism of norquetiapine may contribute to the efficacy in depression and anxiety.
• Neither quetiapine nor norquetiapine have any affinity for benzodiazepine receptors.

Q

THERAPEUTICS

QUETIAPINE

Efficacy Profile
- According to the MDS EBM Committee, quetiapine has been characterized as 'possibly useful' for treating psychosis in Parkinson's disease.
- Quetiapine is considered similarly efficacious to clozapine in treating Parkinson's disease-related psychosis.
- According to a retrospective cohort study directly comparing quetiapine to pimavanserin, the latter may be more clinically useful for the treatment of Parkinson's disease-related psychosis, but quetiapine may carry additional long-term, delayed benefits, including amelioration of agitation or insomnia.

Pharmacokinetics

Absorption and Distribution
- Oral bioavailability: about 100%.
- Food co-ingestion: high-fat meals significantly raise quetiapine Cmax and AUC values when using ER formulations. A marginal effect was found for IR formulations.
- Tmax: about 1.5 h for IR and about 6 h for ER.
- Time to steady state: expected to be achieved within 2 days of initiation.
- Pharmacokinetics: linear for doses up to 800 mg administered once daily.
- Protein binding: about 83%.
- Volume of distribution: 6–14 l/kg.

Metabolism
- Extensively metabolized in the liver, with CYP3A4 being the primary enzyme responsible for producing the active metabolite norquetiapine.
- Quetiapine and several of its metabolites, including norquetiapine, are considered weak inhibitors of CYP1A2, CYP2C9, CYP2C19, CYP2D6, and CYP3A4 at concentrations much higher than those found in Parkinson's disease. Quetiapine is unlikely to cause any clinically significant effects via this mechanism.

Elimination
- Half-life values for IR and ER formulations are 6 h and 7 h, respectively. The half-life of norquetiapine is 12 h.
- Renal excretion: approximately 73% of an administered dose is excreted in the urine and about 21% is found in the faeces with less than 5% excreted unchanged.

Q

Drug Interaction Profile

Pharmacokinetic Drug Interactions

- Effects on quetiapine:
  - CYP450 inducers (e.g. *phenytoin, carbamazepine, rifabutin, rifampin*) may significantly decrease plasma levels of quetiapine.
  - CYP3A4 inhibitors (e.g. *ketoconazole, citalopram, escitalopram*) may significantly increase plasma levels of quetiapine.
- The pharmacokinetics of quetiapine were not markedly affected when co-administered with *fluoxetine* (a CYP3A4 and CYP2D6 inhibitor), *cimetidine* (a non-selective CYP450 inhibitor), the antipsychotics *risperidone* and *haloperidol*.

Pharmacodynamic Drug Interactions

- Co-medication with CNS depressants or alcohol might lead to synergistic sedative effects, including sleep apnoea syndrome.
- Co-medication with drugs exhibiting anticholinergic properties may lead to anticholinergic side effects, including dry mouth, blurred vision, constipation, drowsiness, sedation, hallucinations, memory, and urination problems.
- Co-medication with other neuroleptics or drugs causing electrolyte imbalance or increasing QTc interval (e.g. *amiodarone, azithromycin, buprenorphine, chloroquine, chlorpromazine, citalopram, escitalopram, clarithromycin, donepezil, erythromycin, flecainide, foscarnet, lithium, mirtazapine, moxifloxacin, quinidine, sotalol, trazodone*) might lead to potentially fatal Torsade de Pointes arrhythmias and is considered a risk factor for sudden cardiac death.
- Quetiapine exhibits pharmacodynamic antagonism with dopaminergic drugs (e.g. *levodopa*, dopamine agonists, *bromocriptine*).

ADVERSE EFFECTS

Adverse Effects

How Drug Causes Adverse Effects

- The activity of quetiapine is thought to be mediated by a number of neuronal receptors, mentioned above.
  - The histaminergic antagonistic activity might explain quetiapine-induced somnolence.
  - The α1-adrenergic antagonistic activity might explain quetiapine-induced orthostatic hypotension.
  - Cholinergic adverse reactions might be mediated by the muscarinic effects of norquetiapine.
  - The D2-dopaminergic antagonistic activity probably mediates the extrapyramidal side effects and the pharmacodynamic antagonism with dopaminergic medications.

Common Adverse Effects
- Very common (≥1/10):
  - Decreased haemoglobin, increased triglycerides and total cholesterol (especially LDL), decreased HDL, dizziness, fatigue, somnolence, extrapyramidal symptoms, dry mouth, headache, withdrawal symptoms.
- Common (≥1/100 to <1/10):
  - Neuropsychiatric: abnormal dreams/nightmares, dysarthria.
  - Cardiovascular: palpitations, tachycardia, orthostatic hypotension.
  - Respiratory: dyspnoea, pharyngitis.
  - GI: constipation, dyspepsia, vomiting, increased liver enzymes, abdominal pain.
  - Endocrine: hyperprolactinaemia, decreased total T_4, total T_3 and free T_4, increased TSH.
  - Other: leukopenia (decreased neutrophil count, increased eosinophils) (especially in patients with a history of low WBC or drug-induced neutropenia), increased appetite, increased glucose, blurred vision, peripheral oedema, irritability, pyrexia, back pain/arthralgia/myalgia, rash.
- Uncommon (≥1/1,000 to <1/100):
  - Neuropsychiatric: seizures, RLS, tardive dyskinesia, syncope, confusion.
  - Cardiovascular: QT prolongation, bradycardia.
  - Respiratory: rhinitis.
  - GI: dysphagia.
  - Urinary: urinary retention.
  - Endocrine: decreased free T_3, hypothyroidism.
  - Other: neutropenia, hypersensitivity (e.g. allergic skin reactions), hyponatraemia, sexual dysfunction.

Life-Threatening or Dangerous Adverse Effects
- Common (≥1/100 to <1/10):
  - Suicidal ideation and behaviour.
- Uncommon (≥1/1,000 to <1/100):
  - New-onset/aggravation of diabetes mellitus, ketoacidosis, hyperosmolar coma.
- Rare (≥1/10,000 to <1/1,000):
  - Agranulocytosis.
  - Venous thromboembolism.
  - Pancreatitis, intestinal obstruction/ileus.
  - Hepatitis.
  - Neuroleptic malignant syndrome.
- Very rare (<1/10,000):
  - Anaphylactic reactions.
  - SIADH.
  - Angioedema, Stevens–Johnson syndrome, toxic epidermal necrolysis.
  - Rhabdomyolysis.

Q

- ○ DRESS syndrome, acute generalized exanthematous pustulosis (AGEP), erythema multiforme (appearing during the first 4–6 weeks after quetiapine initiation).
- Unknown frequency:
  - ○ Cardiomyopathy/myocarditis.
  - ○ Stroke.

Rare and Not Life-Threatening Adverse Effects
- Metabolic syndrome.
- Sleep disorders, including sleep talking.
- Breast swelling, menstrual disorder.
- CPK elevation.

Weight Change
- Quetiapine use commonly predisposes to weight gain.

What to Do About Adverse Effects
- Before introducing quetiapine, discuss common or life-threatening adverse effects with patients and/or caregivers, including symptoms that should be reported to the physician.
- Patients and their caregivers should be informed about the possibility of quetiapine causing suicidal ideation/behaviour. If such signs/symptoms emerge, patients should urgently seek for medical advice and be treated accordingly.
- Patients and their caregivers should be informed about the possibility of quetiapine causing orthostatic hypotension, which might lead to falls and injuries, and should be advised to be cautious until they are familiar with the potential effects. If orthostatic hypotension occurs, dose reduction or discontinuation should be considered, especially in patients with underlying cardiovascular disease.
- Consider discontinuation of therapy at first signs of clinically significant decline in WBC ($<1.0 \times 10^9/l$) in absence of other causative factors.
  - Neutropenia should be considered in patients presenting with fever or infection. Patients should be advised to immediately report any signs or symptoms compatible with agranulocytosis or infection (e.g. fever, sore throat, weakness, lethargy) during quetiapine therapy and have a WBC count (including an absolute neutrophil count), especially in the absence of predisposing factors.
- Any worsening in parameters of the metabolic profile, including changes in weight, blood glucose and lipids, should be managed as clinically appropriate.
- Mild or moderate intensity somnolence appearing in the beginning of quetiapine therapy usually subsides. If severe somnolence occurs, close monitoring is required for at least 2 weeks or until symptoms improve. Quetiapine discontinuation might be considered.

- If neuroleptic malignant syndrome occurs, quetiapine should be immediately withdrawn, and appropriate medical treatment should be applied.
- In the case of symptoms suggestive of severe skin reactions (e.g. DRESS syndrome, AGEP), quetiapine should be immediately discontinued and replaced by alternative treatment.
- If adverse effects are persistent or troublesome, including tardive dyskinesias, consider tapering or withdrawing quetiapine.

Dosing and Use

Usual Dosage Range
- In contrast to licensed therapeutic indications, where the maximum daily dose of quetiapine is 750 mg and 800 mg for IR and ER formulations, respectively, quetiapine dosage in the majority of studies in Parkinson's disease ranges from 12.5 mg to a maximum of 300 mg daily.

Available Formulations
- Tablets, immediate release: 25 mg, 50 mg, 100 mg, 200 mg, 300 mg, 400 mg.
- Tablets, extended release: 50 mg, 150 mg, 200 mg, 300 mg, 400 mg.

How to Dose
- An initial dose of 12.5 mg or 25 mg OD at bedtime is suggested.
- Dose can be gradually increased, as tolerated, but optimally should not exceed 100–150 mg/day.

Dosing Tips
- IR formulations can be administered with or without food, while ER formulations should be taken without food.
- Quetiapine is preferably taken in the evening before bedtime to lower the risk of somnolence.
- In persistent cases of Parkinson's disease-related psychosis, quetiapine can be combined with pimavanserin with close monitoring of QT interval.

How to Withdraw Drug
- A gradual withdrawal over a period of at least 1–2 weeks is suggested.
  - Reduce the dose of quetiapine by half every week until the dose of 12.5 mg OD is reached, then discontinue.
- Patients should be closely monitored after quetiapine discontinuation for the occurrence of withdrawal symptoms, including tardive dyskinesias and suicide-related events – especially after abrupt cessation of treatment.

Overdose
- Quetiapine overdose might present with drowsiness and sedation, tachycardia, hypotension, and anti-cholinergic symptoms. In more

Q

severe cases, it can lead to QT prolongation, seizures, rhabdomyolysis, respiratory depression, urinary retention, agitation, confusion, delirium, coma, and death.
- In case of quetiapine ER overdose, a delay in peak symptoms and a prolonged recovery are expected.
- Patients with cardiovascular disease are at an increased risk of the overdose effects.
- There is no specific antidote to quetiapine.
- Supportive measures, close monitoring and maintenance of a clear airway with adequate ventilation are recommended.
- Gastric lavage can be indicated in severe quetiapine intoxication; if possible, perform within 1 h of ingestion.
- Administration of activated charcoal should be considered.
- A laxative can also be used to prevent further drug absorption, if time-appropriate.
- In case of refractory hypotension, consider administering IV fluids and/or sympathomimetic agents.
  - Epinephrine and dopamine should be avoided, as β-stimulation may aggravate hypotension due to quetiapine-induced α-blockade.
- Patients with agitation and delirium presenting with a clear anticholinergic syndrome may be treated with physostigmine 1–2 mg under ECG monitoring.
  - Physostigmine should not be used in case of subjacent dysrhythmias, any degree of heart block, or QRS-widening.
  - Due to the negative effects of physostigmine on cardiac conductance, this is not recommended as a standard treatment.
- Formation of a gastric bezoar has been reported in cases of a quetiapine ER overdose. Appropriate diagnostic imaging is recommended and endoscopic bezoar removal.
  - Routine gastric lavage may not be effective in the bezoar removal due to the sticky consistency of the lesion.
- There are some case reports of patients with quetiapine overdose who were successfully treated with the administration of IV lipid emulsions, after the initial failure of symptomatic management, possibly due to the lipophilic nature of quetiapine.

Tests and Therapeutic Drug Monitoring
- Before initiation of quetiapine therapy:
  - A metabolic panel should be performed, including electrolytes, renal and hepatic function.
  - A baseline ECG should be performed to check for QT prolongation.
  - A fall risk assessment should be performed.
- During quetiapine therapy:
  - Patients' blood pressure should be monitored periodically, including orthostatic vital signs, especially in susceptible patients (e.g. elderly, patients treated with antihypertensives, patients with hypovolaemia or dehydration).

DOSING AND USE

Q

QUETIAPINE

- Patients' weight should be monitored periodically.
- A blood panel with specific focus on complete blood count, fasting glucose, electrolytes, cholesterol, triglyceride levels should be periodically performed, especially in patients with diabetes mellitus to avoid hyperosmolar coma.
- Patients should receive a lens examination every 6 months to monitor for cataract occurrence.

Other Warnings/Precautions
- There is a black box warning for patients (young adults) with major depressive disorders or other psychiatric conditions taking antidepressants, because quetiapine use might predispose to suicidality and associated behaviours despite appropriate therapy.
- Due to the moderate to strong affinity of norquetiapine for muscarinic receptor subtypes, special caution is advised when using quetiapine in patients with a current diagnosis or prior history of urinary retention, clinically significant prostatic hypertrophy, intestinal obstruction or related conditions, increased intra-ocular pressure, or narrow-angle glaucoma.
- Caution is advised when administering quetiapine in patients at high risk of prolonged cardiac repolarization (e.g. co-medication with drugs increasing QT interval, patients with cardiovascular disease, family history of QT prolongation, congenital long QT syndrome, congestive heart failure, heart hypertrophy, hypokalaemia, or hypomagnesaemia), especially in the elderly.
- Use with caution in patients with cardiovascular or cerebrovascular disease or hypotension.
- Use with caution in patients with breast cancer or history of seizures.
- Use with caution in patients with diabetes mellitus or at risk for diabetes.
- Co-administration of quetiapine with anticholinergic (muscarinic) effects, other CNS depressants or alcohol should be avoided.
- In patients treated with hepatic enzyme inducers (e.g. *carbamazepine*, *phenytoin*), quetiapine should only be initiated if the potential benefits outweigh the risks of removing the former agents or replacing them with a non-inducer (e.g. *sodium valproate*).

Do Not Use (Contraindications)
- Known sensitivity to the active substance of quetiapine or to any of its excipients.
- Quetiapine should not be used in elderly patients with dementia-related psychosis, as its use has been associated with an increased risk of death (cardiovascular, cerebrovascular or infectious aetiology) (black box warning).
- Co-medication with CYP3A4 inhibitors (e.g. *ketoconazole*).
- Patients should not consume grapefruit while on quetiapine.

Q

Special Populations

Renal Impairment
• Dosage adjustments are not necessary.

Hepatic Impairment
• Quetiapine is extensively metabolized in the liver and therefore should be used with caution in patients with known hepatic impairment, especially during the initial dosing period. Patients with known hepatic impairment should start on a dosage of 25 mg/day. The dosage should be increased daily with increments of 25–50 mg/day until an effective level is reached, depending on the clinical response and tolerability of the individual patient.

Elderly
• The average clearance of quetiapine is about 30–50% lower in those over 65 compared to younger individuals.
• The elderly are more prone to side effects from quetiapine use. The rate of dose titration may need to be slower, and the daily therapeutic dose lower than that used in younger patients, depending on the clinical response and tolerability of the individual patient.

Pregnancy
• Quetiapine should not be used during pregnancy unless the benefits outweigh the potential risks.
• There have been reports of agitation, hypertonia, hypotonia, tremor, somnolence, respiratory distress, or feeding disorder in newborns who have been exposed to quetiapine during the third trimester.
• Reports on the effect of quetiapine during the first trimester are controversial.

Breastfeeding
• There are no consistent adverse events reported in infants exposed to quetiapine through breast milk.
• There is no information on effects of quetiapine on milk production in humans.
• Breastfeeding benefits should be considered along with mother's need for therapy and any potential side effects on breastfed child.

COSTS

Costs
NHS indicative costs accessed 15 August 2022:
• IR tablets:
• Seroquel 25 mg tablets (Luye Pharma Ltd) – 60 × 25 mg: £48.60; 60 × 100 mg: £135.72; 60 × 200 mg: £135.72; 60 × 300 mg: £204.00.
  • Generic formulations – 60 × 25 mg: £1.16–£48.60; 60 × 100 mg: £2.03–£135.71; 60 × 150 mg: £2.19–£113.10; 60 × 200 mg: £3.05–£135.72; 60 × 300 mg: £3.89–£204.

Q

- MR tablets:
  - Seroquel XL tablets (Luye Pharma Ltd) – 60 × 50 mg: £67.66; 60 × 150 mg: £113.10; 60 × 200 mg: £113.10.
  - Generic formulations – 60 × 50 mg: £8.99–£67.65; 60 × 150 mg: £19.49–£107.45; 60 × 200 mg: £25.99–£169.99.

The Overall Place of Quetiapine in the Treatment of Parkinson's Disease

Quetiapine is an atypical antipsychotic, which, along with its active metabolite, norquetiapine, interact with a broad range of neurotransmitter receptors. They both exhibit higher selectivity for 5-HT2 serotonergic receptors compared to D2 dopaminergic receptors and this combination is speculated to mediate the clinical antipsychotic properties and the low extrapyramidal adverse reactions. These properties render quetiapine unique among other antipsychotic agents and allow its use in low dosage in Parkinson's disease-related psychosis, although off-label. More specifically, several open-label studies and one RCT have supported the efficacy of quetiapine in Parkinson's disease-related psychosis, but this was not confirmed in three double-blind RCTs. Quetiapine remains the most commonly used antipsychotic agent in Parkinson's disease-related psychosis, as it is considered safer than clozapine in routine clinical practice. However, a variety of side effects have been associated with its use, including somnolence and orthostatic hypotension, especially among the elderly or those with subjacent cardiovascular disease, so vigilance is required.

Potential Advantages
- Better safety profile when compared to clozapine, which is also a first-line option in Parkinson's disease-related psychosis.
  - Compared to clozapine, it does not require intensive blood monitoring.
- Compared to other antipsychotics (such as olanzapine or risperidone), quetiapine is believed to improve Parkinson's disease-related psychosis with little propensity to aggravate parkinsonian features.
- Although pimavanserin constitutes a first choice in patients with Parkinson's disease-related psychosis, quetiapine use might be reasonable when psychotic symptoms are intolerable and need to be managed acutely due to its rapid onset of action.
- In contrast to pimavanserin, it is globally available.

Potential Disadvantages
- Not formally established as efficacious in Parkinson's disease-related psychosis due to lack of relevant RCTs.
- Quetiapine use has been associated with increased morbidity and mortality, especially among the elderly and those with dementia or cardiovascular disease.
- Quetiapine use among elderly patients (over 65) with Parkinson's disease has been associated with an increased risk of death.

QUETIAPINE

Clinical Box

A 62-year old man with a 10-year history of Parkinson's disease without cognitive impairment was admitted to the Orthopaedic ward due to surgery after a distal radius fracture of the right arm. His current medication included levodopa/benserazide 200 mg/50 mg QID and pramipexole ER 0.52 mg OD. The rest of his medical history was unremarkable. During his admission, the patient became agitated, developed visual hallucinations, and had difficulty sleeping during the night. The fracture and the surgery were acknowledged as potential contributing factors, although other possible causes, including infections or metabolic abnormalities, were excluded and the patient's neurological examination was similar to his baseline. Non-pharmacological measures were suggested (including support of sleep–wake cycle, early mobilization, and contact with familiar persons), pramipexole was gradually withdrawn over 2 days and a low dose of quetiapine 25 mg OD was initiated at bedtime, which was increased to 50 mg the next day with gradual improvement of symptoms within a few days. ECG monitoring for QT interval prolongation was also undertaken. No deterioration of the patient's parkinsonism was observed before his discharge and his levodopa regimen was maintained as it was. After 2 months, during his follow-up visit with his treating neurologist, and while the patient was free of hallucinations, quetiapine was gradually discontinued.

Q

Suggested Reading

Klein C, T Prokhorov, A Miniovich, E Dobronevsky, JM Rabey. Long-term follow-up (24 months) of quetiapine treatment in drug-induced Parkinson disease psychosis. *Clin Neuropharmacol* 2006; 29(4): 215–219.

Kyle K, JM Bronstein. Treatment of psychosis in Parkinson's disease and dementia with Lewy bodies: a review. *Parkinsonism Relat Disord* 2020; 75: 55–62.

Weintraub D, C Chiang, HM Kim, J Wilkinson, C Marras, B Stanislawski, E Mamikonyan, HC Kales. Association of antipsychotic use with mortality risk in patients with Parkinson disease. *JAMA Neurol* 2016; 73(5): 535–541.

References

AHFS Drug information, 2012. Bethesda: American Society of Health-System Pharmacists. Accessed on 15 August 2022 via www.medicinescomplete.com.

Arslan ED, A Demit, F Yilmaz, C Kavalci, E Karakilic, E Çelikel. Treatment of quetiapine overdose with intravenous lipid emulsion. *Keio J Med* 2013; 62(2): 53–57.

Fernandez HH, MS Okun, RL Rodriguez, IA Malaty, J Romrell, A Sun, SS Wu, S Pillarisetty, A Nyathappa, S Eisenschenk. Quetiapine improves visual hallucinations in Parkinson disease but not through normalization of sleep architecture: results from a double-blind clinical-polysomnography study. *Int J Neurosci* 2009; 119(12): 2196–2205.

Joint Formulary Committee. British National Formulary (online). London: BMJ Group and Pharmaceutical Press. Accessed on 15 August 2022 www.medicinescomplete.com.

Lizarraga KJ, SH Fox, AP Strafella, AE Lang. Hallucinations, delusions and impulse control disorders in Parkinson disease. *Clin Geriatr Med* 2020; 36(1): 105–118.

Ondo WG, R Tintner, KD Voung, D Lai, G Ringholz. Double-blind, placebo-controlled, unforced titration parallel trial of quetiapine for dopaminergic-induced hallucinations in Parkinson's disease. *Mov Disord* 2005; 20(8): 958–963.

Quetiapine. In: Brayfield A (Ed.), *Martindale: The Complete Drug Reference*. London: The Royal Pharmaceutical Society of Great Britain. Accessed on 15 August 2022 via www.medicinescomplete.com.

Quetiapine. In: DRUGDEX® System (electronic version). Truven Health Analytics, Greenwood Village, Colorado, USA. Accessed on 15 August 2022 via www.micromedexsolutions.com.

Rabey JM, T Prokhorov, A Miniovitz, E Dobronevskyu, C Klein. Effect of quetiapine in psychotic Parkinson's disease patients: a double-blind labeled study of 3 months' duration. *Mov Disord* 2007; 22(3): 313–318.

Reddy S, SA Factor, ES Molho, PJ Feustel. The effect of quetiapine on psychosis and motor function in parkinsonian patients with and without dementia. *Mov Disord* 2002; 17(4): 676–681.

Shotbolt P, M Samuel, C Fox, AS David. A randomized controlled trial of quetiapine for psychosis in Parkinson's disease. *Neuropsychiatr Dis Treat* 2009; 5: 327–332.

Shotbolt P, M Samuel, A David. Quetiapine in the treatment of psychosis in Parkinson's disease. *Ther Adv Neurol Disord* 2010; 3(6): 339–350.

Summary of product characteristics – quetiapine 100 mg film-coated tablets. Electronic Medicines Compendium: Quetiapine 100 mg film-coated tablets – summary of product characteristics (SmPC) – (emc). Accessed on 15 August 2022 via www.medicines.org.uk.

RASAGILINE

Therapeutics

Chemical Name and Structure

Rasagiline mesylate ((R)-N-2-propynyl-1-indanamine methanesulfonate) has a molecular weight of 267.3 and a molecular formula of $C_{12}H_{13}N,CH_4O_3S$.

Brand Names
- **Alziras** (*Australia*); **Altina, Anaxira** (*Spain*); **Asanix** (*Lithuania, Poland*); **Asarkin** (*Greece*); **Azagilin** (*Ukraine*); **Azilect** (*Argentina, Australia, Austria, Belgium, Brazil, Canada, China, Cyprus, Denmark, Estonia, Finland, France, Germany, Greece, Hong Kong, Hungary, Ireland, Israel, Italy, Japan, Lithuania, Mexico, Netherlands, Norway, Philippines, Poland, Portugal, Russian Federation, Singapore, South Africa, Spain, Sweden, Switzerland, Thailand, Turkey, UK, Ukraine, USA*); **Azipar** (*Turkey*); **Azipron** (*Cyprus*).
- **Burnix** (*Argentina*).
- **Dardaren** (*Mexico*); **Detreman** (*Poland*); **Devolina** (*Spain*).
- **Elbrus** (*Argentina*); **Etkinia** (*Turkey*).
- **Glarise** (*Turkey*).
- **Kinect** (*South Africa*).
- **Menuix** (*Chile, Ecuador*).
- **Nervogil** (*Turkey*); **Neuromiol** (*Spain*).
- **Parcilect** (*Estonia, Lithuania*); **Pargix** (*South Africa*); **Parlin** (*Turkey*).
- **Ractilen** (*Greece*); **Ragipar** (*Argentina*); **Ragipax** (*Ecuador*); **Ragitar** (*Ecuador, South Africa*); **Raglysa** (*Spain*); **Ralago** (*Estonia, Greece, Lithuania, Poland*); **Ranzal** (*Greece*); **Rasabon** (*Finland, Italy*); **Rasagea** (*Germany*); **Rasalas** (*Turkey*); **Rasalect, Rasaline** (*Australia*); **Rasapar** (*South Africa*); **Rasaral** (*Italy*); **Rasax** (*Argentina*); **Rasazil** (*Australia*); **Rasigerolan** (*Austria*); **Roldap** (*Italy*).
- **Sagilia** (*Cyprus, Estonia, Greece, Lithuania*); **Saglis** (*Turkey*).
- **Tivel** (*Cyprus*); **Trepar** (*Turkey*).

Generics Available
- Yes.

Licensed Indications for Parkinson's Disease
- Treatment of idiopathic Parkinson's disease as monotherapy or as adjunct therapy to levodopa/DDI preparations or dopamine agonists in patients with end-of-dose fluctuations (FDA, EMA, EMC).

Licensed Indications for Other Conditions
- None.

Non-Licensed Use for Parkinson's Disease
- Symptomatic treatment of fatigue.

R

Non-Licensed Use for Other Conditions
• None.

Ineffective
• Not reported.

Mechanism of Action
• Rasagiline is an irreversible and selective MAO-B inhibitor.
• It increases extracellular levels of dopamine in the striatum.

Efficacy Profile
• According to the MDS EBM Committee:
   ◦ Rasagiline is considered 'efficacious' and 'clinically useful':
      ▪ As a monotherapy in the treatment of motor symptoms in Parkinson's disease (although the effect size is smaller compared to levodopa or dopamine agonists).
      ▪ As an adjunct therapy in early or stable Parkinson's disease patients.
      ▪ For the treatment of motor fluctuations in Parkinson's disease.
   ◦ There is 'insufficient evidence' considering the efficacy of rasagiline to prevent or delay the progression of Parkinson's disease.
• The goal of using rasagiline as an adjunctive therapy is to reduce OFF time for Parkinson's disease patients with motor fluctuations.
• Onset of action is within 1 h.

Pharmacokinetics
Absorption and Distribution
• Oral bioavailability: 36%.
• Time to maximum concentration: 0.5–1 h.
• Food co-ingestion does not affect the Tmax of rasagiline, while Cmax and AUC decrease by approximately 60% and 20%, respectively, when taken with a high-fat meal. The manufacturers state that because the AUC is not substantially affected, rasagiline can be administered with or without food.
• Pharmacokinetics: linear.
• Protein binding: 60–70%.
• Volume of distribution: 87 l.

Metabolism
• Extensive hepatic metabolism by cytochrome P450 isoenzymes, predominantly CYP1A2.
• Two main pathways: N-dealkylation and/or hydroxylation to yield: 1-aminoindan, 3-hydroxy-N-propargyl-1 aminoindan and 3-hydroxy-1-aminoindan.
• Recovery time of MAO-B activity (requiring *de novo* synthesis of the enzyme) is about 40 days.

RASAGILINE

Elimination
- Elimination half-life ranges from 0.6 h to 2 h.
- Rasagiline is primarily excreted via urine (62.6%) and secondarily in faeces (21.8%).
- Less than 1% of a dose is excreted unchanged in the urine.
- The major part (95%) of the product is excreted in the urine as glucuronide conjugates.

Drug Interaction Profile
Pharmacokinetic Drug Interactions
- Effects on rasagiline:
  - Potent CYP1A2 inhibitors (e.g. *ciprofloxacin*) may increase levels of rasagiline.
  - Potential pharmacokinetic interaction (increased rasagiline metabolism) with smoking (induction of CYP1A2).
  - Potential pharmacokinetic interaction with *entacapone* (increased rasagiline oral clearance by 28%).
- Effects by rasagiline:
  - Potential pharmacokinetic interaction with drugs metabolized by CYP2C9 (e.g. *warfarin*, where INR has shown increases of up to 20% in studies).

Pharmacodynamic Drug Interactions
- Co-medication with *pethidine* and other opioids might lead to life-threatening reactions, like serotonin syndrome.
- Co-administration with tricyclic or tetracyclic antidepressants or SSRIs/SNRIs (e.g. *fluoxetine*, *paroxetine*, *sertraline*, and *venlafaxine*) can lead to sweating, flushing, hyperthermia, diarrhoea, hypertension or hypotension, seizures, palpitations, dizziness, mental changes, such as agitation, confusion, hallucinations, delirium and coma, ataxia, myoclonus, hyperreflexia, tremor, and serotonin syndrome.
- Co-medication with non-selective MAOIs (including medicinal and natural products without prescription, e.g. St. John's Wort) may lead to a hypertensive crisis.
- Co-medication with serotonin agonists used to treat migraine, including *rizatriptan*, *sumatriptan*, and *zolmitriptan*, may also lead to serotonin syndrome despite metabolism via MAO-A (although they are considered unlikely to interact).
- Co-medication with sympathomimetic agents, including nasal and oral decongestants, containing *ephedrine* or *pseudoephedrine*, may lead to a hypertensive reaction.
- Potential pharmacokinetic interaction with linezolid, leading to an increased risk of a serotonin syndrome.

R

Adverse Effects

How Drug Causes Adverse Effects
- Mainly (but not only) by increasing dopaminergic activity.

Common Adverse Effects
- In monotherapy: headache, flu-like syndrome, melanoma, leukopenia, allergy, depression, hallucinations, conjunctivitis, vertigo, angina pectoris, rhinitis, flatulence, dermatitis, musculoskeletal pain, neck pain, arthritis, urinary urgency, fever, and malaise.
- In adjunctive therapy: dyskinesia, decreased appetite, hallucinations, abnormal dreams, dystonia, carpal tunnel syndrome, balance disorder, orthostatic hypotension, rash, abdominal pain, constipation, nausea and vomiting, dry mouth, rash, arthralgia, neck pain, decreased weight, and falls.
- Possible dopaminergic-induced adverse events, including excessive daytime sleepiness and ICDs, may occur.

Life-Threatening or Dangerous Adverse Effects
- Rare (≥1/10,000 to <1/1,000):
  ○ Cerebrovascular accidents, MI.
  ○ Melanoma.
- If combined with other agents:
  ○ Hypertensive crisis.
  ○ Serotonin syndrome.

Weight Change
- Not reported.

What to Do About Adverse Effects
- Before introducing rasagiline, discuss common adverse effects with patients or caregivers, including symptoms that should be reported to the physician.
- Consider withdrawing therapy if adverse effects are troublesome with concomitant increase in levodopa dosing or alternative levodopa-sparing strategies.

Dosing and Use

Usual Dosage Range
- 500 micrograms to 1 mg daily.

Available Formulations
- Tablets: 1 mg, 500 micrograms

How to Dose
- An initial dose of 1 mg OD is suggested; no dose increases apply.
- In the USA, an initial daily dose of 500 micrograms is recommended for adjunctive therapy.

Dosing Tips
• None.

How to Withdraw Drug
• No specific instructions are needed. Rasagiline can be withdrawn abruptly.

Overdose
• Symptoms of overdose may not appear for up to 12 h and may include irritability, restlessness, dizziness, drowsiness, sweating, severe tachycardia, hypertension, headache, confusion, seizures, and in severe cases, cardiovascular collapse and coma may occur.

Tests and Therapeutic Drug Monitoring
• None.

Other Warnings/Precautions
• Patients and carers should be made aware of the possibility of rasagiline causing ICDs; vigilance is recommended.
• Caution is advised when driving or operating hazardous machinery, as rasagiline may cause dizziness, orthostatic hypotension, excessive daytime sleepiness or episodes of sudden sleep onset. These activities should be avoided until effects have stopped recurring.
• Co-medication with non-selective MAOIs may lead to a hypertensive crisis and these should be avoided.

Do Not Use (Contraindications)
• Hypersensitivity to the active substance or to any of its excipients.
• Severe hepatic impairment.
• Co-medication with serotonin agonists (e.g. triptans), opioids, sympathomimetics, other MAOIs, *linezolid*, antidepressants, including tricyclic/tetracyclic antidepressants and SSRIs/SNRIs, psychostimulants, and central suppressant drugs (e.g. sedatives).

Special Populations
Renal Impairment
• No special precautions are required in patients with renal impairment.

Hepatic Impairment
• Moderate hepatic impairment: rasagiline should be avoided.
• Severe hepatic impairment: contraindicated.

Elderly
• No special warnings or precautions are advised in the elderly.

R

Pregnancy
- No experience from clinical studies of rasagiline use in pregnant women.
- Manufacturer advises that it is preferable to avoid rasagiline use during pregnancy.

Breastfeeding
- Non-clinical data indicate that rasagiline inhibits prolactin secretion and, thus, may inhibit lactation.
- It is not known if rasagiline is excreted in human breast milk. Caution is therefore advised by the manufacturer.

Costs
NHS indicative price accessed 19 March 2022:
- Azilect (Teva UK Ltd) – 28 × 1 mg tablets: £70.72.
- Generic formulations – 28 × 1 mg tablets: £2.55–£70.72.

The Overall Place of Rasagiline in the Treatment of Parkinson's Disease
Rasagiline is a second-generation, oral selective and irreversible MAO-B inhibitor approved for the symptomatic treatment of Parkinson's disease. By irreversibly inhibiting MAO-B, it increases extracellular levels of dopamine in the striatum. It is a well-tolerated drug, used as monotherapy in the early phases of Parkinson's disease or as an add-on therapy to levodopa preparations to address end-of-dose fluctuations. Rasagiline is also considered 'efficacious' for the treatment of fatigue in Parkinson's disease.

Clinical Box
A 65-year-old right-handed man, with a 3-month duration of Parkinson's disease who was drug-naïve, complained of mild and only occasionally troublesome stiffness in his left upper limb and of daytime fatigue. Given the mild severity of his motor symptoms and a non-motor symptom burden dominated by fatigue, rasagiline 1 mg OD was initiated with beneficial effects on both.

Suggested Reading
McCormack PL. Rasagiline: a review of its use in the treatment of idiopathic Parkinson's disease. *CNS Drugs* 2014; 28(11): 1083–1097.

R

References

AHFS Drug Information, 2012. Bethesda: American Society of Health-System Pharmacists. Accessed on 19 March 2022 via www.medicinescomplete.com.

Joint Formulary Committee. British National Formulary (online). London: BMJ Group and Pharmaceutical Press. Accessed on 19 March 2022 via www.medicinescomplete.com.

Rasagiline. In: Brayfield A (Ed.), *Martindale: The Complete Drug Reference*. London: The Royal Pharmaceutical Society of Great Britain. Accessed on 19 March 2022 via www.medicinescomplete.com.

Rasagiline. In: DRUGDEX® System (electronic version). Truven Health Analytics, Greenwood Village, Colorado, USA. Accessed on 10 March 2023 via www.micromedexsolutions.com.

Summary of product characteristics – Azilect 1 mg tablets. Teva Pharmaceuticals Ltd – Electronic Medicines Compendium: Azilect 1 mg tablets – summary of product characteristics (SmPC) – (emc). Accessed on 19 March 2022 via www.medicines.org.uk.

RIVASTIGMINE

R

Therapeutics

Chemical Name and Structure

Rivastigmine ([3-[(1S)-1-(dimethylamino)ethyl]phenyl]N-ethyl-N-methylcarbamate) can be found as an off-white to slightly yellow powder in oral formulations or a viscous, clear, and colourless to yellow to very slightly brown liquid in transdermal formulations. It has a molecular weight of 250.34 (as the base) and an empirical formula of $C_{14}H_{22}N_2O_2$.

Brand Names

- **Alapril** (*Greece*); **Alcenorm** (*Russian Federation*); **Aldemyl** (*Greece*); **Almuriva** (*UK*); **Altigmin** (*Turkey*); **Alzerta** (*Spain*); **Alzest** (*UK*); **Alzigmine** (*Israel*).
- **Balaxon** (*Greece*); **Begusin** (*Poland*).
- **Crista** (*Turkey*).
- **Demelora** (*Italy*); **Divasmin** (*Turkey*).
- **Emerpand** (*Poland*); **Erastig** (*UK*); **Evertas** (*Greece, Poland*); **Exelon** (*Argentina, Australia, Austria, Belgium, Brazil, Canada, Chile, China, Cyprus, Czech Republic, Denmark, Ecuador, Estonia, Finland, France, Germany, Greece, Hong Kong, Hungary, India, Indonesia, Ireland, Israel, Italy, Japan, Lithuania, Malaysia, Mexico, Netherlands, New Zealand, Norway, Philippines, Poland, Portugal, Russian Federation, Singapore, South Africa, Spain, Sweden, Switzerland, Thailand, Turkey, UK, USA, Venezuela*).
- **Immitis** (*Greece*); **Impalon** (*Greece*); **Ivastine** (*Greece*).
- **Kerstipon** (*Greece, Poland*); **Kyriz** (*South Africa*).
- **Lasium** (*Greece*).
- **Mentazac, Mnimoran** (*Greece*).
- **Newvastig** (*Greece*); **Nimvastid** (*Austria, Czech Republic, Denmark, Estonia, Finland, Germany, Ireland, Lithuania, Netherlands, Poland, Spain, Sweden, UK*).
- **Orivast** (*Sweden*).
- **Permente** (*Poland*); **Prometax** (*Brazil, Greece, Italy, Netherlands, Poland, Portugal, Spain, Sweden, UK*).
- **Ralsimina** (*Venezuela*); **Rebetin** (*Cyprus*); **Remizeral** (*Argentina*); **Resymtia** (*Poland*); **Rigmin** (*Sweden*); **Rignyt** (*Venezuela*); **Rilimeba** (*Poland*); **Rimans** (*Turkey*); **Ristart** (*Turkey*); **Ristidic** (*Netherlands, Poland*); **Rivadem** (*Hong Kong*); **Rivagelan** (*Austria*); **Rivagmin** (*Greece*); **Rivaldo** (*Poland*); **Rivamer** (*Venezuela*); **Rivamylan** (*Greece, Poland*); **Rivanel** (*Greece*); **Rivanex** (*Spain*); **Rivarem** (*Turkey*); **Rivarious** (*Greece*); **Rivasan** (*Hong Kong*); **Rivaset** (*Greece*); **Rivasta** (*Thailand*); **Rivastach** (*Japan*); **Rivastelon** (*Brazil*); **Rivastigmelon** (*Australia*); **Rivastinol** (*Greece*); **Rivastiplus** (*Greece*); **Rivaston** (*Hong Kong*); **Rivastor** (*Denmark, Finland, Sweden*); **Rivasvitae** (*Ecuador*); **Rivaxel** (*Tunisia, Turkey*); **Rivazic** (*Ecuador*); **Riveka** (*Poland*);

RIVASTIGMINE

Rivelon (*Greece*); **Rivendo** (*Germany*); **Rivetal** (*Greece, Hong Kong, Tunisia*); **Rivoder** (*Poland*).
- **Signelon** (*Poland*); **Somniton** (*UK*); **Symelon** (*Poland*).
- **Telomens** (*Greece*); **Tigma** (*Brazil*).
- **Vastigma** (*Brazil*); **Vergesin** (*Poland*); **Vialon** (*Cyprus, Greece*); **Vitacholine** (*Tunisia*); **Voleze** (*UK*).

Generics Available
- Yes.

Licensed Indications for Parkinson's Disease
- Mild to moderate Parkinson's disease dementia (FDA, EMA, EMC).

Licensed Indications for Other Conditions
- Alzheimer's disease (oral: mild-to-moderate dementia; transdermal: mild-to-severe dementia) (FDA, EMA, EMC).

Non-Licensed Use for Parkinson's Disease
- Treatment of Parkinson's disease-related apathy and refractory RBD.

Non-Licensed Use for Other Conditions
- Multi-infarct dementia.
- Persistent cognitive impairment – traumatic brain injury.
- Schizophrenia.
- Senile dementia of the Lewy body type.

Ineffective
- MCI and vascular dementia.
- Cognitive impairment in multiple sclerosis.

Mechanism of Action
- A reversible cholinesterase inhibitor, which increases the availability of ACh in cholinergic synapses, enhancing cholinergic transmission.
- Unlike other cholinesterase inhibitors, rivastigmine binds to and inhibits both acetylcholinesterase and butyrylcholinesterase.
  - It is the only cholinesterase inhibitor that significantly inhibits butyrylcholinesterase, although it is not clear how this relates to the clinical effect of rivastigmine.
- Acetylcholinesterase inhibition lasts for approximately 9 h.

Efficacy Profile
- Individual responses to rivastigmine cannot be predicted, although it seems to be more efficacious in moderate dementia.
- According to the MDS EBM Committee, rivastigmine has been labelled as:
  - 'Efficacious' and 'possibly useful' in Parkinson's disease-related dementia and apathy treatment.

THERAPEUTICS

- 'Likely efficacious' and 'possibly useful' as an adjunct therapy for gait and balance impairment in Parkinson's disease, as it has been associated with a reduction in falls.
- Despite the fact that rivastigmine is not recommended in MCI, its use in Parkinson's disease-related MCI was associated with an amelioration in cognition, disease-related health status, anxiety severity, and performance-based measures of cognitive abilities.
- There is preliminary evidence that rivastigmine exerts a beneficial effect on Parkinson's disease-related visual hallucinations and psychosis, especially in patients with dementia, where antipsychotics might not be an optimal choice due to deteriorating cognitive impairment.
- There are some limited indications that rivastigmine might be effective on refractory Parkinson's disease-related RBD (if melatonin, clonazepam, and rotigotine were not effective).
- Perioperative application of rivastigmine patch has been found to reduce the possibility of delirium in cognitively impaired older patients.

Pharmacokinetics

Absorption and Distribution
- Oral bioavailability: 36%.
- Food co-ingestion: food slows absorption, lowers Cmax, and increases AUC.
- Tmax: 1 h (oral), 10–16 h after a single application and 8 h in steady state (transdermal).
- Protein binding: 40%.
- Volume of distribution: 1.8–2.7 l/kg.

Metabolism
- Rapidly and extensively metabolized, primarily by cholinesterases, to the NAP-226-90 metabolite, which may undergo *N*-demethylation and/or sulphate conjugation.

Elimination
- Elimination half-life is 1.5 h for oral and about 3 h for transdermal formulations.
- Renal excretion of the metabolites constitutes the major elimination route, without any unchanged rivastigmine found in urine.
  - Less than 1% of an administered dose of rivastigmine is found in faeces.

Drug Interaction Profile

Pharmacokinetic Drug Interactions
- No pharmacokinetic interactions are expected with agents metabolized by the cytochrome isoenzymes CYP1A2, CYP2D6, CYP3A4/5, CYP2E1, CYP2C9/8/19, and CYP2B6.

- Nicotine may increase rivastigmine clearance, thus, reducing its plasma concentration; the clinical significance of this observation is unclear.

Pharmacodynamic Drug Interactions
- Co-medication with other cholinesterase-blocking agents (e.g. *neostigmine*, *physostigmine*, *oxybutynin*, *tolterodine*) may lead to synergistic effects.
- Rivastigmine may prolong the effects of depolarizing neuromuscular blocking agents (e.g. *suxamethonium*).
- Co-medication with beta-blockers (e.g. *carvedilol*, *metoprolol*, *atenolol*, *propranolol*) and other bradycardia-inducing agents (e.g. class III anti-arrhythmic agents, calcium channel antagonists, *digitalis glycoside*, *pilocarpine*) or drugs predisposing to QT prolongation may increase the risk of bradycardia and syncope.
- Co-medication with antipsychotics (e.g. *chlorpromazine*, *levomepromazine*, *sulpiride*, *amisulpride*, *tiapride*, *pimozide*, *haloperidol*, *droperidol*), *cisapride*, *citalopram*, *diphemanil*, *erythromycin*, *halofantrine*, *mizolastin*, *pentamidine*, and *moxifloxacin* might predispose to bradycardia and Torsade de Pointes.

Adverse Effects
How Drug Causes Adverse Effects
- Most of the adverse effects are cholinergic in nature.
- Local reactions may occur at the site of patch application.

Common Adverse Effects (Oral Formulations)
- Very common (≥1/10):
  ○ Nausea, vomiting, tremor, falls.
- Common (≥1/100 to <1/10):
  ○ Neuropsychiatric: insomnia, anxiety, restlessness, visual hallucinations, depression, dizziness, somnolence, headache, worsening of parkinsonian features (e.g. bradykinesia, rigidity, gait impairment), and/or dyskinesia.
  ○ Cardiovascular: bradycardia, hypertension.
  ○ GI: diarrhoea, abdominal pain, dyspepsia, salivary hypersecretion.
  ○ Other: decreased appetite, dehydration, hyperhidrosis, fatigue, asthenia.
- Uncommon (≥1/1,000 to <1/100):
  ○ Nervous: dystonia.
  ○ Cardiovascular: atrial fibrillation, atrioventricular block, hypotension.

Common Adverse Effects (Transdermal Formulations)
- Common (≥1/100 to <1/10):
  • Neuropsychiatric: anxiety, depression, delirium, agitation, headache, dizziness, syncope.
  • GI: nausea, vomiting, diarrhoea, dyspepsia, abdominal pain.
  • Renal/urinary: urinary tract infections, urinary incontinence.

R

- Other: anorexia, decreased appetite.
  - Application site reactions (e.g. itching, rash, erythema, pruritus, oedema, dermatitis, irritation).
- Uncommon (≥1/1,000 to <1/100):
  - Nervous: aggression.
  - Cardiovascular: bradycardia.
  - GI: gastric ulcer.
  - Other: dehydration.

Life-Threatening or Dangerous Adverse Effects (Mostly with Oral Formulations)
- Seizures.
- Angina pectoris, cardiac arrhythmias.
- Oesophageal rupture after severe and prolonged vomiting.
- Gastric and duodenal ulcers, gastrointestinal haemorrhage.
- Stevens–Johnson syndrome.

Rare and Not Life-Threatening Adverse Effects
- Deterioration of parkinsonian features and falls (transdermal formulations).
- Pancreatitis (oral formulations).
- Pisa syndrome (oral formulations).

Weight Change
- Rivastigmine might induce weight loss.
- Weight loss might necessitate dose reductions or even rivastigmine discontinuation.
- Caution is advised in patients weighing less than 50 kg (especially for those using the 13.3 mg/24 h patch), as they might be more vulnerable to adverse effects.
  - The rivastigmine steady-state concentrations of a patient weighing 65 kg are expected to be double compared to someone weighing 35 kg and half compared to someone weighing 100 kg.

What to Do About Adverse Effects
- Before introducing rivastigmine, discuss common or life-threatening adverse effects with patients and/or caregivers, including symptoms that should be reported to the treating physician.
- Rivastigmine should only be prescribed if a caregiver is available to regularly monitor the drug intake for the patient and the occurrence of adverse effects.
- Adverse effects might occur shortly after dose titration (e.g. tremor in Parkinson's disease-related dementia). If they do not respond to dose reduction, consider discontinuing rivastigmine therapy.
- Some adverse effects (e.g. nausea, vomiting, abdominal pain, appetite/weight loss, worsening of parkinsonian features, like tremor) may respond to omitting one or more doses. If not, consider reducing the

RIVASTIGMINE

THE MOVEMENT DISORDERS PRESCRIBER'S GUIDE TO PARKINSON'S DISEASE

dose to the previously well-tolerated dose of rivastigmine or withdrawing treatment.
  • GI reactions, in particular, are usually dose-related and may occur
    during treatment initiation or dosage increase.
• Dehydration following prolonged vomiting or diarrhoea can be associated with serious sequelae, especially in the elderly; consider management with IV fluids.
• The most common local dermatological adverse effects usually subside within 48 h after patch removal.
• Allergic contact dermatitis should be suspected if application site
  reactions spread beyond the patch size, in case of intense local reactions and if symptoms persist beyond 48 h after patch removal. Under
  these circumstances, rivastigmine therapy should be discontinued.
  • These patients could potentially be switched to oral formulations
    of rivastigmine following a negative allergy testing and under close
    medical supervision, although some patients might not be able to
    tolerate any type of rivastigmine formulation.
• The ability of patients on rivastigmine to drive or operate machinery should be regularly monitored, not only because rivastigmine can
  cause fatigue, dizziness, and somnolence, but also due to the patients'
  background of dementia.
• Patients and/or caregivers should be aware of the potential vagotonic
  effects of rivastigmine (e.g. bradycardia), as there might be synergistic
  effects with the antiparkinsonian drugs (e.g. orthostatic hypotension).
  • If loss of consciousness occurs, consider excluding the above vag-
    otonic phenomena, but also the possibility of seizures (increased
    seizure risk in demented patients).
  • Rivastigmine was found to more beneficial on cognition for
    patients with PDD and orthostatic hypotension, possibly due to a
    direct antihypotensive effect of rivastigmine.
• If troublesome adverse effects persist, considering lowering the dose
  of rivastigmine or completely withdrawing the drug.

Dosing and Use
Usual Dosage Range
• Oral: 3–12 mg daily.
• Transdermal: 4.6–13.3 mg/24 h.

Available Formulations
• Capsules: 1.5 mg, 3 mg, 4.5 mg, 6 mg.
• Transdermal patch: 4.6 mg/24 h, 9.5 mg/24 h, 13.3 mg/24 h.

How to Dose
• Oral:
  • Initial dose of 1.5 mg BID; increase, if needed and well-tolerated,
    by 1.5 mg BID every 2 weeks (EMA, EMC) or 4 weeks (FDA); not
    to exceed 6 mg BID.

R

DOSING AND USE

R

- Transdermal:
  - Initial dose of 4.6 mg/24 h; increase, if needed and well-tolerated, to 9.5 mg/24 h after a minimum of 4 weeks.
  - A further increase to 13.3 mg/24 h after another 4 weeks may be considered (FDA).
  - A dose increase from 9.5 mg/24 h to 13.3 mg/24 h may be considered after 6 months of treatment in patients with an objective cognitive deterioration (e.g. MMSE) and/or function decline based on clinical judgement (EMA, EMC).
  - The daily recommended effective dose is 9.5 mg/24 h (EMA, EMC).

Dosing Tips
- Rivastigmine capsules should be administered with food to reduce the risk for any GI issues.
- The adhesive side of the transdermal patch should be applied to clean, dry, intact healthy skin, which will not be rubbed by tight clothing or under a waistband and skin folds, and won't be directly exposed to the sun or other external sources of direct heat.
- Patches should not be applied to the thigh or the abdomen due to reduced bioavailability of rivastigmine at these sites.
  - Creams, lotions, oils, ointments, or powders should not be applied to the sites of the patch placement.
  - The patch should be pressed firmly in place for at least 30 s until the edges stick well.
  - The patient/caregiver should wash their hands with soap before and after applying the patch and not touch their eyes after applying the patch.
- The patch should be applied at approximately the same time every day, at a convenient time for the patient (preferably after exercise and shower to avoid patch detachment). The previous patch should be removed before the new one is applied.
- Sites of the patch application should rotate every day; the patch should not be applied to the same site more than once every 14 days.
- The patch can be used while the patient bathes/swims or during hot weather.
- In case the patient forgets to apply the patch or the patch is dislodged, a new patch should be applied for the remainder of the day, which will be replaced by a new one the next day according to the patient's regular time schedule.
- If dosing is interrupted for less than 3 days, patients should be instructed to resume treatment at the same or lower dose. If dosing is interrupted for more than 3 days, a gradual titration scheme starting again from 1.5 mg BID (oral) or 4.6 mg/24 h (transdermal) should be applied.

R

- Switching from oral to transdermal: if oral dose is less than 6 mg/day, switch to 4.6 mg/24 h. If oral dose is more than 6 mg/day, switch to 9.5 mg/24 h.
  - The patch should be applied the day following the last oral dose.
- Maintenance therapy can be continued for as long as there is a therapeutic benefit and the drug is well-tolerated.

How to Withdraw Drug
- Abrupt discontinuation of rivastigmine in patients has been associated with cognitive and behavioural decline; thus, a gradual withdrawal is suggested.
- A dose reduction to the next available formulation every 4 weeks is suggested according to the following schemes:
  - Oral formulations: 6 mg BID → 4.5 mg BID → 3 mg BID → 1.5 mg BID → 1.5 mg OD → cease.
  - Transdermal formulations: 13.3 mg/24 h → 9.5 mg/24 h → 4.6 mg/24 h → cease.
- The recommended tapering schedule may be tailored according to circumstances. In case of severe adverse events, rivastigmine can be discontinued without tapering.

Overdose
- Most cases of accidental overdose were asymptomatic and almost all patients were able to resume their treatment 24 h afterwards.
- If asymptomatic overdose occurs, all rivastigmine patches should be removed immediately and no patch should be applied for the next 24 h.
- Overdose with cholinesterase inhibitors, including rivastigmine, can lead to a cholinergic crisis with muscarinic symptoms at first, such as miosis, flushing, abdominal pain, nausea, vomiting, salivation, increased bronchial secretions, lacrimation, sweating, hypotension, bradycardia, involuntary urination and/or defaecation, and, in more severe cases, to nicotinic symptoms, such as muscular weakness, fasciculations, seizures, and respiratory arrest, which might be life-threatening.
- General supportive measures are suggested.
- If severe nausea and vomiting occur, consider administering antiemetics.
- Anticholinergics, like atropine, might serve as an antidote in severely symptomatic overdose.
  - Scopolamine use, as an antidote, is not recommended.
- Haemodialysis, peritoneal dialysis, or haemofiltration are not recommended.

Tests and Therapeutic Drug Monitoring
- Before initiation of rivastigmine therapy:
  - An ECG should be performed to check for QT prolongation.
- During rivastigmine therapy:
  - Monitoring of objective scoring of cognitive performance.
  - Monitoring of body weight.

DOSING AND USE

405

R

Other Warnings / Precautions
• Due to rivastigmine's cholinomimetic actions, caution is advised in patients with pre-existing seizures disorder, urinary tract obstruction, cardiac conduction abnormalities or respiratory disease, including COPD and asthma and those at risk of cardiac repolarization (e.g. uncompensated heart failure, recent myocardial infarction, predisposition to hyper- or hypokalaemia, medications that predispose to QT prolongation).
• Rivastigmine can increase gastric acid secretion and caution is advised for individuals at risk of ulcer disease or gastrointestinal bleeding (e.g. co-medication with NSAIDs).
• Cholinesterase inhibitors, including rivastigmine, might enhance succinylcholine-type muscle relaxation during anaesthesia; consider dose adjustments or temporarily withdrawing rivastigmine.

Do Not Use (Contraindications)
• Known hypersensitivity to rivastigmine or any of the formulation excipients.
• Known history of application site reaction with rivastigmine patch.
• Co-medication with metoclopramide, cholinomimetic, or anticholinergic substances.
• Rivastigmine administration in patients at high risk of prolonged cardiac repolarization (e.g. co-medication with drugs increasing QT interval) should be avoided.

Special Populations
Renal Impairment
• No dose adjustments are recommended; titrate according to patients' tolerability.

Hepatic Impairment
• No dose adjustments are required for mild to moderate hepatic impairment; however, clearance may be reduced, therefore cautious dosage titration according to patients' tolerability is advised.
• Severe hepatic impairment: not recommended.

Elderly
• No dosage adjustments are recommended.

Pregnancy
• Although in animal studies rivastigmine crosses the placenta, such data are not available in humans.
• Rivastigmine should not be used during pregnancy.

Breastfeeding
• Rivastigmine is found in the milk of rats. Data on humans are insufficient.
• Women on rivastigmine should not breastfeed.

Costs

NHS indicative cost (accessed 22 June 2022):

- Capsules:
  - Nimvastid (Consilient Health Ltd) – 28 × 1.5 mg capsules: £28.26; 28 × 3 mg capsules: £28.26; 28 × 4.5 mg capsules: £28.26; 28 × 6 mg capsules £28.26.
  - Generic formulations – 28 × 1.5 mg capsules: £1.91–£28.26; 28 × 3 mg capsules: £2.44–£33.25; 28 × 4.5 mg capsules: £23.51–£33.25; 28 × 6 mg capsules: £26.58–£33.18.
- Oral solution:
  - Generic formulations – 120ml × 2 mg/ml solution: £85.00–£96.82.
- Patches:
  - Almuriva transdermal patches (Sandoz Ltd) – 30 × 4.6 mg/24 h patches: £77.97; 30 × 9.5 mg/24 h patches: £77.97.
  - Alzest transdermal patches (Dr Reddy's Laboratories (UK) Ltd) – 30 × 4.6 mg/24 h patches: £35.10; 30 × 9.5 mg/24 h patches: £19.97; 30 × 13.3 mg/24 h patches: £54.58.
  - Erastig transdermal patches (Teva UK Ltd) – 30 × 13.3 mg/24 h patches: £73.90.
  - Exelon transdermal patches (Novartis Pharmaceuticals UK Ltd) – 30 × 4.6 mg/24 h patches: £77.97, 30 × 9.5 mg/24 h patches: £77.97, 30 × 13.3 mg/24 h patches: £77.97.
  - Prometax transdermal patches (Sandoz Ltd) – 30 × 4.6 mg/24 h patches: £77.97; 30 × 9.5 mg/24 h patches: £77.97.

The Overall Place of Rivastigmine in the Treatment of Parkinson's Disease

Rivastigmine is a pseudo-irreversible and dual inhibitor of both acetyl-cholinesterase and butyrylcholinesterase in the CNS. It is the only officially approved therapy for mild-to-moderate dementia in Parkinson's disease, either in oral or transdermal formulations, while preliminary evidence suggests that it might be useful in Parkinson's disease-related MCI. Considering other non-motor features of Parkinson's disease, rivastigmine is considered an efficacious therapy in Parkinson's disease-related apathy, and there are indications that it might be beneficial in Parkinson's disease-related visual hallucinations and refractory RBD. It is generally considered a safe therapeutic option, especially in the transdermal formulation.

Potential Advantages

- Rivastigmine is the only cholinesterase inhibitor with a licensed indication for the treatment of dementia in Parkinson's disease.
- The option of transdermal application of rivastigmine might favour its use in cognitively impaired patients and patients with swallowing difficulties or GI complications.

R

RIVASTIGMINE

- Once daily application of the transdermal patch allows for better adherence in patients with complicated drug regimens.
- In contrast to other cholinesterase inhibitors, the hepatic cytochrome CYP450 system is not involved in rivastigmine metabolism and fewer drug–drug interactions are expected.

Potential Disadvantages
- Adverse skin and GI reactions are relatively common with transdermal and oral formulations, respectively.

Clinical Box

A 72-year-old man with a 5-year history of Parkinson's disease presented at the Neurology Department Outpatient Clinic with his son, who was concerned because during the past few months his father seemed to have lost interest in his surroundings or any motivation to participate in everyday activities. He had also become more dependent on his routine activities (although still mostly independent) and was not interested in getting out or seeing friends and relatives. The patient did not report any feelings of anxiety or depression. Both he and his caregiver were satisfied with his motor performance. His current medication included levodopa/carbidopa/entacapone 125 mg/31.25 mg/200 mg TID, rasagiline 1 mg OD, and escitalopram 10 mg OD. The rest of his medical history included atrial fibrillation with the patient receiving apixaban 5 mg BID. During the assessment, the patient was diagnosed with mild to moderate cognitive impairment, along with significant apathy. The patient was scheduled for a brain MRI scan, which detected mild generalized brain atrophy. Rivastigmine 1.5 mg BID was prescribed. During the first few days, the patient complained about persistent abdominal pain and vomiting, which was addressed by switching to a transdermal rivastigmine patch of 4.6 mg/24 h and a dose increase to 9.5 mg/24 h after 4 weeks.

Suggested Reading

Burn D, M Emre, I McKeith, PP De Deyn, D Aarsland, C Hsu, R Lane. Effects of rivastigmine in patients with and without visual hallucinations in dementia associated with Parkinson's disease. *Mov Disord* 2006; 21(11): 1899–1907.

Devos D, C Moreau, D Maltête, R Lefaucheur, A Kreisler, A Eusebio, G Defer, T Ouk, JP Azulay, P Krystkowiak, T Witjas, M Dalliaux, A Destée, A Duhamel, R Bordt, L Defebvre, K Dujardin. Rivastigmine in apathetic but dementia and depression-free patients with Parkinson's disease: a double-blind, placebo-controlled, randomised clinical trial. *J Neurol Neurosurg Psychiatry* 2014; 85(6): 668–674.

Di Giacopo R, A Fasano, D Quaranta, G Della Marca, F Bove, AR Bentiglio. Rivastigmine as alternative treatment for refractory REM behavior disorder in Parkinson's disease. *Mov Disord* 2012; 27(4): 559–561.

Emre M, W Poewe, PP De Deyn, P Barone, J Kulisevsky, E Pourcher, T van Laar, A Storch, F Micheli, D Burn, F Durif, R Pahwa, F Callegari, N Tenenbaum, C Strohmaier. Long-term safety of rivastigmine in Parkinson disease dementia: an open-label, randomized study. *Clin Neuropharmacol* 2014; 37(1): 9–16.

Henderson EJ, SR Lord, MA Brodie, DM Gaunt, AD Lawrence, JCT Close, AL Whone, Y Ben-Shlomo. Rivastigmine for gait stability in patients with Parkinson's disease (ReSPonD): a randomised, double-blind, placebo-controlled, phase 2 trial. *Lancet Neurol* 2016; 15(3): 249–258.

Mamikonyan E, SX Xie, E Melvin, D Weintraub. Rivastigmine for mild cognitive impairment in Parkinson disease: a placebo-controlled study. *Mov Disord* 2015; 30(7): 912–918.

References

AHFS Drug information, 2012. Bethesda: American Society of Health-System Pharmacists. Accessed on 22 June 2022 via www.medicinescomplete.com.

Battle CE, AH Abdul-Rassim, SD Shenkin, J Hewitt, TJ Quinn. Cholinesterase inhibitors for vascular dementia and other vascular cognitive impairments: a network meta-analysis. *Cochrane Database Syst Rev* 2021; 2(2): CD013306.

Bullock R, A Cameron. Rivastigmine for the treatment of dementia and visual hallucinations associated with Parkinson's disease: a case series. *Curr Med Res Opin* 2002; 18(5): 258–264.

Espay AJ, L Marsili, A Mahajan, A Sturchio, R Pathan, DS Elango, N Pezous, M Masellis, B Gomez-Mancilla. Rivastigmine in Parkinson's disease dementia with orthostatic hypotension. *Ann Neurol* 2021; 89(1): 91–98.

Jann, MW, KL Shirley, GW Small. Clinical pharmacokinetics and pharmacodynamics of cholinesterase inhibitors. *Clin Pharmacokinet* 2002; 41(10): 719–739.

Joint Formulary Committee. British National Formulary (online). London: BMJ Group and Pharmaceutical Press. Accessed on 22 June 2022 via www.medicinescomplete.com.

Matsunaga S, H Fujishiro, H Takechi. Efficacy and safety of cholinesterase inhibitors for mild cognitive impairment: a systematic review and meta-analysis. *J Alzheimers Dis* 2019: 71(2): 513–523.

McDonald J, E Pourcher, A Nadeau, P Corbeil. A randomized trial of oral and transdermal rivastigmine for postural instability in Parkinson disease dementia. *Clin Neuropharmacol* 2018; 41(3): 87–93.

R

Rivastigmine. In: Brayfield A (Ed.), *Martindale: The Complete Drug Reference*. London: The Royal Pharmaceutical Society of Great Britain. Accessed on 22 June 2022 via www.medicinescomplete.com.

Rivastigmine. In: DRUGDEX® System (electronic version). Truven Health Analytics, Greenwood Village, Colorado, USA. Accessed on 22 June 2022 via www.micromedexsolutions.com.

Ruangritchankul S, P Chantharit, S Srisuma, LC Gray. Adverse drug reactions of acetylcholinesterase inhibitors in older people living with dementia: a comprehensive literature review. *Ther Clin Risk Manag* 2021; 17: 927–949.

Summary of product characteristics – Nimvastid 3 mg hard capsules. Krka UK Ltd – Electronic Medicines Compendium: Nimvastid 3 mg hard capsules – summary of product characteristics (SmPC) – (emc). Accessed on 22 June 2022 via www.medicines.org.uk.

Yan J, A Liu, J Huang, J Wu, R Shen, H Ma, J Yang. Pharmacological interventions for REM sleep behavior disorder in Parkinson's disease: a systematic review. *Front Aging Neurosci* 2021. 13: 709878.

Youn YC, HW Shin, BS Choi, SY Kim, JY Lee, YC Ha. Rivastigmine patch reduces the incidence of postoperative delirium in older patients with cognitive impairment. *Int J Geriatr Psychiatry* 2017; 32(10): 1079–1084.

ROPINIROLE

R

Therapeutics

Chemical Name and Structure

Ropinirole hydrochloride (4-[2-(dipropylamino)ethyl]-2-indolinone hydrochloride) is a white to yellow solid, with a molecular weight of 296.8 and an empirical formula of $C_{16}H_{24}N_2O,HCl$.

Brand Names

- **Appese** (*Australia*); **Adartrel** (*Germany, Greece, France, Netherlands, Norway, Poland, Portugal, Spain, Sweden, Switzerland, UK*); **Aimpart** (*UK*); **Alzorol** (*Estonia, Lithuania*); **Aparxon** (*Poland*); **ApoRopin** (*Poland*); **Aropilo** (*Poland*); **Aropilos** (*Czech Republic*).
- **Ceurolex** (*Poland*).
- **Evecet** (*Greece, Hong Kong*).
- **Ippinnia** (*UK*).
- **Medoquip** (*Cyprus, Estonia*).
- **Nironovo** (*Poland*).
- **Parnirol** (*Poland*); **Parsonil** (*Poland*); **Polpix** (*Poland*).
- **Ralnea** (*Germany, Hungary, UK*); **Raponer** (*Poland, UK*); **Repinex** (*UK*); **Repirol** (*Poland*); **Repreve** (Australia); **Requip** (*Argentina, Austria, Belgium, Chile, China, Czech Republic, Estonia, Finland, France, Germany, Greece, Hong Kong, Hungary, Indonesia, Ireland, Israel, Italy, Japan, Lithuania, Malaysia, Mexico, Netherlands, Norway, Philippines, Poland, Portugal, Russian Federation, Singapore, South Africa, Spain, Sweden, Switzerland, Thailand, Turkey, UK, US*); **Resure** (*South Africa*); **Rolpryna** (*Estonia, Hong Kong, Ireland, Lithuania, Poland, Spain*); **Ropilynz** (*UK*); **Ropin** (*New Zealand*); **Ropinostad** (*Denmark, Finland*); **Ropiqual** (*UK*); **Ropiral** (*Italy*); **Ropitor** (*Lithuania*); **Ropodrin** (*Poland*); **Roprima** (*Italy*); **Rolpryna** (*Czech Republic, Hong Kong, Ireland, Poland, Russian Federation, Spain*); **Roteq** (*Cyprus*).
- **Sindranol** (*Russian Federation*); **Spiroco** (*UK*).
- **Valzorol** (*Poland*); **Vidant** (*Turkey*).

Generics Available

- Yes.

Licensed Indications for Parkinson's Disease

- As a monotherapy in early-stage Parkinson's disease (FDA, EMA, EMC).
- As an adjunctive therapy to levodopa over the course of Parkinson's disease, when the effect of levodopa wears off or becomes inconsistent and end-of-dose or 'on–off'-type fluctuations appear (FDA, EMA, EMC).

Licensed Indications for Other Conditions

- Moderate to severe RLS (only immediate release formulation, UK SPC, EMA, FDA).

THERAPEUTICS

R

Non-Licensed Use for Parkinson's Disease
• None.

Non-Licensed Use for Other Conditions
• Limited and controversial data on cocaine dependence management.
• Preliminary studies on the role of ropinirole in ALS.

Ineffective
• Neuroleptic–induced akathisia.
• Secondary RLS (e.g. caused by renal failure, iron deficiency anaemia, pregnancy).
• As an add-on to antidepressants in depression.

Mechanism of Action
• A non-ergot dopamine agonist with high binding specificity for and intrinsic activity at D_2 and D_3 dopamine receptors ($D_3 > D_2 > D_4$).
• Moderate affinity to opiate receptors.
• Little or no affinity for α_1-, α_2- or β-adrenergic, D_1 dopamine, benzo-diazepine, γ-aminobutyric acid (GABA), 5-HT_1 or 5-HT_2 serotonin, or muscarinic receptors.
• Ropinirole acts in the hypothalamus and pituitary to inhibit prolac-tin secretion.
• Ropinirole acts mainly by directly stimulating post-synaptic D_2 dopa-mine receptors in the corpus striatum.
• The mechanism of action in RLS is largely unknown, although it is suggested to be primarily dopaminergic in nature.

Efficacy Profile
• According to the MDS EBM Committee:
   • Ropinirole IR is 'efficacious' and 'clinically useful' as a symptomatic monotherapy in Parkinson's disease, while ropinirole ER is 'likely efficacious' and 'possibly useful'.
   • Ropinirole IR is 'efficacious' and 'clinically useful' for symptomatic adjunct therapy in early or stable Parkinson's disease patients.
   • Ropinirole IR is 'efficacious' and 'clinically useful' in preventing or delaying dyskinesias, while there is insufficient evidence for pre-venting or delaying motor fluctuations.
   • Both ropinirole IR and ER are 'efficacious' and 'clinically useful' in the treatment of motor fluctuations in Parkinson's disease.
• The efficacy of ropinirole ER may continue for 2 years.
• The systemic exposure to ropinirole is comparable for IR and ER tablets of the same total daily dose.
• Ropinirole is likely to be effective in Parkinson's disease-related depression and apathy.

R

DRUG INTERACTION PROFILE

Pharmacokinetics

Absorption and Distribution
- Oral bioavailability: 45–55%.
- Food co-ingestion: the rate, but not extent, of absorption may be reduced with food consumption. A high-fat diet may prolong Tmax and shorten Cmax.
- Tmax: 1.5 h for IR and 6–10 h for ER formulations after oral administration.
- Time to steady state: within 4 days of therapy initiation with ER preparations.
- Pharmacokinetics: linear kinetics over the therapeutic dosing range of 1–8 mg TID (IR).
- Protein binding: 10–40%.
- Volume of distribution: 7.5 l/kg.

Metabolism
- Extensively metabolized in the liver by cytochrome P450 by *N*-despropylation and hydroxylation to form inactive metabolites.
- Mainly metabolized by CYP1A2.

Elimination
- A mean half-life of approximately 6 h for both ropinirole IR and ER.
- Renal excretion: less than 10% of an administered dose is excreted unchanged in urine. The remainder is excreted as inactive metabolites.
  - *N*-despropyl ropinirole is the primary metabolite found in urine (40%), followed by the carboxylic acid metabolite (10%) and the glucuronide of the hydroxy metabolite (10%).

Drug Interaction Profile

Pharmacokinetic Drug Interactions
- Effects on ropinirole:
  - Inhibitors (e.g. fluoroquinolones, *fluvoxamine, mexiletine, cimetidine*) or inducers (e.g. *omeprazole, carbamazepine*) of the CYP1A2 enzyme might increase or decrease ropinirole plasma concentration, respectively.
    - Because smoking induces CYP1A2, it is expected to increase ropinirole clearance.
- High doses of oestrogens can increase ropinirole plasma levels.

Pharmacodynamic Drug Interactions
- Co-medication with dopamine antagonists (e.g. phenothiazines, thioxanthenes, butyrophenones, *metoclopramide*) can reduce the efficacy of ropinirole.
- Co-medication with anti-hypertensives (e.g. *captopril*) might act synergistically, lowering the blood pressure.

R

- Co-medication with CNS depressants or alcohol might lead to additive effects (e.g. increased sedation or respiratory depression).
- Cases of unbalanced INR have been reported in co-medication with vitamin K antagonists (e.g. *warfarin*).

Adverse Effects

How Drug Causes Adverse Effects

- Mainly, but not solely, through increasing dopaminergic activity.
- Postural hypotension is thought to be caused by a D_2-mediated blunting of the noradrenergic response to standing and a subsequent decrease in peripheral vascular resistance.

Common Adverse Effects

- Very common (≥1/10):
  - Syncope (monotherapy), dyskinesia (adjunct therapy), somnolence, nausea, viral infections, dyspepsia, falls.
- Common (≥1/100 to <1/10):
  - Neuropsychiatric: confusion (adjunct therapy), hallucinations, dizziness, vertigo, sudden onset of sleep (even without warning signs).
  - Eye: abnormal vision, xerophthalmia.
  - Cardiovascular: (postural) hypotension (adjunct therapy), hypertension, chest pain, palpitation.
  - GI: abdominal pain (monotherapy), constipation, heartburn, flatulence.
  - Other: peripheral oedema, flushing, hyperhidrosis, anorexia, malaise, fatigue, urinary tract infections, impotence.
- Uncommon (≥1/1,000 to <1/100):
  - Neuropsychiatric: psychotic reactions, delirium, ICDs (e.g. pathological gambling, compulsive shopping, binge eating, hypersexuality, DDS).
  - Cardiovascular: (postural) hypotension (monotherapy).
  - Respiratory, thoracic, and mediastinal disorders: hiccups.

Life-Threatening or Dangerous Adverse Effects

- Hypersensitivity reactions (urticaria, angioedema, rash, pruritus).
  - The 4 mg ER tablets contain the azo colouring agent sunset yellow, which may cause allergic reactions.
- NMS, DWAS.
- Fibrotic complications, such as pleural effusion/thickening, interstitial lung disease and cardiac valvulopathy (causal association has not been confirmed).

Rare and Not Life-Threatening Adverse Effects

- Dermal eruptions.
- Retinal degeneration.
- Anterocollis, Pisa syndrome.
- Mania.

R

Weight Change
• Not reported.

What to Do About Adverse Effects
• Before introducing ropinirole, discuss common or life-threatening adverse effects with patients and/or caregivers, including symptoms that should be reported to the physician.
  • Before therapy initiation, patients should be asked for somnolence or other factors that increase somnolence risk (e.g. CNS depressants, sleep disorders).
• On a regular basis, monitor for sleepiness (which might occur without preceding warning signs, even later in therapy, e.g. after 1 year), drowsiness, hypotension (especially during dosing escalation), ICDs, mania, hallucinations, or psychotic-like behaviours with focused and direct questions to patients and caregivers, as patients might not acknowledge such symptoms as abnormal to report them.
• If patients taking ropinirole experience somnolence and/or episodes of sudden-onset sleep during activities that require active participation, they should refrain from driving or operating machines and inform their treating physician. Therapy discontinuation is generally advised, as dose reduction might not eliminate episodes of falling asleep while engaged in activities of daily living.
• Patients and their caregivers should be made aware of the possibility of developing ICDs or mania/delirium. In this case, a reduction of ropinirole dose or discontinuation of therapy should be considered.
• Patients taking ropinirole should avoid rising rapidly after sitting or lying down, especially if they have been in a seated or recumbent position for prolonged time periods or if they have just started ropinirole therapy, especially if it is co-administered with levodopa.
• If dyskinesias occur in advanced Parkinson's disease patients taking ropinirole as an add-on to levodopa, consider gradually reducing the total levodopa dose as an initial step, especially if this happens during the initial titration phase of ropinirole.
• If dystonia/postural deformities occur, dopaminergic medications should be reviewed and a ropinirole dosage reduction or even discontinuation should be considered.
• If peripheral oedema occurs as a side effect of ropinirole, consider lowering the dose or discontinuing therapy. The use of diuretics is not recommended due to the risk of aggravating orthostatic hypotension.
• Periodic assessment for augmentation is advised in RLS cases.

Dosing and Use
Usual Dosage Range
• IR: 0.75–24 mg per day in three equally divided doses.
• ER: 2–24 mg per day.

R

ROPINIROLE

Available Formulations
- IR: 0.25 mg, 0.5 mg, 1 mg, 2 mg, 3 mg, 4 mg, 5 mg.
- ER: 2 mg, 4 mg, 6 mg, 8 mg, 12 mg.

How to Dose
- Ropinirole therapy should be initiated at a low dose and gradually titrated upwards according to clinical tolerability and therapeutic effect. The lowest effective dose should be maintained.

Gradual dose increase of ropinirole IR tablets		
Week	Dose (mg)	Total daily dose (mg)
1	3 × 0.25	0.75
2	3 × 0.5	1.50
3	3 × 0.75	2.25
4	3 × 1.0	3.00
5	3 × 1.5	4.50
6	3 × 2.0	6.00
7	3 × 2.5	7.50
8	3 × 3.0	9.00
9	3 × 4.0	12.00
10	3 × 5.0	15.00
11	3 × 6.0 (5.0 + 1.0)	18.00
12	3 × 7.0 (5.0 + 2.0)	21.00
13	3 × 8.0 (5.0 + 3.0)	24.00

- ER formulations: initial dose of 2 mg/day for 1–2 weeks; increase by 2 mg/day at intervals of at least 1 week; not to exceed 24 mg/day.
- Although the maximum recommended dose is 24 mg/day, patients with early and advanced Parkinson's disease are generally treated with doses lower than 12 mg/day and 8 mg/day, respectively.
  - If a therapeutic benefit has not been achieved and the patient does not experience any side effects, consider further increasing the dose.
  - In fixed-dose studies, no therapeutic benefit has been shown with doses higher than 24 mg/day.

Dosing Tips
- Ropinirole may be administered with or without food.
  - If nausea occurs, patients should be advised to take ropinirole with food.

R

- Ropinirole ER tablets should be taken once daily, at a similar time each day.
- Patients who initiate therapy with the lowest dose of 2 mg/day of ropinirole ER and experience non-tolerable adverse effects might benefit from switching to lower total daily doses of ropinirole IR, for example 0.25–0.5 mg TID (total of 0.75–1.5 mg/day).
- Switches between equal doses of ropinirole IR and ER can happen overnight.
- If a dose is skipped in IR formulations, the patient should be advised to take the next dose as scheduled (not a double dose). If therapy is interrupted for more than one day, consider re-initiation by dose titration.
- When ropinirole is added to levodopa regimens, consider gradually lowering the total dose of levodopa, depending on the clinical response, to avoid dyskinesias or other dopaminergic side effects.
- Although domperidone antagonizes the dopaminergic actions of ropinirole peripherally, it does not cross the blood–brain barrier; thus, it can be used as an antiemetic in patients treated with centrally acting dopamine agonists, like ropinirole.
- If Parkinson's disease-related depression does not respond to a maximum of 15 mg ropinirole, other pharmacological options, such as antidepressants, should be used.

How to Withdraw Drug
- Ropinirole withdrawal should be undertaken gradually over a period of 1 week.
- IR formulations (up to a total dose of 3 mg/day): the administration frequency should be reduced from TID to BID for 4 days and then to OD for the remaining 3 days before complete discontinuation.
- Ropinirole can be discontinued by 2 mg every second day until complete cessation.
  - For doses higher than 14 mg/day or 20 mg/day, reduction can start at 6 mg or 8 mg, respectively.
- Withdrawal-emergent hyperpyrexia and confusion (including insomnia, anxiety, apathy, depression, sweating, fatigue, pain) may present during rapid dosage reduction or abrupt withdrawal, which might not respond to levodopa therapy. It might resemble NMS.
- DAWS has been reported with ropinirole cessation, especially if it is discontinued abruptly. Patients may develop neuropsychiatric or autonomic symptoms, which do not respond to levodopa. In severe cases, DAWS can be life-threatening.
  - Limited data suggest that patients with ICDs and those on higher ropinirole doses may be at greater risk for developing DAWS.
  - In case of severe or persistent DAWS, temporary re-administration of ropinirole at the lowest effective dose may be considered.

DOSING AND USE

R

Overdose
- Ropinirole overdose symptoms are generally related to dopaminergic activity.
- Symptoms related to doses higher than 24 mg/day are nausea/vomiting, dizziness, hyperhidrosis, visual hallucinations, claustrophobia, palpitations, agitation, chorea, dyskinesia, nightmares, somnolence, orthostatic hypotension, syncope, and confusion.
- There is no known antidote for dopamine agonist overdose. Close monitoring of vital signs and general supportive measures are suggested.
- If severe symptoms are present, consider administering dopamine antagonists, such as neuroleptics or metoclopramide.

Tests and Therapeutic Drug Monitoring
- Monitoring of blood pressure is advised when ropinirole is co-administered with antihypertensive agents.
- Periodic skin examinations by qualified clinicians should be performed to monitor for melanoma.

Other Warnings / Precautions
- Patients should be advised that ropinirole may cause somnolence and they should not drive a car or operate complex machinery until they have gained sufficient experience with the drug to determine whether it affects their mental and/or motor performance.
- Ropinirole is considered as possibly porphyrinogenic (Norwegian Porphyria Center – NAPOS, Porphyria Center Sweden); therefore, it should only be used when no safer alternative is available. Precautions are advised in vulnerable patients.
- Adjustments in ropinirole dose might be necessary if co-administered with CYP1A2 inhibitors or inducers or with high doses of oestrogen therapy, especially if these medications are initiated or withdrawn during ropinirole treatment.
- Close monitoring of INR is advised when co-administering with vitamin K antagonists.

Do Not Use (Contraindications)
- Hypersensitivity to the active substance or to any of the excipients, including lactose.
  - Patients with rare hereditary problems of galactose intolerance, total lactase deficiency, or glucose–galactose malabsorption should not be treated with ropinirole.
- Co-medication with CNS depressants or alcohol should be avoided due to additive sedative effects.
- Co-administration with antipsychotics, including *clozapine* and *quetiapine*, and other dopamine antagonists (e.g. *metoclopramide*) should be avoided.

Special Populations
Renal Impairment
- CrCl 30–50 ml/min: no dose adjustments are necessary.
- CrCl < 30 ml/min:
  - Ropinirole should not be used in patients with severe renal impairment without regular haemodialysis (EMA, EMC).
  - IR preparations can be with caution, as safety and efficacy have not been established (FDA). ER preparations are not recommended.
- End-stage renal disease on haemodialysis: use with caution, 18 mg/day is the maximum recommended dose in Parkinson's disease.
  - Supplemental doses after dialysis are not required.

Hepatic Impairment
- Use with caution, as safety and efficacy have not been established.
- Ropinirole use is not recommended in patients with severe hepatic impairment.

Elderly
- Oral clearance is reduced by 30% in those over 65 compared to younger patients.
- Aging leads to a relative increase in body fat stores, thus increasing the volume of distribution and half-life of lipophilic drugs, such as ropinirole.
- No dose adjustments are necessary for those over 65 years of age, as ropinirole dose is individually titrated according to clinical response.
- Geriatric patients might be more prone to developing hallucinations or psychotic-like behaviour on ropinirole therapy.

Pregnancy
- There are not enough robust data considering ropinirole use during pregnancy; ropinirole concentrations may gradually increase during pregnancy.
- Ropinirole should not be used during pregnancy unless the potential benefit outweighs the potential risk to the fetus.

Breastfeeding
- According to rat models, ropinirole is found in breast milk.
- There are no adequate data considering the presence of ropinirole or its metabolites in human milks, their effects on breastfed infant, or milk production; lactation inhibition is expected due to ropinirole inhibiting the secretion of prolactin in humans.
- Ropinirole should not be used by nursing mothers.

R

Costs

NHS indicative costs (accessed 23 June 2022):

- IR tablets:
  - Adartrel tablets (GlaxoSmithKline UK Ltd) – 12 × 0.25 mg: £3.94; 28 × 0.5 mg: £15.75; 28 × 2 mg: £31.51.
  - ReQuip tablets (GlaxoSmithKline UK Ltd) – 21 × 0.25 mg: £5.70; 84 × 1 mg: £56.71; 84 × 2 mg: £113.44; 84 × 5 mg: £195.92.
  - Generic formulations – 12 × 0.25 mg: £3.62–£15.00; 28 × 0.5 mg: £6.52–£25.00; 84 × 1 mg: £48.20–£59.38; 84 × 2 mg: £33.25–£67.42; 84 × 5 mg: £200.35–£217.22.
- ER tablets:
  - Ippinia XL tablets (Ethypharm UK Ltd) – 28 × 2 mg: £5.64; 28 × 3 mg: £8.46; 28 × 4 mg: £11.29; 28 × 6 mg: £15.32; 28 × 8 mg: £18.95.
  - Ralnea XL tablets (Consilient Health Ltd) – 28 × 2 mg: £10.65; 28×4 mg: £21.32; 28 × 8 mg: £35.79.
  - Raponer XL tablets (Accord Healthcare Ltd) – 28 × 2 mg: £12.54; 28 × 4 mg: £25.09; 28 × 8 mg: £42.11.
  - ReQuip XL tablets (GlaxoSmithKline UK Ltd) – 28 × 2 mg: £12.54; 28 × 4 mg: £25.09; 28 × 8 mg: £42.11.
  - Repinex XL tablets (Aspire Pharma Ltd) – 28 × 2 mg: £6.20; 28 × 4 mg £12.50; 28 × 8 mg: £21.00.
  - Ropiqual XL tablets (Milpharm Ltd) – 28 × 2 mg: £12.54; 28 × 4 mg £25.09; 28 × 8 mg: £42.11.
  - Generic formulations – 28 × 2 mg: £10.66; 28 × 4 mg: £21.33; 28 × 8 mg: £35.79.

The Overall Place of Ropinirole in the Treatment of Parkinson's Disease

Ropinirole use has been approved for all stages of Parkinson's disease, either early as a monotherapy or as an adjunct to levodopa preparations in early or advanced Parkinson's disease. It is considered efficacious for the management of 'end-of-dose' or 'on–off'-type fluctuations. There are also indications that ropinirole may be effective in the treatment of Parkinson's disease-related depression and apathy. Data on using ropinirole for sleep-related issues in Parkinson's disease are currently scarce, although ER formulations were found to be superior to IR formulations in treating Parkinson's disease-related nocturnal disturbances. Ropinirole is generally well tolerated. However, patients, their caregivers, and treating physicians should be aware of specific side effects, including ICDs, somnolence and sleep attacks, hallucinations, psychotic-like behaviour, and orthostatic hypotension, especially when ropinirole is used as an add-on to levodopa. Ropinirole also has a role in the management of RLS.

Potential Advantages
- Both IR and ER formulations are available, with the latter contributing to patients' adherence, especially in those with complicated treatment regimens.

Potential Disadvantages
- Similarly to other dopamine agonists, development of ICDs, hallucinations or psychotic-like behaviour, sudden sleep attacks, and orthostatic hypotension are a possibility in patients treated with ropinirole and might lead to life-changing consequences (e.g. financial difficulties, injuries). Somnolence is a particular issue among older patients taking dopamine agonists.

Clinical Box

A 60-year-old man with a 7-year history of Parkinson's disease presented at the Movement Disorders Outpatient Clinic with his wife due to end-of-dose deterioration. He did not report any dyskinesia and he was satisfied with his ON state during the day. His current medication included levodopa/carbidopa/entacapone 150 mg/37.5 mg/200 mg TID and rasagiline 1 mg OD. The patient was also being treated for depression with escitalopram 20 mg OD, although mild depressive symptoms were detected during his current assessment. According to his medical records, he was initially treated with pramipexole monotherapy for a few months when he was first diagnosed with Parkinson's disease. However, he had to discontinue therapy due to visual hallucinations. His medical history included hypothyroidism. After a thorough discussion with the patient and his caregiver, considering potential side effects, including his past history of hallucinations, a low dose of ropinirole ER 2 mg OD was prescribed and instructions were given about the potential for dose increases of 2 mg/day every week up to a maximum of 8 mg/day. At a dose of 6 mg/day the patient reported a clear improvement of his symptoms with disappearance of OFF phenomena.

Suggested Reading

Binde CD, IF Tvete, JI Gåsemyr, B Natvig, M Klemp. Comparative effectiveness of dopamine agonists and monoamine oxidase type-B inhibitors for Parkinson's disease: a multiple treatment comparison meta-analysis. *Eur J Clin Pharmacol* 2020; 76(12): 1731–1743.

Mizuno Y, M Nomoto, K Hasegawa, N Hattori, T Kondo, M Murata, M Takeuchi, M Takahashi, T Tomida ; Rotigotine Trial Group. Rotigotine vs ropinirole in advanced stage Parkinson's disease: a double-blind study. *Parkinsonism Relat Disord* 2014;. 20(12): 1388–1393.

Pahwa R, MA Stacy, SA Factor, KE Lyons, F Stocchi, BP Hersh, LW Elmer, DD Truong, NL Earl ; EASE-PD Adjunct Study Investigators.

R

Ropinirole 24-hour prolonged release: randomized, controlled study in advanced Parkinson disease. *Neurology* 2007; 68(14): 1108–1115.

Rektorova I, M Balaz, J Svatova, K Zarubova, I Honig, V Dostal, S Sedlackova, I Nestrasil, J Mastik, M Bares, J Veliskova, L Duseck. Effects of ropinirole on nonmotor symptoms of Parkinson disease: a prospective multicenter study. *Clin Neuropharmacol* 2008; 31(5): 261–266.

Watts RL, KE Lyons, R Pahwa, K Sethi, M Stern, RA Hauser, W Olanow, AM Gray, B Adams, NL Earl ; 228 Study Investigators. Onset of dyskinesia with adjunct ropinirole prolonged-release or additional levodopa in early Parkinson's disease. *Mov Disord* 2010; 25(7): 858–866.

References

Agüera-Ortiz L, R García-Ramos, FLG Pérez, J López-Álvarez, JMM Rodríguez, FJO Rodríguez, JO Pueyo, CP Valero, J Porto-Etessam. Focus on depression in Parkinson's disease: a Delphi consensus of experts in psychiatry, neurology, and geriatrics. *Parkinsons Dis* 2021; 2021: 6621991.

AHFS Drug information, 2012. Bethesda: American Society of Health-System Pharmacists. Accessed on 23 June 2022 via www.medicinescomplete.com.

Dusek P, J Busková, E Růzicka, V Majerová, A Srp, R Jech, J Roth, K Sonka. Effects of ropinirole prolonged-release on sleep disturbances and daytime sleepiness in Parkinson disease. *Clin Neuropharmacol* 2010; 33(4): 186–190.

Gershon AA, R Amiaz, H Shem-David, L Grunhaus. Ropinirole augmentation for depression: a randomized controlled trial pilot study. *J Clin Psychopharmacol* 2019; 39(1): 78–81.

Joint Formulary Committee. British National Formulary (online). London: BMJ Group and Pharmaceutical Press. Accessed on 23 June 2022 via www.medicinescomplete.com.

Koschel J, KR Chaudhuri, L Tönges, M Thiel, V Raeder, WH Jost. Implications of dopaminergic medication withdrawal in Parkinson's disease. *J Neural Transm (Vienna)* 2022; 129(9): 1169–1178.

Latt MD, S Lewis, O Zekry, VSC Fung. Factors to consider in the selection of dopamine agonists for older persons with Parkinson's disease. *Drugs Aging* 2019; 36(3): 189–202.

Okano H, D Yasuda, K Fujimori, S Morimoto, S Takahashi. Ropinirole, a new ALS drug candidate developed using iPSCs. *Trends Pharmacol Sci* 2020; 41(2): 99–109.

Ray Chaudhuri K, P Martinez-Martin, KA Rolfe, J Cooper, CB Rockett, L Giorgi, WG Ondo. Improvements in nocturnal symptoms with ropinirole prolonged release in patients with advanced Parkinson's disease. *Eur J Neurol* 2012; 19(1): 105–113.

ROPINIROLE

Ropinirole. In: Brayfield A (Ed.), *Martindale: The Complete Drug Reference*. London: The Royal Pharmaceutical Society of Great Britain. Accessed on 23 June 2022 via www.medicinescomplete.com.

Ropinirole. In: DRUGDEX® System (electronic version). Truven Health Analytics, Greenwood Village, Colorado, USA. Accessed on 23 June 2022 via www.micromedexsolutions.com.

Rota S, I Boura, L Batzu, N Titova, P Jenner, C Falup-Pecurariu, KR Chaudhuri. "Dopamine agonist phobia" in Parkinson's disease: when does it matter? Implications for non-motor symptoms and personalized medicine. *Expert Rev Neurother* 2020; 20(9): 953–965.

Schmitz JM, R Suchting, CE Green, HE Webber, J Vincent, FG Moeller, SD Lane. The effects of combination levodopa-ropinirole on cognitive improvement and treatment outcome in individuals with cocaine use disorder: a Bayesian mediation analysis. *Drug Alcohol Depend* 2021; 225: 108800.

Summary of Product Characteristics – Requip XL 4 mg prolonged-release tablets. GlaxoSmithKline UK. Electronic Medicines Compendium: Requip XL 4 mg prolonged-release tablets – summary of product characteristics (SmPC) – (emc). Accessed on 23 June 2022 via www.medicines.org.uk.

Tulloch IF. Pharmacologic profile of ropinirole: a nonergoline dopamine agonist. *Neurology* 1997; 49(1 Suppl 1): S58–S62.

R

ROTIGOTINE

Therapeutics

Chemical Name and Structure

Rotigotine ((−)-(*S*)-5,6,7,8-tetrahydro-6-{propyl[2-(2-thienyl)ethyl] amino}-1-naphthol or (6*S*)-6-(propyl[2-(-thienyl)ethyl]amino)-5,6,7, 8-tetrahydro-1-naphthalenol) is a white to off-white crystalline powder, lipophilic and poorly water-soluble at neutral pH, whereas solubility increases at more acidic pH. It has a molecular weight of 315.5 and an empirical formula of $C_{19}H_{25}NOS$.

Brand Names
- **Leganto** (*Austria, Estonia, Germany, Lithuania, Netherlands, Poland*).
- **Neupro** (*Argentina, Australia, Austria, Belgium, Brazil, Canada, Chile, China, Cyprus, Czech Republic, Denmark, Estonia, Finland, France, Germany, Greece, Hong Kong, Hungary, Ireland, Israel, Italy, Japan, Lithuania, Malaysia, Netherlands, Norway, Philippines, Poland, Portugal, Russian Federation, Singapore, Spain, Sweden, Switzerland, Thailand, Turkey, UK, Ukraine, USA, Venezuela*).
- **Nubrenza** (*Mexico*).

Generics Available
- No.

Licensed Indications for Parkinson's Disease
- As a monotherapy in early stage Parkinson's disease (FDA, EMA, EMC).
- As an adjunct therapy to levodopa preparations from early to late Parkinson's disease stages when levodopa efficacy is considered inadequate and fluctuations appear (FDA, EMA, EMC).

Licensed Indications for Other Conditions
- Moderate to severe idiopathic RLS (FDA, EMA, EMC).

Non-Licensed Use for Parkinson's Disease
- As an adjunct therapy to levodopa to treat dyskinesias in Parkinson's disease.
- Troublesome early-morning dystonia and OFF symptoms (RECOVER study).
- Sleep disorders in Parkinson's disease (MDS EBM Committee), including difficulty falling asleep, feeling immobile or stiff during the night, limb restlessness, breathing problems/snoring, feeling tired/sleepy in the morning, sleep fragmentation (RECOVER study).
- In patients with non-motor fluctuations dominated by pain and in nocturnal pain (MDS EBM Committee).

Non-Licensed Use for Other Conditions
- Not reported.

Ineffective
- Not reported.

Mechanism of Action
- A non-ergot full agonist active at all dopamine receptor subtypes. In particular, rotigotine interacts with D_1, D_2, and D_3 receptors. Rotigotine also has antagonistic effects at adrenergic (α_{2B} receptor) and agonistic effects at serotonergic ($5\text{-}HT_{1A}$) receptor sites.
- Rotigotine is delivered continuously through the skin (transdermal route), using a silicone-based patch, which is replaced every 24 h, maintaining stable plasma levels of unconjugated active parent drug over a 24-h time period with a single daily application.
- The drug has no oral bioavailability due to extensive first-pass metabolism.

Efficacy Profile
- According to the MDS EBM Committee:
  - Rotigotine is 'efficacious' and 'clinically useful' as a symptomatic monotherapy, an add-on therapy in early or stable Parkinson's disease patients, and as treatment for motor fluctuations.
- Long-term benefit may last from 1 to 6 years.

Pharmacokinetics

Absorption and Distribution
- Transdermal bioavailability: an average of 45% of the active substance is released within 24 h after a single application with absolute bioavailability being about 37%.
  - Poor oral bioavailability due to extensive first-pass metabolism in the gut and liver.
  - The application site might affect bioavailability with shoulder application presenting the highest bioavailability. This may lead to day-to-day variation in plasma levels although without any clinically significant effects.
- Food co-ingestion: due to transdermal application, food does not affect absorption.
- Tmax: typically 15–18 h after a single dose administration (range 4–27 h).
- Time to steady state: 24–72 h.
- Pharmacokinetics: linear for doses of 1–24 mg/24 h.
  - There is an average of 3 h (1–8 h) before rotigotine is detected in plasma after a single transdermal application (8 mg/24 h).
- Protein binding: about 92% in vitro and 89.5% in vivo.
- Volume of distribution: about 84 l/kg.

R

Metabolism
- Rotigotine is extensively metabolized via *N*-dealkylation and conjugation to form biologically inactive metabolites.
- Rotigotine is metabolized by multiple CYP-450 isoenzymes, sulfotransferases, and the uridine diphosphate-glucuronosyl-transferases UGT1A9 and UGT2B15.
  - If any individual metabolic pathway is inhibited, including any CYP isoenzyme, plasma levels will not be substantially affected.
  - According to in vitro studies, there is a low risk of inhibition of CYP2C19 and CYP2D6 at therapeutic rotigotine concentrations.

Elimination
- Following removal of the transdermal patch, a biphasic elimination is observed, with an initial half-life of 2–3 h, followed by a terminal half-life of 5–7 h.
- About 71% and 23% of the administered dose is excreted as metabolites in the urine and faeces, respectively, after a single IV rotigotine dose.
  - Urinary metabolites include rotigotine sulphate, rotigotine glucuronide, *N*-despropyl-rotigotine sulphate, and *N*-desthienylethyl-rotigotine sulphate.
  - Less than 1% is excreted unchanged in the urine.

Drug Interaction Profile
Pharmacokinetic Drug Interactions
- No interactions reported.

Pharmacodynamic Drug Interactions
- Co-administration with other CNS depressants, such as sedatives, anxiolytics, antipsychotics, opiates, antidepressants, baclofen, triptans, *dihydroergotamine*, antiepileptics, or alcohol, may lead to possible additive effects, including somnolence and falling asleep during activities of daily living.
- Co-administration with other dopamine agonists or levodopa preparations might potentiate their therapeutic and/or adverse dopaminergic effects, including dyskinesia.
- Co-administration with dopamine receptor antagonists, including *amisulpride*, may lead to opposing effects.
- Co-administration with calcium/magnesium/potassium/sodium oxybates may increase the risk for sedation, respiratory depression, coma, and death via pharmacodynamic synergism.
- Co-medication with *captopril* may increase the risk of hypotension due to pharmacodynamic synergism.

ROTIGOTINE

R

Adverse Effects
How Drug Causes Adverse Effects
- Mainly (but not solely) through increasing dopaminergic activity.
- Adverse events are more common with higher therapeutic doses of rotigotine.
- Local reactions, usually of mild or moderate intensity, may occur at the site of the patch application.

Common Adverse Effects
- Very common (≥1/10):
  ○ Headache, somnolence, dizziness, nausea, vomiting.
  ○ Local reactions (e.g. erythema, pruritus, irritation, rash, dermatitis, vesicles, pain, eczema, inflammation, swelling, discolouration, urticaria, hypersensitivity).
- Common (≥1/100 to <1/10):
  ○ Neuropsychiatric: dyskinesia and hallucinations (in advanced Parkinson's disease, dose-related), sleep attacks, sleep disorders (e.g. insomnia, abnormal dreams), ICDs (e.g. urge to gamble, increased sexual urges, uncontrolled spending, binge eating, dopamine dysregulation syndrome), loss of consciousness/syncope, lethargy, tremor.
  ○ Eye/ear: vertigo.
  ○ Cardiovascular: orthostatic hypotension, hypertension, palpitations.
  ○ Respiratory: hiccups, cough, nasal or sinus congestion.
  ○ GI: constipation, diarrhoea, dry mouth, dyspepsia.
  ○ Other: fatigue, malaise, peripheral oedema, anorexia, falls.
- Uncommon (≥1/1,000 to <1/100):
  ○ Nervous/psychiatric: agitation, confusion.
  ○ Eye/ear: visual impairment (e.g. blurred vision, photopsia).
  ○ Cardiovascular: atrial fibrillation.
  ○ GI: abdominal pain.
  ○ Other: generalized pruritus or rash, erectile dysfunction, hepatic enzymes, or CPK increase.

Life-Threatening or Dangerous Adverse Effects
- Sleep attacks during activities of daily living, including operating a motor vehicle, without any warning signs, even after 1 year of rotigotine therapy.
- Hypersensitivity, including angioedema, tongue or lip oedema, especially due to sulphate sensitivity.
- NMS (hyperpyrexia, muscular rigidity, altered consciousness, rhabdomyolysis and/or autonomic instability).
- DAWS (although it is considered the safest option among dopamine agonists).
- Delirium.
- Convulsions.
- Rhabdomyolysis.

ADVERSE EFFECTS

R

Rare and Not Life-Threatening Adverse Effects
- Aggression, paranoid ideation, psychotic-like behaviour.

Weight Change
- Rotigotine might predispose to weight gain (more than 10% of base-line), especially in patients receiving the highest recommended dose or in advanced Parkinson's disease.
  - Weight gain has been associated with fluid retention and peripheral oedema.
- Weight loss has also been reported as an uncommon complication.

What to Do About Adverse Effects
- Before introducing rotigotine, discuss common or life-threatening adverse effects with patients and/or caregivers, including symptoms that should be reported to the physician.
  - Before therapy initiation, patients should be asked about somnolence or other factors that increase the risk of somnolence (e.g. CNS depressants, sleep disorders).
- On a regular basis, monitor for sleepiness, drowsiness, ICDs, hallucinations, or psychotic-like behaviours with focused and direct questions to patients/caregivers, as patients may not acknowledge such symptoms as abnormal.
- Most application site reactions are transient, of mild or moderate intensity, and might be well tolerated by the patient without any dosage reduction. If they are troublesome to the patient, persistent (lasting more than a few days), they increase in severity or they spread outside the application site, consider lowering the dose or withdrawing rotigotine.
  - In case of local reactions, clinicians should make sure that manufacturer's instructions considering application method and day-to-day site rotation are properly followed.
  - In case of generalized skin reactions, transdermal rotigotine should be discontinued.
- Dopaminergic reactions, such as nausea and vomiting, are usually mild or moderate in intensity and might be transient if treatment is continued.
- If troublesome adverse events occur, including dyskinesia (either new-onset or exacerbation of pre-existing), symptomatic orthostatic hypotension, hypertension, tachycardia, syncope, peripheral oedema, ICDs, hallucinations, or psychotic-like behaviour, consider lowering the rotigotine dose or discontinuing the drug altogether.
- If daytime sleepiness develops or episodes of falling asleep during activities that require active participation (e.g. conversations, eating) occur, rotigotine should be discontinued.
  - Patients on rotigotine should be advised to be cautious while driving, operating hazardous machinery, or working at heights.

ROTIGOTINE

- If peripheral oedema occurs as a side effect of rotigotine use, consider lowering the dose or discontinuing therapy. The use of diuretics is not recommended due to an increased risk of aggravating orthostatic hypotension.
- Periodic assessment of efficacy is advised, along with safety evaluation, including augmentation in case of RLS (relatively low augmentation rates in the first 18 months of rotigotine therapy).

Dosing and Use

Usual Dosage Range
- As monotherapy: 2–8 mg/day.
- As an add-on to levodopa: 4–16 mg/day.

Available Formulations
- Transdermal patch: 1 mg, 2 mg, 3 mg, 4 mg, 6 mg, 8 mg per 24 h.

How to Dose
- In early-stage Parkinson's disease, a single daily dose should be initiated at 2 mg/24 h, while in advanced Parkinson's disease a single daily initial dose of 4 mg/h can be applied.
- Gradual dosage increase of 2 mg/week is recommended until the desired therapeutic effect is achieved or the maximum therapeutic dosage is reached, without any significant adverse effects.
- The maximum recommended dose for early-stage Parkinson's disease is either 8 mg/24 h (EMA, EMC) or 6 mg/24 h (FDA); for advanced-stage Parkinson's disease it is 16 mg/24 h (EMA, EMC) or 8 mg/24 h (FDA).

Dosing Tips
- For doses higher than 8 mg/24 h, multiple patches can be used to achieve the total dose (e.g. 12 mg/24 h may be reached by a combination of 8 mg/24 h and 4 mg/24 h or two 6 mg/24 h patches).
- The patch should be applied immediately after opening the pouch and removing the protective liner. It should be pressed firmly in place for 30 s, especially around the edges.
  - In case of difficulties in patch adhesion, it can be stabilized in place with bandage tapes around the edges.
- The adhesive side of the transdermal patch should be applied to clean, dry, intact healthy skin, which will not be rubbed by tight clothing or under a waistband and skin folds and won't be directly exposed to the sun or other external sources of direct heat.
  - Creams, lotions, oils, ointments, or powders should not be applied to the sites of the patch placement.
- The patch should be applied at approximately the same time every day, at a convenient time for the patient (preferably after exercise and showering to avoid patch detachment).

R

- In case the patient forgets to apply the patch, or the patch is dislodged, a new patch should be applied for the remainder of the day, which will be replaced by a new patch the next day according to the patient's regular time schedule.
- Sites of the patch application should rotate every day; the patch should not be applied to the same site more than once every 14 days.
  ○ Potential application sites include the shoulder or upper arm, the abdomen, the flank, the hip, or thigh (see Figure 2).
  ○ If the application site is hairy, the area should be shaved at least 3 days before application.

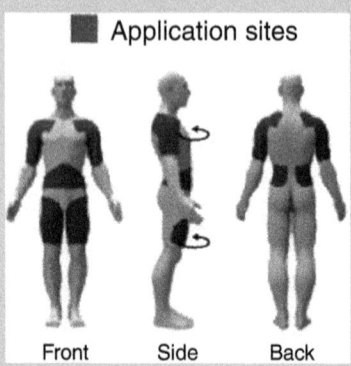

Figure 2 Application sites for the patch. Adapted from: www.medicines
.org.uk/emc/files/pil.1996.pdf

- After handling a rotigotine patch, patients should wash their hands to remove any drug. Patients should be advised to avoid touching their eyes or other objects prior to handwashing.
- If Parkinson's disease is inadequately controlled by rotigotine, switching to another dopamine agonist might be of benefit.

How to Withdraw Drug
- A slow tapering of rotigotine dosage is recommended in order to lower the risk of adverse events, including NMS and DAWS.
- For Parkinson's disease patients, the daily dose should be reduced by 2 mg/24 h every other day until complete withdrawal.
- DAWS can occur independently of the rate of dose reduction. Regular monitoring of patients during the withdrawal period is essential.
- A potential deterioration in motor performance following rotigotine reduction may need to be compensated with introducing or increasing the dose of levodopa/DDI preparations.

ROTIGOTINE

R

Overdose
- Rotigotine overdose might lead to manifestations of central dopaminergic stimulation, including nausea, vomiting, hypotension, hallucinations, confusion, involuntary movements, and convulsions.
- In case of suspected overdose, consider removing the transdermal rotigotine patch to ease the active substance input. Rotigotine plasma levels are expected to decrease rapidly.
- There is no known antidote for dopamine agonists overdose. Close monitoring is advised, including heart rate/rhythm and blood pressure, along with general supportive measures.

Tests and Therapeutic Drug Monitoring
- Periodic skin examinations by qualified clinicians should be performed to monitor for melanoma.
- Ophthalmologic monitoring is recommended at regular intervals or if vision abnormalities occur.
- Careful monitoring of blood pressure and heart rate is advised in patients with severe cardiovascular disease to ensure rapid detection of any relevant complications.
- Monitoring of weight gain and fluid retention is advised in vulnerable patients, such as those with congestive heart failure or renal insufficiency.

Other Warnings / Precautions
- Caution is advised for patients with congestive heart failure or renal insufficiency, as rotigotine might lead to fluid retention.
- Caution is advised for patients with severe cardiovascular disease, as rotigotine might cause (orthostatic) hypotension, hypertension, syncope or tachycardia, especially during dose titration.
- Caution is advised in co-medication of rotigotine and other CNS depressants, including alcohol.

Do Not Use (Contraindications)
- Known hypersensitivity to rotigotine or any of the formulation excipients, including sodium metabisulphite.
- Patients with a history of a major psychotic disorder due to increased risk of exacerbating psychosis.
- Because the backing layer of the rotigotine patch contains aluminium, it should be removed prior to MRI or cardioversion to avoid skin burns.
- Co-administration of dopamine antagonists (e.g. neuroleptics, *metoclopramide*).

DOSING AND USE

431

R

Special Populations

Renal Impairment
- No dosage adjustments required in mild to severe renal impairment, including those with end-stage disease undergoing haemodialysis.

Hepatic Impairment
- No dosage adjustment required in mild or moderate hepatic impairment (Child–Pugh class A or B).
- Rotigotine use has not been evaluated in individuals with severe hepatic impairment. Dosage reduction might be needed in case of worsening liver function.

Elderly
- Aging leads to a relative increase in body fat stores, thus increasing the volume of distribution and half-life of lipophilic drugs, such as rotigotine.
- No specific dosage recommendations are provided, as no overall differences in safety or efficacy have been observed. Rotigotine can be a beneficial option, especially if no other dopamine agonists can be used.
- The possibility of age-related complications cannot be ruled out, especially considering behavioural changes or worsening of mental status.

Pregnancy
- Rotigotine should not be used during pregnancy.
- Embryo-toxicity has been observed in animal studies.

Breastfeeding
- In case of rotigotine use, breastfeeding should be discontinued.
- Rotigotine decreases prolactin secretion and is therefore expected to inhibit lactation.
- Both rotigotine and its metabolites appear in rats' milk.

Costs

NHS indicative prices (as per BNF, accessed 20 June 2021):
- Neupro Transdermal patches (UCB Pharma Ltd) – 28 × 1 mg/24 h patches: £7.24; 28 × 2 mg/24 h patches: £81.10; 28 × 3 mg/24 h patches: £102.35; 28 × 4 mg/24 h patches: £123.60; 28 × 6 mg/24 h patches: £149.93; 28 × 8 mg/24 h patches: £149.93.

The Overall Place of Rotigotine in the Treatment of Parkinson's Disease

Rotigotine is used in Parkinson's disease, both as a monotherapy in early stages and as adjunctive therapy to levodopa preparations in advanced disease. Rotigotine is applied as a transdermal patch, constituting an alternative option to conventional oral treatments for Parkinson's disease and, thus, offering numerous advantages under particular situations, including acute medical emergencies, nil-by-mouth scenarios, or perioperative management. Its efficacy on motor aspects throughout the course of Parkinson's disease, along with its safety and tolerability profile, even in the long term, are well-established. The effect of rotigotine on non-motor symptoms of Parkinson's disease is currently being investigated with encouraging results in the management of sleep-related problems, including insomnia, feeling immobile during the night, and early morning OFF phenomena. Moreover, the combination of infusion therapies and overnight transdermal rotigotine application can be a beneficial and safe option in advanced Parkinson's disease patients in the context of personalized medicine. Rotigotine has demonstrated non-inferiority to ropinirole ER tablets, without significant safety issues, in a double-blind, parallel-group RCT. Finally, it has a role in the management of idiopathic RLS; although no conclusive evidence is available on Parkinson's disease-related RLS, rotigotine would not be discouraged in such a case.

Potential Advantages
- Once daily application, allowing for better adherence in patients with complicated drug schemes.
- In contrast to other dopamine agonists, which predominantly act at D_2- and D_3-R, rotigotine, also acts on D_1-R, suggesting a closer resemblance to dopamine or apomorphine.
- It can be applied irrespective of meal timings.
- The only anti-parkinsonian drug delivered using transdermal system, offering key advantages over oral preparations, including:
  ○ Direct entry into systemic circulation, avoiding gut absorption and 'first-pass' effects of the liver. This allows a drug effect unrelated to food interactions, impaired GI motility, or disorders of the GI tract.
  ○ Administration in nil-by-mouth scenarios (e.g. in severe dysphagia or in acutely ill patients), in pre- or post-surgical management or during hospitalization, emergency situations, or intensive care environments. Under these circumstances, switching from oral dopamine agonists to rotigotine can be undertaken safely, even overnight, although achieving dose equivalence is essential.
- Despite the fact that dopamine agonists can disrupt sleep in a dose-dependent manner and cause somnolence and sudden-onset sleep, these effects are less pronounced with rotigotine. Rotigotine can improve sleep-related problems in Parkinson's disease, including a beneficial effect on sleep structure as shown by polysomnography

studies. The improvement in sleep quality is also, at least partially, through improved motor symptom management at night.

- The 24-h continuous transdermal delivery of rotigotine exerts a beneficial effect on motor parameters even during sleep overnight.
  ○ In the context of personalized medicine, a combination of intrajejunal levodopa or apomorphine infusion with overnight rotigotine transdermal patch is well tolerated, extends the beneficial effects of infusion therapies, and is maintained for up to 1 or 2 years, respectively, in advanced Parkinson's disease patients.
- Rotigotine is considered the less likely among dopamine agonists to cause ICDs. Therefore, it should be the first option among this drug category in patients with a history of ICD or when there is a higher risk for DAWS.

Potential Disadvantages
- Sweating can lead to the rotigotine patch falling off. This may be an issue for those living in hot climates or for those exercising regularly during the day, or for those undertaking manual labour.
- Similar to other dopamine agonists, the development of ICDs, hallucinations or psychotic-like behaviour, sudden sleep attacks, and orthostatic hypotension is a possibility for some patients with potential to have life-changing consequences (e.g. financial difficulties, injuries). Rotigotine is thought to have a better safety profile with regard to somnolence compared to other dopamine agonists.

Clinical Box

A 65-year-old man with a 6-year history of Parkinson's disease presented with early morning OFF and end-of-dose, motor, and non-motor (pain) OFF phenomena. He also reported sleep impairment with frequent sleep awakenings during the night, possibly due to feeling immobile and rigid. His current medications included levodopa/carbidopa/entacapone 125 mg/31.25 mg/200 mg QID. His medical history included well-controlled hypertension and diabetes mellitus. A transdermal rotigotine patch of 4 mg/24 h OD was prescribed and the patient was given instructions of gradual weekly dose increases by 2 mg/24 h and follow-up assessments via phone appointments. At a dose of 8 mg/24 h the patient reported improvement of his symptoms; however, mild-to-moderate generalized dyskinesia developed. This was addressed by reducing levodopa/carbidopa/entacapone dose from 125 mg/31.25 mg/200 mg QID to 100 mg/25 mg/200 mg QID.

R

Suggested Reading

Lau YH, V Leta, K Rukavina, M Parry, JA Natividad, V Metta, G Chung-Faye, KR CHaudhuri. Tolerability of overnight rotigotine transdermal patch combined with intrajejunal levodopa infusion at 1 year: a 24-h treatment option in Parkinson's disease. *J Neural Transm (Vienna)* 2022; 129(7): 889–894.

Raeder V, I Boura, V Leta, P Jenner, H Reichmann, C Trenkwalder, L Klingelhoefer, KR Chaudhuri. Rotigotine transdermal patch for motor and non-motor Parkinson's disease: a review of 12 years' clinical experience. *CNS Drugs* 2021; 35(2): 215–231.

Ray Chaudhuri K, P Martinez-Martin, A Antonini, RG Brown, JH Friedman, M Onofrj, E Surmann, L Ghys, C Trenkwalder. Rotigotine and specific non-motor symptoms of Parkinson's disease: post hoc analysis of RECOVER. *Parkinsonism Relat Disord* 2013; 19(7): 660–665.

Rosa-Grilo M, MA Qamar, RN Taddei, J Pagonabarraga, J Kulisevsky, A Sauerbier, KR Chaudhuri. Rotigotine transdermal patch and sleep in Parkinson's disease: where are we now? *NPJ Parkinsons Dis* 2017; 3: 28.

Todorova A, P Martinez-Martin, A Martin, A Rizos, P Reddy, KR Chaudhuri. Daytime apomorphine infusion combined with transdermal Rotigotine patch therapy is tolerated at 2 years: a 24-h treatment option in Parkinson's disease. *Basal Ganglia* 2013; 3(2): 127–130.

Trenkwalder C, B Kies, M Rudzinska, J Fine, J Nikl, K Honczarenko, P Dioszeghy, D Hill, T Anderson, V Myllyla, J Kassubek, M Stieger, M Zucconi, E Tolosa, W Poewe, E Surmann, J Whitesides, B Boroojerdi, KR Chaudhuri; Recover Study Group. Rotigotine effects on early morning motor function and sleep in Parkinson's disease: a double-blind, randomized, placebo-controlled study (RECOVER). *Mov Disord* 2011; 26(1): 90–99.

References

AHFS Drug information, 2012. Bethesda: American Society of Health-System Pharmacists. Accessed on 31 May 2022 via www.medicinescomplete.com.

Chung SJ, JM Kim, JW Kim, BS Jeon, P Singh, S Thierfelder, J Ikeda, L Bauer; Asia Pacific Rotigotine Switching Study Group. Switch from oral pramipexole or ropinirole to rotigotine transdermal system in advanced Parkinson's disease: an open-label study. *Expert Opin Pharmacother* 2015; 16(7): 961–970.

Elmer LW, E Surmann, B Boroojerdi, J Jankovic. Long-term safety and tolerability of rotigotine transdermal system in patients with early-stage idiopathic Parkinson's disease: a prospective, open-label extension study. *Parkinsonism Relat Disord* 2012; 18(5): 488–493.

R

Hattori N, H Mochizuki, K Hasegawa, M Nomoto, E Uchida, T Terahara, K Okawa, HR Fukuta. Ropinirole patch versus placebo, ropinirole extended-release tablet in advanced Parkinson's disease. *Mov Disord* 2020; 35(9): 1565–1573.

Ibrahim H, Z Woodward, J Pooley, EW Richfield. Rotigotine patch prescription in inpatients with Parkinson's disease: evaluating prescription accuracy, delirium and end-of-life use. *Age Ageing* 2021; 50(4): 1397–1401.

Joint Formulary Committee. British National Formulary (online). London: BMJ Group and Pharmaceutical Press. Accessed on 31 May 2022 via www.medicinescomplete.com.

Koschel J, KR Chaudhuri, L Tönges, M Thiel, V Raeder, WH Jott. Implications of dopaminergic medication withdrawal in Parkinson's disease. *J Neural Transm (Vienna)* 2022; 129(9): 1169–1178.

Latt MD, S Lewis, O Zekry, VSC Fung. Factors to consider in the selection of dopamine agonists for older persons with Parkinson's disease. *Drugs Aging* 2019; 36(3): 189–202.

LeWitt PA, B Boroojerdi, E Surmann, W Poewe; SP716 Study Group; SP715 Study Group. Rotigotine transdermal system for long-term treatment of patients with advanced Parkinson's disease: results of two open-label extension studies, CLEOPATRA-PD and PREFER. *J Neural Transm (Vienna)* 2013; 120(7): 1069–1081.

Pierantozzi M, F Placidi, C Liguori, M Albanese, P Imbriani, MG Marciani, NB Mercuri, P Stanzione, A Stefani. Rotigotine may improve sleep architecture in Parkinson's disease: a double-blind, randomized, placebo-controlled polysomnographic study. *Sleep Med* 2016; 21: 140–144.

Rotigotine. In: Brayfield A (Ed.), *Martindale: The Complete Drug Reference*. London: The Royal Pharmaceutical Society of Great Britain. Accessed on 31 May 2022 via www.medicinescomplete.com.

Summary of product characteristics – Neupro 4 mg/24 h transdermal patch. UCB Pharma Limited. Electronic Medicines Compendium: Neupro 4 mg/24 h transdermal patch – summary of product characteristics (SmPC) – (emc). Accessed on 31 May 2022 via www.medicines.org.uk.

Taguchi S, H Koide, H Oiwa, M Hayashi, K Ogawa, C Ito, K Nakashima, T Yuasa, A Yasumoto, H Ando, A Fujikake, T Fukuoka, K Tokui, M Izuma, Y Tsunoda, Y Kawagashira, Y Okada, JI Niwa, M Doyu. Antiparkinsonian drugs as potent contributors to nocturnal sleep in patients with Parkinson's disease. *PLoS One* 2021; 16(7): e0255274.

Trenkwalder, C., B Kies, P Dioszeghy, D Hill, E Surmann, B Boroojerdi, J Whitesides, KR Chaudhuri. Rotigotine transdermal system for the management of motor function and sleep disturbances in Parkinson's disease: results from a 1-year, open-label extension of the RECOVER study. *Basal Ganglia* 2012; 2(2): 79–85

ROTIGOTINE

SAFINAMIDE

Therapeutics

Chemical Name and Structure
Safinamide ((+)-(S)-2-({p-[(m-fluorobenzyl)oxy]benzyl}amino)propi-
onamide) has a molecular weight of 302.3 and a molecular formula of
$C_{17}H_{19}FN_2O_2$.

Brand Names
- **Xadago** (*Australia, Belgium, Czech Republic, Denmark, Finland, France,
  Germany, Ireland, Netherlands, Norway, Poland, Portugal, Spain, Sweden,
  Switzerland*, UK, *USA*).

Generics Available
- No.

Licensed Indications for Parkinson's Disease
- As an add-on therapy for Parkinson's disease patients who are already
  taking levodopa/carbidopa preparations and experience OFF episodes (FDA).
- As an add-on therapy to stable doses of levodopa alone or in combination with other anti-Parkinson's disease medicinal products in
  mid-to-late stage fluctuating patients with idiopathic Parkinson's disease (EMA, EMC).

Licensed Indications for Other Conditions
- None.

Non-Licensed Use for Parkinson's Disease
- As an add-on therapy to dopamine agonists in Parkinson's disease
  patients with wearing OFF phenomena.

Non-Licensed Use for Other Conditions
- None.

Ineffective
- As a monotherapy in Parkinson's disease.

Mechanism of Action
- Safinamide is a highly selective, long-acting, and fully reversible
  MAO-B inhibitor causing an increase in extracellular dopamine lev-
  els in the striatum.
  - There is full recovery of MAO-B activity within 5 days of safina-
    mide withdrawal.
- Safinamide is also a state-dependent inhibitor of voltage-gated
  sodium channels, with consequent modulation of calcium channels
  and inhibition of excess glutamate release from presynaptic terminals.

S

SAFINAMIDE

- The exact mechanism of action of safinamide in Parkinson's disease remains unknown. The extent of non-dopaminergic effects on symptoms of Parkinson's disease remains to be established.

Efficacy Profile
- Safinamide has been characterized as 'efficacious' and 'clinically useful' in the treatment of motor fluctuations in Parkinson's disease (MDS EBM Committee).
- Three high-quality studies with a follow-up of 24 weeks have found that safinamide 50 mg and 100 mg daily can be effectively used as an adjunct to levodopa preparations in Parkinson's disease patients with motor fluctuations. These results were corroborated by a recent systematic review and meta-analysis.
- A 2-year extension study of one of the above trials has demonstrated a beneficial effect of safinamide on Parkinson's disease patients with motor fluctuations, including an improvement of dyskinesias (at least in patients with moderate to marked dyskinesia at baseline and at a dose of 100 mg), ON time without troublesome dyskinesias, OFF time, ADL, motor symptoms, quality of life, and depression symptoms.
- According to a double-blind RCT, the 100 mg dose of safinamide was found efficacious as an add-on therapy to a stable dose of a dopamine agonist in early-stage Parkinson's disease patients. These results are still considered exploratory.
- Post-hoc analyses, along with observations from 'real-world' clinical data, suggest a beneficial effect of safinamide on non-motor symptoms overall, and specifically on mood, cognition, pain, and sleep impairment, including night-time sleep and daytime sleepiness.
- Doses higher than 100 mg/day are not expected to show additional benefit.

Pharmacokinetics
Absorption and Distribution
- Oral bioavailability: about 95%.
- Food co-ingestion is not expected to alter safinamide pharmacokinetics.
- Tmax: 1.8–2.8 h.
- Time to steady state: within 7 days.
- Pharmacokinetics: linear.
- Protein binding: 88–90%.
- Volume of distribution: 165 l.

Metabolism
- Safinamide undergoes hydrolytic oxidation of the amide moiety leading to the production of safinamide acid, the primary metabolite.
- O-debenzylated safinamide is also produced by oxidative cleavage of the ether bond.

- Oxidative cleavage of the amine bond of either safinamide or safinamide acid to form N-dealkylated acid also takes place; this is further conjugated with glucuronic acid to yield its acyl glucuronide.

Elimination
- Elimination half-life ranges between 20 h and 30 h.
- Safinamide is mainly excreted in the urine, mostly in the form of inactive metabolites (76%). About 5% of the parent drug is excreted unchanged in the urine.

Drug Interaction Profile
Pharmacokinetic Drug Interactions
- Effects by safinamide:
  - Safinamide may increase levels and effects of intestinal breast cancer resistance protein (BCRP) substrates, including statins (e.g. *atorvastatin, pitavastatin, rosuvastatin*), *chlorothiazide, cimetidine, imatinib, methotrexate, pantoprazole, sulfasalazine* due to inhibition of intestinal BCRP.
  - Safinamide may increase levels of OCT1 substrates, which have similar Tmax to safinamide (e.g. *metformin, acyclovir, ganciclovir*), due to exhibiting inhibitory action of OCT1 in vitro at clinically relevant portal vein concentrations.

Pharmacodynamic Drug Interactions
- Co-administration with tricyclic/tetracyclic antidepressants (e.g. *amitriptyline*), SSRIs/SNRIs (e.g. *fluoxetine, paroxetine, sertraline*, and *venlafaxine*), MAOIs (e.g. *amoxapine*), opiates (e.g. *fentanyl, tramadol*), *isoniazid* can lead to increased toxicity, including a potentially fatal serotonin syndrome, due to elevated serotonin levels.
- Co-administration with agents exhibiting sympathetic (adrenergic) effects (e.g. *methylphenidate, midodrine*) may lead to pharmacodynamic synergism and increased risk of an acute hypertensive episode.
- Dopamine antagonists (e.g. neuroleptics, *metoclopramide*) may decrease safinamide effects by pharmacodynamic antagonism and aggravate parkinsonian symptoms.
- Co-administration with *dextromethorphan* may cause psychosis or bizarre behaviour.

Adverse Effects
How Drug Causes Adverse Effects
- Mainly (but not only) by increasing dopaminergic activity.

Common Adverse Effects
- Very common (≥1/10):
  - Dyskinesia.

S

ADVERSE EFFECTS

- Common (≥1/100 to <1/10):
  - Neuropsychiatric: insomnia, anxiety, somnolence, headache.
  - Eye/ear: cataract.
  - Cardiovascular: hypertension, orthostatic hypotension.
  - Respiratory: cough.
  - GI: nausea, dyspepsia.
  - Other: increased liver enzyme values, falls.
- Uncommon (≥1/1,000 to <1/100):
  - Neuropsychiatric: hallucinations, depression, abnormal dreams, anxiety, paraesthesia, dystonia, balance impairment, dysarthria, cognitive impairment.
  - Eye/ear: blurred vision, scotoma, diplopia, photophobia, retinal disorder, conjunctivitis, glaucoma, vertigo.
  - Cardiovascular: palpitations, tachycardia, sinus bradycardia, arrhythmia, varicose vein, prolonged QT.
  - Respiratory: cough, dyspnoea, rhinorrhoea.
  - GI: constipation, vomiting, dry mouth, diarrhoea, abdominal pain, gastritis, flatulence, abdominal distension, salivary hypersecretion, gastroesophageal reflux disease, aphthous stomatitis.
  - Renal/urinary: urinary tract infection, nocturia, dysuria, abnormal urine analysis.
  - Skin: hyperhidrosis, generalised pruritus, erythema, photosensitivity reaction.
  - Musculoskeletal: back pain, arthralgia, muscle spasms, muscle rigidity, pain in extremity, muscular weakness, foot fractures.
  - Other: anaemia, leukopenia, red blood cell abnormality, decreased/increased appetite, hypertriglyceridaemia, hypercholesterolaemia, hyperglycaemia, syncope, fatigue, asthenia, peripheral oedema, increased CPK/triglycerides/glucose/urea/alkaline phosphatase/bicarbonate/creatinine, abnormal liver function tests.

Life-Threatening or Dangerous Adverse Effects
- Uncommon (≥1/1,000 to <1/100):
  - Basal cell carcinoma.
- Rare (≥1/10,000 to <1/1,000):
  - Bronchopneumonia.
  - Hyperkalaemia, decreased blood calcium/potassium.
  - Delirium.
  - Suicidal ideation.
  - Sleep attacks.
  - Eye haemorrhage.
  - MI.
  - Arterial spasm, arteriosclerosis, hypertensive crisis.
  - Bronchospasm, oropharyngeal spasm.
  - Peptic ulcer, upper GI haemorrhage.
- Unknown frequency:
  - Hypersensitivity, including swelling of tongue/gingiva and dyspnoea.

Rare and Not Life-Threatening Adverse Effects
- Rash.
- Nasopharyngitis, rhinitis, pyoderma, tooth infection, viral infection.
- ICDs.
- Loss of libido, premature ejaculation.
- Social phobia.
- Abnormal coordination, attention impairment, hyporeflexia, dysgeusia, radicular pain.
- Amblyopia, diabetic retinopathy, eye pain, eyelid oedema, hypermetropia, keratitis, increased lacrimation, night blindness, papilledema, presbyopia, strabismus.
- Dysphonia, oropharyngeal pain.
- Alopecia, blister, contact dermatitis, ecchymosis, night sweats, pigmentation disorder, psoriasis, seborrheic dermatitis, acrochordon, melanocytic naevus, seborrheic keratosis, skin papilloma.
- Joint swelling, musculoskeletal pain, myalgia, neck pain, osteoarthritis.
- Micturition urgency, polyuria, urinary hesitation.
- Benign prostatic hyperplasia, breast pain.
- Decreased blood cholesterol/haematocrit/haemoglobin.
- Increased body temperature.

Weight Change
- Increased or decreased weight may be an uncommon complication of safinamide.

What to Do About Adverse Effects
- Before introducing safinamide, discuss common adverse effects with patients or caregivers, including symptoms that should be reported to the physician.
  - Patients should be directly questioned about drowsiness or sleepiness during specific activities or ICDs, as they might not acknowledge these symptoms until specifically asked.
- If safinamide causes new-onset dyskinesia or aggravates pre-existing dyskinesia, consider a levodopa dose reduction to mitigate this effect.
- If hallucinations, psychotic behaviour, or development of ICDs occur, consider a reduction of safinamide dose or complete withdrawal of therapy.

Dosing and Use
Usual Dosage Range
- 50–100 mg daily.

Available Formulations
- Tablets: 50 mg, 100 mg.

S

DOSING AND USE

S

How to dose
• An initial dose of 50 mg OD is suggested; dose can be increased to 100 mg OD after 2 weeks, according to patient's tolerability and clinical needs.

Dosing Tips
• Safinamide can be taken with or without food.
• It should be taken at approximately the same time each day.
• If a dose is missed, patients should be advised to take the next dose at the same time the next day.
• An overnight switch from rasagiline to safinamide was found to be safe and well tolerated (no blood pressure changes or serotonin-related symptoms).

How to Withdraw Drug
• The dose of 50 mg/day can be abruptly discontinued.
• The dose of 100 mg/day should be reduced to 50 mg/day for 1 week before cessation.

Overdose
• Excessive MAO-B inhibition through overdose would be expected to lead to increased dopamine levels and symptoms including postural hypotension, hallucinations, agitation, nausea, vomiting, and dyskinesia.
• There is no known antidote to safinamide.
• Close monitoring and supportive measures should be applied.

Tests and Therapeutic Drug Monitoring
• During safinamide therapy:
  • Regular measurement of blood pressure is recommended.
  • Periodic assessment of visual changes is advised in patients with a history of retinal/macular degeneration, uveitis, inherited retinal conditions, family history of hereditary retinal disease, albinism, retinitis pigmentosa, or any active retinopathy due to reported retinal degeneration and loss of photoreceptor cells in animal studies.

Other Warnings/Precautions
• Safinamide therapy may lead to new-onset hypertension or exacerbate existing hypertension; vigilance is recommended.
• At least 14 days should elapse between discontinuation/initiation of safinamide and other drugs that may increase serotonin levels, such as tricyclic/tetracyclic antidepressants, SNRIS, triptans, *dihydroergotamine*, opiates, neuroleptics, *linezolid, lithium, isoniazid*, or other drugs that exhibit pharmacodynamic synergism with MAOIs, including sympathomimetic agents.
  • Close monitoring is recommended if co-administered with SSRIs (fluoxetine and fluvoxamine should be avoided). The lowest effective dose of safinamide should be used.

SAFINAMIDE

- A washout period of five half-lives of the SSRI previously used should be considered prior to initiating safinamide treatment.
- Caution is advised if co-administered with dopamine antagonists, such as neuroleptics; alternative therapeutic options are suggested.
- Close monitoring is advised if co-administered with intestinal BCRP substrates due to potential increased pharmacologic effect or side effects.
- Patients are advised not to drive or use dangerous machinery until they know how safinamide affects them (e.g. dizziness, daytime sleepiness, impairment of reaction capacity).

Do Not Use (Contraindicated)
- Known hypersensitivity to safinamide or any of the formulation excipients.
- Patients with albinism, retinal degeneration, uveitis, inherited retinopathy, or severe progressive diabetic retinopathy.
- Co-medication with serotonin agonists (e.g. triptans), opioids (e.g. pethidine, methadone, tramadol, dextropropoxyphene), sympathomimetics (including over-the-counter decongestants and cold remedies), other MAOIs, antidepressants, tricyclic/tetracyclic antidepressants and SNRIs, psychostimulants, central suppressant drugs (e.g. sedatives), and oral contraceptives.
- Co-administration with dextromethorphan.

Special Populations
Renal Impairment
- No dosage modifications are necessary.

Hepatic Impairment
- Mild hepatic impairment (Child–Pugh A): no dosage modifications needed.
- Moderate hepatic impairment (Child–Pugh B): a maximum dose of 50 mg OD is recommended.
- Severe hepatic impairment (Child–Pugh C): contraindicated.

Elderly
- No dosage modifications are necessary.
- Limited experience on the use of safinamide in patients older than 75 years old.

Pregnancy
- No adequate and well-controlled studies are available at the moment considering the use of safinamide among pregnant women.
- Animal studies have demonstrated developmental toxicity, including teratogenic effects.
- Safinamide use is not recommended during pregnancy.
- Safinamide should not be prescribed to women of childbearing potential, unless adequate contraception is in place.

S

Breastfeeding
- According to animal studies, safinamide is excreted in milk, although it is not known whether it is excreted in human milk.
- Safinamide use is not recommended during breastfeeding, as potential adverse effects on the nursing infant cannot be excluded.

Costs
NHS indicative price (accessed 15 April 23):
- Xadago Tablets (Zambon UK Ltd) – 30 × 50 mg tablets: £69.00; 30 × 100 mg tablets: £69.00.

The Overall Place of Safinamide in the Treatment of Parkinson's Disease

Safinamide is approved for the treatment of motor fluctuations in Parkinson's disease. It can only be used as an adjunctive therapy to levodopa preparations. It has a unique pharmacological profile with a dual mechanism of action, being a selective and reversible MAO-B inhibitor, but also a glutamate release modulator through sodium channel blockade. This action is believed to mediate its beneficial effect on dyskinesia. High-quality studies have demonstrated a positive effect of safinamide as an add-on therapy to levodopa preparations in mid- to late-stage Parkinson's disease patients with motor fluctuations. These results were also confirmed in a post-hoc analysis, which showed a favourable effect of safinamide on ON and OFF time, irrespective of concomitant use of other anti-parkinsonian agents (such as dopamine agonists, COMT inhibitors, and amantadine). Safinamide also diminished parkinsonian motor features of bradykinesia, rigidity, tremor, and gait impairment. Post-hoc analyses, along with observations from 'real-world' clinical data, have shown a beneficial effect of safinamide both on non-motor symptoms overall and specifically on mood, cognition, pain, and sleep impairment, including night-time sleep and daytime sleepiness. Although these results are encouraging, further investigation is required. Preliminary results have suggested a beneficial effect of safinamide when co-administered with a stable dose of a dopamine agonist, although this remains an off-label use. Safinamide is generally considered a well-tolerated drug, even for older patients, although caution is recommended to avoid co-administration with drugs increasing serotonin levels.

Potential Advantages
- In contrast to rasagiline and selegiline, which are irreversible MAO-B inhibitors, safinamide is a reversible MAO-B inhibitor; therefore, any potential side effects may rapidly regress after safinamide discontinuation.

- In contrast to rasagiline and selegiline, co-administration with SSRIs is possible, if administered at minimum doses needed and with increased vigilance for side effects.
- Unlike other MAO-B inhibitors, a low dose of safinamide is allowed in moderate hepatic impairment.
- Unlike rasagiline and selegiline, safinamide may also modulate glutamatergic transmission.

Potential Disadvantages
- Safinamide is not globally available.

Clinical Box
A 60-year-old woman with a 9-year history of Parkinson's disease presented at the Movement Disorders Outpatient Clinic due to end-of-dose OFF phenomena and non-troublesome dyskinesia. She had a recent history of troublesome dyskinesia, which was addressed by reducing levodopa dose and introducing pramipexole ER. The patient also reported non-specific pain symptoms, which seemed to improve with dopaminergic drugs, plus a decreased mood. She was receiving levodopa/benserazide 200 mg/50 mg ¾ QID and pramipexole 1.05 mg OD. The rest of her medical history included well-controlled hypertension and diabetes mellitus with mild renal impairment. MAOIs were considered as a good initial option to mildly increase dopaminergic activity in order to address OFF phenomena without aggravating dyskinesia. A trial of safinamide 50 mg OD was suggested due to the concurrent non-motor symptoms of pain and low mood. She was also given specific instructions for regular blood pressure monitoring.

Suggested Reading
Abbruzzese G, P Barone, L Lopiano, F Stocchi. The current evidence for the use of safinamide for the treatment of Parkinson's disease. *Drug Des Devel Ther* 2021; 15: 2507–2517.

Bianchi MLE, G Riboldazzi, M Mauri, M Versino. Efficacy of safinamide on non-motor symptoms in a cohort of patients affected by idiopathic Parkinson's disease. *Neurol Sci* 2019; 40(2): 275–279.

Borgohain R, J Szasz, P Stanzione, C Meshram, M Bhatt, D Chirilineau, F Stocchi, V Lucini, R Giuliani, E Forrest, P Rice, R Anand. Randomized trial of safinamide add-on to levodopa in Parkinson's disease with motor fluctuations. *Mov Disord* 2014; 29(2): 229–237.

Hattori N, Y Tsuboi, A Yamamoto, Y Sasagawa, M Nomoto. Efficacy and safety of safinamide as an add-on therapy to L-DOPA for patients with Parkinson's disease: a randomized, double-blind, placebo-controlled, phase II/III study. *Parkinsonism Relat Disord* 2020; 75: 17–23.

S

SUGGESTED READING

S

Schapira AH, SH Fox, RA Hauser, J Jankovic, WH Jost, C Kenney, J Kulisevsky, R Pahwa, W Poewe, R Anand. Assessment of safety and efficacy of safinamide as a levodopa adjunct in patients with Parkinson disease and motor fluctuations: a randomized clinical trial. *JAMA Neurol* 2017; 74(2): 216–224.

References

AHFS Drug information, 2012. Bethesda: American Society of Health-System Pharmacists. Accessed on 9 October 2021 via www .medicinescomplete.com.

Alborghetti M, F Nicoletti. Different generations of type-B monoamine oxidase inhibitors in Parkinson's disease: from bench to bedside. *Curr Neuropharmacol* 2019; 17(9): 861–873.

Borgohain R, J Szasz, P Stanzione, C Meshram, MH Bhatt, D Chirilineau, F Stocchi, V Lucini, R Giuliani, E Forrest, P Rice, R Anand. Two-year, randomized, controlled study of safinamide as add-on to levodopa in mid to late Parkinson's disease. *Mov Disord* 2014; 29(10): 1273–1280.

Cattaneo C, M Sardina, E Bonizzoni. Safinamide as add-on therapy to levodopa in mid- to late-stage Parkinson's disease fluctuating patients: post hoc analyses of Studies 016 and SETTLE. *J Parkinsons Dis* 2016; 6(1): 165–173.

Cattaneo C, RL Ferla, E Bonizzoni, M Sardina. Long-term effects of safinamide on dyskinesia in mid- to late-stage Parkinson's disease: a post-hoc analysis. *J Parkinsons Dis* 2015; 5(3): 475–481.

Geroin C, IA DiVico, G Squintani, A Segatti, T Bovi, M Tinazzi. Effects of safinamide on pain in Parkinson's disease with motor fluctuations: an exploratory study. *J Neural Transm (Vienna)* 2020; 127(8): 1143–1152.

Giossi R, F Carrara, M Mazzari, F Lo Re, M Senatore, A Schicchi, F Corrù, VA Fittipaldo, A Pani, I Tramacere, AE Elia, F Scaglione. Overall efficacy and safety of safinamide in Parkinson's disease: a systematic review and a meta-analysis. *Clin Drug Investig* 2021; 41(4): 321–339.

Joint Formulary Committee. British National Formulary (online). London: BMJ Group and Pharmaceutical Press. Accessed on 9 October 2021 via www.medicinescomplete.com.

Liguori C, A Stefani, R Ruffini, NB Mercuri, M Pierantozzi. Safinamide effect on sleep disturbances and daytime sleepiness in motor fluctuating Parkinson's disease patients: a validated questionnaires-controlled study. *Parkinsonism Relat Disord* 2018; 57: 80–81.

Rinaldi D, M Sforza, F Assogna, C Savini, M Salvetti, C Caltagirone, G Spalletta, FE Pontieri. Safinamide improves executive functions in fluctuating Parkinson's disease patients: an exploratory study. *J Neural Transm (Vienna)* 2021; 128(2): 273–277.

SAFINAMIDE

Safinamide. In: Brayfield A (Ed.), *Martindale: The Complete Drug Reference*. London: The Royal Pharmaceutical Society of Great Britain. Accessed on 9 October 2021 via www.medicinescomplete.com.

Stocchi F, L Vacca, P Grassini, C Tomino, G Caminiti, M Casali, V D'Antoni, M Volterrani, M Torti. Overnight switch from rasagiline to safinamide in Parkinson's disease patients with motor fluctuations: a tolerability and safety study. *Eur J Neurol* 2021; 28(1): 349–354.

Summary of product characteristics – Xadago 50 mg film-coated tablets. Zambon UK Limited (Formerly Profile Pharma Ltd). Electronic Medicines Compendium: Xadago 50 mg film-coated tablets – summary of product characteristics (SmPC) – (emc). Accessed on 9 October 2021 via www.medicines.org.uk.

S

SELEGILINE

Therapeutics

Chemical Name and Structure

Selegiline hydrochloride ((R)-(−)-N,α-dimethyl-N-2-propynylphene-thylamine hydrochloride) and commonly referred to as L-deprenyl, is a white to near-white crystalline powder, freely soluble in water, with a molecular weight of 223.75 and an empirical formula of $C_{13}H_{17}N•HCl$.

Brand Names
- **Antiparkin** (*Germany*); **Atapryl** (*USA*).
- **Brintenal** (*Argentina*).
- **Cosmopril** (*Greece*).
- **Deprenyl** (*France*); **Deprilan** (*Brazil*).
- **Egibren** (*Italy*); **Eldepryl** (*Australia, Belgium, China, Denmark, Finland, India, Ireland, Norway, South Africa, Sweden, Switzerland, UK, Ukraine*); **Elegelin** (*India*); **Emsam** (*USA*).
- **Feliselin** (*Greece*); **Fu An** (*China*).
- **Jinsiping** (*China*); **Julab** (*Thailand*); **Jumax** (*India*); **Jumex** (*Argentina, Cyprus, Hungary, India, Italy, Malaysia, Russian Federation, Ukraine, Venezuela*); **Jumexil** (*Brazil*).
- **Legil** (*Greece*).
- **Moverdin** (*Turkey*).
- **Niar** (*Brazil, Mexico*).
- **Parkilyne** (*South Africa*); **Plurimen** (*Spain*); **Procythol** (*Greece*).
- **Resostyl** (*Greece*).
- **Sefmex** (*Hong Kong, Thailand*); **Segan** (*Poland, Ukraine*); **Selecom** (*Italy*); **Seledat** (*Italy*); **Selegos** (*Cyprus, Czech Republic, Hong Kong, Philippines, Singapore*); **Selerin** (*India*); **Selex** (*Cyprus*); **Selgin** (*India, Israel*); **Selgina** (*Chile*); **Selgene** (*Australia*); **Selgres** (*Poland*).
- **Xilopar** (*Italy, Portugal*).
- **Zelapar** (*USA*).

Generics Available
- Yes.

Licensed Indications for Parkinson's Disease
- As monotherapy for early, symptomatic Parkinson's disease (EMC).
- As an adjunct therapy to levodopa in early or stable Parkinson's disease (EMC).
- As an adjunct therapy to levodopa in Parkinson's disease patients who exhibit a deterioration of their response to treatment, especially in motor fluctuations, such as end-of-dose fluctuations, ON–OFF symptoms, or other dyskinesias (FDA, EMA, EMC).

S

Licensed Indications for Other Conditions
• Symptomatic parkinsonism, dopa-responsive (EMC).
• Major depressive disorder (transdermal patch, only available in the USA) (FDA).

Non-Licensed Use for Parkinson's Disease
• Early symptomatic Parkinson's disease (USA).

Non-Licensed Use for Other Conditions
• Palliative treatment of mild to moderate dementia in Alzheimer's disease (equivocal results).
• Treatment of cocaine abuse and dependence (transdermal patch, equivocal results).
• Attention-deficit/hyperactivity disorder.

Ineffective
• To prevent/delay disease progression in Parkinson's disease (MDS EBM Committee).
• To prevent/delay motor fluctuations in Parkinson's disease (MDS EBM Committee).
• Bipolar disorder.

Mechanism of Action
• An irreversible, selective and potent MAO-B inhibitor, which prevents dopamine degradation in the brain, facilitating and prolonging the effect of exogenous and endogenous dopamine in the striatum. It may also elevate dopaminergic activity through inhibition of presynaptic dopamine reuptake.
• After a single 10 mg dose of selegiline, the marked inhibitory effect on platelet MAO-B activity lasts for more than 24 h and only returns to normal after approximately 2 weeks when new MAO-B enzyme has been synthesized.
• Although dietary restrictions are not necessary, MAO-B inhibition in blood platelets might lead to a potentiation of the effects of tyramine not broken down by GI MAO-A during absorption.
• In higher doses, selegiline becomes a non-selective MAOI, inhibiting both MAO-A and MAO-B, allowing it to be used in the treatment of depression.
• It has been suggested that amphetamine metabolites of selegiline may act to increase the release of monoamine neurotransmitters and give rise to sympathomimetic effects of the drug.

Efficacy Profile
• According to the MDS EBM Committee:
  • Selegiline is 'efficacious' and 'clinically useful' as a monotherapy for early, symptomatic Parkinson's disease.
    • This effect is smaller compared to levodopa and dopamine agonists.

THERAPEUTICS

- There is insufficient evidence to support its role as an adjunct therapy to levodopa in early Parkinson's disease.
- There is insufficient evidence to support its role in the management of motor fluctuations.
- There is insufficient evidence to support selegiline use in treating depressive symptoms in Parkinson's disease.
- Selegiline monotherapy in early Parkinson's disease is expected to be efficient in the long term.
- The addition of selegiline to levodopa regimens is expected to reduce levodopa dosage by an average of 10–30%.
- The addition of selegiline to levodopa might not be beneficial in patients experiencing non-dose-dependent fluctuations.
- Peak response to selegiline is expected after 7 days.

Pharmacokinetics

Absorption and Distribution

- Bioavailability: about 10% (oral route, large interindividual variation); about 30% (oral transmucosal and transdermal route).
- Tmax: 30–45 min after oral administration in fasting state.
- Time to steady state: 4 days (10 mg of oral dose).
- Pharmacokinetics: non-linear increase of selegiline concentration after multiple oral doses with serum accumulation of selegiline and L-N-desmethyl-selegiline, probably due to MAO-B binding site saturation or decrease in the first-past metabolism of selegiline. This accumulation is not harmful due to the MAO-B selectivity of selegiline.
- Protein binding: 75–85% at therapeutic concentrations.
- Volume of distribution: 26 l/kg.

Metabolism

- Rapidly metabolized to L-N-desmethyl-selegiline ($T_{1/2}$=2.1 h), L-methamphetamine ($T_{1/2}$=20.5 h), and L-amphetamine ($T_{1/2}$=17.7 h), mainly in the liver (CYP system), with the latter being the primary metabolite.
- In vitro studies show CYP2B6 is the main enzyme involved in selegiline metabolism with a possible contribution from CYP3A4 and CYP2A6.
- All metabolites are found in the serum, CSF and urine.

Elimination

- Mean elimination half-life in adults is about 1.5–3.5 h after a single oral dose.
  - At steady state the elimination half-life is about 10 h.
- Selegiline metabolites are excreted mainly via urine with about 15% found in faeces.
  - 75% of a conventional oral dose is excreted in the urine as amphetamine metabolites.

Drug Interaction Profile

Pharmacokinetic Drug Interactions
- Effects on selegiline:
  - *Oral contraceptives* significantly increase selegiline bioavailability.
  - *Rifampin* will decrease levels and effects of selegiline by affecting hepatic enzyme CYP2B6 metabolism.

Pharmacodynamic Drug Interactions
- Co-medication with opioids (e.g. *pethidine*), triptans, *dihydroergotamine*, neuroleptics (e.g. *aripiprazole*, *quetiapine*, *clozapine*), *isoniazid*, or *lithium* may increase serotonin levels and lead to life-threatening serotonin syndrome.
- Co-administration with tricyclic/tetracyclic antidepressants or SSRIs/SNRIs (e.g. *fluoxetine*, *paroxetine*, *sertraline*, and *venlafaxine*) can lead to sweating, flushing, hyperthermia, diarrhoea, hypertension or hypotension, seizures, palpitations, dizziness, mental changes, such as agitation, confusion, hallucinations, delirium and coma, ataxia, myoclonus, hyperreflexia, tremor, and serotonin syndrome, even after a drug-free period, due to increased serotonin levels.
- Co-administration with non-selective MAO inhibitors might lead to severe orthostatic hypotension (*iproniazid*) or a hypertensive crisis as a response to tyramine (*moclobemide*).
- Co-administration with sympathomimetic agents, including *ephedrine*, may lead to an acute hypertensive crisis.
- Co-administration with *midodrine* or *modafinil* may lead to a hypertensive reaction.
- Co-administration with *dextromethorphan* may result in bizarre behaviour or psychosis.
  - Selegiline may increase the hypoglycaemic effect of antidiabetic agents, such as *metformin* and *insulin*.
  - *Carbamazepine* may increase toxicity of selegiline by an unknown mechanism.
  - Selegiline may increase the hypotensive effects of antihypertensive agents, such as *captopril* and *isoproterenol*.
  - *Pregabalin* may increase the therapeutic effect of selegiline.

Adverse Effects

How Drug Causes Adverse Effects
- Mainly (but not only) by increasing dopaminergic activity.
- Most reported adverse events, with the exception of dyskinesias and arrhythmias, have been seen with selegiline administered both as monotherapy and adjunct therapy.
- The amphetamine metabolites may mediate some adverse effects, including insomnia and abnormal dreams.
- In higher doses of selegiline (which are not recommended in clinical practice), MAO selectivity is lost and adverse events could be attributed to the non-selective MAO inhibitory activity.

S

ADVERSE EFFECTS

Common Adverse Effects
- Very common (≥1/10):
  - Stomatitis, nausea.
- Common (≥1/100 to <1/10):
  - Neuropsychiatric: sleep disorders (including somnolence, especially in the elderly), confusion, hallucinations, depression, abnormal movements (dyskinesia, akinesia/bradykinesia), tremor, impaired balance, dizziness, falls, headache.
  - Eye/ear: vertigo.
  - Cardiovascular: bradycardia, hypotension (sometimes sudden in onset), hypertension.
  - Respiratory: nasal congestion, sore throat.
  - GI: abdominal pain, constipation, diarrhoea, dry mouth/ulceration.
  - Musculoskeletal: arthralgia, back pain, cramps.
  - Other: increased sweating, fatigue, mild hepatic enzymes increase.
- Uncommon (≥1/1,000 to <1/100):
  - Neuropsychiatric: abnormal dreams, agitation, anxiety, psychoses, mood change.
  - Eye/ear: blurred vision.
  - Cardiovascular: arrhythmias, palpitations, angina pectoris, supraventricular tachycardia.
  - Respiratory: dyspnoea.
  - Musculoskeletal: myopathy.
  - Renal/urinary: micturition disorders.
  - Other: pharyngitis, leukocytopenia, thrombocytopenia, loss of appetite, hair loss, skin eruptions, ankle oedema.

Life-Threatening or Dangerous Adverse Effects
- Serotonin syndrome.
- Suicidal thoughts/behaviour.

Rare and Not Life-Threatening Adverse Effects
- ICDs.

Weight Change
- Rare reports of anorexia and weight decrease.

What to Do About Adverse Effects
- Before introducing selegiline, discuss common adverse effects with patients or caregivers, including symptoms that should be reported to the physician.
  - Patients should be directly questioned about drowsiness or sleepiness during specific activities, as they might not acknowledge these symptoms until specifically asked.
- Because selegiline potentiates the effect of levodopa, many adverse events are considered dopaminergic in origin and a reduction in co-administered levodopa dose might improve them. Consider reducing

total levodopa dose or adjusting dosage of/withdraw other dopaminergic agents (e.g. dopamine agonists) in case of relevant complications, such as dyskinesias, somnolence, hypotension, nausea, hallucinations, confusion, or ICDs. If adverse effects are still troublesome or persist, consider discontinuing therapy completely.
- If new adverse effects appear, consider interactions with other medications.
- Consider discontinuing selegiline in individuals with a greater than 20 mmHg fall in blood pressure on standing for 2 min.
- If a serotonin syndrome is suspected, close monitoring and discontinuation of selegiline or other interacting agents should be considered.

Dosing and Use
Usual Dosage Range
- Tablets/capsules: 2.5–10 mg/day.
- ODT: 1.25–2.5 mg/day.

Available Formulations
- Tablets: 5 mg.
- Capsules: 5 mg.
- ODT tablets: 1.25 mg (only in the USA).
- Transdermal film, extended release: 6 mg/24 h, 9 mg/24 h, 12 mg/24 h.

How to Dose
- Conventional formulations: either as a single dose of 10 mg in the morning or in two divided doses of 5 mg at breakfast and lunch; maximum dose of 10 mg per day.
- ODT: a single dose of 1.25 mg in the morning before breakfast; may increase to 2.5 mg/day after 6 weeks, if inadequate response; maximum dose of 2.5 mg per day.

Dosing Tips
- After 2–3 days of selegiline therapy, tapering of levodopa dose can begin by 10–30%, as tolerated (if applicable). Tapering can be continued according to patient's response.
- Due to the formation of amphetamine metabolites an evening dose of selegiline is not recommended.
- ODT formulations are preferred in Parkinson's disease patients with swallowing difficulties.
- If selegiline needs to be discontinued (e.g. due to side effects), another selective MAO inhibitor may be introduced.
- Although ODT exhibit a better pharmacokinetic profile (improved bioavailability, lower selegiline dose, lower exposure to amphetamine metabolites), their clinical efficacy and safety profile are comparable to conventional formulations.

DOSING AND USE

- Patients should avoid ingesting any foods or liquid for 5 min before and after administration of ODT.
- With dry hands, ODT formulations should be placed on the tongue (where dissolution occurs in seconds) immediately after the original packaging is removed.

How to Withdraw Drug
- A gradual reduction of selegiline dose by 2.5 mg every third day is recommended.

Overdose
- Reports of hypotension and psychomotor agitation with doses of 600 mg/day.
- Selegiline overdose might lead to non-selective MAO inhibition activity, which may progress over 24 h, including CNS and cardiovascular symptoms.
- There is no specific antidote and the treatment is symptomatic.
- Patient should be under observation for 24–48 h.

Tests and Therapeutic Drug Monitoring
- Blood pressure should be measured at baseline and regularly during selegiline therapy.

Other Warnings / Precautions
- Caution is recommended for patients with labile hypertension, cardiac arrhythmias, severe angina pectoris, psychosis, or a history of peptic ulcerations, as these conditions might be aggravated during selegiline therapy.
- With doses higher than 10 mg/day there is a theoretical risk of hypertension after ingestion of tyramine-rich food.
- For transdermal preparations, dietary restrictions are necessary at doses of 9 mg and above: patients should be warned not to eat any tyramine-rich foods during selegiline treatment and for at least 14 days after discontinuation of therapy or after dose reduction to 6 mg daily.
- Each 1.25 mg ODT formulation contains 1.25 mg phenylalanine; thus, consider combined daily amount of phenylalanine from all sources in phenylketonuria patients.
- Caution is advised in patients with a history of hepatic dysfunction, although severe hepatotoxicity has not been reported.
- Selegiline is classified as probably porphyrinogenic.
- MAOIs, including selegiline, may potentiate the effects of CNS depressants used in general anaesthesia; therefore, caution is advised.
- At least 14 days should elapse between discontinuation/initiation of selegiline and drugs that may increase serotonin levels, such as tricyclic/tetracyclic antidepressants, SSRIs/SNRIS (5 weeks for *fluoxetine*

due to long $T_{1/2}$), triptans, *dihydroergotamine*, opiates, neuroleptics, *linezolid*, *lithium*, *isoniazid*, and others.
- At least 14 days should elapse between discontinuation/initiation of selegiline and carbamazepine.
- Co-administration with metformin, insulin, or other antidiabetic agents should be avoided.
- Close monitoring is advised in case of co-administration with antihypertensive agents.
- Patients are advised not to drive or use dangerous machinery until they know how selegiline affects them (e.g. dizziness, somnolence, cognitive impairment, impairment of reaction capacity).
- Alcohol intake should be avoided.

Do Not Use (Contraindications)
- Known hypersensitivity (including severe dizziness or hypotension) to selegiline or any of the formulation excipients.
- Parkinsonism not related to dopamine deficiency.
- Active duodenal or gastric ulcer.
- Severe cardiovascular disease, arterial hypertension, tachycardia, arrhythmias, severe angina pectoris, and phaeochromocytoma.
- Hyperthyroidism, thyrotoxicosis.
- Narrow-angle glaucoma.
- Prostatic adenoma with appearance of residual urine.
- Psychosis, advanced dementia.
- Co-administration with serotonin agonists (e.g. triptans), opioids (e.g. *pethidine*, *methadone*, *tramadol*, *dextropropoxyphene*), sympathomimetics, other MAOIs, antidepressants, including tricyclic/tetracyclic antidepressants and SSRIs/SNRIs, psychostimulants, central suppressant drugs (e.g. sedatives) and oral contraceptives.

Special Populations
Renal Impairment
- Tablets/capsules: no dosage adjustment is required in mild or moderate renal impairment. Caution is advised in severe renal impairment.
- ODT: not recommended in severe renal impairment (CrCl < 30 ml/min) or end-stage renal disease.

Hepatic Impairment
- Tablets/capsules: no dosage adjustment is required in mild or moderate hepatic impairment. Caution is advised in severe hepatic impairment.
- ODT: in mild-to-moderate hepatic disease, daily dose should be reduced from 2.5 mg to 1.25 mg, depending on clinical response and tolerability. Not recommended in severe hepatic impairment.

Elderly
- No special warnings or precautions are advised.

Pregnancy
- Insufficient data to support selegiline use during pregnancy – avoid usage.

Breastfeeding
- Insufficient data to support selegiline use during breastfeeding – avoid usage.
- Selegiline is probably excreted in breast milk due to low molecular weight.
- Significant neurotoxicity in animal studies.

Costs
NHS indicative price (accessed 15 May 2022):
- Eldepryl, Orion Pharma UK Ltd – 100 × 5 mg tablets: £16.52; 100 × 10 mg tablets: £32.23.

The Overall Place of Selegiline in the Treatment of Parkinson's Disease

MAO-B inhibitors are used in clinical practice to alleviate parkinsonian symptoms by reducing MAO-catalysed breakdown of dopamine in the brain. Selegiline was the first selective MAO-B inhibitor therapeutically used in Parkinson's disease, either as monotherapy in the early stages or as an add-on therapy to levodopa preparations throughout the disease course. Its established role in Parkinson's disease therapy has declined after the introduction of newer generation MAO-B inhibitors, such as rasagiline and safinamide, with the former exhibiting high evidence-based efficacy both as a monotherapy and as a complementary treatment to levodopa in early and advanced Parkinson's disease. Despite initial indications of a potential neuroprotective/disease-modifying effect of selegiline from experimental studies, there is insufficient evidence of this in humans.

Potential Advantages
- No need for dietary restrictions in therapeutic doses.
- A levodopa-sparing strategy.

Potential Disadvantages
- Insufficient evidence of an effect of selegiline as an add-on therapy to levodopa in early Parkinson's disease and motor fluctuations compared to other MAO-B inhibitors.
- Insufficient evidence on the effect of selegiline on non-motor symptoms of Parkinson's disease.
- The amphetamine metabolites of selegiline have potential sympathomimetic effects and might worsen sleep quality.

S

- Risk of 'cheese reaction' and toxic effects on the cardiovascular system, especially if selegiline is combined with other MAOIs.
- Cannot be safely co-administered with antidepressants, which might be problematic, as depression is quite prevalent among Parkinson's disease patients.
- Not a good therapeutic option in patients with postural hypotension, cardiovascular diseases, or hallucinations.

Clinical Box

A 65-year-old man was referred to the Neurology Outpatient Clinic due to bilateral, gradually deteriorating, slight to mild bradykinesia and rigidity, more pronounced in the right side, along with a long history of constipation and anosmia. His medical history was otherwise unremarkable. After a thorough assessment, a clinical diagnosis of early stage Parkinson's disease was made and, as the patient had no contraindications, therapy with selegiline 10 mg OD was initiated. After 4 weeks of treatment the patient reported improvement of his symptoms without any troublesome complications and a follow-up assessment was set at 6 months.

REFERENCES

Suggested Reading

Cereda E, R Cilia, M Canesi, S Tesei, CB Mariani, AL Zecchinelli, G Pezzoli. Efficacy of rasagiline and selegiline in Parkinson's disease: a head-to-head 3-year retrospective case–control study. *J Neurol* 2017; 264(6): 1254–1263.

Fabbrini G, G Abbruzzese, S Marconi, M Zappia. Selegiline: a reappraisal of its role in Parkinson disease. *Clin Neuropharmacol* 2012; 35(3): 134–140.

Mizuno Y, N Hattori, T Kondo, M Nomoto, H Origasa, R Takahashi, M Yamamoto, N Yanagisawa. Long-term selegiline monotherapy for the treatment of early Parkinson disease. *Clin Neuropharmacol* 2019; 42(4): 123–130.

Tan Y-Y, P Jenner, S-D Chen. Monoamine oxidase-B inhibitors for the treatment of Parkinson's disease: past, present, and future. *J Parkinsons Dis* 2022; 12(2): 477–493.

References

AHFS Drug information, 2012. Bethesda: American Society of Health-System Pharmacists. Accessed on 15 May 2022 via www .medicinescomplete.com.

Binde CD, IF Tvete, JI Gåsemyr, B Natvig, M Klemp. Comparative effectiveness of dopamine agonists and monoamine oxidase type-B inhibitors for Parkinson's disease: a multiple treatment comparison meta-analysis. *Eur J Clin Pharmacol* 2020; 76(12): 1731–1743.

S

Deleu D, MG Northway, Y Hanssens. Clinical pharmacokinetic and pharmacodynamic properties of drugs used in the treatment of Parkinson's disease. *Clin Pharmacokinet* 2002; 41(4): 261–309.

Joint Formulary Committee. British National Formulary (online). London: BMJ Group and Pharmaceutical Press. Accessed on 15 May 2022 via www.medicinescomplete.com.

Koschel J, KR Chaudhuri, L Tönges, M Thiel, V Raeder, WH Jost. Implications of dopaminergic medication withdrawal in Parkinson's disease. *J Neural Transm (Vienna)*, 2022; 129(9): 1169–1178.

Laine K, M Anttila, R Huopponen, O Mäki-Ikola, E Heinonen. Multiple-dose pharmacokinetics of selegiline and desmethylselegiline suggest saturable tissue binding. *Clin Neuropharmacol* 2000; 23(1): 22–27.

Nagatsu T, M Sawada. Molecular mechanism of the relation of monoamine oxidase B and its inhibitors to Parkinson's disease: possible implications of glial cells. *J Neural Transm Suppl* 2006; 2006(71): 53–65.

Selegiline. In: Brayfield A (Ed.), *Martindale: The Complete Drug Reference*. London: The Royal Pharmaceutical Society of Great Britain. Accessed on 15 May 2022 via www.medicinescomplete.com.

Summary of product characteristics – Eldepryl 10 m tablets. Orion Pharma (UK) Ltd. Electronic Medicines Compendium: Eldepryl 10mg tablets – summary of product characteristics (SmPC) – (emc). Accessed on 15 May 2022 via www.medicines.org.uk.

Tábi T, E Szökő, L Vécsei, K Magyar. The pharmacokinetic evaluation of selegiline ODT for the treatment of Parkinson's disease. *Expert Opin Drug Metab Toxicol* 2013; 9(5): 629–636.

SILDENAFIL

S

Therapeutics

Chemical Name and Structure

Sildenafil citrate (5-[2-ethoxy-5-(4-methylpiperazin-1-ylsulfonyl)phe-nyl]-1,6-dihydro-1-methyl-3-propylpyrazolo[4,3-*d*]pyrimidin-7-one cit-rate; 1-{[3-(6,7-dihydro-1-methyl-7-*oxo*-3-propyl-1*H*-pyrazolo[4,3-*d*] pyrimidin-5-yl)-4-ethoxyphenyl]sulfonyl}-4-methylpiperazone citrate) is a phosphodiesterase-5 inhibitor with a molecular weight of 666.7 and a molecular formula of $C_{22}H_{30}N_6O_4S,C_6H_8O_7$.

Brand Names

*Some products may only be approved for a specific indication (e.g. Revatio in the USA is only approved for pulmonary arterial hypertension).

- **Actigra** (*Poland, South Africa*); **Activil** (*Argentina*); **Adams Delite** (*India*); **Adenafil** (*Tunisia*); **Afilon** (*Netherlands*); **Ah–Zul** (*Brazil*); **Air Bus** (*India*); **Aktor** (*Ecuador*); **Alfin** (*Chile*); **Almaximo** (*Argentina, Ecuador*); **Alsigra** (*India*); **Amfidor** (*Czech Republic, Lithuania, Portugal*); **Andros** (*Philippines*); **Androz** (*India, Singapore*); **Apodefil** (*Mexico*); **Aronix** (*UK*); **As-One** (*Tunisia*); **Avigra** (*New Zealand, South Africa*); **Avixar** (*Estonia, Lithuania*); **Azulsix** (*Netherlands, Spain*); **Azurvig** (*Poland*).

- **Balcoga** (*Czech Republic, Italy, Netherlands, Spain*); **Bandol** (*Spain*); **Be-Force** (*India*); **Believe** (*Ecuador*); **Bifort** (*Argentina*); **Bison** (*India*); **Blugral** (*Cyprus, Greece, Ireland*); **Bluozi** (*Greece*); **Blupill** (*Brazil*); **Bullenza** (*Mexico*); **Buster** (*Ecuador*).

- **Caprenafil** (*Indonesia*); **Caverta** (*Ecuador, India*); **Cetinor** (*France*); **C-Gra** (*India*); **Cilafil** (*Austria*); **Clavupen** (*Ecuador*); **Combo** (*Turkey*); **Conegra** (*Ukraine*); **Cupid** (*Philippines*).

- **Darculin** (*Philippines*); **Defil** (*Ecuador*); **Degra** (*Turkey*); **Dejavu** (*Brazil*); **Denargra** (*Hong Kong*); **Dialex** (*Greece*); **Dionixol** (*Mexico*); **Direktan** (*Austria*); **Dirtop** (*Chile*); **Disilden** (*Chile*); **DoppelSil** (*Poland*); **Dragul** (*Spain*); **Duraforte** (*Hong Kong*); **Duramet** (*Ecuador*); **Duraviril** (*Germany*); **Durofil** (*Ecuador*); **Duroval** (*Venezuela*); **Dynafil** (*South Africa*); **Dynamico** (*Russian Federation*).

- **Echarge** (*India*); **Ecriten** (*Czech Republic, Hungary, Lithuania*); **Edegra** (*India, Mexico, Singapore*); **Edyfil** (*Hong Kong, Malaysia*); **Egira** (*Turkey*); **Egomax** (*Argentina*); **Elonza** (*Hong Kong, Malaysia, Thailand*); **Emposil** (*Indonesia*); **Endurax** (*Ecuador*); **Enthusia** (*India*); **Entranin** (*Netherlands*); **Equis X** (*Ecuador*); **Eraflex** (*South Africa*); **Erasilton** (*Hungary*); **Eratec** (*Tunisia*); **Erduro** (*Poland*); **Erec** (*India*); **Erecor** (*Hong Kong*); **Erecstar** (*Ecuador*); **Erecta** (*Tunisia*); **Erectimax** (*India*); **Erecto** (*Hong Kong*); **Erectol** (*Argentina*); **Erektil** (*Ukraine*); **Erectron** (*Ecuador*); **Erexesil** (*Russian Federation*); **Ergos** (*Ukraine*); **Ericfil** (*Hong Kong*); **Ernafil** (*Hong Kong, Singapore*); **Ero-Life** (*Ukraine*); **Erosfil** (*Chile*); **Erosil** (*Ukraine*); **Erotil** (*Ecuador*); **Eroton** (*Ukraine*); **Esantop** (*Chile*); **Euro-Vaga** (*Hong Kong*); **Exagra**

S

SILDENAFIL

(*Netherlands*); **Exifol** (*Chile*); **Expit** (*Argentina, Ecuador*); **Extement** (*Greece*); **Falic** (*Argentina*); **Falsigra** (*Poland*); **Fexion** (*Spain*); **Figral** (*Mexico*); **Filagra** (*Philippines*); **Filap** (*Ukraine*); **Fildlata** (*Estonia*); **File** (*Argentina*); **Filtrin** (*South Africa*); **Finegra** (*Hong Kong*); **Firmel** (*Argentina*); **Fogo** (*Ecuador*); **Forsage** (*Ukraine*); **Forzak** (*Argentina*); **Fulove** (*Hong Kong*); **Funcional** (*Ecuador*); **Funtoosh** (*India*).

- **G4** (*Mexico*); **Galotam** (*Spain*); **Gavia** (*South Africa*); **Gimonte Sildenafil** (*Argentina*); **Go** (*Mexico*); **Gramax** (*Indonesia*); **Granpidam** (*Austria, Cyprus, Czech Republic, Denmark, Estonia, Finland, France, Germany, Ireland, Italy, Lithuania, Netherlands, Norway, Poland, Spain, Sweden, UK*).
- **Hewon** (*India*); **Hippigra** (*Hong Kong*); **Honygra** (*India*); **Hydenex** (*Philippines*).
- **Idilico** (*Austria, Netherlands, Sweden*); **Idoka** (*Spain*); **Infors** (*Ukraine*); **Innogra** (*South Africa*); **Intagra** (*India, Ukraine*); **Integra** (*India*); **Inventum** (*Poland*); **Invida** (*Russian Federation*); **Iqnyde** (*Malaysia*); **Itaka** (*Venezuela*).
- **Jean Siagra** (*India*); **Jeligra** (*Turkey*); **Jenagra** (*Ukraine*); **Josh-IN** (*India*); **Juan** (*India*); **Juvena** (*Russian Federation*); **Juvigor** (*Argentina*).
- **Kamagra** (*India, Philippines*); **Kamasut** (*Ecuador*); **Katora** (*Czech Republic*); **Kohagra** (*Philippines*); **Kopigra** (*New Zealand*).
- **Labsamax** (*Argentina*); **Leegra** (*India*); **Lekap** (*Cyprus, Poland*); **Lerk** (*Mexico*); **Le-Roma** (*Hong Kong*); **Levitrin** (*Argentina*); **Liberize** (*UK*); **Licosil** (*Austria, Greece, Poland*); **Lifaned** (*South Africa*); **Lifter** (*Chile*); **Lonisar** (*South Africa*); **Lovegra** (*India*); **Lovera** (*United Arab Emirates*); **Lupigra** (*India*).
- **Maclitio** (*South Africa*); **Magnus** (*Argentina*); **Manforce** (*India*); **Manpower** (*India*); **Maxdura** (*Hong Kong*); **Maxigra** (*Hong Kong, Poland, Russian Federation, Ukraine*); **Maxking** (*Hong Kong*); **Maxon** (*Poland*); **Mazzogran** (*Mexico*); **Medovigor** (*Hong Kong, Poland*); **Megaforte** (*Hong Kong*); **Mensil** (*Poland*); **Merewin** (*Hungary*); **Meriday** (*India*); **Modrasil** (*Czech Republic*); **Moginin** (*Ukraine*); **Moragara** (*India*); **Myedra** (*South Africa*); **Mysildecard** (*Austria, Estonia, France, Germany, Ireland, Italy, Lithuania, Netherlands, Poland, Spain, Sweden*).
- **Neoben** (*Ecuador*); **Neogra** (*India*); **Neo-Up** (*Philippines*); **Nexofil** (*Argentina*); **N-Gra** (*India*); **Niagra** (*India*); **Nipatra** (*UK*); **Novagra** (*Ukraine*); **Novalif** (*Chile*); **Nyte** (*India*).
- **Olmax** (*Russian Federation*); **Olvion** (*Cyprus, Czech Republic, Estonia, Greece, Lithuania, Singapore*); **Orisild** (*Finland, Norway, Sweden*); **Osidea** (*Mexico*); **Oximun** (*Spain*).
- **Paramen** (*Argentina*); **Patrex** (*Mexico*); **Penegra** (*India, Philippines*); **Penimex** (*Ukraine*); **Permitil** (*Argentina*); **Persex** (*Ecuador*); **Plusefec** (*Chile*); **Pluspen** (*Argentina*); **Potentiale** (*Ukraine*); **Powergra** (*Hong Kong*); **Prilo** (*Brazil*); **Primax** (*Venezuela*); **Princex** (*Poland*); **Pseueva** (*Hong Kong*); **Psiliber** (*Spain*); **Pularter** (*Turkey*); **Pulmolan** (*Austria*); **Pulmopresil** (*Austria*); **Pulmova** (*Hong Kong*).

- **Rabestrom** (*Italy*); **Raviag** (*South Africa*); **Reejump** (*Russian Federation*); **Religra** (*South Africa*); **Remenafil** (*Singapore*); **Remidia** (*Poland*); **Restomin** (*Turkey*); **Revastad** (*Denmark, Finland, Netherlands, Sweden*); **Revatio** (*Australia, Austria, Belgium, Brazil, Canada, Cyprus, Czech Republic, Denmark, Estonia, Finland, France, Germany, Greece, Hong Kong, Hungary, Ireland, Israel, Italy, Japan, Malaysia, Netherlands, Norway, Poland, Portugal, Russian Federation, Singapore, South Africa, Spain, Sweden, Switzerland, Thailand, Turkey, UK, Ukraine, USA, Venezuela*); **Rinemak** (*South Africa*); **Ripol** (*Chile, Venezuela*); **Rosytona** (*Netherlands*); **Roveta** (*South Africa*); **Rovost** (*New Zealand*); **Rozgra** (*Indonesia*).
- **Sanbenafil** (*Indonesia*); **Segurex** (*Argentina*); **Sempavox** (*Austria, Estonia, Lithuania, Netherlands*); **Senagra** (*Hong Kong*); **Seregra** (*Philippines*); **Siafil** (*Chile*); **Sidegra** (*Thailand*); **Sidena** (*Ireland*); **Sife** (*Singapore*); **Silafil** (*Russian Federation*); **Silagra** (*Hong Kong, India, New Zealand, South Africa*); **Silandyl** (*Netherlands, Poland*); **Silaplus** (*Tunisia*); **Silaran** (*Australia*); **Silatio** (*Hong Kong, Thailand*); **Silcarfil** (*Ireland*); **Silchemo** (*Austria*); **Silcontrol** (*Poland*); **Sildaccord** (*Australia*); **Sildalic** (*Hong Kong*); **Sildanil** (*Australia*); **Sildara** (*Brazil*); **Sildatio PHT** (*Australia*); **Sildavee** (*South Africa*); **Sildeagil** (*Germany*); **Sildegra** (*Hungary, Singapore, Turkey*); **Sildehexal** (*Germany*); **Sildenamed** (*Netherlands*); **Sildenax** (*Switzerland*); **Sildenon** (*Belgium*); **Sildera** (*Thailand*); **Silderec** (*Hungary*); **Silderos** (*Poland*); **Sildex** (*Israel, Philippines, Venezuela*); **Sildojub** (*Hong Kong*); **Sildora** (*Philippines*); **Siler** (*Italy*); **Silerec** (*Australia*); **Silfect** (*Turkey*); **Silungo** (*Estonia, Lithuania, Poland*); **Silvasta** (*New Zealand*); **Silvie** (*Hong Kong*); **Silwin** (*South Africa*); **Silvir** (*Switzerland*); **Sinafil** (*Hong Kong*); **Sinegra** (*Turkey, Ukraine*); **Slider** (*Israel*); **Solira** (*South Africa*); **Sollevare** (*Brazil*); **Speedgra** (*Philippines*); **Stigmax** (*Venezuela*); **Stronde** (*Ukraine*); **Strondem** (*Greece*); **Super-O** (*Argentina*); **Superviga** (*Ukraine*); **Suvvia** (*Brazil*); **Sylecta** (*South Africa*).
- **Tarim** (*Israel*); **Taxier** (*Hungary, Lithuania, Russian Federation*); **Tecnomax** (*Argentina*); **Tegrum** (*Ukraine*); **Theogra** (*Hong Kong*); **Tigerfil** (*Hong Kong, Philippines*); **Tonafil** (*Thailand*); **Topgra** (*Indonesia*); **Tornetis** (*Netherlands, Russian Federation*); **Trectyl** (*Mexico*).
- **Uni-Jetup** (*Hong Kong*); **Uprima** (*Hong Kong*).
- **Valinger** (*Poland*); **Valpez** (*South Africa*); **Vasafil** (*Australia*); **Vasifil** (*Brazil*); **Vasofil** (*Hong Kong*); **Vedafil** (*Australia, New Zealand*); **Veligo** (*Hong Kong*); **Verventi** (*Belgium*); **Via-Avenir** (*Israel*); **Viadis** (*Tunisia*); **Viagra** (*Argentina, Australia, Austria, Belgium, Brazil, Canada, Chile, China, Cyprus, Czech Republic, Denmark, Estonia, Finland, France, Germany, Greece, Hong Kong, Hungary, India, Indonesia, Ireland, Israel, Italy, Japan, Lithuania, Malaysia, Mexico, Netherlands, New Zealand, Norway, Philippines, Poland, Portugal, Russian Federation, Singapore, South Africa, Spain, Sweden, Switzerland, Thailand, Tunisia, Turkey, UK, Ukraine, USA, Venezuela*); **Viajoy** (*Indonesia*); **Viamax** (*Tunisia*); **Viandros**

S

(*Hungary*); **Viasan-LF** (*Russian Federation*); **Viasek** (*Venezuela*); **Viasil** (*Brazil, Ukraine, Venezuela*); **Viatec** (*Tunisia*); **Viatile** (*Russian Federation*); **Viaxon** (*Tunisia*); **Videna** (*South Africa*); **Videnfil** (*Brazil*); **Vigaroo** (*Turkey*); **Vigorex** (*Chile*); **Vigrande** (*Russian Federation, Turkey*); **Vigrasol** (*Venezuela*); **Vilakra** (*Hong Kong*); **Vildegra** (*Russian Federation*); **Vimax** (*Argentina, Chile*); **Viosex** (*Venezuela*); **Viridil** (*Venezuela*); **Virineo** (*Brazil*); **Viripotens** (*Argentina*); **Vitarfil** (*Argentina*); **Vitramax** (*Hong Kong*); **Vitrixa** (*South Africa*); **Vivayra** (*Russian Federation*); **Vivic** (*Hong Kong, Malaysia, Singapore*); **Vizarsin** (*Austria, Czech Republic, Cyprus, Denmark, Estonia, Finland, France, Greece, Hungary, Ireland, Lithuania, Netherlands, Poland, Russian Federation, Spain, UK, Ukraine*); **Voguel** (*Mexico*); **Vorst** (*Argentina*); **Voltin** (*Hong Kong*).
- **Wafesil** (*Australia*); **Willmon** (*Hong Kong*); **Wingora** (*Philippines*).
- **Xcite** (*Hong Kong*); **Xirect** (*Poland*); **Xybilun** (*France*).
- **Zeldina** (*South Africa*); **Zenegra** (*South Africa*); **Zenera** (*Philippines*); **Zilden** (*Philippines*); **Zilfic** (*Chile*); **Zost** (*Venezuela*); **Zuandol** (*Spain*); **Zyforma** (*South Africa*); **Zygra** (*Hong Kong*).

Generics Available
- Yes.

Licensed Indications for Parkinson's Disease
- None.

Licensed Indications for Other Conditions
- Erectile dysfunction in adult men (FDA, EMA, EMC).
  - Because of safety issues, sildenafil is not recommended for simply enhancing erections in men who are not impotent.
- Pulmonary arterial hypertension (FDA, EMA, EMC).

Non-Licensed Use for Parkinson's Disease
- Erectile dysfunction in male Parkinson's disease patients.

Non-Licensed Use for Other Conditions
- Female sexual arousal disorder.
- Antidepressant agent-induced sexual dysfunction in both men and women (limited evidence).
- Antipsychotic agent-induced erectile dysfunction (including olanzapine) in men.
- Depression-related erectile dysfunction in men.
- Diabetes mellitus-related erectile dysfunction in men.
- Erectile dysfunction in male patients on chronic dialysis.
- Erectile dysfunction in male patients with stable CAD.
- Erectile dysfunction associated with Peyronie disease.
- Erectile dysfunction after prostatectomy with nerve-sparing procedures.

SILDENAFIL

- Erectile dysfunction associated with radiation therapy for prostate carcinoma.
- Erectile dysfunction in young male patients with spina bifida.
- Erectile dysfunction in male patients associated with spinal cord injury and spina bifida.
- Secondary Reynaud phenomenon.
- Advanced idiopathic pulmonary fibrosis.
- As an adjunct in the treatment of altitude-induced hypoxaemia.

Ineffective
- Fatigue in Parkinson's disease.
- Neuroprotective action in Parkinson's disease.

Mechanism of Action
- Sildenafil restores impaired erectile function by increasing blood flow to the penis. Erection involves the release of nitric oxide in the corpus cavernosum during sexual stimulation, which then activates the enzyme guanylate cyclase, leading to increased concentration of cyclic guanosine monophosphate (cGMP); this latter compound mediates smooth muscle relaxation in the corpus cavernosum, allowing blood inflow.
- Sildenafil is a potent and selective inhibitor of cGMP-specific phosphodiesterase type 5 (PDE5) in the corpus cavernosum, where PDE5 mediates cGMP degradation.
  - Sildenafil has no direct relaxant effect on human corpus cavernosum, but potentially enhances the relaxant effect of nitric oxide on this tissue. The nitric oxide/cGMP pathway is activated through sexual stimulation, which is, therefore, a prerequisite for sildenafil use.

Efficacy Profile
- Sildenafil has been characterized as 'efficacious' and 'clinically useful' for the management of sexual dysfunction in Parkinson's disease patients (MDS EBM Committee).
- One small, double-blind, crossover RCT has assessed the effect of sildenafil on male Parkinson's disease patients with erectile dysfunction; researchers concluded that sildenafil (25–100 mg stat) was safe and significantly improved erectile dysfunction, although quality of life was not affected.
- Another small, double-blind, crossover RCT has assessed the effect of sildenafil on an equal number of male Parkinson's disease and MSA patients with erectile dysfunction; it was concluded that sildenafil (50 mg) is an efficacious drug in both conditions.
- A small, open-label, prospective (2-month follow-up) study found that sildenafil significantly improved selected sexual health parameters, including overall sexual satisfaction, ability to achieve/maintain erection, and ability to reach orgasm in male Parkinson's disease patients.

- Finally, an open-label, prospective (4-month follow-up) study found that sildenafil (50 mg) significantly increased the ability of depressed male Parkinson's disease patients (H&Y ≤ 3) to achieve and maintain an erection. An indirect amelioration of depressive symptoms was also noted, alongside improvement in patients' overall sexual satisfaction.
- Sildenafil per se does not cause erection. Sexual stimulation is necessary for sildenafil to be effective, which means the patient has to stay concentrated on sexual activity or the erection will fade away.
- There are limited data on long-term efficacy of sildenafil. In long-term and open-label studies, it was found to remain effective for a minimum period of 3 years with current evidence supporting that continued sildenafil therapy is justifiable as long as the relevant indication persists and no contraindications arise. The possibility that prolonged sildenafil use may mask the progression of a serious subjacent disorder should also be considered.

Pharmacokinetics

Absorption and Distribution

- Oral bioavailability: about 40% (range of 25–63%).
- Food co-ingestion, especially high-fat meals, may delay sildenafil effect compared to the fasted state due to delay in GI absorption.
- Tmax: 30–120 min.
- Time to steady state: not applicable.
- Pharmacokinetics: dose-proportional over the single-dose range of 1.25–200 mg.
- Protein binding: about 96% bound to plasma proteins.
- Volume of distribution: about 105 l.

Metabolism

- Sildenafil undergoes hepatic metabolism mainly by CYP3A4 and by CYP2C9 in lower amounts.
- The active metabolite N-desmethyl derivative is produced in the liver and has a phosphodiesterase selectivity profile similar to sildenafil (~50% PDE5 potency of the parent drug, ~20% of sildenafil pharmacologic activity).

Elimination

- Half-life is 3–5 h and 10–70 min for the parent drug and the active metabolite, respectively.
- About 80% of an administered dose is found as metabolites in faeces and about 13% is excreted in the urine.

S

Drug Interaction Profile
Pharmacokinetic Drug Interactions
- Effects on sildenafil:
  - CYP3A4 inhibitors (e.g. *chloramphenicol, clarithromycin, cyclosporine, diltiazem, isoniazid, istradefylline*) may increase levels and effects of sildenafil.
  - CYP3A4 inducers (e.g. *oxcarbazepine, phenobarbital, phenytoin, primidone, dexamethasone*) may decrease levels and effects of sildenafil.

Pharmacodynamic Drug Interactions
- Co-medication with drugs causing vasodilation (e.g. *isosorbide, nitroglycerin, ketoconazole*) has synergistic action, which may lead to fatal hypotension and/or haemodynamic compromise.
- Co-medication with antihypertensive medications (e.g. beta-blockers, ACE inhibitors, calcium channel blockers, angiotensin II receptor blockers) has additive effects in lowering blood pressure.

Adverse Effects
How Drug Causes Adverse Effects
- The most common adverse effects of sildenafil result from the pharmacologic activity of the drug as a phosphodiesterase inhibitor, including those secondary to (a) vascular smooth muscle relaxation and vasodilation (PDE5), (b) relaxation of the lower oesophageal sphincter (PDE5), (c) mucosal hyperaemia (PDE5), and (d) ocular PDE6 inhibition, which is involved in the phototransduction pathway in the retina.
  - Sildenafil exhibits modest peripheral vasodilation at usual dosage and can decrease systemic and pulmonary arterial pressure, and cardiac output due to inhibition of PDE5 present in vascular smooth muscle (e.g. flushing, headache, hypotension).
- Adverse effects are more common with higher doses.

Common Adverse Effects
- Very common (≥1/10):
  - Headache, flushing, dyspepsia.
- Common (≥1/100 to <1/10):
  - Neuropsychiatric: dizziness.
  - Eye/ear: visual colour distortion, blurred/abnormal vision.
  - Respiratory: nasal congestion.
- Uncommon (≥1/1,000 to <1/100):
  - Neuropsychiatric: somnolence, hypoaesthesia.
  - Eye/ear: lacrimation disorders, eye pain, photophobia, photopsia, ocular hyperaemia, visual brightness, conjunctivitis, vertigo, tinnitus.
  - Cardiovascular: tachycardia, palpitations, hypertension, hypotension, chest pain.
  - Respiratory: rhinitis, epistaxis, sinus congestion.

ADVERSE EFFECTS

S

SILDENAFIL

- ○ GI: gastro–oesophageal reflux disease, vomiting, abdominal pain, dry mouth.
- ○ Other: hypersensitivity, rash, myalgia, pain in extremity, fatigue, feeling hot.

Life-Threatening or Dangerous Adverse Effects
- Rare (≥1/10,000 to <1/1,000):
  - ○ Cerebrovascular accident, transient ischaemic attack.
  - ○ Sudden cardiac death.
  - ○ Myocardial infarction, unstable angina.
  - ○ Ventricular arrhythmia, atrial fibrillation.
  - ○ Seizures.
  - ○ NAION.
  - ○ Retinal vascular occlusion, retinal haemorrhage, arteriosclerotic retinopathy.
  - ○ Glaucoma.
  - ○ Stevens–Johnson syndrome, toxic epidermal necrolysis.
  - ○ Penile haemorrhage, priapism.

Rare and Not Life-Threatening Adverse Effects
- Syncope.
- Visual field defects, reduced visual acuity, diplopia, myopia, asthenopia, vitreous floaters, iris disorder, mydriasis, halo vision, eye/eyelid oedema, conjunctival hyperaemia, eye irritation, abnormal sensation in eye, scleral discoloration.
- Deafness.
- Throat tightness, nasal oedema, nasal dryness.
- Oral hypoesthesia.
- Irritability.

Weight Change
- Not reported.

What to Do About Adverse Effects
- Before introducing sildenafil, discuss common or life-threatening adverse effects with patients and/or caregivers, including symptoms that should be reported to the physician. Adverse effects are mostly transitory and of minor intensity.
- In case of sudden loss of vision in one or both eyes, patients should immediately seek medical care, as it may be a sign of NAION.
- In case of a sildenafil-induced erection that persists for more than 4 h or is extremely painful, the patient should seek immediate medical assistance, as priapism may lead to penile tissue damage and permanent loss of potency if left untreated.
- In case of clinically significant sildenafil-induced hypotension, consider placing the patient in the Trendelenburg position and initiating fluid resuscitation. In case of severe hypotensive episodes, vasopressors/adrenergic agonists should be used judiciously.

Dosing and Use

Usual Dosage Range
- 25–100 mg daily.

Available Formulations
- Tablets: 20 mg, 25 mg, 50 mg, 100 mg.
- Injectable solution: 10 mg/12.5 ml.
- Oral suspension: 10 mg/ml.

How to Dose
- An initial dose of 50 mg should be taken about 1 h before sexual activity. Sildenafil effects are expected between 30 min and 4–6 h after ingestion.
- Sildenafil dose can range from 25 mg to 100 mg based on effectiveness and tolerance.
- Maximum dosing frequency is once per day.
- Sildenafil can be used repeatedly, although a maximum frequency of once or twice per week is suggested.

Dosing Tips
- Sildenafil can be consumed with or without food.
- Patients are advised not to consume more than 2 alcoholic drinks within 1 h of anticipated sexual activity and sildenafil use.
- For patients who are physically active and can achieve levels of moderate exercise on an exercise treadmill test without demonstrating ischaemia, the risk of ischaemia during coitus with a familiar partner in a familiar setting and without the added stress of heavy meal or alcohol ingestion is probably low.

How to Withdraw Drug
- No special instructions needed.

Overdose
- In case of overdose, an increased incidence of sildenafil reported adverse events is expected, including headache, flushing, dizziness, dyspepsia, nasal congestion, and altered vision.
- Standard supportive measures should be applied.

Tests and Therapeutic Drug Monitoring
- Before initiation of sildenafil therapy:
- A baseline measurement of blood pressure is recommended (BP > 90/50 mmHg).
- Patients should be assessed for orthostatic hypotension.

Other Warnings/Precautions
- Caution is advised in case of prescribing sildenafil in Parkinson's disease patients with orthostatic hypotension.

S

DOSING AND USE

S

SILDENAFIL

- A precipitous reduction in blood pressure may occur over the initial 24 h after taking sildenafil; however, this risk may be prolonged in patients with hepatic dysfunction, severe renal impairment, geriatric patients, or those receiving potent CYP3A4 inhibitors.
- Care should be taken to identify patients with a diagnosis of MSA, which may mimic Parkinson's disease, as sildenafil may cause a significant blood pressure drop in these vulnerable patients.
- Caution is advised in the case of patients with pre-existing cardiovascular disease (e.g. recent (at least 6 months) history of myocardial infarction or stroke, unstable angina, heart failure, life-threatening arrhythmia), especially in men for whom sexual activity is inadvisable due to their subjacent cardiovascular status. More specifically, prior to introducing sildenafil, physicians should consider the cardiovascular status of their patients, as there is a degree of cardiac risk related to sexual activity per se, which can be enhanced when combined with the vasodilatory effect of sildenafil.
- Use with caution in patients with anatomic deformation of penis (e.g. angulation, cavernosal fibrosis, or Peyronie disease), conditions predisposing to priapism (e.g. sickle cell anaemia, multiple myeloma, leukaemia), hypotension or hypertension, bleeding disorders, active peptic ulcer disease, liver disease, or renal impairment.
- Caution is advised in retinitis pigmentosa, as sildenafil may cause dose-related impairment of colour discrimination.
- Caution is advised in patients with a 'crowded' optic disc, as they may be at increased risk of NAION.
- Close monitoring is recommended when administering sildenafil to patients taking antihypertensive medications due to additive effects in lowering blood pressure, especially in patients with renal impairment.
- Co-administration of pulmonary vasodilators may significantly worsen cardiovascular status of patients with pulmonary veno-occlusive disease.
- Patients on alpha-blockers should be stabilized before introducing sildenafil; the latter should be given at the lowest possible dose. If sildenafil therapy is already optimized before administering an alpha-blocker, the latter should be initiated at the lowest possible dose.

Do Not Use (Contraindications)
- Known sensitivity to sildenafil or to any of its excipients, including lactose.
  - Patients with rare hereditary problems of galactose intolerance, total lactase deficiency, or glucose–galactose malabsorption.
- Patients who have vision loss in one eye due to NAION, regardless of whether the episode was associated with the use of a PDE-5 inhibitor, as sildenafil may precipitate a similar episode in the other eye.
- Co-administration with drugs causing vasodilation, including nitrates in any form and soluble guanylate cyclase stimulators (e.g. *riociguat*), is contraindicated due to potentially fatal hypotension and/or haemodynamic compromise.

S

- Co-administration with CYP3A4 inhibitors/inducers should be avoided.
  - If sildenafil use is absolutely necessary, an initial lower dose of 25 mg should be considered (with the exception of ritonavir).
- Co-administration with other PDE-5 inhibitors is contraindicated.

Special Populations

Renal Impairment
- Mild–moderate impairment (CrCl 30–80 ml/min): no dosage modification required.
- Severe impairment (CrCl < 30 ml/min): an initial dose of 25 mg is suggested (based on efficacy and tolerance, the dose can be further increased to 50 mg or 100 mg).

Hepatic Impairment
- In case of mild to moderate hepatic impairment, an initial dose of 25 mg is recommended.
- Severe impairment (Child–Pugh class C): sildenafil safety has not been established, so sildenafil is contraindicated in this group of patients.

Elderly
- No dosage adjustments required.
- Clearance may be reduced and plasma concentrations may be increased in geriatric patients.

Pregnancy
- Not applicable.

Breastfeeding
- Not applicable.

COSTS

Costs
NHS indicative costs (accessed 30 December 2022):
- Grandipam tablets (Accord Healthcare Ltd) – 90 × 20 mg tablets: £424.01.
- Revatio tablets (Viatris Healthcare Ltd) – 90 × 20 mg tablets: £446.33.
- Revatio 10 mg/ml oral suspension (Viatris UK Healthcare Ltd) – 112 ml: £186.75.
- Revatio 10 mg/12.5 ml solution for injection vials (Viatris UK Healthcare Ltd): £45.28.
- Viagra tablets (Viatris UK Healthcare Ltd) – 4 × 25 mg tablets: £0.76; 8 × 25 mg tablets: £33.19; 4 × 50 mg tablets: £0.81; 8 × 50 mg tablets: £42.54; 4 × 100 mg tablets: £23.50; 8 × 100 mg tablets: £46.99.
- Vizarsin tablets (Consilient Health Ltd) – 4 × 25 mg tablets: £14.10; 4 × 50 mg tablets: £0.81; 4 × 100 mg tablets: £19.97.

S

- Sildenafil 20 mg tablets – 90 × 20 mg tablets: £50.00–£446.33.
- Sildenafil 25 mg tablets – 4 × 25 mg tablets: £0.78–£16.59; 8 × 25 mg tablets: £1.16–£33.19.
- Sildenafil 50 mg tablets – 4 × 50 mg tablets: £0.63–£18.08; 8 × 50 mg tablets: £0.94–£42.54.
- Sildenafil 100 mg tablets – 4 × 100 mg tablets: £0.72–£23.50; 8 × 100 mg tablets: £2.00–£46.99.
- Sildenafil 10 mg/ml oral suspension – 122 ml suspension: £186.75.

SILDENAFIL

The Overall Place of Sildenafil in the Treatment of Parkinson's Disease

Sildenafil is a phosphodiesterase type 5 inhibitor, which enhances blood flow in the cavernous bodies of the penis, promoting an enhanced response to sexual arousal and maintenance of erection. There are two double-blind, crossover RCTs and two open-label studies specifically addressing the use of sildenafil in male Parkinson's disease patients with erectile dysfunction, with all of them finding a beneficial effect. Although sildenafil action is expected between 30 min and 6 h following its consumption, Parkinson's disease patients have reported a longer time to onset for successful intercourse, which may be explained by potential slowed GI motility in Parkinson's disease. In the context of dysautonomia, extra caution is advised when prescribing sildenafil, as these patients are particularly vulnerable to vasodilatory effects, especially during sexual activity. Sildenafil may exacerbate or unmask hypotension, although this is more common in MSA rather than Parkinson's disease. The most common safety issues include headaches, flushing, and dyspepsia, and patients should be informed beforehand. Temporary visual symptoms, such as impairment in colour perception, may occur with higher doses.

Potential Advantages
- Studies have shown an indirect beneficial effect of sildenafil on patients' depressive symptoms.

Potential Disadvantages
- Sildenafil is not recommended for women with sexual dysfunction.
- Significant safety issues may arise in patients with cardiovascular problems.

Clinical Box

A 47-year-old man with a 3-year history of Parkinson's disease presented at the Neurology Department Outpatient Clinic with his wife for his regular follow-up appointment. Considering his motor performance, the patient was relatively stable and satisfied with a scheme of long-acting levodopa/carbidopa, pramipexole, and rasagiline. However, he mentioned an increased libido (probably in the context of the recently introduced dopamine agonist), which was accompanied by an inability to maintain an erection or achieve an orgasm and occasional episodes of premature ejaculation. All the above had a negative impact on his self-image and increased marital tension. The patient had no other co-morbidities. He was initially prescribed sildenafil 50 mg but due to a poor response, the higher dose of 100 mg was subsequently administered with satisfactory results.

Suggested Reading

Bernard BA, LV Metman, L Levine, B Ouyang, S Leurgans, CG Goetz. Sildenafil in the treatment of erectile dysfunction in Parkinson's disease. *Mov Disord Clin Pract* 2017; 4(3): 412–415.

Hussain IF, CM Brady, MJ Swinn, CJ Mathias, CJ Fowler. Treatment of erectile dysfunction with sildenafil citrate (Viagra) in parkinsonism due to Parkinson's disease or multiple system atrophy with observations on orthostatic hypotension. *J Neurol Neurosurg Psychiatry* 2001; 71(3): 371–374.

Raffaele R, I Vecchio, B Giammusso, G Morgia, MB Brunetto, L Rampello. Efficacy and safety of fixed-dose oral sildenafil in the treatment of sexual dysfunction in depressed patients with idiopathic Parkinson's disease. *Eur Urol* 2002; 41(4): 382–386.

Zesiewicz TA, M Helal, RA Hauser. Sildenafil citrate (Viagra) for the treatment of erectile dysfunction in men with Parkinson's disease. *Mov Disord* 2000; 15(2): 305–308.

References

AHFS Drug information, 2012. Bethesda: American Society of Health-System Pharmacists. Accessed on 31 December 2022 via www.medicinescomplete.com.

Bronner G, DB Vodušek. Management of sexual dysfunction in Parkinson's disease. *Ther Adv Neurol Disord* 2011; 4(6): 375–383.

Joint Formulary Committee. British National Formulary (online). London: BMJ Group and Pharmaceutical Press. Accessed on 31 December 2022 via www.medicinescomplete.com.

Salonia A, P Rigatti, F Montorsi. Sildenafil in erectile dysfunction: a critical review. *Curr Med Res Opin* 2003; 19(4): 241–262.

Sildenafil. In: Brayfield A (Ed.), *Martindale: The Complete Drug Reference*. London: The Royal Pharmaceutical Society of Great Britain. Accessed on 31 December 2022 via www.medicinescomplete.com.

Sildenafil. In: DRUGDEX® System (electronic version). Truven Health Analytics, Greenwood Village, Colorado, USA. Accessed on 31 December 2022 via www.micromedexsolutions.com.

S

Smith BP, M Babos. Sildenafil. In: *StatPearls*. 2022, StatPearls Publishing. Copyright © 2022, Treasure Island (FL): StatPearls Publishing LLC.
Summary of product characteristics – Viagra 25 mg film-coated tablets. Upjohn UK Limited. Electronic Medicines Compendium: Viagra 25 mg film-coated tablets – summary of product characteristics (SmPC) – (emc). Accessed on 31 December 2022 via www.medicines.org.uk.

SILDENAFIL

SOLIFENACIN

S

Therapeutics
*Solifenacin dosage mentioned below refers to solifenacin succinate.

Chemical Name and Structure
Solifenacin succinate ((3*R*)-1-azabicyclo[2.2.2]oct-3-yl (1*S*)-1-phenyl-3,4-dihydroisoquinoline-2(1H)-carboxylate compound with butane-odioic acid (1:1)) has a molecular weight of 480.6 and a molecular formula of $C_{23}H_{26}N_2O_2,C_4H_6O_4$. Solifenacin succinate 5 mg is equivalent to solifenacin 3.8 mg. Dosage of solifenacin succinate is expressed in terms of the salt.

Brand Names
- **Adablok** (*Poland*); **Afenix** (*Poland*); **ApoSoli** (Poland); **Asolfena** (*Czech Republic, Estonia, Hong Kong, Lithuania, Poland*); **Aurosolin** (*Poland*).
- **Belmacina** (*Austria, Germany, Spain*); **Beloflow** (*Poland*); **Bladiton** (*Singapore*); **Bladocad** (*South Africa*); **Bulapt** (*South Africa*).
- **Cecure** (*Greece*); **Cistil** (*Argentina*); **Continental** (*Equador*).
- **Dicrisol** (*Spain*).
- **Elysion** (*Thailand*); **Enirlad** (*South Africa*).
- **Fluriva** (*South Africa*); **Folinar** (*Czech Republic*); **Furlin** (*South Africa*).
- **Giraxine** (*UK*).
- **Impere** (*Brazil*); **Incoves** (*Italy*).
- **Jubsolifen** (*Hong Kong*).
- **Mivago** (*Poland*); **Muscarisan** (*Czech Republic*).
- **Nacerfin** (*Greece*); **Natysin** (*Turkey*); **Nifelox** (*Poland*); **Novurit** (*Argentina*).
- **Samile** (*Brazil*); **Saprax** (*Cyprus*); **Silamil** (*Poland*); **Sincal** (*Spain*); **Sivenacin** (*Greece*); **Sofcare** (*Hong Kong, Thailand*); **Solfesire** (*Turkey*); **Solicare** (*Czech Republic, Greece, Tunisia*); **Solicin** (*Greece, Hong Kong*); **Solifas** (*Turkey*); **Solifemin** (*Germany*); **Solifen** (*Argentina*); **Soliflow** (*Czech Republic*); **Solifurin** (*Poland*); **Solinco** (*Poland*); **Solirest** (*South Africa*); **Soliron** (*Turkey*); **Solixa** (*Czech Republic*); **Solnatec** (*Greece*); **Soluro** (*Poland*); **Solvicyd** (*South Africa*); **Solysin** (*Turkey*); **Soreca** (*Poland*); **Symcare** (*Poland*).
- **Tamisten** (*Estonia, Lithuania, Spain*); **Trunace** (*South Africa*).
- **Uriquil** (*South Africa*); **Urocare** (*Poland*); **Uronorm** (*Poland*).
- **Veloxsol** (*Netherlands, Poland*); **Vesicare** (*Argentina, Australia, Austria, Belgium, Brazil, Canada, Chile, China, Czech Republic, Cyprus, Denmark, Estonia, Finland, France, Germany, Greece, Hong Kong, Hungary, Israel, Japan, Lithuania, Malaysia, Mexico, Netherlands, New Zealand, Norway, Philippines, Poland, Portugal, Russian Federation, Singapore, South Africa, Spain, Sweden, Switzerland, Thailand, Tunisia, Turkey, UK, Ukraine, USA*); **Vesifix** (*Turkey*); **Vesigamp** (*Russian Federation*); **Vesiker** (*Italy*); **Vesikur** (*Germany*); **Vesinorm** (*South Africa*); **Vesisol** (*Austria,*

S

Poland, Turkey); **Vesitirim** (*Ireland*); **Vesoligo** (*Poland*); **Vesurol** (*Spain*); **Vezimed** (*Cyprus*); **Viland** (*Greece*).
* **Xinity** (*South Africa*).
* **Zebcare** (*Czech Republic*); **Zevesin** (*Czech Republic, Lithuania, Poland, Turkey, Ukraine*).

Generics Available
* Yes.

Licensed Indications for Parkinson's Disease
* None.

Licensed Indications for Other Conditions
* Overactive bladder (symptoms of urge urinary incontinence, urgency, and urinary frequency) (FDA, EMA, EMC).

Non-Licensed Use for Parkinson's Disease
* Overactive bladder.

Non-Licensed Use for Other Conditions
* Ureteral stent-related symptoms – prophylaxis.

Ineffective
* Not reported.

Mechanism of Action
* Solifenacin is a competitive, specific muscarinic receptor antagonist (M3 subtype receptor).
* Acetylcholine contracts the detrusor smooth muscle through muscarinic receptors, with M3 subtype being predominantly involved; therefore, solifenacin inhibits this contraction, leading to reduced bladder activity (a genito-urinary antispasmodic agent).
* Solifenacin selectivity for muscarinic M3 receptors in vitro allows functional selectivity for urinary bladder over secretory glands (e.g. salivary).
* Solifenacin demonstrates a moderate ability to cross the blood–brain barrier.

Efficacy Profile
* Solifenacin has been characterized as 'possibly useful' in the treatment of urinary urgency and/or urge incontinence in Parkinson's disease (MDS EBM Committee).
* An RCT study, consisting of a double-blind 12-week phase and an open-label 8-week phase, has found that solifenacin therapy was significantly associated with improved urinary incontinence and nocturia episodes during the open-label phase. However, the primary

SOLIFENACIN

outcome measure of the study, which was the daily number of micturitions, was not reached.
- Based on data from an open-label, long-term extension study, the efficacy of solifenacin was maintained for up to 52 weeks for symptoms of urinary frequency, urgency, or urge incontinence.

Pharmacokinetics
Absorption and Distribution
- Oral bioavailability: about 90%.
- Food co-ingestion does not affect solifenacin serum concentration.
- Tmax: 3 h (5-mg dose), 8 h (10-mg dose).
- Pharmacokinetics: linear in the therapeutic dose range.
- Protein binding: about 98% (mainly to α1-acid glycoprotein).
- Volume of distribution: 600 l (following IV administration).

Metabolism
- Solifenacin undergoes extensive hepatic metabolism, mainly by CYP3A4, producing one active metabolite (4R-hydroxy solifenacin) and numerous non-active metabolites.

Elimination
- Half-life ranges between 45 h and 68 h.
- About 69% of an administered dose is excreted in urine (approximately 11% unchanged) and 23% is found in faeces.

Drug Interaction Profile
Pharmacokinetic Drug Interactions
- Effects by solifenacin:
  - Solifenacin decreases levels of *aripiprazole, clozapine, haloperidol, olanzapine, quetiapine, risperidone* by inhibition of GI absorption.
- Effects on solifenacin:
  - CYP3A4 inhibitors (e.g. *acetazolamide, clarithromycin, diltiazem, itraconazole, ketoconazole, verapamil*) will increase levels and effects of solifenacin.
  - CYP3A4 inducers (e.g. *carbamazepine, cortisone, dexamethasone, fosphenytoin, phenytoin, prednisone, rifampin, topiramate*), including grapefruit, will decrease levels and effects of solifenacin.

Pharmacodynamic Drug Interactions
- Co-administration with neuroleptics or drugs causing electrolyte imbalance or increasing QT interval (e.g. *amiodarone, azithromycin, buprenorphine, chloroquine, chlorpromazine, citalopram, clarithromycin, donepezil, erythromycin, escitalopram, flecainide, foscarnet, lithium, moxifloxacin,*

S

pimozide, quetiapine, quinidine, siponimod, sotalol, trazodone, venlafaxine) might lead to potentially fatal Torsade de Pointes arrhythmias.
- Co-administration with *abobotulinumtoxinA*, *onabotulinumtoxinA*, *amantadine*, tricyclic antidepressants, neuroleptics, and other agents with anticholinergic properties (e.g. *trazodone*) may enhance potential systemic anticholinergic effects (synergistic action).
- Co-medication with cholinergic receptor agonists may reduce solifenacin efficacy.
- Solifenacin may reduce the effect of medicinal products, which stimulate GI motility (e.g. *metoclopramide, cisapride*).

Adverse Effects
How Drug Causes Adverse Effects
- Solifenacin adverse effects are mostly mediated by its antimuscarinic activity.

Common Adverse Effects
- Very common (≥1/10):
  - Dry mouth, constipation.
- Common (≥1/100 to <1/10):
  - Neuropsychiatric: dizziness, depression.
  - Eye/ear: blurred vision, dry eyes.
  - Cardiovascular: hypertension, peripheral oedema.
  - Respiratory: cough.
  - Renal/urinary: urinary tract infections.
  - GI: dyspepsia, nausea/vomiting, abdominal pain.
  - Other: influenza, fatigue.
- Uncommon (≥1/1,000 to <1/100):
  - Neuropsychiatric: somnolence, dysgeusia.
  - Renal/urinary: cystitis, difficulty in micturition.
  - GI: gastro-oesophageal reflux disease, dry throat.
  - Skin: dry skin.
  - Other: peripheral oedema.

Life-Threatening or Dangerous Adverse Effects
- Rare (≥1/10,000 to <1/1,000):
  - Anaphylactic reaction.
  - Urinary retention.
  - Colonic obstruction, faecal impaction.
- Very rare (<1/10,000):
  - Angioedema, erythema multiforme.
- Unknown frequency:
  - Delirium.
  - Glaucoma.
  - Ileus.
  - QT prolongation/arrhythmias.

- Information of the licensed product, although causality and frequency could not be determined.

Rare and Not Life-Threatening Adverse Effects
- Hallucinations, confusion.
- Headache.
- Pruritus, rash, urticaria.

Weight Change
- Not reported.

What to Do About Adverse Effects
- Before introducing solifenacin, discuss common or life-threatening adverse effects with patients and/or caregivers, including symptoms that should be reported to the physician.
  - Patients should be particularly aware of potential antimuscarinic CNS adverse reactions, especially after solifenacin initiation or after dose increase. If such side effects occur, consider dose reduction or complete cessation of therapy.
  - Patients should also know that solifenacin might increase the risk of heat prostration during hot weather due to decreased sweating.
  - Due to high risk for narrow-angle glaucoma, patients should be advised to seek medical help immediately if they have sudden loss of visual acuity or ocular pain.
- If angioedema or anaphylactic shock occur, which may be after the initial dose or after multiple doses, solifenacin therapy should be discontinued and appropriate treatment should be applied to ensure a patent airway.
- Regular dental check-ups are advisable during solifenacin therapy due to high risk of causing dry mouth, which predisposes to dental caries, parodontosis, or oral candidiasis.
- If patients are concomitantly treated with medicinal products administered sublingually (e.g. sublingual nitrates), they should know that absorption might be impaired due to high risk of solifenacin causing dry mouth. Patients should be advised to moisten their mouth with a little water before taking a sublingual tablet.

Dosing and Use
Usual Dosage Range
- 5 mg daily.

Available Formulations
- Tablets: 5 mg, 10 mg.
- Oral suspension: 1 mg/1 ml.

S

DOSING AND USE

S

SOLIFENACIN

How to Dose
- An initial dose of 5 mg OD is suggested; it may be increased to 10 mg OD according to clinical response and if well tolerated.
- Maintenance dose should be the lowest effective for the shortest possible duration due to potential anticholinergic effects.

Dosing Tips
- Solifenacin tablets may be taken with or without food.
- At least 4 weeks of solifenacin therapy is needed before the drug demonstrates its full potential.
- In case of oral suspension, shake bottle well before administration of each dose.
- Oral suspension ingestion should be followed by liquid consumption (e.g. water or milk) after each dose.

How to Withdraw Drug
- If the maximum 10 mg dose is used, consider reducing to the 5 mg dose for 4 weeks before complete discontinuation of solifenacin.
- If intolerable symptoms recur or withdrawal effects are felt, consider resuming the previous lowest tolerated dose and recommence weaning after 6–12 weeks.
- Withdrawal symptoms, including irritability, anxiety, insomnia, sweating and GI effects, are usually mild and can last up to 6–8 weeks.

Overdose
- Consider activated charcoal or gastric lavage if applied within 1 h after solifenacin ingestion. Vomiting should not be induced.
- Supportive measures, close monitoring of core temperature, vital signs and mental status, and maintenance of a clear airway with adequate ventilation are recommended.
  - Protect airway early in patients with severe intoxication.
- Solifenacin overdose can potentially present with severe anticholinergic effects (anticholinergic poisoning); clinical manifestations may be prolonged due to delayed absorption in the setting of anticholinergic ileus.
- If hallucinations or severe excitation occurs, consider treatment with physostigmine or carbachol.
- Severe delirium may develop, requiring large doses of benzodiazepines for sedation.
- If seizures occur, consider aggressive use of benzodiazepines and propofol, as they may progress to status epilepticus.
- If tachycardia occurs, consider treatment with beta-blockers, although it is usually mild and well tolerated without any specific intervention.
- If mydriasis occurs, consider administration of pilocarpine eye drops; patient should be placed in a dark room.
- If urinary retention occurs, catheterization should be applied.
- If hyperthermia occurs, control agitation with benzodiazepines and introduce aggressive external cooling measures.

S

- Physostigmine is indicated to reverse potential CNS effects in toxic dosages of anticholinergic agents; however, its action is relatively short (45–60 min).
- Physostigmine is often used diagnostically to distinguish anticholinergic delirium from other causes of altered mental status.
  - If co-administered with tricyclic antidepressants, physostigmine may precipitate seizures and dysrhythmias.

Tests and Therapeutic Drug Monitoring
- Before initiation of solifenacin therapy:
- A baseline ECG should be performed to check for QT prolongation.
- Test for a potential urinary tract infection and treat with appropriate antibacterial therapy if necessary.

Other Warnings / Precautions
- Close monitoring is advised in case of significant bladder outflow obstruction (risk for urinary retention).
- Close monitoring is advised if decreased GI motility or GI obstructive disorders occur due to high risk for gastric retention.
- Caution is advised if hiatus hernia/gastro-oesophageal reflux occurs or in those concurrently treated with medicinal products that may trigger or aggravate oesophagitis.
- Caution is advised if there is a known history of QT prolongation or taking medications known to prolong QT interval or cause electrolyte imbalance, particularly hypokalaemia.
  - Close monitoring is advised if co-administered with *apomorphine* due to QT prolongation.
- Caution is advised if autonomic neuropathy occurs, as solifenacin may exacerbate symptoms of decreased GI motility.
- Solifenacin use should be avoided in elderly patients with delirium or at high risk of delirium, or in patients with dementia or cognitive impairment.
- Caution is advised in male patients with lower urinary tract symptoms or benign prostatic hyperplasia, as solifenacin may cause reduced urinary flow and urinary retention.
- Co-administration with strong CYP3A4 inhibitors/inducers should be avoided.
  - If co-administered with strong CYP3A4 inhibitors, a maximum dose of solifenacin 5 mg/day is recommended.
- Caution is advised if co-administered with other drugs with anticholinergic properties due to additive effects. A one-week interval is suggested after discontinuation of solifenacin therapy before introducing another anticholinergic agent.
- Solifenacin may cause blurred vision and somnolence; therefore, driving or operating dangerous machinery is not advised, at least until patients know how therapy affects them.

DOSING AND USE

S

Do Not Use (Contraindications)
- Known sensitivity to solifenacin or to any of the excipients, including lactose.
  - Patients with rare hereditary problems of galactose intolerance, total lactase deficiency, or glucose–galactose malabsorption.
- Gastric or urinary retention.
- Severe GI condition (including toxic megacolon).
- Myasthenia gravis.
- Uncontrolled narrow-angle glaucoma.
- Co-administration with drugs that predispose to QT prolongation, such as Class IA and III antiarrhythmics, antipsychotics (e.g. *haloperidol*, *phenothiazine* derivatives, pimozide), tricyclic antidepressants, certain antimicrobial agents (e.g. *moxifloxacin*, *erythromycin*, *fluconazole*), certain antihistamines (e.g. *astemizole*, *mizolastine*), and others.

Special Populations
Renal Impairment
- Mild-to-moderate impairment (CrCl ≥ 30 ml/min): no dosage modifications needed.
- Severe (CrCl < 30 ml/min): maximum dose of 5 mg/day is recommended.
- Patients on haemodialysis: not recommended.

Hepatic Impairment
- Mild impairment (Child–Pugh A): no dosage modifications needed.
- Moderate impairment (Child–Pugh B): maximum dose of 5 mg/day is recommended.
- Severe (Child–Pugh C): solifenacin therapy is not recommended.

Elderly
- According to a systemic review of placebo-controlled trials examining the effect of solifenacin on overactive bladder symptoms in a geriatric population (over 65 years of age) for 4–12 weeks, solifenacin use was found to be associated with an increased risk of both anticholinergic (e.g. dry mouth, constipation) and non-anticholinergic adverse events (e.g. dyspepsia, dizziness, headache, urinary tract infections) compared to control groups.
- Solifenacin elimination half-life increased by 20–25% in geriatric patients.
- No dosage adjustments are needed.

Pregnancy
- Category C.
- No data are available on the use of solifenacin during pregnancy in humans.

- Results from animal studies have not demonstrated any direct negative effects of solifenacin on fetal development or parturition.
- Caution is advised in case of administering solifenacin during pregnancy, as potential risks for the fetus cannot be excluded.

Breastfeeding
- It is not known whether solifenacin is excreted in human milk.
- No data are available on the effect of solifenacin on nursing infants or milk production.
- Solifenacin use is not recommended during breastfeeding, as potential risks for the nursing infant cannot be excluded.

Costs
NHS indicative price (accessed on 31 December 2022):
- Vesicare tablets (Astellas Pharma Ltd) – 30 × 5 mg tablets: £27.62.
- Vesicare 1 mg/ml oral suspension (Astellas Pharma Ltd) – 150 ml: £27.62.
- Solifenacin 5 mg tablets – 30 × 5 mg tablets: £1.23–£27.62.
- Solifenacin 10 mg tablets – 30 × 10 mg tablets: £1.19–£35.91.
- Solifenacin 5 mg/5 ml oral solution – 150 ml solution: £27.62–£112.85.

The Overall Place of Solifenacin in the Treatment of Parkinson's Disease
Solifenacin succinate is a muscarinic receptor antagonist, approved for the treatment of overactive bladder symptoms in the general population. There is only one randomized control pilot study exploring the effect of solifenacin in urinary symptoms specifically in Parkinson's disease patients for a total of 20 weeks. This showed a significant decrease in the number of urinary incontinence and nocturia episodes. Among other antimuscarinic agents, which are typically used to manage urinary symptoms, solifenacin is the only one included in the MDS EBM Committee recommendations for use in Parkinson's disease. Notably, its efficacy and safety in patients over 65 years of age has been demonstrated. However, antimuscarinic agents may add to the total anticholinergic burden when used with other medicinal products occasionally employed in Parkinson's disease, which also exhibit anticholinergic properties, such as amantadine, trihexyphenidyl, tricyclic antidepressants, neuroleptics, or botulinum toxin. The increased burden may precipitate symptoms such as agitation, confusion, somnolence, or hallucinations. Finally, solifenacin therapy may affect cognitive performance and Parkinson's disease-related autonomic features, such as constipation or orthostasis, so caution and close monitoring is advised.

S

SOLIFENACIN

Potential Advantages
- Compared to oxybutynin IR in a head-to-head double-blind RCT outside the context of Parkinson's disease, solifenacin use was associated with a lower rate of therapy discontinuation and treatment-related adverse events, including occurrence of dry mouth.
- In contrast to most other anticholinergic drugs used for the management of overactive bladder, solifenacin is selective for M3 receptors.
- Among major antimuscarinic agents, solifenacin has been associated with the highest rate of compliance.
- In selected patients with residual urgency after treatment with tolterodine ER, subsequent treatment with solifenacin was associated with significant improvement in overactive bladder symptoms and health-related quality of life.

Potential Disadvantages
- Among antimuscarinic agents used for overactive bladder, solifenacin use has been associated with high rates of constipation and urinary tract infections.
- Solifenacin use has been associated with conflicting results considering its effect on cognitive performance of older people. A recent network meta-analysis concluded that, among oral antimuscarinic drugs, it was the least related to cognitive impairment.

Clinical Box
A 55-year-old man with a 5-year diagnosis of Parkinson's disease presented to the Neurology Outpatient Clinic for his follow-up appointment. He was recently examined by a urologist due to urinary urgency, increased urinary frequency, and involuntary loss of urine. The patient was diagnosed with an overactive bladder with predominant storage symptoms. Prostatic hyperplasia was excluded and his symptoms were attributed to Parkinson's disease. The patient had already been started on solifenacin 5 mg OD by his urologist about 5 weeks previously. Due to persistent symptoms, a dose of 10 mg OD was introduced with a good response after 3 weeks.

Suggested Reading
Wagg A, JJ Wyndaele, P Sieber. Efficacy and tolerability of solifenacin in elderly subjects with overactive bladder syndrome: a pooled analysis. *Am J Geriatr Pharmacother* 2006; 4(1): 14–24.
Zesiewicz TA, M Evatt, CP Vaughan, I Jahan, C Singer, R Ordorica, JL Salemi, JD Shaw, KL Sullivan. Randomized, controlled pilot trial of solifenacin succinate for overactive bladder in Parkinson's disease. *Parkinsonism Relat Disord* 2015; 21(5): 514–520.

References

AHFS Drug information, 2012. Bethesda: American Society of Health-System Pharmacists. Accessed on 31 December 2022 via www.medicinescomplete.com.

Chancellor MB, N Zinner, K Whitmore, K Kobashi, JA Snyder, P Siami, M Karram, C Laramée, JP Capo, Jr, R Seifeldin, S Forero-Schwanhaeuser, I Nandy. Efficacy of solifenacin in patients previously treated with tolterodine extended release 4 mg: results of a 12-week, multicenter, open-label, flexible-dose study. *Clin Ther* 2008; 30(10): 1766–1781.

Haab F, L Cardozo, C Chapple, AM Ridder. Long-term open-label solifenacin treatment associated with persistence with therapy in patients with overactive bladder syndrome. *Eur Urol* 2005; 47(3): 376–384.

Herschorn S, P Pommerville, L Stothers, B Egerdie, J Gajewski, K Carlson, S Radomski, H Drutz, J Schulz, J Barkin, E Hirshberg, J Corcos. Tolerability of solifenacin and oxybutynin immediate release in older (> 65 years) and younger (≤ 65 years) patients with overactive bladder: sub-analysis from a Canadian, randomized, double-blind study. *Curr Med Res Opin* 2011; 27(2): 375–382.

Joint Formulary Committee. British National Formulary (online). London: BMJ Group and Pharmaceutical Press. Accessed on 31 December 2022 via www.medicinescomplete.com.

Lua LL, P Pathak, V Dandolu. Comparing anticholinergic persistence and adherence profiles in overactive bladder patients based on gender, obesity, and major anticholinergic agents. *Neurourol Urodyn* 2017; 36(8): 2123–2131.

Malcher MF, S Droupy, C Berr, A Ziad, H Huguet, JL Faillie, C Serrand, T Mura. Dementia associated with anticholinergic drugs used for overactive bladder: a nested case-control study using the French national medical-administrative database. *J Urol* 2022; 208(4): 863–871.

Solifenacin. Brayfield A (Ed.), *Martindale: The Complete Drug Reference*. London: The Royal Pharmaceutical Society of Great Britain. Accessed on 31 December 2022 via www.medicinescomplete.com.

Solifenacin. In: DRUGDEX® System (electronic version). Truven Health Analytics, Greenwood Village, Colorado, USA. Accessed on 31 December 2022 via www.micromedexsolutions.com.

Summary of Product Characteristics – Vesicare 10 m film-coated tablets. Astellas Pharma Ltd. Electronic Medicines Compendium: Vesicare 10 mg film-coated tablets – summary of product characteristics (SmPC) – (emc). Accessed on 31 December 2022 via www.medicines.org.uk.

Vouri SM, CD Kebodeaux, PM Stranges, BF Teshome. Adverse events and treatment discontinuations of antimuscarinics for the treatment of overactive bladder in older adults: a systematic review and meta-analysis. *Arch Gerontol Geriatr* 2017; 69: 77–96.

S

Wagg A, W Gibson, J Ostaszkiewicz, T Johnson, 3rd, A Markland, MH Palmer, G Kuchel, G Szonyi, R Kirschner-Hermanns. Urinary incontinence in frail elderly persons: report from the 5th International Consultation on Incontinence. *Neurourol Urodyn* 2015; 34(5): 398–406.

Yang N, Q Wu, F Xu, X Zhang. Comparisons of the therapeutic safety of seven oral antimuscarinic drugs in patients with overactive bladder: a network meta-analysis. *J Int Med Res* 2021; 49(9): 3000605211042994.

SOLIFENACIN

TOLCAPONE

T

Therapeutics

Chemical Name and Structure

Tolcapone (3,4–dihydroxy-4′-methyl-5-nitrobenzophenone or (3,4–dihydroxy-5-nitrophenyl)(4-methylphenyl)methanone) is a yellow, odourless, crystalline, lipophilic compound with a molecular weight of 273.24 and an empirical formula of $C_{14}H_{11}NO_5$.

Brand Names
- **Sen De Ning** (*China*).
- **Tasmar** (*Argentina, Austria, Brazil, Chile, China, Cyprus, Czech Republic, Estonia, France, Germany, Greece, Hungary, Ireland, Italy, Netherlands, New Zealand, Poland, South Africa, Spain, Sweden, Switzerland, Turkey, UK, USA*).

Generics Available
- No.

Licensed Indications for Parkinson's Disease
- As an adjunct therapy to levodopa preparations in patients with advanced Parkinson's disease with motor fluctuations and an inadequate response or intolerance to other COMT inhibitors (FDA, EMA, EMC).

Licensed Indications for Other Conditions
- None.

Non-Licensed Use for Parkinson's Disease
- As an adjunct therapy in early or stable Parkinson's disease patients.

Non-Licensed Use for Other Conditions
- None.

Ineffective
- Patients not receiving levodopa therapy.

Mechanism of Action
- Tolcapone is a selective and reversible inhibitor of COMT that mediates metabolism of levodopa to 3-methoxy-4-hydroxy-L-phenylalanine (3-OMD). It inhibits both peripheral and central COMT, although the contribution of central inhibition to the therapeutic effects is unknown. When co-administered with levodopa and a DDI, tolcapone leads to more stable plasma levodopa levels.
  ○ No anti-parkinsonian activity when administered alone.
- Maximum COMT inhibition following a single 200 mg oral dose of tolcapone is reported to exceed 80%.

THERAPEUTICS

T

Efficacy Profile
- According to the MDS EBM Committee, tolcapone:
  ○ Was considered 'efficacious' and 'clinically useful' in the management of motor fluctuations.
  ○ Although characterized as an 'efficacious' add-on therapy to levodopa preparations in early or stable Parkinson's disease patients, it has also been considered 'unlikely useful' in clinical practice due to potentially fatal complications.

Pharmacokinetics
Absorption and Distribution
- (Oral) bioavailability: about 65–68%.
- Food co-ingestion: food delays and decreases absorption.
- Tmax: 2 h (oral route of 5–800 mg).
- Pharmacokinetics: linear pharmacokinetics for the dosage range of 50–400 mg, independently of levodopa co-administration.
- Protein binding: >99%.
- Volume of distribution: 9 l.

Metabolism
- Extensively metabolised, mainly by conjugation to the inactive glucuronide, but also through methylation to 3-O-methyltolcapone and through hydroxylation to a primary alcohol, which is then oxidized to the carboxylic acid.
- Oxidation is by hepatic CYP450 isoenzymes (CYP3A4 and CYP2A6).

Elimination
- The elimination half-life is about 2–3 h.
- About 60% of an administered dose is excreted in urine. The remainder appears in the faeces.
- About 13% of the oral dose is excreted in the urine as the glucuronide metabolite (also appearing in the faeces), 2% as the carboxylic acid metabolite, and less than 0.5% as unchanged drug.

Drug Interaction Profile
Pharmacokinetic Drug Interactions
- Effects by tolcapone:
  ○ Tolcapone may increase levels and effects of *dobutamine, epinephrine, isoproterenol, norepinephrine, dopamine, methyldopa* by decreasing their metabolism via COMT inhibition.

Pharmacodynamic Drug Interactions
- Co-administration with non-selective MAO inhibitors (e.g. *phenelzine, tranylcypromine, isocarboxazid*) might lead to inhibition of the

principal pathways involved in metabolism of catecholamines, leading to high blood pressure or heart rate; thus, this combination should be avoided.
  ○ Co-administration with selective MAO-B inhibitors (e.g. *selegiline*) is not discouraged.
- Co-administration with drugs affecting the brain monoaminergic system, including non-selective MAO inhibitors (or simultaneous administration of both selective MAO-A and MAO-B inhibitors), tricyclic antidepressants and SSRIs, or the cholinergic system might cause a constellation of symptoms mimicking NMS; therefore, caution is advised.
- Co-administration with CNS depressants (e.g. *lorazepam*, *tramadol*, *metoclopramide*) might lead to additive sedative effects.
- An affinity of tolcapone to CYP2C9 has been found in vitro; however, clinically relevant interactions involving CYP2C9 appear unlikely.
- No important interactions have been found between tolcapone and substrates of CYP2A6 (e.g. *warfarin*), CYP3A4 (e.g. *cyclosporine*, *midazolam*, *terfenadine*), CYP1A2 (e.g. *caffeine*), CYP2C19 (e.g. S-*mephenytoin*), or CYP2D6 (e.g. *desipramine*).
- Co-administration with certain antipsychotic agents may aggravate parkinsonian symptoms and lead to reduced tolcapone efficacy.
- Caution is advised in co-medication of tolcapone with benserazide, as it might lead to increased levels of the latter and dose-related adverse effects.

T

ADVERSE EFFECTS

Adverse Effects
How Drug Causes Adverse Effects
- Some adverse effects might be dopaminergic in origin caused by its effect on levodopa levels.

Common Adverse Effects
- Very common (≥1/10):
  ○ Neuropsychiatric: dyskinesia, insomnia, somnolence, hallucinations (more common in those >75 years), confusion, excessive dreaming, dystonia (less common in those >75 years), headache.
  ○ Cardiovascular: orthostatic hypotension.
  ○ GI: nausea, diarrhoea.
    ▪ Diarrhoea, which usually occurs during the first 6–12 weeks of therapy initiation, is one of the main reasons for tolcapone discontinuation.
- Common (≥1/100 to <1/10):
  ○ Neuropsychiatric: fatigue, loss of balance, falls, hyper/hypokinesia, paraesthesia.
  ○ Cardiovascular: syncope, hypotension, peripheral oedema, palpitations.
  ○ Respiratory: dyspnoea, upper respiratory infection, sinus congestion.

- GI: vomiting, constipation, abdominal pain, xerostomia.
- Renal/urinary: urinary tract infection, haematuria, urine discoloration (yellow intensification of urine).
- Musculoskeletal: neck pain.
- Other: increased transaminases, increased sweating, rash, chest pain, influenza-like illness.
- Uncommon (≥1/1,000 to <1/100):
  - Cardiovascular: hypertension, angina pectoris, arteriospasm, heart failure, atrial fibrillation, bradycardia, arrhythmia, MI, pulmonary embolus, cerebral haemorrhage.
  - Respiratory: increased cough, rhinitis, laryngitis, hiccups.
  - GI: dysphagia, GI haemorrhage, gastroenteritis, mouth ulceration, esophagitis, cholelithiasis, colitis
  - Renal/urinary: dysuria, nocturia, polyuria, oliguria.
  - Other: prostatic disorder, vaginitis, hepatocellular injury/liver failure.

Life-Threatening or Dangerous Adverse Effects
- Acute, potentially fatal, liver injury.
  - Most cases of elevated hepatic enzymes occurred between 6 weeks and 6 months after tolcapone initiation with enzyme levels returning to baseline within 1–3 months in half of the patients who remained on tolcapone treatment and within 2 weeks to 2 months in patients who discontinued tolcapone.
  - Liver failure may be rapid despite discontinuation of tolcapone.
  - Hepatic changes may not be visible on ultrasound.
  - Higher risk among women.
- Isolated cases of NMS (fever, muscular rigidity, altered consciousness) have been described after dose reduction or abrupt discontinuation of tolcapone.
- Severe rhabdomyolysis and multi-organ system failure, potentially fatal, have been reported in few cases, sometimes as a complication of NMS.

Rare and Not Life-Threatening Adverse Effects
- ICDs.

Weight Change
- Not reported.

What to Do About Adverse Effects
- Discuss common adverse events with patients or caregivers before starting medication, including symptoms that should be reported to the physician.
- In general, many tolcapone-induced adverse events are levodopa-associated and dopaminergic in nature. Reducing the levodopa dosage may mitigate these complications.

- Tolcapone discontinuation is strongly suggested if ALT/SGPT or AST/SGOT concentrations exceed the upper limit of normal or if clinical picture suggests an onset of hepatic dysfunction (e.g. jaundice, dark urine, persistent nausea, anorexia, fatigue, lethargy, pruritus, tenderness in the right upper abdomen).
  - Periodic monitoring of liver enzymes cannot reliably predict fulminant hepatitis; however, it is believed that early detection of hepatic dysfunction along with immediate tolcapone withdrawal enhances the chances of recovery.
  - If patients recover after evidence of acute liver injury with tolcapone, they should not be considered for tolcapone re-treatment.
- Dyskinesia usually occurs within 24 h of tolcapone initiation and can be controlled by reducing levodopa dosage by 20–30%. If dyskinesia persists, consider discontinuation of tolcapone.
- Hallucinations generally manifest within the first 2 weeks of tolcapone initiation and may be responsive to levodopa dosage reduction. If persistent, consider tolcapone discontinuation.
- Anorexia usually resolves with time, without tolcapone discontinuation. If persistent, consider tolcapone withdrawal.
- In case of ICD, consider reducing the dosage or discontinuing tolcapone or other ICD-related dopaminergic agents (e.g. dopamine agonists, levodopa).

Dosing and Use

Usual Dosage Range
- 300–600 mg daily.

Available Formulations
- Tablets: 100 mg.

How to Dose
- An initial dose of 100 mg TID is suggested; may increase to 200 mg TID, as required.
- The maximum dose of 600 mg should not be exceeded, as there is no evidence of additional efficacy at higher doses.

Dosing Tips
- The first dose of tolcapone for the day should be administered at the same time as the levodopa/DDI preparation. The second one should be administered after 6 h and the third tablet after 12 h.
- Tolcapone may be taken with or without food.
- Tolcapone tablets should be swallowed whole due to their bitter taste.
- Tolcapone may be administered with conventional or ER levodopa/DDI preparations.

DOSING AND USE

T

T

- If the patient does not exhibit an adequate beneficial clinical response within 3 weeks of tolcapone therapy initiation, treatment should be withdrawn due to potential severe complications.
- Most patients starting tolcapone will need a reduction in their levodopa dosage (an average of 30%), especially in regimens including more than 600 mg of levodopa.

How to Withdraw Drug
- Tapering of tolcapone dosage has not been systematically evaluated. Reducing the administration frequency to BID or OD may not prevent potential adverse reactions, because the duration of tolcapone-related COMT inhibition is 5–6 h or longer.
- The patient should be closely monitored after tolcapone withdrawal.
- Levodopa dosage may have to be increased after tolcapone discontinuation to levels equal to or greater than before tolcapone initiation. Adjustments in levodopa are usually required within 1–2 days of tolcapone discontinuation.
- In case of NMS after tolcapone discontinuation, consider increasing the patient's levodopa dose.

Overdose
- Tolcapone overdose in Parkinson's disease patients has not been clearly described.
- Symptoms of nausea, vomiting, and dizziness have been observed with doses of 800 mg TID in healthy volunteers.
- General supportive care and hospitalization is advised.

Tests and Therapeutic Drug Monitoring
- Before initiation of therapy:
  - Test liver function (liver enzymes levels); if abnormal values are found, tolcapone is not recommended.
- During therapy:
  - Liver function should be monitored every 2 weeks for the first year of therapy, every 4 weeks for the next 6 months, and every 8 weeks thereafter.
  - Liver enzymes should be tested before every increase in tolcapone dosage. The above scheme should be followed again after increasing tolcapone dose.
  - If co-administered with warfarin, coagulation parameters (preferably INR) should be regularly monitored.

Other Warnings/Precautions
- Although falling asleep while engaged in activities of daily living usually occurs in the context of pre-existing somnolence, some patients might not experience warning signs (sudden sleep onset).
- Patients should be regularly monitored for the development of ICDs.

TOLCAPONE

T

Do Not Use (Contraindications)
- Hypersensitivity to the active substance or to any of the formulation excipients.
- Tolcapone therapy should not be initiated in patients with clinical evidence of active liver disease, or ALT/SGPT or AST/SGOT values exceeding the upper normal limit, or any other evidence of hepato-cellular dysfunction.
- Patients with severe dyskinesia.
- History of NMS or non-traumatic rhabdomyolysis or hyperthermia.

Special Populations
Renal Impairment
- CrCl 30–130 ml/min: no dosage adjustments needed.
- Severe renal impairment (CrCl < 30 ml/min): use with caution.

Hepatic Impairment
- Any degree of hepatic impairment or liver disease or increased liver enzymes contraindicates tolcapone therapy.
- In moderate cirrhotic liver disorders (Child–Pugh class B) tolcapone clearance may be reduced by 50%.

Elderly
- No age-related differences in the tolcapone pharmacokinetics.

Pregnancy
- There is insufficient evidence of tolcapone use in pregnant women.
- Tolcapone should only be used during pregnancy if the potential benefit outweighs the potential risk to the fetus.
- Indications of fetal malformation or other pregnancy complications (e.g. reduced fetal weight) in animal studies.

Breastfeeding
- Women should not breastfeed when treated with tolcapone.
- It is not known whether tolcapone is distributed into human milk.
- Excretion of tolcapone into milk has been reported in rats.

COSTS

Costs
NHS indicative price (as per BNF, accessed 20 May 2022):
- 100 × 100 mg tablets: £95.20 + VAT.

T

The Overall Place of Tolcapone in the Treatment of Parkinson's Disease

Tolcapone is a second-line COMT inhibitor, which requires regular hepatic monitoring. Tolcapone is efficacious in the treatment of motor fluctuations in Parkinson's disease and as an adjunct therapy to levodopa preparations in early Parkinson's disease. After the initial introduction of tolcapone to the market in 1997 (Europe) and 1998 (USA), three deaths were reported due to tolcapone-induced liver impairment, leading to the drug being withdrawn from the market in numerous countries (e.g. Australia). Its use globally has been greatly reduced and it has been withdrawn from guidelines in favour of safer options without the risk of a potentially fatal liver injury, such as entacapone or opicapone.

Potential Advantages
• Tolcapone is generally considered more efficacious compared to ent-acapone and has a longer duration of action.

Potential Disadvantages
• Not a first-line therapy due to potentially fatal, acute hepatotoxicity.
• Regular monitoring of hepatic function is required.
• May exacerbate dyskinesia and other levodopa-related adverse reactions (e.g. somnolence, hallucinations).

TOLCAPONE

Clinical Box

A 65-year-old man with a 10-year history of Parkinson's disease reported motor wearing off phenomena, along with mild, not troublesome, dyskinesia. He also reported troublesome sleep fragmentation. His current anti-parkinsonian medications were levodopa/carbidopa 200 mg/50 mg QID and rasagiline 1 mg OD. His medical history consisted of well-controlled hypertension (amlodipine 5 mg OD) and hypercholesterolaemia (atorvastatin 10 mg OD). The patient was initially treated with a gradually increasing dose of rotigotine; however, he developed severe skin reactions on the application site, which necessitated discontinuation of therapy. He was subsequently prescribed increasing doses of pramipexole ER up to 2.1 mg OD, which led to both motor and non-motor symptom improvement. However, the patient developed ICDs (troublesome hypersexuality and binge eating), which were highlighted by his wife and necessitated discontinuation of therapy. Entacapone 200 mg QID was subsequently prescribed, as opicapone formulations were not available in his country. Although the patient's OFF phenomena improved, they did persist, while he also developed severe diarrhoea and abdominal discomfort, leading him to discontinue entacapone therapy. After a detailed discussion with the patient and his caregiver, considering potential risks and the regular liver function monitoring, and after excluding any potential contraindications, tolcapone 100 mg TID was prescribed. OFF phenomena improved significantly, but dyskinesia was aggravated, being troublesome to the patient. Reduction of levodopa/carbidopa dose led to dyskinesia improvement.

Suggested Reading

Artusi CA, L Sarro, G Imbalzano, M Fabbri, L Lopiano. Safety and efficacy of tolcapone in Parkinson's disease: systematic review. *Eur J Clin Pharmacol* 2021; 77(6): 817–829.

Eggert K, WH Oertel, AJ Lees. Safety and efficacy of tolcapone in the long-term use in Parkinson disease: an observational study. *Clin Neuropharmacol* 2014; 37(1): 1–5.

Fabbri M, JJ Ferreira, O Rascol. COMT inhibitors in the management of Parkinson's disease. *CNS Drugs* 2022; 36(3): 261–282.

References

AHFS Drug information, 2012. Bethesda: American Society of Health-System Pharmacists. Accessed on 23 May 2022 via www .medicinescomplete.com.

Coker AR, DN Weinstein, TA Vega, CS Miller, AS Kayser, JM Mitchell. The catechol-*O*-methyltransferase inhibitor tolcapone modulates alcohol consumption and impulsive choice in alcohol use disorder. *Psychopharmacology (Berl)* 2020; 237(10): 3139–3148.

Forsberg M, M Lehtonen, M Heikkinen, J Savolainen, T Järvinen, PT Männstö. Pharmacokinetics and pharmacodynamics of entacapone and tolcapone after acute and repeated administration: a comparative study in the rat. *J Pharmacol Exp Ther* 2003; 304(2): 498–506.

Joint Formulary Committee. British National Formulary (online). London: BMJ Group and Pharmaceutical Press. Accessed on 23 May 2022 via www.medicinescomplete.com.

Summary of product characteristics – Tasmar 100 m film-coated tablets. Mylan. Electronic Medicines Compendium: Tasmar 100 mg film-coated tablets – summary of product characteristics (SmPC) – (emc). Accessed on 23 May 2022 via www.medicines.org.uk.

Tolcapone. In: Brayfield A (Ed.), *Martindale: The Complete Drug Reference*. London: The Royal Pharmaceutical Society of Great Britain. Accessed on 23 May 2022 via www.medicinescomplete.com.

TOLTERODINE

Therapeutics
*Tolterodine dosage mentioned below refers to tolterodine tartrate.

Chemical Name and Structure
Tolterodine tartrate ((+)-(R)-2-{α-[2-(di-isopropylamino)ethyl]benzyl}–p-cresol tartrate) is the tartrate salt form of tolterodine. It has a molecular weight of 475.6 and a molecular formula of $C_{22}H_{31}NO,C_4H_6O_6$. One milligram of tolterodine tartrate corresponds to 0.68 mg of tolterodine.

Brand Names
- **BeiKe** (*China*); **Blerone** (*UK*); **Breminal** (*Argentina*); **Bu Mai Ding** (*China*).
- **Caristenol** (*Ireland, Poland*); **Cinterol** (*Greece*).
- **Defur** (*Poland*); **Detrol** (*Canada, USA*); **Detrulet** (*Greece*); **Detrulon** (*Greece*); **Detrusitol** (*Argentina, Australia, Austria, Belgium, Brazil, Chile, China, Cyprus, Czech Republic, Denmark, Ecuador, Estonia, Finland, France, Germany, Greece, Hong Kong, India, Indonesia, Ireland, Israel, Italy, Japan, Lithuania, Malaysia, Mexico, Netherlands, New Zealand, Norway, Singapore, South Africa, Spain, Sweden, Switzerland, Thailand, Tunisia, Turkey, UK, Ukraine, Venezuela*); **Dezrol** (*India*).
- **Eltoven** (*Chile*).
- **Flochek** (*India*).
- **Inconex** (*UK*).
- **Le Zai** (*China*).
- **Mariosea** (*UK*).
- **Neditol** (*UK*); **NeiQing** (*China*).
- Preblacon (*UK*).
- **Ranolteril** (*Poland*); **Roliten** (*Russian Federation, Ukraine*).
- **Santizor** (*Austria*); **SheNiTing** (*China*).
- **Tendrotil** (*Ireland*); **Terol** (*India*); **Te Su An** (*China*); **Titlodine** (*Poland*); **Tolbasadin** (*Poland*); **Toldelo** (*UK*); **Toldesor** (*Greece*); **Toldin** (*Turkey*); **Tolteccord** (*New Zealand*); **Toltem** (*Argentina*); **Tolterana** (*Cyprus*); **Tolterma** (*UK*); **Toltertan** (*Ireland*); **Tolthen** (*UK*); **Toltex** (*Turkey*); **Tolusitol** (*Ireland*); **Tolzurin** (*Poland*); **Trudenia** (*Greece*); **Trusitev** (*Ireland*).
- **Urginol** (*Argentina*); **Urimper** (*Lithuania, Poland*); **Uroflex** (*Russian Federation*); **Uroflow** (*Czech Republic, Estonia, Lithuania, Poland*); **Uroline** (*Netherlands*); **Urostop** (*Chile*); **Urotol** (*Russian Federation, Ukraine*); **Urotrol** (*Mexico, Spain*).

Generics Available
- Yes.

Licensed Indications for Parkinson's Disease
- None.

Licensed Indications for Other Conditions
- Overactive bladder symptoms, including urge incontinence and/or increased urinary frequency/urgency (FDA, EMA, EMC).

Non-Licensed Use for Parkinson's Disease
- Overactive bladder symptoms.

Non-Licensed Use for Other Conditions
- Not reported.

Ineffective
- Not reported.

Mechanism of Action
- Tolterodine is a competitive muscarinic receptor antagonist that decreases bladder contraction. According to animal studies, it displays a selectivity for activity on the bladder over salivary glands.
- According to in vitro studies, tolterodine has no selectivity for any subtype of muscarinic receptors.
- Tolterodine demonstrates a moderate ability to cross the blood–brain barrier.

Efficacy Profile
- Up to now, there are no published studies investigating the effect of tolterodine on Parkinson's disease-related urinary symptoms. High-quality studies concerning tolterodine efficacy on overactive bladder symptoms in the general population, including elderly patients, have been used by regulatory authorities to grant approval for its use in Parkinson's disease for the management of overactive bladder symptoms.
- The peak effect of tolterodine is expected after 2–4 weeks of therapy.
- Limited data suggest that tolterodine efficacy can be maintained for up to 12 months of therapy.

Pharmacokinetics
Absorption and Distribution
- Oral bioavailability: approximately 17% (about 65% in poor CYP2D6 metabolizers).
- Food co-ingestion may increase levels of tolterodine, although clinically relevant changes are not typically expected.
- Tmax: 1–3 h (IR preparations), 2–6 h (ER preparations).
- Time to steady state: about 2 days (IR preparations).
- Pharmacokinetics: linear in the therapeutic dosage range.
- Protein binding: highly bound (approximately 96%) to plasma proteins, mainly to α1-acid glycoprotein. About 64% of the active metabolite is bound to protein.
- Volume of distribution: 113 ± 26.7 l.

PHARMACOKINETICS

T

T

Metabolism
- Tolterodine undergoes hepatic metabolism mainly by CYP2D6, producing the active metabolite 5-hydroxymethyl tolterodine. The latter exhibits a similar pharmacological profile to the parent compound.
- In a minority of poor CYP2D6 metabolizers, tolterodine is metabolized by CYP3A4 isoenzymes producing the inactive *N*-dealkylated derivative. These differences in metabolism are not clinically significant.

Elimination
- Plasma half-life is 1.9–3.7 h for the parent drug (about 10 h in poor CYP2D6 metabolizers) and 3 h for the active metabolite.
- About 77% of an administered dose is excreted in the urine and about 17% is found in faeces. Less than 1% of tolterodine is excreted as unchanged drug.

Drug Interaction Profile
Pharmacokinetic Drug Interactions
- Effects by tolterodine:
  - Tolterodine decreases levels of *aripiprazole, clozapine, haloperidol, olanzapine, quetiapine, risperidone* by inhibition of GI absorption.
- Effects on tolterodine:
  - CYP3A4 inhibitors (e.g. *acetazolamide, clarithromycin, chloramphenicol, diltiazem, erythromycin, istradefylline, itraconazole, ketoconazole, marijuana, verapamil*) will increase levels and effects of tolterodine.
  - CYP2D6 inhibitors (e.g. *bupropion, clobazam, fluoxetine, mirabegron, paroxetine*) will increase levels and effects of tolterodine.
  - CYP3A4 inducers (e.g. *carbamazepine, cortisone, dexamethasone, fosphenytoin, phenytoin, prednisone, rifampin, topiramate*), including grapefruit, will decrease levels and effects of tolterodine.

Pharmacodynamic Drug Interactions
- Co-administration with *abobotulinumtoxinA, onabotulinumtoxinA, amantadine*, tricyclic antidepressants, and other agents with anticholinergic properties (e.g. *trazodone*) may enhance potential systemic anticholinergic effects (synergistic action).
- Co-administration with cholinergic agents (e.g. cholinesterase inhibitors, *pilocarpine, pyridostigmine*) leads to opposing results; effect of interaction is not clear.
- Tolterodine may reduce the effect of medicinal products that stimulate GI motility (e.g. *metoclopramide, cisapride*).

Adverse Effects

How Drug Causes Adverse Effects
- Tolterodine adverse effects are mostly mediated by its antimuscarinic activity.

Common Adverse Effects
- Very common (≥1/10):
  ○ Dry mouth, headache.
- Common (≥1/100 to <1/10):
  ○ Neuropsychiatric: dizziness, drowsiness, somnolence, paraesthesia.
  ○ Eye/ear: abnormal vision, accommodation disturbances, xerophthalmia, vertigo.
  ○ Cardiovascular: palpitations, chest pain.
  ○ Respiratory: bronchitis.
  ○ GI: constipation, dyspepsia, abdominal pain, flatulence, vomiting, diarrhoea.
  ○ Renal/urinary: dysuria, urinary retention.
  ○ Other: dry skin, fatigue, peripheral oedema.
- Uncommon (≥1/1,000 to <1/100):
  ○ Neuropsychiatric: nervousness, memory impairment.
  ○ Cardiovascular: tachycardia, arrhythmia, cardiac failure.
  ○ GI: gastroesophageal reflux.
  ○ Other: hypersensitivity reactions.

Life-Threatening or Dangerous Adverse Effects
- Anaphylactoid reactions.
- Angioedema.

Rare and Not Life-Threatening Adverse Effects
- Confusion, hallucinations, disorientation.
- Flushing.

Weight Change
- Increased weight is a common adverse effect of tolterodine.

What to Do About Adverse Effects
- Before introducing tolterodine, discuss common or life-threatening adverse effects with patients and/or caregivers, including symptoms that should be reported to the physician.
  - Patients should be particularly aware of potential antimuscarinic CNS adverse reactions, especially after tolterodine initiation or dose increase. In case of such side effects, consider dose reduction or complete cessation of therapy.
  - Due to high risk of narrow-angle glaucoma, patients should be advised to immediately ask for medical help in case of sudden loss of visual acuity or ocular pain.

T

ADVERSE EFFECTS

T

- Tolterodine may cause blurred vision and somnolence; therefore, driving or operating dangerous machinery is not advised, at least until patients know how therapy affects them.
- In case of angioedema or anaphylactic shock (e.g. hypotension, difficulty breathing), which may occur after the initial dose or after multiple doses, tolterodine therapy should be immediately discontinued and appropriate treatment should be applied to ensure a patent airway.

Dosing and Use

Usual Dosage Range
- 2–4 mg daily.

Available Formulations
- Tablets, IR: 1 mg, 2 mg.
- Capsules, ER: 2 mg, 4 mg.

How to Dose
- IR: initial dose of 2 mg BID; may lower dose to 1 mg BID based on clinical response and tolerability.
- ER: initial dose of 2–4 mg OD; may lower dose to 1 mg OD based on clinical response and tolerability.
- Tolterodine efficacy should be reassessed after 2–3 months of therapy.

Dosing Tips
- Oral preparations can be taken with or without food.
- IR preparations are usually taken in the morning and in the evening (12 h gap).
- ER preparations should be consumed with an adequate amount of fluid.
- There are indications that ER preparations may be slightly more effective in improving certain symptoms (e.g. urge incontinence) compared to IR preparations and have been associated with a better safety profile (e.g. dry mouth).

How to Withdraw Drug
- A gradual discontinuation is suggested by 25–50% of the daily dose every 1–4 weeks.
- Consider a faster tapering in case of adverse events.

Overdose
- There are limited data on tolterodine overdose, with the most common reported manifestations being accommodation disturbances, micturition difficulties, and QT prolongation. However, potential anticholinergic effects should be anticipated.

TOLTERODINE

- In case of tolterodine overdose, consider treatment with activated charcoal or gastric lavage, if close to tolterodine consumption.
  - Haemodialysis or peritoneal dialysis are not expected to be beneficial due to extensive protein binding of tolterodine.
- Supportive measures, close monitoring of core temperature, vital signs, ECG and mental status, and maintenance of a clear airway with adequate ventilation are recommended.
  - Protect airway early in patients with severe intoxication.
- In case of central anticholinergic effects (e.g. hallucinations, severe excitation), consider treatment with physostigmine.
  - Physostigmine should not be routinely used due to potential adverse effects.
- In case of seizures or pronounced excitation, consider treatment with benzodiazepines.
- In case of tachycardia, consider treatment with beta-blockers.
- In case of mydriasis, consider conjunctival application of pilocarpine eye drops; patient should be placed in a dark room.
- In case of urinary retention, catheterization should be applied.

Tests and Therapeutic Drug Monitoring
- Before initiation of tolterodine therapy:
  - A baseline ECG should be performed to check for QT prolongation.

Other Warnings/Precautions
- Close monitoring is advised in the case of significant bladder outflow obstruction due to a high risk for urinary retention.
- Caution is advised in male patients with lower urinary tract symptoms or benign prostatic hyperplasia, as tolterodine may cause reduced urinary flow and urinary retention.
- Close monitoring is advised where there is decreased GI motility or GI obstructive disorders (e.g. pyloric stenosis) due to high risk for gastric retention.
- Caution is advised in hiatus hernia/gastro-oesophageal reflux or for those concurrently treated with medicinal products that may trigger or aggravate oesophagitis.
- Caution is advised in patients with narrow-angle glaucoma (risk of increased intra-ocular pressure).
- Caution is advised in autonomic neuropathy, as tolterodine may exacerbate symptoms of decreased GI motility.
- Tolterodine use should be avoided in elderly patients with delirium or at high risk of delirium, or in patients with dementia or cognitive impairment due to increased risk of adverse events and potential to worsen symptoms.
- Caution is advised when using tolterodine in patients with a history of congenital or documented acquired QT prolongation or other conditions predisposing to QT prolongation, such as electrolyte disturbances (e.g. hypokalaemia, hypomagnesaemia, hypocalcaemia),

T

DOSING AND USE

T

bradycardia, relevant pre-existing cardiac conditions, or concurrent administration of QT-prolonging drugs, due to reports of tolterodine causing QT prolongation in high doses (4–8 mg daily).
- Co-administration with strong CYP3A4 inhibitors should be avoided due to risk of overdose.
  - A maximum dose of 1 mg BID (IR preparations) or 2 mg (ER preparations) is recommended in case of co-administration with strong CYP3A4 inhibitors.
- Close monitoring is advised if prescribing tolterodine in patients with dementia receiving cholinesterase inhibitors, as it might affect their cognitive status and their functional abilities and predispose to problematic behaviours.
- Caution is advised if co-administering with other drugs with anticholinergic properties due to additive effects.
- Although no clinically significant interactions are expected, increases in INR have been reported in individuals concomitantly receiving tolterodine and warfarin.
- Tolterodine may cause blurred vision due to impairment of accommodation and increase reaction time, which might affect ability to drive or operate machinery.

Do Not Use (Contraindications)
- Known sensitivity to tolterodine or to any of its excipients or to fesoterodine fumarate, which is metabolized to 5-hydroxymethyl tolterodine.
- Urinary or gastric retention.
- Severe ulcerative colitis, toxic megacolon.
- Myasthenia gravis, due to decreased cholinergic activity at neuromuscular junction (risk of paralysis).
- Uncontrolled narrow-angle glaucoma.
- Co-administration with strong CYP3A4 inhibitors in moderate hepatic or renal impairment.

Special Populations
Renal Impairment
- CrCl 10–30 ml/min: a maximum dose of 1 mg BID (IR preparations) or 2 mg (ER preparations) is recommended.
- CrCl < 10 ml/min: not recommended.

Hepatic Impairment
- Mild-to-moderate impairment (Child–Pugh class A or B): a maximum dose of 1 mg BID (IR preparations) or 2 mg (ER preparations) is recommended.
- Severe impairment (Child–Pugh class C): not recommended.

Elderly
- Dose adjustments are not necessary based solely on age.

Pregnancy
- No data are available on the use of tolterodine during pregnancy in humans.
- Tolterodine is not recommended during pregnancy, as potential risks for the fetus cannot be excluded.

Breastfeeding
- Tolterodine may be excreted in milk in low amounts according to animal studies.
- No data are available on the effect of tolterodine on nursing infants or milk production.
- Tolterodine use should better be avoided during breastfeeding.

Costs
NHS indicative pricing (accessed on 1 January 2023):
- Detrusitol tablets (Viatris UK Healthcare Ltd) – 56 × 1 mg tablets: £29.03; 56 × 2 mg tablets: £30.56.
- Mariosea XL capsules (Teva UK Ltd) – 28 × 2 mg capsules: £11.59; 28 × 4 mg capsules: £12.79.
- Neditol XL capsules (Aspire Pharma Ltd) – 28 × 2 mg capsules: £11.60; 28 × 4 mg capsules: £12.89.
- Toldelo XL capsules (Morningside Healthcare Ltd) – 28 × 2 mg capsules: £6.99; 28 × 4 mg capsules: £4.89.
- Tolterma XL capsules (Macleods Pharma UK Ltd) – 28 × 2 mg capsules: £24.36; 28 × 4 mg capsules: £25.78.
- Tolthen XL capsules (Northumbria Pharma Ltd) – 28 × 2 mg capsules: £6.99; 28 × 4 mg capsules: £6.99.
- Blerone XL capsules (Zentiva Pharma UK Ltd) – 28 × 4 mg capsules: £9.59.
- Detrusitol XL capsules (Viatris UK Healthcare Ltd) – 30 × 4 mg capsules: £25.78.
- Peblacon XL capsules (Accord Healthcare Ltd) – 28 × 4 mg capsules: £25.78.
- Tolterodine 1 mg tablets – 56 × 1 mg tablets: £1.46–£29.03.
- Tolterodine 2 mg tablets – 56 × 2 mg tablets: £1.68–£30.56.

The Overall Place of Tolterodine in the Treatment of Parkinson's Disease
Tolterodine was the first antimuscarinic agent designed for the targeted management and treatment of overactive bladder symptoms and is still very commonly used in routine clinical practice. More specifically, it is a muscarinic receptor antagonist, possessing both antimuscarinic and antispasmodic properties, which result in increasing residual urine in the bladder and reducing pressure of the detrusor muscle. Although it is not specific for any muscarinic subtypes, it is believed to exhibit selectivity

T

for the bladder compared to salivary glands according to animal studies. Among other antimuscarinic agents, particularly oxybutynin, tolterodine is believed to have a better safety profile, especially in terms of causing dry mouth, constipation, dizziness, or urinary retention. However, when deciding between solifenacin and IR tolterodine, the former might be preferred for better efficacy and less risk of xerostomia.

There are no specific trials assessing the effect of tolterodine on overactive bladder symptoms in Parkinson's disease patients. However, safety and efficacy of tolterodine have been confirmed in multiple high-quality studies in the general population, including geriatric patients. It is also considered suitable for long-term therapy. Tolterodine ER preparation offers some advantages in terms of fewer side effects (e.g. dry mouth), along with the convenience of once-daily administration, which is expected to improve patients' adherence and may be preferred if available. Similarly, to other antimuscarinic agents, it may add to the total anticholinergic burden of other medicinal products with such properties commonly used in Parkinson's disease. Finally, it may affect cognitive performance and Parkinson's disease-related autonomic features, so caution and close monitoring is advised.

Potential Advantages
- As a result of direct comparisons, tolterodine has similar efficacy to oxybutynin (both IR and ER preparations); however, patients on tolterodine are more likely to adhere to long-term treatment due to fewer side effects.
- Compared to solifenacin, tolterodine may decrease the rate of constipation after 12 weeks of therapy.
- Tolterodine is believed to have the most favourable overall safety profile among antimuscarinic agents.

Potential Disadvantages
- Similarly to oxybutynin, tolterodine use has been associated with significant cognitive deterioration and should be used with caution in geriatric patients.
- Compared to solifenacin, tolterodine was found to be less beneficial in the management of leakage/urgency episodes, in terms of reported cure/improvement and patients' quality of life.

Clinical Box
A 55-year-old cognitively intact woman with a 5-year history of Parkinson's disease presented at the Neurology Department Outpatient Clinic for a follow-up assessment. The patient recently complained of overactive bladder symptoms and the urodynamic tests revealed detrusor overactivity. Due to concurrent troublesome constipation, the patient was given the option of tolterodine IR 2 mg BID among other antimuscarinic agents. She exhibited a good response of her symptoms

after 3 weeks of therapy. However, due to development of *de novo* significant xerostomia the dose was reduced to 1 mg BID with improvement of dry mouth, while efficacy on overactive bladder symptoms was maintained. An alternative option replacing the IR preparation with the ER preparation would also be justified.

Suggested Reading

Abrams P, R Freeman, C Anderström, A Mattiasson. Tolterodine, a new antimuscarinic agent: as effective but better tolerated than oxybutynin in patients with an overactive bladder. *Br J Urol* 1998; 81(6): 801–810.

Appell RA. Clinical efficacy and safety of tolterodine in the treatment of overactive bladder: a pooled analysis. *Urology* 1997; 50(6A Suppl): 90–96; discussion 97–99.

Rovner ES. Tolterodine for the treatment of overactive bladder: a review. *Expert Opin Pharmacother* 2005; 6(4): 653–666.

Van Kerrebroeck P, K Kreder, U Jonas, N Zinner, A Wein. Tolterodine once-daily: superior efficacy and tolerability in the treatment of the overactive bladder. *Urology* 2001; 57(3): 414–421.

References

AHFS Drug information, 2012. Bethesda: American Society of Health-System Pharmacists. Accessed on 29 December 2022 via www.medicinescomplete.com.

Appell RA, P Abrams, HP Drutz, PE Van Kerrebroeck, R Millard, A Wein. Treatment of overactive bladder: long-term tolerability and efficacy of tolterodine. *World J Urol* 2001; 19(2): 141–147.

Chung DE, AE Te. Tolterodine extended-release for overactive bladder. *Expert Opin Pharmacother* 2009; 10(13): 2181–2194.

Duong V, A Iwamoto, J Pennycuff, B Kudish, C Iglesia. A systematic review of neurocognitive dysfunction with overactive bladder medications. *Int Urogynecol J* 2021; 32(10): 2693–2702.

Joint Formulary Committee. British National Formulary (online). London: BMJ Group and Pharmaceutical Press. Accessed on 29 December 2022 via www.medicinescomplete.com.

Madhuvrata P, JD Cody, G Ellis, GP Herbison, EJ Hay-Smith. Which anticholinergic drug for overactive bladder symptoms in adults. *Cochrane Database Syst Rev* 2012; 1: CD005429.

Malone-Lee JG, JB Walsh, MF Maugourd. Tolterodine: a safe and effective treatment for older patients with overactive bladder. *J Am Geriatr Soc* 2001; 49(6): 700–705.

Stahl MM, B Ekström, B Sparf, A Mattiasson, KE Andersson. Urodynamic and other effects of tolterodine: a novel antimuscarinic drug for the treatment of detrusor overactivity. *Neurourol Urodyn* 1995; 14(6): 647–655.

T

Summary of product characteristics – Detrusitol 2 mg film-coated tablets. Upjohn UK Ltd. Electronic Medicines Compendium: Detrusitol 2 mg film-coated tablets – summary of product characteristics (SmPC) – (emc). Accessed on 24 February 2023 via www.medicines.org.uk.

Takei M, Y Homma. Long-term safety, tolerability and efficacy of extended-release tolterodine in the treatment of overactive bladder in Japanese patients. *Int J Urol* 2005; 12(5): 456–464.

Tolterodine. In: Brayfield A (Ed.), *Martindale: The Complete Drug Reference*. London: The Royal Pharmaceutical Society of Great Britain. Accessed on 1 January 2023 via www.medicinescomplete.com.

Tolterodine. In: DRUGDEX® System (electronic version). Truven Health Analytics, Greenwood Village, Colorado, USA. Accessed on 29 December 2022 via www.micromedexsolutions.com.

Wang HT, M Xia. Comparisons of therapeutic efficacy and safety of solifenacin versus tolterodine in patients with overactive bladder: a meta-analysis. *Urol Int* 2019; 103(2): 187–194.

Yang N, Q Wu, F Xu, X Zhang. Comparisons of the therapeutic safety of seven oral antimuscarinic drugs in patients with overactive bladder: a network meta-analysis. *J Int Med Res* 2021; 49(9): 3000605211042994.

Zinner NR, A Mattiasson, SL Stanton. Efficacy, safety, and tolerability of extended-release once-daily tolterodine treatment for overactive bladder in older versus younger patients. *J Am Geriatr Soc* 2002; 50(5): 799–807.

TOLTERODINE

TRIHEXYPHENIDYL

Therapeutics

Chemical Name and Structure

Trihexyphenidyl hydrochloride (1-cyclohexyl-1-phenyl-3-piperidi-nopropan-1-ol hydrochloride) is an anticholinergic and antispasmodic agent with a molecular weight of 337.9 and a molecular formula of $C_{20}H_{31}NO$, HCl. Dosage of trihexyphenidyl hydrochloride is expressed in terms of the salt.

Brand Names

- **Aca** (*Malaysia, Thailand*); **Acamed** (*Thailand*); **Apo-Trihex** (*Hong Kong, Malaysia, Singapore*); **Arkine** (*Indonesia*); **Artandyl** (*Hong Kong*); **Artane** (*Argentina, Australia, Belgium, Brazil, France, Germany, Greece, Hong Kong, Italy, Japan, Netherlands, Philippines, Portugal, Spain, Thailand, UK, USA*).
- **Barohexy** (*India*); **Beahexol** (*Singapore*); **Benzhexol** (*Thailand*); **Bexol** (*India*).
- **Cyclodol** (*Estonia, Lithuania, Russian Federation, Ukraine*).
- **Dyskinil** (*India*); **Dystonil** (*India*).
- **Hexymer** (*Indonesia*); **Hipokinon** (*Mexico*).
- **Lahexy** (*India*).
- **Manohexy** (*India*).
- **Pacitane** (*India*); **Parales** (*India*); **Parkinal** (*Indonesia*); **Parkinane** (*France*); **Parkisonal** (*Japan*); **Parkizol** (*Tunisia*); **Parkoran** (*Germany, Greece, Lithuania, Russian Federation, Ukraine*); **Parnon** (*India*); **Partane** (*Israel*); **Pozhexol** (*Thailand*); **Rodenal** (*Israel*); **Sedrena** (*Japan*).
- **Tonaril** (*Chile*); **Tremin** (*Japan*); **Tridyl** (*Thailand*); **Triexidyl** (*Brazil*); **Trihexy** (*France*).

Generics Available

- Yes.

Licensed Indications for Parkinson's Disease

- Alleviation of parkinsonism in Parkinson's disease (FDA, EMA, EMC).

Licensed Indications for Other Conditions

- Drug-induced extrapyramidal symptoms (e.g. *reserpine, phenothiazines*) (FDA, EMA, EMC).
- Symptomatic therapy in all forms of parkinsonism (postencephalitic, arteriosclerotic, and idiopathic), either as a monotherapy or as adjuvant therapy to levodopa (EMA, EMC).

Non-Licensed Use for Parkinson's Disease

- None.

T

Non-Licensed Use for Other Conditions
• Dystonia.
• Nystagmus.

Ineffective
• Drug-related tardive dyskinesias.
• Spasticity in cerebral palsy or hemiplegia.

Mechanism of Action
• Trihexyphenidyl hydrochloride is a tertiary amine with antimuscarinic actions similar to atropine on parasympathetic–innervated peripheral systems including smooth muscle.
• It also has a direct antispasmodic action on smooth muscle.
• The exact mechanism of action in Parkinson's disease is not clear, but it may result from blockade of efferent impulses and from central inhibition of cerebral motor centres.

Efficacy Profile
• Anticholinergics, including trihexyphenidyl, have been labelled as 'likely efficacious' and 'clinically useful' when used for symptomatic monotherapy or for symptomatic adjunct therapy in early or stable Parkinson's disease patients (MDS EBM Committee).
• Trihexyphenidyl is effective in reducing the rigidity of muscle spasm, tremor, and excessive salivation associated with parkinsonism.
• Trihexyphenidyl's effect starts about 1 h after ingestion and lasts for about 6–12 h.
• A small prospective study found that trihexyphenidyl had a beneficial effect on axial symptoms which had developed after STN-DBS in Parkinson's disease patients.

Pharmacokinetics
Absorption and Distribution
There is limited information available on the pharmacokinetics of anticholinergic antiparkinsonian agents, including trihexyphenidyl.
• Oral bioavailability: high.
• Tmax: about 1.3 h.
• Volume of distribution: relatively high.

Metabolism
• No information available.

Elimination
• Elimination half-life is about 33 h.
• Trihexyphenidyl is excreted both in the urine (~76%) and the bile, probably as unchanged drug.

T

Drug Interaction Profile

Pharmacodynamic Drug Interactions

- Co-medication with *abobotulinumtoxinA*, *onabotulinumtoxinA*, *amantadine*, tricyclic antidepressants, neuroleptics, antimuscarinic agents used for overactive bladder (e.g. *solifenacin, oxybutynin*), antihistamines, MAO inhibitors, and other agents with anticholinergic properties (e.g. *trazodone*) may enhance potential systemic anticholinergic effects (synergistic action), particularly in terms of inhibiting GI motility.
- Co-medication with cholinergic agents (e.g. anticholinesterase inhibitors, *pilocarpine, pyridostigmine*) leads to opposing results; the effect of interaction is not clear.
- In case of co-administration with levodopa, trihexyphenidyl may enhance the therapeutic effects of levodopa, but it may also exacerbate dyskinesia.
- Trihexyphenidyl may reduce the effect of drugs that stimulate GI motility (e.g. *metoclopramide, cisapride*).

Adverse Effects

How Drug Causes Adverse Effects

- Trihexyphenidyl side effects are mostly mediated by its anticholinergic activity.
- It exhibits weak mydriatic, antisialogogue, and cardiovagal blocking activity.

Common Adverse Effects

- Very common ($\geq 1/10$):
  - Rash, xerostomia, constipation, blurring of vision, dizziness, mild nausea, nervousness.
- Common ($\geq 1/100$ to $<1/10$) or uncommon ($\geq 1/1,000$ to $<1/100$):
  - Immune: hypersensitivity.
  - Neuropsychiatric: restlessness, confusion, agitation, delusions, hallucinations, insomnia, impairment of immediate and short-term memory function, euphoria.
  - Eye: mydriasis/loss of accommodation/photophobia, increased intra-ocular pressure.
  - Cardiovascular: tachycardia.
  - Respiratory: decreased bronchial secretions.
  - GI: vomiting.
  - Skin: flushing, dry skin.
  - Renal/urinary: urinary retention, difficulty in micturition.
  - Other: thirst, pyrexia, suppurative parotitis.

Life-Threatening or Dangerous Adverse Effects

- Angle-closure glaucoma.
- Delirium.
- Paralytic ileus.
- Hypersensitivity reactions.

Weight Change
• Not reported.

What to Do About Adverse Effects
• Before introducing trihexyphenidyl, discuss common or life-threatening adverse effects with patients, including symptoms that should be reported to the physician.
  • Patients should be particularly aware of potential anticholinergic adverse reactions or memory impairment, especially after trihexyphenidyl initiation or after dose increase. In case of such side effects, consider dose reduction or complete cessation of therapy.
  • Due to a high risk of narrow-angle glaucoma, patients should be advised to immediately ask for medical help in case of sudden loss of visual acuity or ocular pain.
• Trihexyphenidyl may increase the risk of heat prostration during hot weather due to decreased sweating, especially if administered concomitantly with anticholinergic agents (also predisposing to decreased sweating).
• Adverse effects tend to become less pronounced as treatment continues; low initial dose and gradual dose increases allow patients to develop tolerance until an effective level is reached.
  • In case of a severe reaction, which requires discontinuation of trihexyphenidyl, resuming at a lower dose after a few days may be considered.
• Adverse effects are usually reversible on stopping trihexyphenidyl treatment.

Dosing and Use
Usual Dosage Range
• 1–15 mg daily.

Available Formulations
• Tablets: 2 mg, 5 mg.
• Oral solution: 0.4 mg/ml.

How to Dose
• Initial dose of 1 mg; subsequent dose increases by 1–2 mg every 3–5 days may be introduced to reach optimal effect. Total maintenance daily dose usually ranges between 6 mg and 10 mg divided in 2–4 doses given at mealtimes.
  • Selected patients (e.g. post-encephalitic parkinsonism) may require higher doses up to 12–15 mg per day.
• Due to potential safety issues, the lowest effective dose should be used.
• Optimal dosage is determined empirically, usually by introducing trihexyphenidyl at a low dose and by subsequent graduated increments (personalized scheme).

Dosing Tips
- Trihexyphenidyl may be taken before or after food, although it is usually taken with meals.
- In the case of co-administration with levodopa preparations, the usual dose of each drug may need to be reduced; depending on side effects and the degree of symptom control, (a total daily dose of trihexyphenidyl 3–6 mg is usually sufficient).

How to Withdraw Drug
- Except in the case of complications requiring urgent trihexyphenidyl discontinuation, trihexyphenidyl therapy should be gradually discontinued over a period of several days.
- Abrupt cessation or rapid dose reduction may lead to exacerbation of parkinsonism, the onset of a NMS or withdrawal symptoms, including anxiety, orthostatic hypotension, and tachycardia.

Overdose
- Similarly to other anticholinergic agents, trihexyphenidyl may be the subject of abuse (based on its hallucinogenic or euphoriant properties).
- Trihexyphenidyl overdose can potentially present with severe anticholinergic effects, including CNS disturbances (from restlessness to excitement, confusion and psychotic behaviour, delirium or seizures or incoordination), circulatory changes (flushing, hypotension), respiratory failure, paralysis, and coma.
- Supportive measures, close monitoring of core temperature, vital signs and mental status, and maintenance of a clear airway with adequate ventilation are recommended.
  - Protect airway early in patients with severe intoxication, as these individuals may develop paralysis of respiratory muscles.
- In pronounced restless/excitation or convulsions, consider administering IV diazepam (risk of CNS or respiratory depression).
- Anti-arrhythmic drugs are not recommended in case of dysrhythmia.

Tests and Therapeutic Drug Monitoring
- Before initiation of trihexyphenidyl therapy:
  - Measurement of intra-ocular pressure (gonioscopic examination).
- During trihexyphenidyl therapy:
  - Regular monitoring of intra-ocular pressure is recommended.

Other Warnings / Precautions
- Trihexyphenidyl use should be avoided in patients with delirium or at high risk of delirium or hallucinations, or in patients with dementia or cognitive impairment, as it may trigger or aggravate these symptoms, especially when administered in high doses.
- Close monitoring is recommended in the case of subjacent hypertension or cardiovascular disorders.
- Caution is advised in male patients with lower urinary tract symptoms or benign prostatic hyperplasia/prostatic hypertrophy (especially

T

TRIHEXYPHENIDYL

in the elderly), as trihexyphenidyl may cause reduced urinary flow and urinary retention.
- Close monitoring is advised in patients with obstructive disease of the GI or the genitourinary tract, as trihexyphenidyl may aggravate these conditions.
- Trihexyphenidyl use is not recommended for treatment in tardive dyskinesias, as it may aggravate involuntary movements unless they exist concomitantly with Parkinson's disease.
- Great caution is recommended in case of myasthenia gravis due to decreased cholinergic activity at the neuromuscular junction (risk of paralysis); trihexyphenidyl should be avoided.
- Close monitoring is advised when co-administered with other drugs exhibiting anticholinergic properties due to synergistic effects.
  - In patients who are already on antidepressant therapy with tricyclic antidepressants, the lowest dose of trihexyphenidyl should be administered and the patient should be regularly reviewed.
- Caution is advised in case of co-administration with cholinergic agents due to opposing effects and doubtful therapeutic benefits.
- Trihexyphenidyl may cause blurred vision, dizziness, and somnolence; thus, driving or operating dangerous machinery is not advised, at least until patients know how therapy affects them.

Do Not Use (Contraindications)
- Known sensitivity to trihexyphenidyl or to any of its excipients.
- Angle-closure glaucoma.

Special Populations
Renal Impairment
- Close monitoring is recommended.

Hepatic Impairment
- Close monitoring is recommended.

Elderly
- Patients over 65 years old require lower doses.
- Elderly patients may be more vulnerable to developing cognitive deficits/memory impairment, delirium, confusion, or hallucinations when prescribed trihexyphenidyl.
- Geriatric patients develop increased sensitivity to parasympathetic drugs and may be more prone to presenting with glaucoma.

Pregnancy
- Pregnancy category C.
- No data are available on the use of trihexyphenidyl during pregnancy in humans.
- Trihexyphenidyl should not be used during pregnancy, unless clearly necessary, as potential risks to the fetus cannot be excluded.

Breastfeeding
- No data are available on the effect of trihexyphenidyl on nursing infants.
- Trihexyphenidyl may inhibit lactation.
- It is not recommended during breastfeeding.

Costs
NHS indicative costs (accessed on 1 January 2023):
- Trihexyphenidyl 2 mg tablets – 84 × 2 mg tablets: £3.53–£6.17.
- Trihexyphenidyl 5 mg tablets – 84 × 5 mg tablets: £17.91–£20.62.
- Trihexyphenidyl 5 mg/5 ml oral solution – 200 ml: £94.00.
- Trihexyphenidyl 5 mg/5 ml syrup – 200 ml: £94.00.

The Overall Place of Trihexyphenidyl in the Treatment of Parkinson's Disease
Anticholinergic agents, including trihexyphenidyl, are the oldest type of medication used for the treatment of Parkinson's disease. After the establishment of levodopa as the cornerstone of Parkinson's disease treatment, the role of trihexyphenidyl was re-evaluated and is used both as monotherapy and as adjunctive therapy to levodopa. It is often administered during the early Parkinson's disease stages and is believed to be more beneficial on Parkinson's disease-related tremor than on other parkinsonian motor features; however, this notion is largely anecdotal and not supported by RCTs. Due to the effect on tremor and its rapid onset and short duration of action, patients may occasionally use a low dose of trihexyphenidyl on demand before engaging in a task requiring fine motor skills or before social events in order to control rest tremor. Trihexyphenidyl may also be considered as a levodopa-sparing therapeutic option, particularly in younger patients with mild and tolerable clinical manifestations. Tolerance to trihexyphenidyl may develop with prolonged use. Caution is advised, as trihexyphenidyl is the most recorded anticholinergic drug of abuse due to its euphorigenic potential, usually among patients with psychiatric disorders. Potential safety issues may arise from the anticholinergic properties of trihexyphenidyl (unfavourable neuropsychiatric tolerance profile and long-term risk of memory impairment), with older and cognitively impaired patients being at higher risk.

Potential Advantages
- It may have a beneficial effect on tremor, which is commonly a drug-resistant symptom.
- It is a levodopa-sparing therapy in Parkinson's disease.

T

Potential Disadvantages
- It is not well tolerated by the elderly or those with memory problems and who comprise a significant portion of the Parkinson's disease population.
- It requires multiple dosing during the day.

Clinical Box

A 43-year-old woman presented at the Neurology Department Outpatient Clinic due to new-onset tremor of the right hand. The rest of her medical history was unremarkable. After a thorough clinical evaluation, a diagnosis of Parkinson's disease was considered possible, which was further supported by DaTscan results. Due to prominent tremor with only mild manifestations of bradykinesia and rigidity, the patient, who was cognitively intact, was offered the therapeutic option of trihexyphenidyl. She was initially prescribed a low dose of 1 mg BID, and gradually increased by 1 mg increments every 5 days. The patient reported an adequate response of her tremor at a dose of 2 mg TID.

Suggested Reading

Hughes RC, JG Polgar, D Weightman, JN Walton. Levodopa in Parkinsonism: the effects of withdrawal of anticholinergic drugs. *Br Med J* 1971; 2(5760): 487–491.

Martin WE, RB Loewenson, JA Resch, AB Baker. A controlled study comparing trihexyphenidyl hydrochloride plus levodopa with placebo plus levodopa in patients with Parkinson's disease. *Neurology* 1974; 24(10): 912–919.

References

AHFS Drug information, 2012. Bethesda: American Society of Health-System Pharmacists. Accessed on 2 January 2023 via www.medicinescomplete.com.

Baba Y, MA Higuchi, H Abe, K Fukuyama, R Onozawa, Y Uehara, T Inoue, T Yamada. Anti-cholinergics for axial symptoms in Parkinson's disease after subthalamic stimulation. *Clin Neurol Neurosurg* 2012; 114(10): 1308–1311.

Joint Formulary Committee. British National Formulary (online). London: BMJ Group and Pharmaceutical Press. Accessed on 2 January 2023 via www.medicinescomplete.com.

Summary of product characteristics –trihexyphenidyl 2 mg tablets. Genus Pharmaceuticals. Electronic Medicines Compendium: trihexyphenidyl 2 mg tablets – summary of product characteristics (SmPC) – (emc). Accessed on 2 January 2023 via www.medicines.org.uk.

Trihexyphenidyl. In: Brayfield A (Ed.), *Martindale: The Complete Drug Reference*. London: The Royal Pharmaceutical Society of Great Britain. Accessed on 2 January 2023 via www.medicinescomplete.com.

Trihexyphenidyl. In: DRUGDEX® System (electronic version). Truven Health Analytics, Greenwood Village, Colorado, USA. Accessed on 2 January 2023 via www.micromedexsolutions.com.

T

REFERENCES

VENLAFAXINE

Therapeutics

Chemical Name and Structure

Venlafaxine (1-[2-(dimethylamino)-1-(4-methoxyphenyl)ethyl]cyclohexan-1-ol) is a bicyclic antidepressant with a molecular weight of 277.4 and an empirical formula of $C_{17}H_{27}NO_2$. Each ER capsule of venlafaxine hydrochloride 85 mg is equivalent to 75 mg of venlafaxine free base.

Brand Names

- **Adefaxin** (*Ecuador, Mexico*); **Alenthus** (*Brazil*); **Alventa** (*Estonia, Lithuania, Poland, Russian Federation, UK*); **Amphero** (*UK*); **Arafaxina** (*Spain*); **Argofan** (*Czech Republic, Estonia, Greece*); **Arvifax** (*Greece*); **Axone** (*Chile*); **Axyven** (*Poland*).
- **Benolaxe** (*Mexico*).
- **Dalium** (*India*); **Dapfix** (*Russian Federation*); **Depefex** (*UK*); **Deprevix** (*Greece, Hong Kong, Singapore*); **Depurol** (*Chile*); **Desinax** (*Portugal*); **Dislaven** (*Spain*); **Dobupal** (*Spain*); **Doxural** (*Cyprus*).
- **Ectien** (*Chile*); **Efastad** (*Denmark, Sweden*); **Efaxine** (*Cyprus, Greece*); **Efectin** (*Austria, Czech Republic, Poland, Russian Federation*); **Efegen** (*South Africa*); **Efevelon** (*Poland*); **Efexor** (*Argentina, Australia, Belgium, Brazil, Chile, Cyprus, Denmark, Ecuador, Estonia, Finland, Greece, Hong Kong, Indonesia, Ireland, Israel, Italy, Japan, Lithuania, Malaysia, Mexico, Netherlands, New Zealand, Norway, Philippines, Portugal, Singapore, South Africa, Sweden, Switzerland, Thailand, Tunisia, Turkey, UK, Venezuela*); **Efevelon** (*Poland, Russian Federation*); **Effexine** (*Hong Kong, Tunisia*); **Effexor** (*Canada, France, Tunisia, USA*); **Elafax** (*Argentina*); **Elaxine** (*Australia*); **Elify** (*Cyprus, Czech Republic, Lithuania*); **Emlev** (*South Africa*); **Enlafax** (*Australia, New Zealand*); **Envelaf** (*India*).
- **Falven** (*Hungary*); **Faxigen** (*Poland*); **Faxine** (*Italy*); **Faxiprol** (*Hungary*); **Faxiven** (*India, Turkey*); **Faxolet** (*Poland*); **Flavix** (*India*); **Foraven** (*UK*).
- **Galinex** (*South Africa*); **Ganavax** (*Argentina*); **Genexin** (*Portugal*).
- **Idoxen** (*Venezuela*); **Illovex** (*South Africa*); **Ireven** (*Ireland*); **Ixilania** (*Italy*).
- **Lafactin** (*Poland*); **Lafaxin** (*Chile*); **Lafeks** (*South Africa*); **Lanvexin** (*Estonia, Lithuania*); **Levest** (*Spain*); **Linexel** (*Mexico*).
- **Majoven** (*Ireland, UK*); **Maxibral XR** (*Argentina*); **MaXine** (*Philippines*); **Mazda** (*Mexico*); **Mebolex** (*South Africa*); **Melocin** (*Greece*); **Memomax-S** (*Greece*); **Myletin** (*Brazil*); **Myprax** (*New Zealand*).
- **Newvelong** (*Russian Federation*); **Nezel** (*Ecuador*); **Norafexine** (*Greece*); **Norezor** (*Greece*); **Norpilen** (*Chile*); **Novidat** (*Brazil*).
- **Odiven** (*South Africa*); **Odven SBK** (*Mexico*); **Olwexya** (*Czech Republic, Hungary, Poland*); **Oriven** (*Poland*); **Oxialpress** (*Ecuador*).
- **Politid** (*UK*); **Pracet** (*Portugal*); **Prefaxine** (*Poland*); **Psiseven** (*Argentina*).
- **Quilarex** (*Argentina*).

V

- **Senexon** (*Chile*); **Sentidol** (*Chile*); **Serosmine** (*Greece*); **Sesaren** (*Argentina, Venezuela*); **Subelan** (*Chile, Ecuador*); **Sulinex** (*Turkey*); **Sunveniz** (*UK*); **Sunvex** (*Argentina, Ecuador*); **Symfaxin** (*Poland*).
- **Tedema** (*Tunisia*); **Tifaxin** (*UK*); **Tonpular** (*Poland*); **Trevilor** (*Germany, Hong Kong*); **Tudor** (*Greece*).
- **Valexor** (*South Africa*); **Valosine** (*Hong Kong, Thailand*); **Vandral** (*Spain*); **Vedixal** (*Ireland, Portugal*); **Vefax** (*South Africa*); **Velafax** (*Poland, Russian Federation*); **Velaxin** (*Czech Republic, Lithuania, Hungary, Poland, Russian Federation, Ukraine*); **Velept** (*Greece*); **Velostad** (*Austria*); **Velpine** (*Greece*); **Venaxx, Vencarm** (*UK*); **Vencontrol** (*Chile*); **Venegis** (*Turkey*); **Venex** (*Ireland*); **Venexor** (*Hong Kong, South Africa*); **Venfalex** (*Netherlands*); **Ven-Fax** (*Greece*); **Venforin** (*Brazil*); **Veniba** (*Turkey*); **Veniz** (*Brazil, Venezuela*); **Venla** (*Australia, Israel*); **Venlablue** (*Ireland, UK*); **Venlabrain** (*Spain*); **Venladep** (*Turkey*); **Venladex** (*UK*); **Venladoz** (*Netherlands*); **Venlafab** (*Austria*); **Venlafex** (*Ireland*); **Venlagamma** (*Estonia, Germany*); **Venlalic** (*UK*); **Venlamylan** (*Spain*); **Venlapine** (*Spain*); **Venlasan** (*Greece*); **Venlasand** (*Netherlands*); **Venlasov** (*UK*); **Venlatev** (*Ireland*); **Venlavitae** (*Ecuador*); **Venlax** (*Chile, Switzerland*); **Venlaxin** (*Brazil, Cyprus, Greece*); **Venlaxor** (*Russian Federation, Ukraine*); **Venlazid** (*Norway*); **Venlectine** (*Poland*); **Venlex** (*Singapore*); **Venlifax** (*Argentina*); **Venlift** (*Brazil, Hong Kong, Russian Federation*); **Venlofex** (*Ireland*); **Venlor** (*Hong Kong, India, South Africa*); **Venorion** (*Norway*); **Vensate** (*Brazil*); **Vensir** (*Ireland, UK*); **Vensuert** (*Russian Federation*); **Venxin** (*Portugal*); **Venxor** (*Hong Kong, Malaysia*); **Venzip** (*UK*); **Vessril** (*Turkey*); **Vexor** (*Hong Kong, India*); **Vextor** (*Mexico*); **Viepax** (*Israel, Singapore, UK*); **Voxafen** (*Greece*); **Voxemel** (*Russian Federation*).
- **Winfex** (*UK*).
- **Xadevil** (*Greece*).
- **Zacalen** (*Greece*); **Zaredrop** (*Greece, Portugal*); **Zarelis** (*Italy, Spain*); **Zarelix** (*Portugal*); **Zenexor** (*Tunisia*).

Generics Available
- Yes.

Licensed Indications for Parkinson's Disease
- None.

Licensed Indications for Other Conditions
- Major depressive disorder – treatment, recurrence prevention (FDA, EMA, EMC).
- Generalized anxiety disorder (FDA, EMA, EMC).
- Social anxiety disorder (FDA, EMA, EMC).
- Panic disorder (FDA, EMA, EMC).

Non-Licensed Use for Parkinson's Disease
- Moderate to severe depression in Parkinson's disease.

THERAPEUTICS

VENLAFAXINE

Non-Licensed Use for Other Conditions
- Hot flushes due to hormonal haemotherapy.
- Post-traumatic stress disorder.
- Attention deficit disorder.
- Neuropathic pain.
- Fibromyalgia.

Ineffective
- Not recommended for weight loss either as a monotherapy or in combination with other products.

Mechanism of Action
- A potent inhibitor of serotonin and norepinephrine reuptake (SNRI).
  - It reduces β-adrenergic responsiveness.
- A weak inhibitor of dopamine reuptake.
- Venlafaxine does not exhibit any MAOI activity or activity for H1 histaminergic, muscarinic, cholinergic, or alpha2-adrenergic receptors. It has no affinity for opiate- or benzodiazepine-sensitive receptors.
- O-desmethylvenlafaxine, the active metabolite of venlafaxine, exhibits a similar pharmacological and pharmacokinetic profile to the parent compound.

Efficacy Profile
- According to the MDS EBM Committee, venlafaxine has been characterized as 'efficacious' and 'clinically useful' for the treatment of depression in Parkinson's disease.
- Extended release venlafaxine may be more effective than paroxetine in women with Parkinson's disease, in co-administration with dopamine agonists, and in patients with longer disease duration.
- There have been case reports of venlafaxine being successfully used in the treatment of hallucinations in Parkinson's disease patients, either alone or combined with clozapine.

Pharmacokinetics
Absorption and Distribution
- Oral bioavailability: 40–45%.
- Food co-ingestion: no effect on venlafaxine bioavailability.
- Tmax: 2–3 h (IR preparation), 5.5–9 h (ER preparation).
- Time to steady state: within 3 days.
- Pharmacokinetics: linear over the therapeutic dose range.
- Protein binding: 27–30%.
- Volume of distribution: 7.5 l/kg.

Metabolism
- Venlafaxine undergoes extensive hepatic metabolism, mostly by CYP2D6 and to a lesser extent by CYP3A4, producing its major active metabolite, O-desmethylvenlafaxine.

Elimination
- Half-life is 5 h for venlafaxine and 11 h for O-desmethylvenlafaxine.
- Renal excretion: 87% of an administered dose is excreted in the urine either unchanged (5%) or as (un)conjugated O-desmethylvenlafaxine or other minor inactive compounds.

Drug Interaction Profile
Pharmacokinetic Drug Interactions
- Effects by venlafaxine:
  - Venlafaxine is a weak inhibitor of CYP2D6.
- Effects on venlafaxine:
  - CYP3A4 inhibitors (e.g. *clarithromycin, indinavir, itraconazole, ketoconazole* might increase levels of venlafaxine and O-desmethylvenlafaxine.

Pharmacodynamic Drug Interactions
- Co-administration with other serotonergic agents, including SSRIs/SNRIs, tricyclic/tetracyclic antidepressants, opioids, *lithium, buspirone,* amphetamines, and triptans, can lead to a potentially life-threatening serotonin syndrome.
- Co-administration with agents affecting platelet function, including antiplatelet (e.g. *aspirin*), anticoagulants (e.g. *warfarin*), and NSAIDs, increases the risk of bleeding events, including life-threatening haemorrhage.
- Co-administration with diuretics might increase the risk of hyponatraemia.
- Co-administration with CNS depressants (e.g. benzodiazepines, most antipsychotics, antihistamines H1 antagonists, opioids) or alcohol might lead to synergistic sedative effects, including somnolence and dizziness.
- Co-administration with drugs causing electrolyte imbalance or increasing QT interval, such as Class IA and III anti-arrhythmics, antipsychotics (e.g. *haloperidol, phenothiazine derivatives, pimozide*), tricyclic antidepressants, certain antimicrobial agents (e.g. *moxifloxacin, erythromycin*), certain antihistamines (e.g. *astemizole, mizolastine*), and others may lead to potentially fatal Torsade de Pointes arrhythmias and is considered a risk factor for sudden cardiac death.

Adverse Effects
How Drug Causes Adverse Effects
- Venlafaxine (and its active metabolite, O-desmethylyvenlafaxine (ODV)) are potent inhibitors of neuronal serotonin and norepineph-rine reuptake and weak inhibitors of dopamine reuptake.

ADVERSE EFFECTS

V

V

VENLAFAXINE

Common Adverse Effects
- Very common (≥1/10):
  - Dry mouth, nausea, constipation, headache, sweating (including night sweats), insomnia, dizziness, sedation.
- Common (≥1/100 to <1/10):
  - Neuropsychiatric: confusion, depersonalization, abnormal dreams, nervousness, agitation, decreased libido, anorgasmia, akathisia/psychomotor restlessness, tremor, paraesthesia, dysgeusia, hypertonia.
  - Eye/ear disorders: visual impairment, accommodation disorder (including blurred vision), mydriasis, tinnitus.
  - Cardiovascular: palpitations, tachycardia, hypertension, hot flushes.
  - Respiratory: dyspnoea, yawning.
  - GI: diarrhoea, vomiting.
  - Skin: rash, pruritus.
  - Renal/urinary: urinary hesitation/retention, pollakiuria.
  - Reproductive: menorrhagia, metrorrhagia, erectile dysfunction, ejaculation disorder.
  - Other: decreased appetite, fatigue, chills, increased cholesterol.
- Uncommon (≥1/1,000 to <1/100):
  - Neuropsychiatric: mania, hypomania, hallucinations, derealization, abnormal orgasm, bruxism, apathy, syncope, myoclonus, abnormal coordination, dyskinesia, balance problems.
  - Cardiovascular: (orthostatic) hypotension.
  - GI: gastrointestinal haemorrhage, abnormal liver function tests.
  - Skin: urticaria, alopecia, angioedema, photosensitivity reaction.
  - Renal/urinary: urinary incontinence.

Life-Threatening or Dangerous Adverse Effects
- Rare (≥1/10,000 to <1/1,000):
  - Serotonin syndrome.
  - Interstitial lung disease, eosinophilic pneumonia.
  - SIADH.
  - Agranulocytosis, aplastic anaemia, pancytopenia, neutropenia.
  - Anaphylactic reaction.
  - Steven–Johnson syndrome, toxic epidermal necrolysis.
  - Delirium.
  - Seizures.
  - Pancreatitis, hepatitis.
  - Rhabdomyolysis.
- Very rare (<1/10,000):
  - Thrombocytopenia.

Rare and Not Life-Threatening Adverse Effects
- Dystonia.
- Erythema multiforme.
- Tardive dyskinesia.

Weight Change
- Increase or decrease of weight are common with venlafaxine.

What to Do About Adverse Effects
- Before introducing venlafaxine, discuss common or life-threatening adverse effects with patients and/or caregivers, including symptoms that should be reported to the physician.
- Most venlafaxine-related symptoms appear during the first weeks of therapy and are mild and self-resolving.
- Patients and their caregivers should be informed about the possibility of venlafaxine causing suicidal ideation/behaviour; such a risk might persist until significant remission of depression occurs. If such signs/symptoms emerge, patients should urgently seek medical advice and be treated accordingly; venlafaxine should be discontinued.
- If a serotonin syndrome is suspected, close monitoring and discontinuation of venlafaxine or other interacting agents should be considered.
- Treatment with venlafaxine should be discontinued if a patient presents with seizures.
- Before treatment initiation, patients should be informed about the possibility of venlafaxine causing sexual dysfunction, as patients may not spontaneously report it.
  - In case of sexual dysfunction, a detailed history should be obtained to exclude other causes, including psychiatric disorders.
  - Sexual dysfunction might persist despite treatment discontinuation.
- In case a patient using venlafaxine reports:
  - Bone pain, the possibility of a subjacent bone fracture should be excluded.
  - Dyspnoea, cough, or chest discomfort, the possibility of interstitial lung disease and eosinophilic pneumonia should be excluded. Consider venlafaxine discontinuation.
- Because of the high probability of venlafaxine causing dry mouth, the importance of dental hygiene should be highlighted to patients.
- SNRIs, including venlafaxine, might aggravate RBD in Parkinson's disease patients; consider removing it before initiating treatment for RBD.
- In case of venlafaxine-related nausea, consider taking it with or after food and avoid rich or spicy food.

Dosing and Use
Usual Dosage Range
- ER preparations: 37.5–225 mg daily.
- IR preparations: 75–375 mg daily.

Available Formulations
- Tablets, IR: 25 mg, 37.5 mg, 50 mg, 75 mg, 100 mg.
- Tablets, ER: 37.5 mg, 75 mg, 150 mg, 225 mg.
- Capsules, ER: 37.5 mg, 75 mg, 150 mg.
- Tablets, ER (besylate salt): 112.5 mg.
- Oral solution: 37.5 mg/ml, 75 mg/ml.

V

DOSING AND USE

V

How to Dose
- ER preparations: initial dose of 37.5–75 mg OD; may be increased by 75 mg/day every 4 days to 2 weeks; not to exceed 225 mg/day.
- IR preparations: initial dose of 75 mg per day divided in 2 or 3 doses (every 12 or 8 h, respectively); may be increased by a maximum of 75 mg/day every 4 days to 2 weeks; not to exceed 225 mg/day (moderate depression) or 375 mg/day (severe depression).
- Dosage increases can be made at a minimum of 2-week intervals.
  - In urgent cases, dosage increases can be made more frequently, but not more frequently than every 4 days.
  - Clinical evaluation is advised before any dosage increase due to dose-related side effects.
- The lowest effective dose should be maintained.

Dosing Tips
- ER formulations are administered as a single dose at the same time each day (morning or evening). If the patient reports any sleeping problems, venlafaxine should be administered in the morning.
- Long-term treatment of several months (or longer) is usually necessary, although venlafaxine should be discontinued if no longer required to avoid adverse effects.
- In Parkinson's disease patients with depression and neuropathic pain who need antidepressant therapy consider venlafaxine as an initial choice.

How to Withdraw Drug
- Dosage tapering is necessary to lower the risk of withdrawal symptoms, which is affected by duration and dose of venlafaxine therapy.
- Common withdrawal symptoms include dizziness, sensory disturbances, sleep problems (e.g. insomnia, intense dreams), agitation/anxiety, nausea/vomiting, tremor, headache, visual impairment, hypertension, vertigo and flu-like symptoms.
- Withdrawal symptoms are usually mild to moderate and resolve within 2 weeks without any intervention needed.
- In case of severe or prolonged (more than 2–3 months) symptoms during dosage reduction or withdrawal, consider resuming the previously prescribed dose and follow a longer tapering period.
- The tapering scheme should be personalized according to each patient's needs and may take months to achieve.

Overdose
- Venlafaxine overdose might present with changes in level of consciousness (somnolence to coma), vomiting, vertigo, mydriasis, hypotension, tachycardia/bradycardia, hypotension, electrocardiographic changes, seizures.
- Venlafaxine overdose is usually encountered in combination with alcohol or other medicinal products and might be fatal.

- There is no specific antidote to venlafaxine overdose.
- Supportive measures, close monitoring, and maintenance of a clear airway with adequate ventilation are recommended.
- Gastric lavage can be helpful if performed soon after ingestion or in a symptomatic patient. Activated charcoal may also be of use.

Tests and Therapeutic Drug Monitoring
- Before initiation of venlafaxine therapy:
  - Hypertension should be controlled.
  - A baseline ECG should be performed to check for QT prolongation.
  - A metabolic panel should be performed, including electrolytes, renal and hepatic function.
- During venlafaxine therapy:
  - Blood pressure should be monitored regularly, especially after dose increases.
  - Patients should be evaluated regularly for worsening of depression, suicidality, behaviour changes, or other common adverse effects, especially after introducing therapy or during dose modifications.

Other Warnings/Precautions
- There is a black box warning for young adults (less than 24 years old) who take venlafaxine for depression and other psychiatric disorders concerning suicidal thinking and behaviour.
  - A slight increase in suicidal thinking has also been seen in the elderly (>65 years old) receiving venlafaxine.
  - Patients with a history of suicide-related events are at higher risk and careful monitoring during treatment is required, especially early in therapy and following changes in dosage.
- Close monitoring is recommended in patients with a history of bipolar disorder, as venlafaxine may trigger a manic episode.
  - Venlafaxine should be withdrawn in any patient entering a manic phase.
  - Avoid monotherapy in bipolar disorder.
- Close monitoring is recommended in patients with a history of seizures or cardiovascular disease.
- Caution and careful monitoring is advised in patients at high risk of prolonged cardiac repolarization (e.g. co-administration with drugs increasing QT interval, patients with cardiovascular disease, family history of QT prolongation, congenital long QT syndrome, congestive heart failure, heart hypertrophy, hypokalaemia or hypomagnesaemia), especially the elderly.
- An angle-closure attack may be triggered in patients with high intraocular pressure or those at risk of angle-closure glaucoma.
- Hyponatraemia and/or SIADH has been reported with venlafaxine therapy, especially in dehydrated or volume-depleted patients.
- Venlafaxine might alter glycaemic control in patients with diabetes and antidiabetic treatment might need to be modified accordingly.

- Venlafaxine might cause CNS depression, affecting the ability to drive or operate dangerous machinery.
  - Co-administration with CNS depressants or alcohol should be avoided.
- Venlafaxine use might cause false-positive urine immunoassay screening test for phencyclidine (PCP) and amphetamine.

Do Not Use (Contraindications)
- Known sensitivity to venlafaxine or to any of the excipients.
- Co-administration with MAOIs or within 2 weeks after their discontinuation due to increased risk of potentially fatal serotonin syndrome.
- Co-administration with linezolid or methylene blue IV.
  - In case linezolid administration is necessary, venlafaxine should be discontinued immediately, and the patient should be monitored for CNS toxicity. Venlafaxine therapy can be resumed 24 h after last linezolid dose or after 2 weeks of monitoring, whichever applies first.
- Co-administration with serotonin precursors (e.g. tryptophan supplements) is not recommended.
- Co-administration with weight loss agents.

Special Populations
Renal Impairment
- Mild or moderate impairment (CrCl 30–89 ml/min):
  - Total venlafaxine dosage should be decreased by 25–50% (FDA).
  - No dosage change is necessary, although caution is advised (EMA, EMC).
- Severe impairment (CrCl < 30 ml/min) or haemodialysis: total venlafaxine dosage should be decreased by at least 50%.
- A maximum of 112 mg per day is suggested for patients treated with ER tablets.
- Due to inter-individual variability in clearance, dose individualization is suggested.

Hepatic Impairment
- Mild or moderate impairment (Child–Pugh 5–9): total venlafaxine dosage should be decreased by 50%.
- Severe impairment (Child–Pugh 10–15) or cirrhosis: total venlafaxine dosage should be decreased by at least 50%.
- In case of hepatic impairment, a maximum of 112 mg per day is suggested for patients treated with ER tablets.
- Due to inter-individual variability in clearance, dose individualization is suggested.

Elderly
- No specific dose adjustments are suggested.
- Careful monitoring is advised during dose increments.
- Older patients might be at greater risk of hyponatraemia.

VENLAFAXINE

V

Pregnancy
- Neonates exposed to SNRIs or SSRIs late in the third trimester might develop complications, requiring hospitalization, respiratory support, and tube feeding.
- An increased risk for preeclampsia has been reported when pregnant women use venlafaxine during mid-to-late pregnancy.
- An increased risk for postpartum haemorrhage has been reported when pregnant women use venlafaxine near delivery.
- Consider risk of untreated depression in case of discontinuation or change of treatment during pregnancy. Venlafaxine must only be used during pregnancy if the expected benefits outweigh any potential risks.

Breastfeeding
- Venlafaxine and its active metabolite have been identified in human milk.
- Breastfed infants might develop irritability, crying, and abnormal sleep patterns, while symptoms consistent with venlafaxine withdrawal have also been reported after discontinuation of breastfeeding.
- Health benefits of breastfeeding should be considered along with mother's need for venlafaxine therapy and any potential effects on the breastfed infant, either from the drug or from mother's underlying condition.

COSTS

Costs
NHS indicative costs (accessed 1 November 2022):
- Venlafaxine tablets – 56 × 37.5 mg tablets: £2.25–£7.95; 56 × 75 mg tablets: £12.86–£21.24.
- Venlafaxine modified-release tablets – 28 × 150 mg tablets: £3.64–£18.70.
- Venlafaxine modified-release capsules – 28 × 225 mg capsules: £44.75.
- Venlafaxine oral solution – 150 ml × 37.5 mg/ml: £158.76; 150 ml × 75 mg/5 ml: £207.37.
- Venlalic XL tablets (Ethypharm UK Ltd) – 30 × 37.5 mg tablets: £6.60; 30 × 75 mg tablets: £2.60; 30 × 150 mg tablets: £3.90; 30 × 225 mg tablets: £33.60; 30 × 300 mg tablets: £35.00.
- Sunveniz XL tablets (Sun Pharmaceutical Industries Europe B.V.) – 30 × 75 mg tablets: £11.14; 30 × 150 mg tablets: £18.64.
- Venladex XL tablets (Dexcel-Pharma Ltd) – 28 × 75 mg tablets: £11.20; 28 × 150 mg tablets: £18.70; 28 × 225 mg tablets: £31.36.
- ViePax XL tablets (Dexcel-Pharma Ltd) – 28 × 75 mg tablets: £2.60; 28 × 150 mg tablets £3.90; 28 × 225 mg tablets: £31.36.
- Majoven XL capsules (Bristol Laboratories Ltd) – 28 × 37.5 mg capsules: £5.25; 28 × 75 mg capsules: £22.08; 28 × 150 mg capsules: £36.81.

- Vencarm XL capsules (Aspire Pharma Ltd) – 28 × 37.5 mg capsules: £3.30; 28 × 75 mg capsules: £2.59; 28 × 150 mg capsules: £3.89; 28 × 225 mg capsules: £9.90.
- Venlablue XL capsules (Zentiva Pharma UK Ltd) – 28 × 37.5 mg capsules: £5.25; 28 × 75 mg: £6.95; 28 × 150 mg capsules: £9.95.
- Alventa XL capsules (Consilient Health Ltd) – 28 × 75 mg capsules: £19.12; 28 × 150 mg capsules: £31.88.
- Efexor XL capsules (Viatris UK Healthcare Ltd) – 28 × 75 mg capsules: £22.08; 28 × 150 mg capsules: £36.81; 28 × 225 mg capsules: £47.11.
- Palotid XL capsules (Accord Healthcare Ltd) – 28 × 75 mg capsules: £23.41; 28 × 150 mg capsules: £39.03.
- Venaxx XL capsules (Advanz Pharma) – 28 × 75 mg capsules: £10.40; 28 × 150 mg capsules: £17.40.
- Venlasov XL capsules (Sovereign Medical Ltd) – 28 × 75 mg capsules: £2.98; 28 × 150 mg capsules: £3.97.
- Vensir XL capsules (Morningside Healthcare Ltd) – 28 × 75 mg capsules: £2.86; 28 × 150 mg capsules: £4.10; 28 × 225 mg capsules: £25.19.
- Venzip XL capsules (Milpharm Ltd) – 28 × 75 mg capsules: £22.08; 28 × 150 mg capsules: £36.81.

The Overall Place of Venlafaxine in the Treatment of Parkinson's Disease

Venlafaxine, a dual norepinephrine and serotonin reuptake inhibitor (SNRI), is a well-studied and widely used agent in the treatment of major depression. According to preclinical studies, the antidepressant activity occurs in lower doses, possibly due to enhancement of serotonergic transmission, while higher doses have been associated with a simultaneous serotonergic and noradrenergic effect. Although it appears to be among the most effective options in major depression, its use might be limited to some extent due to tolerance issues. The effectiveness of venlafaxine in Parkinson's disease-related moderate-to-severe depression has been demonstrated in a large RCT over a course of 12 weeks. Although this study involves ER venlafaxine up to a dose of 225 mg/day, the use of IR formulations and higher dosage in severe major depressive disorder in Parkinson's disease patients can also be justified in everyday clinical practice. In depressed Parkinson's disease patients, venlafaxine has been shown to address primarily the affective symptoms, but also the somatic and cognitive symptoms later in the treatment course. It is generally well tolerated and has been associated with a reduced cardiotoxicity and fewer anticholinergic and CNS-related complications than tricyclic antidepressants.

Potential Advantages
- Venlafaxine is the only one among the antidepressants (SSRIs, SNRIs, tricyclic or other antidepressants) considered to be 'efficacious' and 'clinically useful' in the treatment of Parkinson's disease-related depression (MDS EBM Committee).
- It has a quicker onset of action compared to other antidepressants.

Potential Disadvantages
- The use of venlafaxine has not been extensively studied in Parkinson's disease patients.
- Venlafaxine carries a greater suicide risk compared to SSRIs.

Clinical Box
A 75-year-old woman with a recent diagnosis of Parkinson's disease presented at the Neurology Department Outpatient Clinic for her regular follow-up appointment. The patient was taking levodopa/benserazide 100 mg/25 mg TID. The rest of her medical history included well-controlled hypertension and a recent diagnosis of diabetes mellitus and diabetic neuropathy due to poor glycaemic control. For this latter diagnosis, the patient had been treated with gabapentin, although without significant improvement. She was relatively stable on her motor performance; however, she mentioned low mood, loss of interest, and occasional crying during the past few months, which significantly impaired her social functioning. A diagnosis of moderate depression was made, and initiation of therapy was considered necessary. Due to the concomitant, insufficiently treated diabetic neuropathy, gabapentin was discontinued and a low dose of venlafaxine ER 75 mg OD was prescribed.

Suggested Reading
Bauer M, P Tharmanathan, HP Volz, HJ Moeller, N Freemantle. The effect of venlafaxine compared with other antidepressants and placebo in the treatment of major depression: a meta-analysis. *Eur Arch Psychiatry Clin Neurosci* 2009; 259(3): 172–185.

Richard IH, MP McDermott, R Kurlan, JM Lyness, PG Como, N Pearson, SA Factor, J Juncos, C Serrano Ramos, M Brodsky, C Manning, L Marsh, L Shulman, HH Fernandez, KJ Black, M Panisset, CW Christine, W Jiang, C Singer, … W McDonald. A randomized, double-blind, placebo-controlled trial of antidepressants in Parkinson disease. *Neurology* 2012; 78(16): 1229–1236.

Starkstein SE, S Brockman. Management of depression in Parkinson's disease: a systematic review. *Mov Disord Clin Pract* 2017; 4(4): 470–477.

V

SUGGESTED READING

References

AHFS Drug information, 2012. Bethesda: American Society of Health-System Pharmacists. Accessed on 1 November 2022 via www.medicinescomplete.com.

Broen MP, AF Leentjens, S Köhler, ML Kuijf, WM McDonald, IH Richard. Trajectories of recovery in depressed Parkinson's disease patients treated with paroxetine or venlafaxine. *Parkinsonism Relat Disord* 2016; 23: 80–85.

Coutens B, A Yrondi, C Rampon, BP Guiard. Psychopharmacological properties and therapeutic profile of the antidepressant venlafaxine. *Psychopharmacology (Berl)* 2022; 239(9): 2735–2752.

Joint Formulary Committee. British National Formulary (online). London: BMJ Group and Pharmaceutical Press. Accessed on 1 November 2022 via www.medicinescomplete.com.

Sid-Otmane L, P Huot, M Panisset. Effect of antidepressants on psychotic symptoms in Parkinson disease: a review of case reports and case series. *Clin Neuropharmacol* 2020; 43(3): 61–65.

Summary of product characteristics – venlafaxine 75 mg tablets. Dexcel Pharma Ltd. Electronic Medicines Compendium: venlafaxine 75 mg tablets – summary of product characteristics (SmPC) – (emc). Accessed on 1 November 2022 via www.medicines.org.uk.

Venlafaxine. In: Brayfield A (Ed.), *Martindale: The Complete Drug Reference*. London: The Royal Pharmaceutical Society of Great Britain. Accessed on 1 November 2022 via www.medicinescomplete.com.

Venlafaxine. In: DRUGDEX® System (electronic version). Truven Health Analytics, Greenwood Village, Colorado, USA. Accessed on 1 November 2022 via www.micromedexsolutions.com.

ZONISAMIDE

Therapeutics

Chemical Name and Structure

Zonisamide (1-(1,2-Benzoxazol-3-yl)methanesulphonamide) is a sulphonamide derivative with a molecular weight of 212.2 and a molecular formula of $C_8H_8N_2O_3S$.

Brand Names

- **Cinal** (*Spain*).
- **Desizon** (*UK*).
- **Ersittin** (*Czech Republic*); **Excegran** (*Japan, Turkey*).
- **Kinaplase** (*Argentina*).
- **Nyzol** (*Spain*).
- **Trerief** (*Japan*).
- **Zonegran** (*Australia, Austria, China, Cyprus, Czech Republic, Denmark, Estonia, Finland, France, Germany, Greece, Hungary, Indonesia, Ireland, Italy, Lithuania, Malaysia, Netherlands, Norway, Philippines, Poland, Portugal, Russian Federation, Spain, Sweden, Switzerland, Thailand, UK, USA*); **Zonesme** (*Spain*); **Zonibon** (*Austria, Czech Republic, Hungary*); **Zonisade** (*USA*); **Zonisol** (*Germany*).

Generics Available

- Yes.

Licensed Indications for Parkinson's Disease

- As an adjunctive therapy to levodopa preparations in previously treated Parkinson's disease patients (Japan).

Licensed Indications for Other Conditions

- Partial seizures, either alone or as an adjunctive therapy (FDA, EMA, EMC).
- Partial and generalized seizures (Japan).

Non-Licensed Use for Parkinson's Disease

- Reported as an add-on to current antiparkinsonian therapy to improve motor function and reduce wearing off time mostly in late Parkinson's disease.

Non-Licensed Use for Other Conditions

- Binge-eating disorder.
- Refractory migraine prophylaxis.
- Alcohol withdrawal syndrome/dependence.

Ineffective

- Bipolar disorder.

Z

Mechanism of Action
- Zonisamide's anti-epileptic action is mediated by inhibiting voltage-gated sodium and T-type calcium channels and decreasing presynaptic release of glutamate; whether a link exists between anti-epileptic and antiparkinsonian effects of zonisamide remains unknown.
- The mechanism of action in Parkinson's disease is not clear. It is a weak inhibitor of carbonic anhydrase. It facilitates dopaminergic and serotoninergic transmission in both in vitro and in vivo studies.
- Zonisamide possesses multiple other potential pharmacological actions relevant to Parkinson's disease, including MAO-B inhibition, Na/Ca channel blocking activity, and the inhibition of glutamate release.

Efficacy Profile
- Zonisamide has been characterized as 'efficacious' and 'clinically useful' as an adjunct therapy for the management of early or stable Parkinson's disease patients and for motor fluctuations in Parkinson's disease (MDS EBM Committee).
- There is 'insufficient evidence' considering the use of zonisamide on dyskinesia; its use is considered 'investigational' (MDS EBM Committee).
- Two double-blind RCTs in Parkinson's disease patients in Japan (follow-up period of 10 and 16 weeks) demonstrated a significant improvement in motor symptoms and OFF time when zonisamide was used as an add-on therapy to levodopa preparations.
- A double-blind RCT of zonisamide (as an adjunctive therapy to levodopa preparations) in Japanese DLB patients with a 16-week follow-up showed a significant improvement in motor symptoms without aggravating cognitive impairment or psychiatric symptoms.
- Two meta-analyses have suggested zonisamide is effective for both Parkinson's disease and DLB patients in Japan, although the authors concluded that further investigation was needed.
- A small open-label study found a beneficial effect of zonisamide on Parkinson's disease-related ICDs, which were resistant to dose reductions of levodopa preparations and/or dopamine agonists.

Pharmacokinetics
Absorption and Distribution
- Oral bioavailability: approximately 100%.
- Food co-ingestion decreases the rate of zonisamide absorption, although the extent of absorption remains unaffected.
- Tmax: 2–6 h (capsules); 0.5–5 h (oral suspension).
- Time to steady state: within 2 weeks.
- Pharmacokinetics: almost linear after multiple doses over the range of 100–400 mg.
- Protein binding: 40%.
- Volume of distribution: 1.1–1.7 l/kg.

Metabolism
- Zonisamide undergoes hepatic metabolism via CYP3A4 (reductive cleavage of the benzisoxazole ring) to produce 2-sulfamoylacetylphenol; both the parent compound and the metabolite undergo glucuronidation. Zonisamide is also acetylated to *N*-acetyl zonisamide.
- In vitro studies show zonisamide is also metabolized by CYP2C19 and CYP3A5.

Elimination
- Plasma half-life is about 63 h. However, the drug has a half-life of about 105 h in RBC.
- About 62% of an administered dose is excreted in the urine (35% unchanged) and about 3% is found in the faeces.

Drug Interaction Profile
Pharmacokinetic Drug Interactions
- Effects by zonisamide:
  - Zonisamide decreases levels and effects of *acetaminophen* and *succinylcholine* by increasing metabolism.
  - In vitro studies have shown that zonisamide is a weak inhibitor of p-gp; thus, it may affect the pharmacokinetics of p-gp substrates (e.g. *digoxin, quinidine*).
- Effects on zonisamide:
  - Zonisamide is a CYP3A4 substrate; thus, medication that affects hepatic/intestinal CYP3A4 (e.g. *abametapir, acetazolamide, apalutamide, budesonide, carbamazepine, chloramphenicol, cimetidine, clarithromycin, dexamethasone, erythromycin, fluvoxamine, fosphenytoin, hydrocortisone, istradefylline, itraconazole, ketoconazole, lonafarnib, nefazodone, nifedipine, primidone, prednisone, rifabutin, rifampin, topiramate, verapamil*) and grapefruit may alter zonisamide levels and effects.

Pharmacodynamic Drug Interactions
- Co-medication with CNS depressants (e.g. neuroleptics, benzodiazepines) may lead to additive effects, including increased sedation or respiratory depression.
- Zonisamide may increase toxicity of *metformin* by decreasing serum bicarbonate and inducing non-anion gap and hyperchloraemic metabolic acidosis.
- Zonisamide decreases effects of *onabotulinumtoxinA* by pharmacodynamic antagonism, although this association is considered clinically minor.

Adverse Effects
How Drug Causes Adverse Effects
* Zonisamide contains a sulphonamide group, which may predispose to serious immune-based adverse reactions.

Common Adverse Effects
*Adverse events refer to the general population, not specifically Parkinson's disease patients.
* Very common (≥1/10):
  ○ Somnolence, anorexia, dizziness, agitation, irritability, confusion, depression.
* Common (≥1/100 to <1/10):
  ○ Neuropsychiatric: headache, ataxia, diplopia, insomnia, difficulty concentrating, memory impairment, speech disorder, mental slowing, nystagmus, paraesthesia, anxiety, nervousness, schizophrenic/schizophreniform behaviour.
  ○ GI: nausea, abdominal pain, diarrhoea, dyspepsia, constipation, dry mouth, taste perversion.
  ○ Skin: rash, ecchymosis.
  ○ Other: fatigue, flu-like symptoms, peripheral oedema.
* Uncommon (≥1/1,000 to <1/100):
  ○ Neuropsychiatric: tremor, convulsions, abnormal gait, hyperaesthesia, hypertonia, twitching, abnormal dreams, decreased libido, neuropathy, hyperkinesia, dysarthria, euphoria.
  ○ Eye/ear: amblyopia, conjunctivitis, visual field defect, tinnitus, deafness, vertigo.
  ○ Cardiovascular: palpitations, tachycardia, vascular insufficiency, hypotension, hypertension, thrombophlebitis, bradycardia.
  ○ Respiratory: pharyngitis, increased cough, dyspnoea, pneumonia.
  ○ GI: vomiting, flatulence, gingivitis, gum hyperplasia, gastritis, gastroenteritis, stomatitis, cholelithiasis, glossitis, gastro-duodenal ulcer, dysphagia, gum haemorrhage.
  ○ Renal/urinary: increased urinary frequency, polyuria, nocturia, dysuria, urinary incontinence/retention, haematuria, urinary tract infection, kidney stones.
  ○ Musculoskeletal: leg cramps, myalgia, myasthenia, arthralgia, arthritis.
  ○ Skin: pruritus, acne, alopecia, dry skin, increased sweating, eczema, urticaria, hirsutism.
  ○ Other: syncope, anaemia, lymphadenopathy, thirst, impotence, amenorrhea, hypokalaemia.

Life-Threatening or Dangerous Adverse Effects
*Usually with higher doses used in the context of epilepsy (400–600 mg/day).
* Rare (≥1/10,000 to <1/1,000):
  ○ Atrial fibrillation, heart failure, ventricular extrasystoles.
  ○ Cerebrovascular accident.
  ○ Pulmonary embolus.

Z

- ○ Lupus erythematosus.
- ○ Hypersensitivity reactions, including face oedema, Stevens–Johnson syndrome, toxic epidermal necrolysis, fulminant hepatic necrosis, blood dyscrasias.
- ○ GI haemorrhage.
- ○ Cholangitis, cholecystitis, colitis, duodenitis, oesophagitis.
- ○ Hypoglycaemia, hyponatraemia.
- ○ Encephalopathy.
- ○ Apnoea, haemoptysis.
- ○ Menorrhagia.
- Very rare (<1/10,000):
  - ○ Hepatocellular damage.
  - ○ Thrombocytopenia, leukopenia, aplastic anaemia, agranulocytosis.
  - ○ Metabolic acidosis, renal tubular acidosis.
  - ○ Hydronephrosis, renal failure.
  - ○ NMS.
- Unknown frequency:
  - ○ Acute pancreatitis.
  - ○ Secondary angle-closure glaucoma.
  - ○ Rhabdomyolysis.
  - ○ Drug reaction with eosinophilia and systemic symptoms (DRESS).

Rare and Not Life-Threatening Adverse Effects
- Neck rigidity.
- Faecal incontinence.
- Mouth ulceration.
- Increase LDH/ALT/AST.
- Dyskinesia, dystonia, myoclonus, oculogyric crisis.
- Facial paralysis.
- Photophobia, iritis.
- Enuresis, bladder pain, albuminuria.
- Gynecomastia, mastitis.
- Increased CPK.
- Hallucinations.
- Myopia.

Weight Change
- Weight loss has been reported as a common effect of zonisamide therapy.
- Weight gain has been reported as an uncommon effect of zonisamide therapy.

What to Do About Adverse Effects
- Discuss common adverse effects with patients or caregivers before starting medication, including symptoms that should be reported to the physician.
- Zonisamide administration should be stopped immediately if symptoms of hypersensitivity reactions appear, including rash.

ADVERSE EFFECTS

Z

- Zonisamide therapy may predispose to the formation of kidney stones; increased fluid intake and urine output is advised in zonisamide-treated patients, particularly if other risk factors exist.
- If signs or symptoms of metabolic acidosis are apparent, serum bicarbonate levels should be measured; if metabolic acidosis develops and persists, zonisamide should be withdrawn.
- If signs or symptoms of encephalopathy appear, consider measuring ammonia serum levels; zonisamide therapy should be withdrawn.
- If pancreatitis is present and in the absence of another obvious cause, zonisamide should be discontinued.
- If severe muscle pain and/or weakness is reported, consider measuring markers of muscle damage (e.g. serum CPK, aldolase); if elevated, and in the absence of another obvious cause, zonisamide should be discontinued and appropriate treatment should be applied.

Dosing and Use

Usual Dosage Range
- 25 mg daily.

Available Formulations
- Capsules: 25 mg, 50 mg, 100 mg.
- Oral suspension: 100 mg/5 ml.

How to Dose
- A dose of 25 mg OD is suggested (the only approved dose for Parkinson's disease).
- Doses of 50 mg and 100 mg were no more effective than the dose of 25 mg in clinical studies and were associated with more side effects.

Dosing Tips
- Zonisamide may be administered with or without food.

How to Withdraw Drug
- Zonisamide at a dose of 25 mg/day can be abruptly discontinued.

Overdose
- Overdose may be asymptomatic or may present with somnolence, nausea, gastritis, nystagmus, myoclonus, bradycardia, renal impairment, hypotension, respiratory depression, and coma.
- No specific antidote for zonisamide is available.
- Consider gastric lavage or induction of emesis (with the usual precautions to protect the airway) in case of a suspected recent overdose; haemodialysis may also apply.
- Supportive measures are recommended, including monitoring of vital signs and close observation, as zonisamide has a long half-life and overdose symptoms may persist.

Z

Tests and Therapeutic Drug Monitoring
- Serum bicarbonate levels should be measured prior to and periodically during zonisamide therapy.
- Regular monitoring for new-onset or aggravation of depression, suicidal thoughts/behaviour, and/or unusual changes in mood/behaviour.

Other Warnings/Precautions
- Antiepileptic drugs, including zonisamide, may increase the risk of suicidal thoughts/behaviour in patients taking these drugs for any indication.
- Specific co-morbidities, such as renal disease, severe respiratory disorder, status epilepticus, diarrhoea, ketogenic diet, or specific drugs, may predispose to metabolic acidosis in case of zonisamide therapy; this effect seems to be dose-dependent and can present even at low doses of zonisamide (e.g. 25 mg/day).
- Zonisamide therapy in patients with chronic untreated metabolic acidosis may predispose to nephrolithiasis or nephrocalcinosis.
- Caution is advised in individuals with inborn errors of metabolism or reduced hepatic mitochondrial activity, or when zonisamide is co-administered with drugs that predispose to hyperammonaemia (e.g. *valproic acid*, *topiramate*) due to increased risk of encephalopathy.
- Close monitoring is advised when co-administered with sedative drugs due to additive effects.
- Close monitoring is recommended when co-administered with medication, which are CYP3A4 inducers/inhibitors.
- Close monitoring is recommended when co-administered with metformin due to potential increased toxicity of the latter.
- Caution is advised when co-administered with p-gp substrates.
- Caution is advised while driving or using hazardous machinery, as zonisamide may predispose to drowsiness or impairment of concentrations. Patients may need to refrain from activities requiring a high degree of alertness, at least until they are aware of how zonisamide affects them.

Do Not Use (Contraindications)
- Known sensitivity to zonisamide or to any of its excipients or sulphonamides.
  - Fatalities have occurred as a result of severe reaction to sulphonamides.
- Severe hepatic impairment.

Special Populations
Renal Impairment
- A slower dose titration is recommended with regular monitoring.
- GFR < 50 ml/min: not recommended.
- Zonisamide therapy should be discontinued in case of acute renal failure or clinically significant increase in creatinine/BUN.

SPECIAL POPULATIONS

Z

ZONISAMIDE

Hepatic Impairment
- Zonisamide use has not been studied in any degree of hepatic impairment.
- Mild-to-moderate impairment: use with caution and consider a slower titration.
- Severe impairment: not recommended.

Elderly
- No dosage modifications needed.

Pregnancy
- Zonisamide use is contraindicated during pregnancy.
- Zonisamide use during pregnancy may cause teratogenic effects and has been associated with an increased rate of small-for-gestational-age infants (possible link to metabolic acidosis).
- In case of zonisamide use during pregnancy, dose adjustments may be necessary to maintain clinical response, as physiological changes during pregnancy may affect zonisamide systemic levels and therapeutic effect.
- Women of childbearing potential are advised to use effective contraception if on zonisamide therapy and for one month after zonisamide cessation.

Breastfeeding
- Zonisamide is excreted in human milk.
- No data are available on milk production.
- Infants exposed during breastfeeding should be closely monitored for poor feeding, weight loss, sedation, decreased muscle tone, and elevated temperature.

Costs
NHS indicative costs (accessed on 1 January 2023):
- Zonegran Capsules (Advanz Pharma) – 14 × 25 mg capsules: £8.82; 56 × 50 mg capsules: £47.04; 56 × 100 mg capsules: £62.72.
- Desizon 20 mg/ml oral suspension (Desitin Pharma Ltd) – 250 ml suspension: £181.90
- Zonisamide 25 mg capsules – 14 × 25 mg capsules; £6.50–£12.09; 56 × 50 mg capsules: £33.67–£47.04; 56 × 100 mg capsules: £7.13–£62.72.

Z

The Overall Place of Zonisamide in the Treatment of Parkinson's Disease

Zonisamide is a mixed MAO-B inhibitor, channel blocker, and glutamate release inhibitor. Although it has been used primarily as an anticonvulsant, there is growing interest in other potential applications, including Parkinson's disease. During the past 15 years, large high-quality studies have been performed in the Japanese population, showing a beneficial effect of zonisamide when used as an adjunct therapy to levodopa preparations with significant improvement of motor performance, including tremor, and reduction of OFF time. Zonisamide (daily dose of 25 mg) was officially approved in Japan as an add-on to levodopa in previously treated Parkinson's disease patients. This dose is generally well tolerated. The most commonly reported adverse events in the context of Parkinson's disease are increased CPK, apathy, somnolence, dizziness, decreased appetite, weight decrease, and constipation.

Potential Advantages
- Zonisamide is a levodopa-sparing strategy.

Potential Disadvantages
- Zonisamide is officially approved as an antiparkinsonian agent only in Japan.
- All currently available studies were performed in Japanese Parkinson's disease patients; future studies in other populations are necessary in order to globally expand zonisamide use.

SUGGESTED READING

Clinical Box

A 55-year-old man with a 9-year-history of Parkinson's disease presented at the Movement Disorders Outpatient Clinics due to end-of-dose OFF phenomena. His current medication was levodopa/carbidopa/entacapone 200 mg/50 mg/200 mg 5 times per day, rotigotine 8 mg/24 h, and amantadine 100 mg BID. The rest of his medical history was unremarkable. He was prescribed zonisamide 25 mg OD with a subsequent reduction in OFF time.

Suggested Reading

Goel A, R Sugumaran, SK Narayan. Zonisamide in Parkinson's disease: a current update. *Neurol Sci* 2021; 42(10): 4123–4129.

Murata M, K Hasegawa, I Kanazawa. Zonisamide improves motor function in Parkinson disease: a randomized, double-blind study. *Neurology* 2007; 68(1): 45–50.

Murata M, K Hasegawa, I Kanazawa, J Fukasaka, K Kochi, R Shimazu. Zonisamide improves wearing-off in Parkinson's disease: a randomized, double-blind study. *Mov Disord* 2015; 30(10): 1343–1350.

Z

Murata M, T Odawara, K Hasegawa, S Iiyama, M Nakamura, M Tagawa, K Kosaka. Adjunct zonisamide to levodopa for DLB parkinsonism: a randomized double-blind phase 2 study. *Neurology*2018; 90(8): e664–e672.

References

AHFS Drug information, 2012. Bethesda: American Society of Health-System Pharmacists. Accessed on 2 January 2023 via www.medicinescomplete.com.

Arawaka S, S Fukushima, H Sato, A Sasaki, K Koga, S Koyama, T Kato. Zonisamide attenuates α-synuclein neurotoxicity by an aggregation-independent mechanism in a rat model of familial Parkinson's disease. *PLoS One* 2014; 9(2): e89076.

Bermejo PE, C Ruiz-Huete, B Anciones. Zonisamide in managing impulse control disorders in Parkinson's disease. *J Neurol* 2010; 257(10): 1682–1685.

Gluck MR, LA Santana, H Granson, MD Yahr. Novel dopamine releasing response of an anti-convulsant agent with possible anti-Parkinson's activity. *J Neural Transm (Vienna)* 2004; 111(6): 713–724.

Kong L, J Xi, Z Jiang, X Yu, H Liu, Z Wang. Zonisamide's efficacy and safety on Parkinson's disease and dementia with Lewy bodies: a meta-analysis and systematic review. *Biomed Res Int* 2022; 2022: 4817488.

Joint Formulary Committee. British National Formulary (online). London: BMJ Group and Pharmaceutical Press. Accessed on 2 January 2023 via www.medicinescomplete.com.

Matsunaga S, T Kishi, N Iwata. Combination therapy with zonisamide and antiparkinson drugs for Parkinson's disease: a meta-analysis. *J Alzheimers Dis* 2017; 56(4): 1229–1239.

Summary of product characteristics – zonegran 50 mg hard capsules. Advanz Pharma. Electronic Medicines Compendium: Zonegran 50 mg hard capsules – summary of product characteristics (SmPC) – (emc). Accessed on 2 January 2023 via www.medicines.org.uk.

Yang LP, CM Perry. Zonisamide: in Parkinson's disease. *CNS Drugs* 2009; 23(8): 703–711.

Zonisamide. In: Brayfield A (Ed.), *Martindale: The Complete Drug Reference*. London: The Royal Pharmaceutical Society of Great Britain. Accessed on 2 January 2023 via www.medicinescomplete.com.

Zonisamide. In: DRUGDEX® System (electronic version). Truven Health Analytics, Greenwood Village, Colorado, USA. Accessed on 2 January 2023 via www.micromedexsolutions.com.

ZONISAMIDE

LEVODOPA DOSE EQUIVALENCE IN PARKINSON'S

There are a number of classes of antiparkinsonian medications with different mechanisms of action and routes of administration. To compare dosing of different therapeutic agents across different populations, the concept of the levodopa equivalent dose was introduced. Table 1 shares the estimated equivalence from a systematic review published in 2023.

Table 1 Potential formulae for calculation of levodopa equivalence dose.

Drug class	Drug	Conversion factor/ratio
Levodopa	Levodopa	DD × 1
	Dual-release levodopa	DD × 0.85
	Controlled-release levodopa	DD × 0.75
	Extended-release levodopa	DD × 0.5
	Inhaled levodopa	DD × 0.69 (capsules)
	Intrajejunal levodopa/carbidopa infusion	DD × 1.11
	Intrajejunal levodopa/carbidopa/entacapone infusion	DD × 1.11 (morning dose) + DD × 1.46 (maintenance and extra doses)
	Subcutaneous foslevodopa/foscarbidopa	DD × 0.75
COMT Inhibitors	Entacapone	LD × 0.33
	Tolcapone	LD × 0.5
	Opicapone	LD × 0.5
Irreversible MAO-B inhibitors	Selegiline (oral)	DD × 10
	Selegiline (sublingual)	DD × 80
	Rasagiline	DD × 100

Table 1 (Cont.)

Drug class	Drug	Conversion factor/ratio
Non-ergot-derived dopamine agonists	Pramipexole (extended or immediate release)	DD × 100 (salt), DD × 142.86 (base)
	Ropinirole	DD × 20
	Rotigotine	DD × 30.3
	Piribedil	DD × 1
	Apomorphine hydrochloride (subcutaneous)	DD × 10
	Apomorphine hydrochloride (sublingual)	DD × 1.5
Others	Amantadine hydrochloride (immediate release)	DD × 1
	Amantadine hydrochloride (extended release)	DD × 1.25
	Safinamide	LED = 150 mg
	Zonisamide	LED = 100 mg
	Trihexyphenidyl	LED = 100 mg
	Istradefylline	LD × 0.2

Abbreviations: DD, daily dose of drug being converted to a levodopa equivalent dose; LD, levodopa dose; LED, levodopa equivalent dose.

These estimated conversion factors have also been used to develop calculators to support formulation switches in acute scenarios, for example on admission to hospital if a patient is suddenly unable to swallow or made nil by mouth. While not replacing the need for clinical assessment and judgement, these can be a helpful tool to support patients to receive the dopaminergic replacement therapy they need.

Reference

Jost ST, M-A Kaldenbach, A Antonini, P Martinez-Martin, L Timmermann, P Odin, R Katzenschlager, R Borgohain, A Fasano, F Stocchi, N Hattori, PL Kukkle, M Rodríguez-Violante, C Falup-Pecurariu, S Schade, JN Petry-Schmelzer, V Metta, D Weintraub, G Deuschl, … HS Dafsari ; International Parkinson and Movement Disorders Society Non-Motor Parkinson's Disease Study Group. Levodopa dose equivalency in Parkinson's disease: updated systematic review and proposals. *Mov Disord* 2023; 38: 1236–1252.

SUBCUTANEOUS FOSLEVODOPA FOSCARBIDOPA INFUSION

Therapeutics
Abbvie produced ABBV-951 to provide continuous subcutaneous infusion of levodopa/carbidopa prodrug which is a solution of prodrugs that are rapidly converted to levodopa and carbidopa upon subcutaneous administration in the skin. This product is now marketed as produodopa (Foslevodopa/Fos carbidopa).

Brand Name
• Produodopa.

Licensed Indication for Parkinson's Disease
• Advanced parkinson's disease as judged by clinical decision and use of the Manage -PD tool.
• Non licensed use of relevance.
• Advanced parkinson's disease with significant nighttime and early morning off periods.

Licensed Indication for Other Conditions
• Not relevant.

Mechanism of Action and Pharmacokinetics
• Providing continuous dopaminergic stimulation over 24 hours with a full range of levodopa doses that can be delivered to advanced PD patients over a 24 hours period using a specially designed portable pump in much smaller volumes compared to intrajejunal levodopa infusion. Comparison of 16-hour levodopa carboidopa intrajejunal gel (LCIG) infusion supplemented by two separate nighttime oral LD/CD doses and foslevodopa/foscarbidopa SC infusion generated similar levodopa levels to LCIG infusion over the 16-hour interval but also maintained levodopa levels throughout the nighttime period thus providing real 24 hr cover.

Efficacy Profile
• The licensing trial of Foslevodopa/foscarbidopa was a 12 week randomised, double-blind, double-dummy, active-controlled study (NCT04380142) enrolled 174 patients of whom 141 was randomised to continuous subcutaneous infusion of foslevodopa/foscarbidopa plus oral placebo capsules (n=74) or oral encapsulated immediate-release levodopa-carbidopa plus continuous subcutaneous infusion of placebo solution (n=67). Foslevodopa-foscarbidopa infusion showed a significantly greater increase in on time without troublesome dyskinesia (Good on) of 1·75 h, p=0·0083) and a significantly greater reduction in off time (−1·79 h, p=0·0054). Foslevodopa-foscarbidopa ambulatory drug–device was able to deliver a range of therapeutically effective doses of foslevodopa (approximately 600–4250 mg/day levodopa equivalents) while infusion rates could be adjusted in small increments (approximately 1·7 mg of levodopa per h)

allowing for personalised medicine delivery. Data from a 52-week, open label international phase 3 registrational trial (NCT03781167) showed significant improvement in "On" time without troublesome dyskinesia (3.8 [3.3] hours) as well as reduction in "Off" time (-3.5 [3.1]) compared to baseline. There were improvement in quality of life (QoL) and motor complications noted at week 1 after foslevodopa/foscarbidopa and sustained throughout the 52-week treatment period. At 52 weeks there were approximately 50% fewer patients who reported early morning akinesia or off periods compared to baseline and overall rates of early morning off periods were reduced from 77.7% at baseline to 27.8% at week 52 with a sharp drop noted at week 1 (77.7% to 31%).

Adverse Events
• Most adverse events occur early and stabilise after 3 months . In the pivotal licensing double dummy study of foslevodopa/foscarbidopa adverse events were reported in 63 (85%) foslevodopa-foscarbidopa participants and in 42 (63%) levodopa-carbidopa participants. Incidences of serious adverse events were similar between the groups. Major side effects were related to infusion site adverse events in the foslevodopa/foscarbidopa with erythema [27%], local site pain [26%], cellulitis [19%] and skin oedema [12%]. In the 12 months open label phase 3 study serious adverse events were reported in 25.8% of patients and included infusion site cellulitis (4.1%) and infusion site abscess (3.3%).

What to do about Adverse Effects
• Good patient selection with multidisciplinary backup is important and scrupulous skin care with regular washing of skin with soap as well as changing of subcutaneous infusion line every 3 days is recommended. In case of secondary infection such as cellulitis early use of appropriate antibiotics is recommended and drainage for any abscess and infusion treatment can be continued.

References
Soileau, M. J., Aldred, J., Budur, K., Fisseha, N., Fung, V. S., Jeong, A., et al. (2022). Safety and efficacy of continuous subcutaneous foslevodopa-foscarbidopa in patients with advanced Parkinson's disease: A randomised, double-blind, active-controlled, phase 3 trial. Lancet Neurology, 21(12), 1099-1109.
Aldred, J., Freire-Alvarez, E., Amelin, A. V., Antonini, A., Bergmans, B., Bergquist, F., Chaudhuri KR et al. (2023). Continuous Subcutaneous Foslevodopa/Foscarbidopa in Parkinson's Disease: Safety and Efficacy Results From a 12-Month, Single-Arm, Open-Label, Phase 3 Study. Neurol Ther, 12(6), 1937-1958.

INDEX